Current Topics in
Osteoporosis

Current Topics in
Osteoporosis

Editors

Hong-wen Deng

Creighton University, USA
Xi'an Jiaotong University, P R China &
Hunan Normal University, P R China

Yao-zhong Liu

Creighton University, USA

Associate Editors

Chun-yuan Guo

P&G Pharmaceuticals, USA

Di Chen

University of Rochester Medical Center, USA

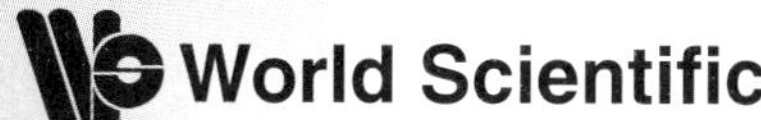

World Scientific

NEW JERSEY • LONDON • SINGAPORE • BEIJING • SHANGHAI • HONG KONG • TAIPEI • CHENNAI

Published by

World Scientific Publishing Co. Pte. Ltd.

5 Toh Tuck Link, Singapore 596224

USA office: 27 Warren Street, Suite 401-402, Hackensack, NJ 07601

UK office: 57 Shelton Street, Covent Garden, London WC2H 9HE

British Library Cataloguing-in-Publication Data
A catalogue record for this book is available from the British Library.

CURRENT TOPICS IN OSTEOPOROSIS

ISBN 981-256-153-6

Printed in Singapore.

FOREWORD

Osteoporosis has been termed a "disease of civilization", although "industrialization" might be more apt. The disease is apparently less common in predominantly agrarian and labor-intensive societies. The reasons are varied and include factors as divergent as shorter life-span, the osteotrophic effect of physical work, and simple medical under-reporting of osteoporotic fractures. Osteoporosis has also been termed a Gompertzian disorder, meaning that risk and prevalence rise geometrically with age. The reasons are that the factors leading to bony fragility are, for the most part, cumulative in their effect. As a result, social or economic changes that lead to increases in life expectancy will increase Gompertzian diseases as well. For this reason alone, if not for others, osteoporosis will become an increasing problem in the nations of East and Southeast Asia. It has been estimated, in fact, that by 2050, there will be 6.3 million hip fractures annually, worldwide, with over half of those in Asia.

Because osteoporotic fractures are disabling and resource-consuming, they create heavy demands on the health care systems of nations with high proportions of elderly. For example, in a country such as Finland, roughly 40% of hospital bed days are accounted for by osteoporotic fractures. Thus, prevention of osteoporotic fractures becomes of paramount importance.

One of the more common medical myths is that, in order to prevent and treat a disorder, one first must understand its cause. But the history of medical advances reveals that this is rarely the case. Instead, empirical approaches that are partially effective develop first, leading to better diagnostic distinctions, better understanding of pathogenesis, and ultimately, to more precise, efficacious therapies. It is a circular, iterative process. That has certainly been the case for osteoporosis.

First recognized as a distinct disease around the turn of the 20th century, osteoporosis was characterized, as its very name indicated, by a decreased amount of bony tissue in skeletal structures. This led to development of sophisticated technology for measurement of bone mass; but widespread application of this technology soon revealed that knowing the mass or density of bone was not enough. In 1990, at the Consensus Conference in Copenhagen, osteoporosis was redefined for the first time in 90 years as a disease, not of low bone mass, but of increased skeletal fragility. Low bone mass was retained in the definition, but relegated to the status of a risk factor, that is, one of several causes of fragility. This redefinition reflected a growing understanding of the importance of factors as varied as fall patterns and bone quality in influencing whether a person might suffer an osteoporotic fracture. Nevertheless, the bone mass paradigm for osteoporosis had enormous momentum, reinforced by the ability to measure mass in the clinic with an accuracy and precision better than found in the corresponding measures available to most other fields of medicine.

The reduced bone mass originally considered integral to the condition was judged to be the result of excessive, unbalanced bone resorption – a model that led naturally to the development and utilization of antiresorptive drugs, most notably the bisphosphonates. As an instance of the iterative character of evolving medical understanding, it soon became apparent that these agents were more efficacious than they should have been, had their action been primarily to alter bone loss. Moreover, as we looked more closely at their effect, we found that the bisphosphonates reduced fracture risk within a few months of starting treatment, before any appreciable mass difference could accumulate. This led to a realization that these agents were acting primarily by reducing bone remodeling activity and that remodeling was, itself, a fragility factor. Up till then, remodeling had been largely ignored, partly because it was difficult to measure in the clinic with any precision, and partly because remodeling had been considered to be a process that strengthened bone by repairing micro-damage, not a source of weakness.

The difficulty in measuring remodeling with precision is still to some extent with us, although the technology of bone remodeling biomarkers is improving steadily and, given time, could rival the accuracy and precision of bone mass measurement. The importance of quantifying remodeling is underscored by recent advances in skeletal histomorphometry, which have revealed that mean bony remodeling rates double across menopause in women, and triple by the time a woman reaches her mid 60s. These increases in remodeling are not related to need for mechanical repair, and their net mechanical effect is a weakening of the skeleton.

Thus osteoporotic fractures are now understood to be occurring in a context of exaggerated remodeling that confers no mechanical benefit. Antiresorptives are precisely the right form of therapy to reverse this abnormal situation. In fact, it has been suggested that osteoporosis be redefined once again, now as a disease of increased bony fragility due to increased remodeling. Low bone mass thus becomes not the cause of the fracture, nor even of the fragility, but a determinant of which individuals with high remodeling will be most prone to fracture.

But even so, the bone mass technological juggernaut continues its unstoppable downhill roll. Four years after the 1990 redefinition, a WHO panel defined treatment cut-off values for osteoporosis exclusively in terms of bone mass measurement. Specifically, the diagnosis "osteoporosis" was applied to individuals with a bone density value (BMD) more than 2.5 standard deviations below the young adult mean. This reflected not so much a turning of the field's back on the 1990 definition as the need to establish international guidelines for diagnosis and treatment in the absence of a well-developed technology for the addition of other undoubted risk factors into the assessment of individual patient risk. Advances in remodeling measurement will almost surely lead to changes in the WHO diagnostic criteria. Already it is recognized that the combination of high remodeling and low bone mass are much more strongly predictive of fracture than is low BMD alone.

But even as the field expands into a better understanding of the pathogenetic role of exaggerated remodeling, the final answer will still elude us. Not every woman experiences an increase in bony remodeling after menopause. Why do some and not others? We do not know. One of the factors hypothesized to underlie the mid-life rise in bone remodeling is a combination of low calcium intake and low vitamin D status. Since both lead to increased parathyroid gland activity, this explanation has considerable face validity. Parathyroid hormone is known to be the principal systemic determinant of the amount of bone remodeling activity. But as we have gained more experience with these problems, it has turned out that not everyone with inadequate vitamin D status develops a parathyroid response. Why do some and not others? We do not know.

As we make finer and finer distinctions, other such questions continue to arise. Hence, as we have gained more experience with this disorder and developed better treatments, it has become clear that osteoporosis is a more complex disorder than we could have imagined.

Robert P. Heaney, M.D.
Creighton University
Omaha, Nebraska, USA

TABLE OF CONTENTS

CHAPTER 1

EPIDEMIOLOGY OF OSTEOPOROSIS

E. M. C. Lau

Department of Community & Family Medicine,
The Chinese University of Hong Kong, 4/F School of Public Health,
Prince of Wales Hospital, Shatin, N.T., Hong Kong

The epidemiology of osteoporosis is reviewed in this article. Attempts were made to answer the following questions:

1. How should osteoporosis be defined?
2. How can risk factors and BMD measurements be applied to diagnose osteoporosis?
3. How do the rates for osteoporotic fractures vary by country, sex, age and time?
4. What are the cost for osteoporosis in terms of direct and indirect cost, morbidity and mortality?

According to the WHO criteria, osteoporosis can be defined as bone mineral density (BMD) of 2.5 standard deviation or more below the young normal mean. BMD measurements are predictive of fracture risks. Hip fracture is by far the most costly of osteoporotic fracture; and the rates are highest in Caucasians, intermediate in Asians and lowest in Blacks. Risk factors could be used to assist in decision in prescribing BMD measurements.

Research agenda

Further studies aimed at refining the use of risk factors and BMD in predicting fractures.

Further study on the cost-effectiveness of primary and secondary prevention of hip and other fractures.

Studies on the various aspects of epidemiology of osteoporosis in Asian populations.

Summary

Bone mineral density measurements and risk factors can be used to predict osteoporotic fractures. The important osteoporotic fractures are hip fracture, vertebral fracture and forearm fracture. The incidence of hip fracture is highest in Caucasians, intermediate in Asians and lowest in Negroid populations. The incidence of hip fracture increases exponentially with age in both sexes, but remains higher in women than men throughout life. Most vertebral fractures are clinically silent but are associated with much morbidity. Hip fracture is associated with extremely high direct cost in developed countries; and the cost is on the rise in developing countries.

Introduction

Osteoporosis can be defined as a "systematic skeletal disease characterized by low bone mass, and microarchitectural deterioration of bony tissue, with a consequent increase in bone fragility and susceptibility to fractures" [1]. As fragility fractures are the main public health consequence of osteoporosis, diagnostic criteria should be such that they are predictive of fractures.

Definition

In 1994, an expert panel of the World Health Organization recommended thresholds of bone mineral density in women to define osteoporosis [2], that have been widely but not universally accepted by the international scientific community and by regulatory agencies [3,4,5]. Osteoporosis in postmenopausal Caucasian women is defined as a value of bone mineral density (BMD) or bone mineral content (BMC) more than 2.5 standard deviations below the young average value (Fig 1). Severe osteoporosis (established osteoporosis) uses the same threshold, but in the presence of one or more fragility fractures.

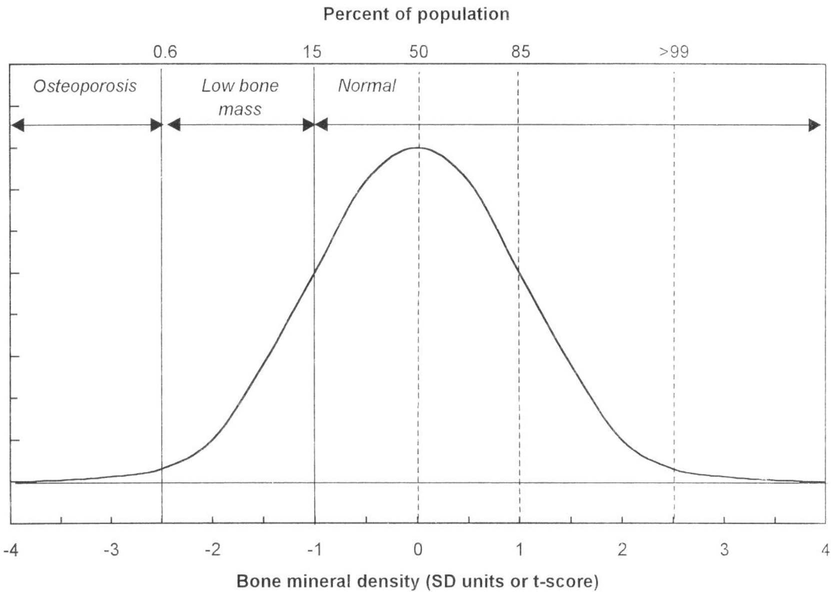

Fig. 1   Diagnostic thresholds for women based on the distribution of bone mineral density in the young healthy female population.

Predicting fracture risk

The association of BMD values and fracture risk has been studied in several large cohort studies. DEXA measurements of the hip, spine, forearm and calcaneus predict the risk of any fragility fracture in older women similarly, each with a relative risk (RR) for any fracture of 1.5, per age-adjusted standard deviation decrease. It is important to note that the risk of specific types of fractures, especially hip fractures, is more strongly predicted by measuring bone density at that site. The results of the Study of Osteoporotic Fracture showed that the RR for hip fracture is 2.6 for each standard deviation decrease in age-adjusted BMD at the femoral neck, while the RR is 1.5 for mid-radius [6].

BMD measurements are less accurate in predicting absolute risk than the relative risk of fracture, for absolute risk changes marked with age [7]. Absolute risks are important for decision making on therapeutic interventions.

The National Osteoporosis Foundation (NOF) has issued clear guidelines concerning the use of risk factors in predicting fracture [8]. It was stated that risk factors for low bone density have limited value in estimating a women's actual bone density [8]. However, risk factors for fracture can be useful in identifying women at high risk of fractures [9-12].

Five factors were selected by the NOF workgroup as being especially useful in a clinical setting, because they are easily assessible and are relatively common [8]. They were:

- Low bone mineral density;
- History of a prior fracture after age 40;
- History of a fracture at the hip, wrist, or vertebra in a first-degree relative ("family history");
- Being in the lowest quartile in weight;
- Current cigarette smoking.

A simple counting method was recommended by the NOF, in which practitioners will only need to determine whether a woman has had a prior fracture, and then count whether she has none, one, two or more of the remaining three clinical risk factors: family history of fracture, relatively low body weight, and smoking [8]. This method is practicable.

There is a general lack of longitudind data on the relationship between BMD measurements, risk factors and the risk of hip fracture among Asian populations. However, cross-sectional studies demonstrated that risk factors for hip fracture are similar to Caucasian [13]. Moreover, the relationship between the relative risk of hip fracture and diminishing BMD in Hong Kong Chinese were found to be similar to Caucasians [14]. Hence much of the above recommendation in Caucasian is probably applicable to Asian populations.

Fracture epidemiology

There is no universal definition of osteoporotic fractures. It is logical to consider low energy fractures as being osteoporotic, for osteoporotic individuals are more likely to fracture than their normal counterparts [15]. Fractures of the hip, vertebra and forearm are considered to be osteoporotic fractures. They share common epidemiological features: the incidences are higher in women than in men, increases exponentially with age, and occur at sites with a large proportion of trabecular bone [16].

It is increasingly being recognized, however, that osteoporosis can lead to fracture at other sites. These include fracture of the humerus, ribs, tibia (in women), pelvis and other femoral fractures. Exclusion of such fractures would lead to considerable underestimates in studying the cost of osteoporosis.

Hip fracture

A. Geographical pattern

There is pronounced geographical variation in the incidence of hip fracture, with rates being highest in Caucasians living in North Europe, followed by rates in Caucasian living in North America. The rates are intermediate in Asians and lowest in Black populations (Table 1) [17]. Moreover, the female to male ratio for hip fracture was 3:1 in Caucasians, but 1:1 in Chinese and Bantu.

 E. M. C. Lau

Table 1. Age-adjusted rate* of hip fracture per 100,000 population for females and males, by ethnic group and year of study

Ethnic group	Site	Year of study	Female	Male	Female to male ratio
Blacks	Maryland, USA	1979-1988	345	191	1.8
	California, USA	1983-1984	241	153	1.6
	Johannesburg, SA	1950-1964	26	29	1.3
Hispanics	California, USA	1983-1984	219	97	2.3
	Texas, USA	1980	305	128	2.4
Asians	Hong Kong	1985	389	196	2.0
	Hong Kong	1965-1967	179	113	1.6
	Tottori, Japan	1986-1987	227	79	2.9
	Okinawa, Japan	1984-1985	325	86	3.8
	California, USA	1983-1984	383	116	3.3
	Hawaii, USA	1979-1981	224	66	3.4
	New Zealand	1973-1976	212	121	1.8
	Singapore	1955-1962	83	111	0.7
Caucasian	Sweden	1972-1981	730	581	1.3
	Kuopio, Finland	1968	280	107	2.6
	Malmo, Sweden	1950-1960	468	153	3.1
	Norway	1983-1984	737	298	2.5
	Edinburgh, Scotland	1978-1979	529	174	3.0
	Oxford, England	1983	603	114	5.3
	California, USA	1983-1984	617	215	2.9
	Hawaii, USA	1979-1981	645	205	3.1
	New Zealand	1973-1976	466	139	3.4

*   Rates were age- and gender-adjusted to the 1990 US non-Hispanic Caucasian population.

Reproduced with permission from Villa ML, Nelson L (Ref 17).

The incidence of hip fracture also varies between subjects of the same origins but living in different countries. In Europe, the incidences of hip fracture vary more than 7 folds from one country to another [18,19].

There is some evidence that the incidence of hip fracture is raising rapidly in developing Asian countries. For instance, in Hong Kong, a highly urbanized city in China, the incidence of hip fracture had increased by 200% in the last 3 decades [20]. A recent multi-national study conducted in four Asian countries showed the incidence of hip fracture to be directly proportional to economic developments. The adjusted rates in Hong Kong and Singapore were almost identical to American Caucasians (at 19 per 10,000), while the rate in Thailand and Malaysia were 2/3 and 1/2 of the Hong Kong rates respectively [21]. With rapid economic development and aging of the population, hip fracture will be a major health problem in Asia.

Indeed, Cooper et al [22] had projected that, by the year 2050, more than half of all hip fractures in the world would occur in Asia. The projected number of fractures will be 6.3 million, with 3.2 million in Asia.

B. Secular trends

Recent research suggested that the incidence of hip fracture has experienced either a leveling off or a slightly downturn in North America and Europe. In Malmo, Sweden, Gullberg described a leveling off of hip fracture incidence during the mid 80's [23]. Nungu reported that the age-adjusted incidence of hip fracture remained at around 6/1000 population in the Uppsala country of Sweden in the same period [24].

In the Canton of Vaud, Switzerland, Jequier et al found a slight increase in hip fracture incidence in Swiss men, but not in women, from 1986 to 1991[25]. In Siena, Italy, the incidence of hip fracture increased slightly in men, but not in women from 1980 to 1991 [26].

The time trends for hip fracture in the UK from 1968 to 1986 was studied by Spector et al, using data from the Hospital In Patient Enquiry [27]. The standardized admission rates for hip fracture increased tremendously from 1968 to 1980 in both sexes, after which the rates

                               E. M. C. Lau

leveled off. A more recent study by Evans et al confirmed these results
[28].

Similar trends have been observed in North America. Melton et al
reported a downturn in hip fracture incidence in Rochester Minnesota,
between 1984 and 1987 [29]. It is not known if such changes are due to
health education, lifestyle changes; or cohort effects. Assuming no
increase in hip fracture incidence, the number of hip fracture patients will
continue to rise in all continents, as a result of population ageing.

C. Incidence by sex and age

As shown in Figure 2, the incidence rates for hip fracture increased
exponentially with ageing in both sexes [30]. The incidence in Rochester
rises from 2 per 100,000 person-years among women less than 35 years
old to 3,032 per 100,000 for women 85 years old and over [30].
Although the annual incidence among young men was similar to young
women, the rates in elderly men were only half of those in elderly
women [30]. These patterns were representative of those in Caucasian
populations.

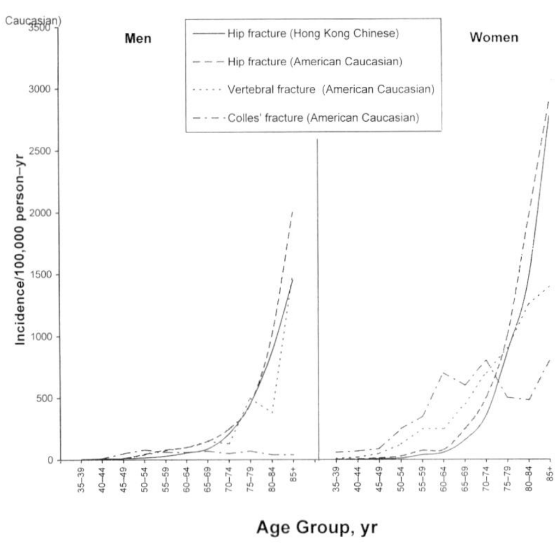

Fig. 2   Estimated numbers of hip fractures in 8 geographic regions in 1990, 2025 and
2050.

The age-specific rates of hip fracture in Hong Kong Chinese in 1995 are also presented in Fig 2 (Lau, unpublished data). The changes in the incidence of hip fracture with age are similar to those observed in Rochester. While the incidence were similar in young men and women, an exponential rise was seen in women from 65 years onwards and in men from 70 years old onwards. The rates in elderly women remained to be twice as high as in elderly men. In general, the incidence rates for hip fracture in elderly Chinese men were 75% of those observed in Rochester, while the rates in elderly women approached 90% of those observed in Rochester.

Vertebral fracture

Epidemiological studies on vertebral fractures are hampered by the lack of universally accepted criteria for the definition of vertebral fracture. Moreover, a substantial proportion of vertebral deformities are clinically silent.

A. Geographical pattern

According to radiographic studies, 19-26% of postmenopausal women have a vertebral deformity [31-34]. Vertebral fractures are as frequent in Asians as in white women [35,36]. However, vertebral fractures are less common in African-American [37] and Hispanic population [38].

The incidence of new vertebral fracture has been estimated to be around three times that of hip fracture, with the female to male ratio to be 2:1 [39].

B. Temporal trends

The temporal trends for vertebral fracture are not as well studied as for hip fracture, and the results are mixed. According to Bengnèr et al [40], the prevalence of vertebral fracture increased in Sweden between the periods 1950-1952 and 1982-1983.

Nevertheless, the temporal trend was found to be stable in Rochester, USA, from 1950 to 1989 [41].

Distal forearm fracture

The change in incidence with age for distal forearm fracture is different from fractures of the hip and vertebra. Study results from the Mayo clinic suggested that incidence rates increased linearly from age 40-65 years and then stabilized [30]. However, in men, the incidence remained relatively constant between 20 to 80 years. The female to male ratio for forearm fracture was 4 to 1. This ratio was much larger than that of 2 to 1 for vertebral and hip fracture.

The reasons why the incidence of forearm fracture plateaus with age are unknown. Nevitt and Cummings [42] proposed that elderly women have a slower gait and impaired neuromuscular coordination, and are hence more likely to fall backwards to land on their hip. On the other hand, younger women tended to fall on their outstretched arms. The changes in the incidence of forearm fracture with age concur with the pattern of age-related bone loss [43].

The international pattern for forearm fracture is not well described. There is some evidence to suggest that forearm fracture is much less frequent in Asian [44] and Black [45] population than Caucasians.

Socio-economic impact of osteoporosis

Mortality

The mortality attributable to osteoporosis results largely from hip fractures. Hip fracture causes a 12% to 20% reduction in expected survival [46]. Hospital-based studies showed that mortality rate was higher in men, older patients and in non-white populations [46]. Such observations can be explained by the difference in the prevalence of co-morbidity in population subgroups [47].

Morbidity and quality of life

Osteoporotic fractures cause varying degrees of morbidity. Colles' fractures have only short-term consequences, while hip fracture causes much disability. Many hip fracture patients become permanently disabled. Up to a third of hip fracture patients become totally independent, necessitating institutionalization [48].

The morbidity caused by vertebral fracture varies with the frequency of fractures. Multiple fractures typically cause the most pain and disability. Ettinger et al, demonstrated that vertebral fracture caused significant back pain, disability and height loss in Americans [49,50].

The effects of vertebral fracture on back pain and low morale were consistently demonstrated in Chinese men and women [51].

Costs of osteoporosis

Studies in various countries showed that the costs of osteoporosis are very substantial. Hip fracture is a major cause of hospital admission in the elderly. The acute care cost associated with hip fracture is tremendous in all developed countries. In the USA, the direct cost of hip fractures was around US$13.8 billion in 1995 [52]. In the UK, the direct for hip fracture was £942 million per year in 1998 [53]. The predicted annual treatment costs in Australia for atraumatic fractures occurring in subjects ≥60 yeas was A$779 million (or approximately A$44 million per million of population per annum) [54]. The majority of direct cost (95%) were incurred by hospitalized patients and related to hospital and rehabilitation cost [54]. In 1996, the acute hospital care cost of hip fracture per annum amounted to 1% of the total hospital budget, or US$17 million, for Hong Kong with a population of 6 million (Lau, unpublished data).

In the United States of America, the average nursing home care cost for each hip fracture patient was as much as US$3,875 in 1995 [52]. This approximated 28% of the total cost for hip fracture. As death due to hip fracture occurs mainly in the elderly, the indirect cost due to reduced productivity is much lower than for other chronic disorders such as ischaemic heart disease; stroke or breast cancer. However, the direct cost is comparable.

REFERENCES

1. Anonymous. Consensus development conference: diagnosis, prophylaxis and treatment of osteoporosis. American Journal of Medicine 1993;94: 646-50.
2. World Health Organization. Assessment of fracture risk and its application to screening for postmenopausal osteoporosis. WHO technical report series 843. Geneva: WHO, 1994.
3. Committee for Proprietary Medicinal Products (CPMP). Note for guidance on involutional osteoporosis in women. London: European Agency for the Evaluation of Medicinal Products (CPMP/EWP/5 52/95), 1997.
4. Orimo H, Sugioka Y, Fukunaga M, Muto Y, Hotokebuchi T, Gorai I, Nakamura T, Kushida K, Tanaka H, Ikai T, Oh-hashi Y. The committee of the Japanese Society for Bone and Mineral Research for the Development of Diagnostic Criteria. Diagnostic criteria of primary osteoporosis. Journal of Bone Mineral Metabolism 1998;16: 139-50.
5. World Health Organization. Guidelines for preclinical evaluation and clinical trials in osteoporosis. Geneva: WHO, 1998.
6. Cummings SR, Black DM, Nevitt MC, Browner W, Cauley J, Ensrud K, Genant HK, Palermo L, Scott J, Vogt TM. Bone density at various sites is predictive of hip fracture. Lancet 1993;341: 72-5.
7. Kanis JA, Delmas P, Burchardt P, Cooper C, Torgerson D on behalf of the European Foundation for Osteoporosis and Bone disease. Guidelines for diagnosis and management of osteoporosis. Osteoporosis International 2000;11: 192-202.
8. National Osteoporosis Foundation. Osteoporosis: Review of the evidence for prevention, diagnosis, and cost-effectiveness analysis. Osteoporosis International 1998;8(suppl 4): S1-S88.
9. Slemenda CW, Hui SL, Longcope C, Wellman H, Johnston JR CC. Predictors of bone mass in perimenopausal women: A prospective study of clinical data using photon absorptiometry. Annals of Internal Medicine 1990;112: 96-101.

10. Orwoll ES, Bauer DC, Vogt TM, Fox KM. Axial bone mass in older women. Annals of Internal Medicine 1996;124: 187-196.

11. Cummings SR. Treatable and untreatable risk factors for hip fracture. Bone 1996;19(suppl 3): 165S-167S.

12. Cummings SR, Nevitt MC, Browner WS, Stone K, Fox KM, Ensrud KE, Cauley J, Black D, Vogt TM, for the Study of Osteoporotic Fractures Research Group. Risk factors for hip fracture in white women. New England Journal of Medicine 1995;332: 767-773.

13. Lau EMC, Suriwongpaisal P, Lee JK, Das De S, Festin MR, Saw SM, Khir A, Torralba A, Sham A, Sambrook P. Risk factors for hip fracture in Asian men and women – the Asian Osteoporosis Study (AOS). Journal of Bone and Mineral Research 2001;16(3):572-580.

14. Lau EMC, Woo J, Leung PC, Leung D. Low bone mineral density, grip strength and skin-fold thickness are important risk factors for hip fracture in Hong Kong Chinese. Osteoporosis International 1993;3(2): 66-70.

15. Sanders KM, Pasco JA, Ugoni AM, Nicholson GC, Seeman E, Martin TJ, Skoric B, Panahi S, Kotowicz MA. The exclusion of high trauma fractures may underestimate the prevalence of bone fragility fractures in the community. The GEELONG osteoporosis study. Journal of Bone and Mineral Research 1998;13: 1447-1342.

16. Melton LJ III. Epidemiology of fractures. In: Riggs BL and Melton LJ III (eds) Osteoporosis: Etiology, Diagnosis and Management. New York: Raven Press, 1995, pp 225-248.

17. Villa ML, Nelson L. Race, Ethnicity, and Osteoporosis. In: Marcus R, Feldman D, Kelsey J (eds) Osteoporosis. California: Academic Press, 1996, pp 435-447.

18. Ellfors I, Allander E, Kanis JA, Gullberg B, Johnell O, Dequeker J, Dilsen G, Gennari C, Lopes Vaz AA, Lyritis G, Mazzuoli GF, Miravet L, Passeri M, Perez Cano R, Rapado A, Ribot C. The variable incidence of hip fracture in Southern Europe; The MEDOS Study. Osteoporosis International 1994;4: 253-263.

19. Johnell O, Gullberg B, Allander E, Kanis JA. The apparent incidence of hip fracture in Europe: A study of national register sources. MEDOS Study Group. Osteoporosis International 1992;2: 298-302.

20. Lau EMC, Cooper C, Fung H, Lam D, Tsang KK. Hip fracture in Hong Kong over the last decade – a comparison with Britain. Journal of Public Health Medicine 1999;21(3): 249-250.

21. Lau EMC, Lee JK, Suriwongpaisal P, Saw SM, Das De S, Khir A, Sambrook P. The incidence of hip fracture in five Asian countries – the Asian Osteoporosis Study (AOS). Osteoporosis International 2000 (in press).

22. Cooper C, Campion G, Melton LJ III. Hip fractures in the elderly: A worldwide projection. Osteoporosis International 1992;2: 285-289.

23. Gulberg B, Duppe H, Nilsson B, Redlund Johnell I, Sernbo I, Obrant K, Johnell O. Incidence of hip fractures in Malmö, Sweden. Bone 1993;14: S23-S29.

24.   Nungu S, Olerud C, Rehnberg L.   The incidence of hip fracture in Uppsala Country. Acta Orthopaedica Scandinavica 1993;64(1): 75-78.

25.   Jéquier V, Burnand B, Vader J-P, Paccaud F.   Hip fracture incidence in the Canton of Vaud, Switzerland, 1986-1991. Osteoporosis International 1995;5: 191-195.

26.   Agnusdei D, Camporeale A, Gerardi D, Rossi S, Bocchi L, Gennari C. Trends in the incidence of hip fracture in Siena, Italy, from 1980 to 1991. Bone 1993;14: S31-34.

27.   Spector TD, Cooper C, Fenton Lewis A. Trends in admission for hip fracture in England and Wales, 1968-85. British Medicine Journal 1990;300: 1173-4.

28.   Evans JG, Seagroatt V, Goldacre MJ.   Secular trends in proximal femur fracture, Oxford record linkage study area and England 1968-86.   Journal Epidemiology and Community Health 1997;51: 424-429.

29.   Melton LJ III, Atkinson EJ, Madhok R.   Downturn in hip fracture incidence. Public Health Reports 1996;111: 146-50.

30.   Cooper C, Melton LJ III.   Epidemiology of osteoporosis.   Trends in Endocrinology and Metabolism 1992;314: 224-229.

31.   Ettinger B, Black DM, Nevitt MC, Rundle AC, Cauley JA, Cummings SR, Genant HK.   The Study of Osteoporotic Fractures Research Group. Contribution of vertebral deformities to chronic back pain and disability. Journal of Bone and Mineral Research 1992;7: 449-56.

32.   Melton LJ III, Lane AW, Cooper C, Eastell R, O'Fallon WM, Rigs B. Prevalence and incidence of vertebral deformities. Osteoporosis International 1993;3: 113-9.

33.   Jones G, White C, Nguyen T, Sambrook PN, Kelly PJ, Eisman JA. Prevalent vertebral deformities: Relationship to bone mineral density and spinal osteophytosis in elderly men and women. Osteoporosis International 1996;6: 233-9.

34.   O'Neill TW, Felsenberg D, Varlow J, Cooper C, Kanis JA, Silman AJ, and The European Vertebral Osteoporosis Study Group. The prevalence of vertebral deformity in European men and women: The European Vertebral Osteoporosis Study. Journal of Bone and Mineral Research 1996;11: 1010-8.

35.   Ross PD, Fujiwara S, Huang C, Davis JW, Epstein RS, Wasnicn RD, Kodama K, Melton LJ III.   Vertebral fracture prevalence in women in Hiroshima compared to Caucasians or Japanese in the U.S.   International Journal of Epidemiology 1995;24: 1171-7.

36.   Lau EMC, Chan HHL, Woo J, Black D, Nevitt M, Leung PC. Normal ranges for vertebral height ratios and prevalence of vertebral fracture in Hong Kong Chinese: A comparison with American Caucasians.   Journal of Bone and Mineral Research 1996;11: 1364-8.

37.   Jacobsen SJ, Cooper C, Gottlieb MS, Goldberg J, Yahnke DP, Melton LJIII. Hospitalization with vertebral fracture among the aged: A national population-based study. 1986-1989. Epidemiology 1992;3: 515-8.

38.   Bauer RL, Deyo RA. Low risk of vertebral fracture in Mexican American women. Archives of Internal Medicine 1987;147: 1437-9.

39. Cooper C, Atkinson EJ, O'Fallon WM, Melton LJ III. The incidence of clinically diagnosed vertebral fracture: A population-based study in Rochester, Minnesota. Journal of Bone Mineral Research 1992;7: 221-7.

40. Bengnèr U, Johnell O, Redlund-Johnell I. Changes in the incidence and prevalence of vertebral fractures during 30 years. Calcified Tissue International 1988;42: 293-296.

41. Cooper C, Atkinson EJ, Kotowicz M, O'Fallon WM, Melton LJ. Secular trends in the incidence of postmenopausal vertebral fractures. Calcified Tissue International 1992;51: 100-104.

42. Nevitt MC, Cummings SR and the Study of Osteoporotic Fractures Research Group (1993) Type of fall and risk of hip and wrist fractures: the study of osteoporotic fractures. Journal of the American Geriatrics Society 1993;41: 1226-1234.

43. Horsman A, Burkinshaw L. Stochastic models of bone loss and fracture risk. In: Ring EFJ, Evan WD, Dixon AS (eds) Osteoporosis and bone mineral measurement. Institute of Physical Sciences in Medicine, York, England, 1989, pp15-30.

44. Hagino H, Yamamoto K, Teshima R, Kishimoto H, Kuranobu K, Nakamura T. The incidence of fractures of the proximal femur and the distal radius in Tottori prefecture, Japan. Archives of Orthopaedic and Trauma Surgery 1989;109: 43-44.

45. Griffin MR, Ray WA, Fought RL, Melton LJ III (1992) Black-white difference in fracture rates. American Journal of Epidemiology 1992;136: 1378-1385.

46. Sexson SB, Lehner JT (1988) Factors affecting hip fracture mortality. Journal of Orthopaedic Trauma 1988;1: 298-305.

47. Magaziner J, Simonsick EM, Kashner TM, Hebel JR, Kenzora JE. Survival experience of aged hip fracture patients. American Journal of Public Health 1989;79: 274-278.

48. Bonar SK, Tinetti ME, Speechley M, Cooney LM (1990) Factors associated with short-versus long-term skilled nursing facility placement among community-living hip fracture patients. Journal of the American Geriatrics Society 1990;38: 1139-1144.

49. Ettinger B, Block JE, Smith R, Cummings SR, Harris ST, Genant HK. An examination of the association among vertebral deformities, physical disabilities and psychosocial problems. Maturitas 1988;10: 283-296.

50. Ettinger B, Black DM, Nevitt MC, Cauley JA, Cummings SR and The Study of Osteoporosis Fractures Research Group. Contribution of vertebral deformity, chronic back pain and disability. Journal of Bone and Miner Research 1992;7(4): 449-456.

51. Lau EMC, Woo J, Chan H, Chan MKF, Griffith J, Chan YH, Leung PC. The Health Consequences of vertebral deformity in elderly Chinese men and women. Calcified Tissue International 1998;63: 1-4.

52. Ray NF, Chan JK, Thamer M, Melton LJ III. Medical expenditures for the treatment of osteoporotic fractures in the United States in 1995: Report from

the National Osteoporosis Foundation. Journal of Bone and Mineral Research 1997;12: 24-35.

53. Torgerson D, Cooper C. Osteoporosis as a candidate for disease management: Epidemiological and cost of illness considerations. Disease Management and Health Outcomes 1998;3: 207-14.

54. Randell A, Sambrook PN, Nguyen TV, Lapsley H, Jones G, Kelly PJ, Eisman JA. Direct clinical and welfare costs of osteoporotic fractures in elderly men and women. Osteoporosis International 1995;5:427-432.

CHAPTER 2

THE SOCIAL AND FINANCIAL COSTS OF OSTEOPOROSIS

Elaine King and Gang Li

Department of Trauma and Orthopaedic Surgery, School of Medicine, Queen's University Belfast, Musgrave Park Hospital, Belfast, BT9 7JB, UK

A brief discussion into the nature of the condition, its prevalence, incidence and its target population was required before the social and financial costs could be stated. Indeed it was crucial to establish the condition as an important financial stress to health services worldwide. Estimations were then made concerning the costs, both economically and socially, with subsequent research to determine the most viable method for reduction of such costs. The possibility of reducing hospitalization periods via the introduction of community care projects, the concept of screening for the condition and an increased awareness of the preventive mechanisms were all considered. It became apparent that, due to limited knowledge concerning the disease and its treatment, it was best to focus attention on preventing the condition.

1. Nature of osteoporosis

Osteoporosis, as defined by WHO in is a systemic skeletal disease characterized by low bone mass and microarchitectural deterioration of bone tissue with a consequent increase in bone fragility and susceptibility to fracture.[1] Osteoporosis may affect the entire skeleton with the most common fracture sites being the hip, wrist and vertebrae. These fractures are a considerable health problem causing substantial morbidity and mortality in the elderly and imposing enormous financial strains on the health service. As indicated by the WHO, Osteoporosis is defined using the measurement of Bone Mineral Density (BMD), where a value of BMD 2.5 SD or more below the young adult reference mean denotes the

17

condition.[2] How common is this condition and whom does it affect? Osteoporosis is a complaint primarily affecting postmenopausal women (Type I osteoporosis), and secondly targeting the elderly (Type II osteoporosis). Its pronounced prevalence in these groups can be attributed to the fact that peak bone mass is usually achieved in the age range from 20 – 30 years, after which a decrease is inevitable. This decrease is much more common in females than in males, due to the onset of the menopause. This is related to the fact that the sex hormones i.e. estrogens are crucial in maintaining and controlling bone turnover. Osteoporosis is also associated with conditions such as Cushing's disease, rheumatoid arthritis, alcohol abuse, scurvy and endocrine disorders. In addition to being more common in the female sex, osteoporosis is more prevalent in Caucasians and Asians; those with a slim body build sedentary lifestyle, low calcium intake and nulliparity. Osteoporosis is a common condition; with the remaining lifetime risk of osteoporotic fracture in a 50 yr old British white female has been estimated at 14% for hip, 14% for spine and 13% for the radius. The comparative values for their North American counterparts are somewhat higher, estimated at 17.5%, 15.6% and 16% respectively.[3] The remaining risk of any fragility fracture approaches 40% in women and 13% in men.[4]

2. Financial costs of osteoporosis

When discussing the cost of osteoporosis, in both human and economic terms, it is most practical to study data concerning hip fractures. Unlike fractures of the vertebrae and wrist, hip fractures almost invariably require hospital admission making data collection most feasible. It is estimated that 2/3 of vertebral fractures are not diagnosed clinically.[4] Osteoporosis, being a condition, which mainly affects the elderly, is more prevalent in developed countries due to the increased life expectancy. Therefore, to formulate accurate assumptions concerning costs, it is necessary to study the statistics from such countries. In the UK there are 6,000 estimated hip fractures, 50,000 fractures of the distal radius, and 40,000 clinically diagnosed vertebral fractures annually.[3] The total cost of osteoporotic fractures in England and Wales (1995) amounts to £742 million with £614 million being attributed to fractures of the hip.[3] In the USA health care expenditures attributable to osteoporotic fractures in 1995 were "estimated at $13.8 billions, of which $10.3 billions were for the treatment of white men, $0.7 billion for non white women, and $0.2 billion for non white men. Of the $13.8 billion, $8.6 billion was spent on impatient care, $3.9 billion on nursing homes, and $1.3 billion on outpatient care.[5] As illustrated by the figures above, it is not simply hospitalization, which costs health services, indeed much aftercare, and attention is required. This is further reinforced by the following data: in New Zealand (population 3 million) the combined total cost of caring for women in the two years after a hip fracture in 1994 was £22 millions[6] and France (excluding vertebral fracture) $740 millions for a population of 57 million people. In Australia it has been suggested that each individual pays $40 annually towards the cost of osteoporotic fractures.[7] As life expectancy has improved and continues to do so in many parts of the world the burden of osteoporotic fractures continues to rise. In 1995 there were about 325 millions individuals in the world 65 years old or more and it is predicted to rise to more than 1500 million by the year 2050. Based on the ageing U.S. population One study has predicted that an annual hip fracture rate greater than 500, 000 by the year 2040 and at 5% inflation rate the total cost of the fractures would be $240 billion by the year 2040.[8]

3. Social costs of osteoporosis

It would be very easy only to consider the financial cost of osteoporosis and to forget about the individual. Loss of independence is the major and most dreaded consequence of fracture in the elderly. Until recently most studies of morbidity were limited to studies of fracture malunion, aseptic necrosis and segmental collapse. More recent studies of human costs of fracture have considered the functional limitations, reduced activities of daily living, limitations in mobility and pain. Other quality of life issues have received less attention. When some fracture survivors return home they have an excellent medical result but they will be so scared at the possibility of falling that their lifestyle will be severely restricted.

Osteoporosis and its associated fractures have, in many ways, as great a human cost as financial. It has been estimated by Doube et al[9], that 1/3 of patients with osteoporotic hip fracture die as a result of the fracture, with a further 1/3 of patients requiring continued institutionalized care and with many of the remaining 1/3 suffering from loss in their independence and ability to perform their daily tasks. These serious social implications can directly lead to a reduced quality of life and an increased incidence of depression. This inevitably leads to further costs for the health service, in terms of psychiatry and social work. Parker et al argues that the mortality of 33% quoted relates to mortality at one year, and that all deaths over this period should not be attributed to the hip fracture. As the population is normally elderly approximately a 10% death rate should be expected annually, a further 10% might be accounted for by associated medical conditions. Parker therefore leaves, in his opinion, a more realistic figure of 10% as appropriate.[6] A main contributor to the costs of osteoporosis is the long hospitalization period associated with hip fractures, it is therefore reasonable to discuss methods that attempt to reduce this time without placing the patient at any potential risks, such as early discharge scheme for fracture patients.

4. Screening program: BMD Vs Bone turnover markers

Diseases of epic cost to the NHS, such as breast cancer are routinely screened for amongst the target population. This attempts to catch susceptible individuals before the condition progresses and treatment costs accumulate. In this respect it is reasonable to question why osteoporosis is not incorporated into a widespread screening program. The WHO acknowledges osteoporosis as a generally asymptotic condition until fracture occurs, it is crucial to examine the criteria necessary for a successful and cost effective screening program. It is essential that the measurement renders a screening test which is highly sensitive i.e. has a definite ability to detect the disease when present, and also highly specific - having the ability to identify healthy individuals as non - diseased giving few false positives. At present, one of the golden diagnostic criteria for osteoporosis is the measurement of bone mineral density (BMD) by DEXA, as indicated by the WHO.

BMD measurement was reported to have a sensitivity of 9% and specificity of 99% at a critical threshold of -2SD below the normal adult mean.[10] Hence, BMD may be an efficient measurement and provides a good assessment of fracture risk as stated that the predicative value of bone mass is similar to blood pressure for stroke, and better than that of serum cholesterol for cardiovascular diseases.[10] Although BMD can be an efficient measure and provides a good assessment of fracture risk it cannot, identify individuals who will have a fracture,[10] since the risk of fracture depends on many other skeletal related and fall related factors, many of which are independent of BMD. Skeletal related factors include femoral geometry, bone mass, microarchitecture, bone mineral structure and bone turnover. Fall related factors include variables such as neuromuscular function, cognitive impairment and visual acuity. In turn the chance of fracture once a fall has occurred is mediated by factors such as age, height, weight, mobility, and a genetic susceptibility to fracture. For these reasons, a universal screening program for osteoporosis, without maximum discretion is neither economically viable nor acceptable by general medics. A selective screening for susceptible individuals such as women with early menopause, who in addition are heavy smokers or alcohol consumers and have an important genetic disposition to the disease, may be a more feasible alternative. However, even such a limited screening initiative meets much opposition such as low compliance rates to the program, and treatment regimes, but more importantly to the effectiveness of reduction in fracture incidence.

It has recently been challenged that bone density alone cannot indicate the risk of fracture. Hui found that for the same BMD the risk of fracture rose from 8 fold to 10 fold from age less than 45 years to greater than 80 years. In a sample of 5,800 man and women over 55 years of age the risk of hip fracture rose 13 fold with age.[11] These observations suggest that something very important in the ageing process influences fracture risk independently of bone density. As indicated by Black et al a study on the association of BMD and fracture risk showed a reduction in the risk of fracture at the hip and spine of more than 50% with a corresponding increase in BMD at these sites of only 5–8%,[12] and it difficult to attribute such a spectacular clinical result to such small increases in bone mass.

Bone turnover markers as indicators of osteoporosis are useful alternatives or should be used in combination with BMD screening. Bone turnover is maintained by two groups of cells – osteoblasts and osteoclasts. Osteoclastic activity is carefully mediated by the action of sex steroids and a co-coordinated physiological balance with the osteoblasts is maintained to ensure no net change of bone during adult life. After the menopause, circulating estrogen concentrations decrease, osteoclastic activity is no longer maintained accelerates far exceeding that of the osteoblasts. This directly implies that the concentration of bone turnover markers in postmenopausal women may be a new diagnostic method for osteoporosis and a better indicator of fracture risk. This concept also has direct implications for treatment i.e. the administration of anti-reabsorptive drugs such as bisphosphonates. Again, the sensitivity and specificity of the serum and urine bone turnover makers to fracture predication is still debatable.

The Royal College of Physicians (England) has recently published clinical guidelines for the prevention and treatment of osteoporosis. These conclude that there is no universally accepted policy for screening and that, although screening strategies may be developed in the future, in their absence a case finding strategy where patients are identified on the basis of fragility fracture or the presence of strong risk factors. It is clearly apparent that even if desired a widespread screening serve is simply not feasible.

5. Public awareness and prevention of osteoporosis

As illustrated, widespread screening for osteoporosis is an undesirable concept, how then can the financial costs of the disease are significantly reduced? Through research it has become apparent that in order to decrease this "silent epidemic" prevention is the key. To reduce the incidence of a condition via preventative mechanisms, the general public, via public health programs must be very aware of the condition and its implications. How well is the general public informed about this condition? A study performed by Keene et al concerned 84 patients who had recently suffered osteoporotic fractures. The results were most disappointing; with only 34 of the patients being aware of the condition and with this knowledge coming from doctors in only 29%.[13] These statistics represent a huge flaw in health education and promotion policies and also serious breakdown in communication between doctors and patients.

Since osteoporosis is thought to be inextricably linked to bone mass, it is reasonable to state that any mechanism increasing bone mass will present a defense to the condition. Peak bone mass occurs between the ages between 20–30 years, after which an inevitable decline is to be expected. Therefore, it is necessary to try and increase the peak bone bass achieved, which is possible only through childhood. The general public also needs further education on the importance of calcium rich and balanced diet on skeletal development. Exercise affects the skeleton in many ways. The direct effect of stress loading can be to increase bone mineral density, and should be regarded as important in the prevention of osteoporosis. Children from primary school age should be systematically taught of the importance of exercise in bone development. Vigorous exercise during growing age increases BMD by 2–20%, and is more beneficial than during adulthood.[14] Studying the BMD of professional athletes reinforces this concept, that a tennis players playing arm can be up to 30% more dense than the non – playing arm.[14] Although excessive weight bearing exercise cannot be recommended for the elderly and infirm, light exercise is thought to decrease the risk of an osteoporotic fracture even in people who are aged over 80. Moderate exercise may further decrease the risk of osteoporosis by improving muscle tone and balance – hence decreasing the likelihood of fall.

6. Conclusion

It is clear that osteoporosis is a huge financial burden to the health services worldwide. With these costs set to rise in the future it is imperative that dramatic interventions occur in an attempt to reduce and limit these costs. As discussed, the possibility of a widespread screening program is not desired, and the advantages of early discharge form hospital have been vague. Attention must therefore be focused on prevention of both the condition and its endpoint i.e. fractures of the wrist, vertebrae and most importantly the hip. Through raising public awareness of the condition it can be hoped that, in general, individuals and families may alter their lifestyles. Children should be encouraged all levels to exercise regularly and consume a healthy diet in an attempt t o increase their peak bone mass. Postmenopausal women should be educated on the importance of HRT, and the increased risk denoted by heavy smoking and alcohol consumption. In addition patients on long-term steroid use should be routinely informed of the risk of osteoporosis and prescribed treatment where necessary. For the elderly, attention should be focused, not on maintaining an already decreased BMD, but on preventing falls.[15] Simple advice such as keeping all areas well lit, fitting down loose edges of carpets, using non – slip mats in the bathroom, and having regular eyesight tests could all reduce the likelihood of fall and hence the cost of the condition. However, it has become most evident, that before it is possible to reduce the costs of this condition; more research into the condition is needed.

REFERENCES

1. Consensus development conference: diagnosis, prophylaxis, and treatment of osteoporosis, *Am. J. Med.*, 94 (1993).
2. WHO study group on assessment of fracture risk and its application to screening for postmenopausal osteoporosis, *WHO technical series*, 843 (1994).
3. L. J. Donaldson, A. Cook and R. G. Thompson, *J. Epidemiol. Com. Health*, 44 (1990).
4. L. J. Melton, E. A. Chinscilles, C. Cooper and A. W. Lane, *B. M. J.*, 92 (1992).
5. N. F. Ray, J. K. Chan, M. Thamer and L. J. Melton, *J. Bone Miner. Res*, 12 (1997).
6. M. J. Parker and J. K. Anand, *Public Health* 105 (1991).
7. E. Barrett-Connor, *Am. J. Med.*, 98 (1995).

8.   R. Lindsay, *Am. J. Med.*, 98 (1995).
9.   Doube, *B. M. J.*, 318 (1999).
10. D. Marshall, O. Johnell and H. Wedel, *B. M. J.*, 312 (1996).
11. S. L. Hui, C. W. Slemenda and J. R. Johston, *J. Clin. Invest.*, 81 (1988).
12. D. M. Black, S. R. Cummings, D. B. Karpf and J. A. Cauley, *N. Engl. J. Med.*, 348 (1996).
13. G. S. Keene, M. J. Parker and G. A. Pryor, *B. M. J.*, 307 (1993).
14. S. Bass, G. Pearce, E. Hendrich and P. Delmas, *J. Bone Miner. Res.*, 13 (1998).
15. P. Kannus, *B. M. J.*, 818 (1999).

CHAPTER 3

PATHOGENESIS OF OSTEOPOROSIS IN ASIAN AND CAUCASIAN WOMEN

Yunbo Duan, M.D.

Department of Medicine and Endocrinology,
Austin Hospital, Austin Health,
The University of Melbourne,
Heidelberg, Victoria, 3084, Australia
Tel: 613 9496 5489, Fax: 613 9496 3365
Email: ybd@unimelb.edu.au

Fragility fractures of the spine and hip are a public health problem in both Asian and Caucasian women. Epidemiological studies have suggested that the vertebral fracture prevalence or incidence is similar or higher, while the hip fracture rate is lower in Asian women than Caucasian women. Most of the comparative studies have been focused on racial differences in areal BMD (aBMD), in which the lower aBMD in Asians than Caucasians is largely due to Asians having smaller bone size. Both growth- and age-related factors may contribute to the pathogenesis of bone fragility at each group and to the racial differences in fractures rates between the two groups. However, the structural basis and the pathophysiologic mechanisms responsible for the purported racial differences in fracture rates are largely unknown. There is very limited data in Asian women regarding the structural basis of bone modelling and remodelling on the periosteal and endosteal surfaces of bone during growth and aging, nor hypothesis-driven studies comparing the racial differences of growth and age-related surface specific changes. Comparative studies between the two groups are needed in almost every aspect of skeletal biology. However, these studies require careful design and attention to methodological issues. The results of these comparative studies will provide important insights into the structural basis and pathophysiology of bone fragility in both groups.

1. Introduction

Reduced bone mass and architectural disruption are the basic features of osteoporotic bone in postmenopausal women with fragility fractures in both Asians and Caucasians. Over the last two decades, there has been progress in understanding of the pathogenesis of osteoporosis in women and men. We recognize that reduced peak bone mass accrual during growth, accelerated bone loss during the early phase of menopause caused by estrogen deficiency, continued slow phase of bone loss in the elderly associated with secondary hyperparathyroidism, impaired bone formation with age, and non skeletal factors such as falls, form the basic features of the pathogenesis of bone fragility and fractures in postmenopausal women.

Although these mechanisms are generally applied to the aetiology of bone fragility in all women, the pathophysiology and structural abnormalities predisposed to the increased bone fragility in old age are likely to be heterogenous, varying in both individuals and race/ethnic groups. Understanding the structural basis of bone fragility requires studies on bone surfaces, as the morphological basis for bone gain during growth and bone loss during aging is a surface-based modelling/remodelling processes. The purpose of this article is to review recent advances in the structural basis and pathophysiologic mechanism for bone fragility in Asian and Caucasian women, and by contrasting the racial differences between the two groups, to gain insight into the pathogenesis of bone fragility in women of both races, and to draw attention to areas that require further study.

2. Epidemiology of fracture

2.1. Vertebral fracture

It is difficult to interpret race specific patterns in vertebral fracture prevalence or incidence because differences in methodology in defining vertebral fractures may contribute to observations. Despite this methodological problem, limited data suggests that the age-specific

                                   Y. Duan

prevalence is similar or lower in Chinese women than in Caucasian women [1-5]. In contrast, both vertebral fracture prevalence and incidence were reported to be higher in Japanese women than American Caucasian women [6, 7] (**Figure 1**). Thus, more attention to standard morphometric definitions of vertebral fracture is required before any conclusions concerning racial differences in vertebral fracture rates can be made with any confidence.

Comparing sexes, vertebral fracture *prevalence* is similar in both Caucasian women and Caucasian men reported by cross-sectional studies [8-12]. However, prospective studies have demonstrated that the incidence of vertebral fractures is higher in Caucasian women than Caucasian men [13-17]. The European Vertebral Osteoporosis Study reported that the vertebral fracture rate was about two-fold higher in women than in men, being 9.3 and 4.5 per 1000 person-years in women and men aged 50 to 79 years, respectively [16]. It has also been reported that the prevalence of vertebral fractures is similar or only modestly higher in Chinese women than Chinese men [1-5] (**Figure 1**). *Incidence* figures have not been documented in Chinese but a recent study in Japan showed that vertebral fracture incidence is as twice as high in women than in men (23 vs. 9 /1000 person-years) [7].

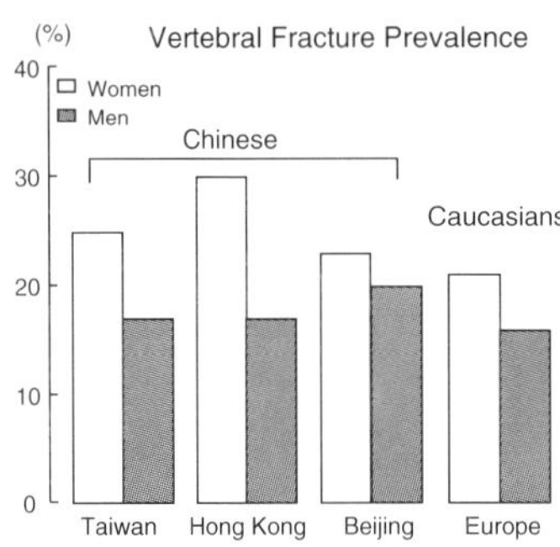

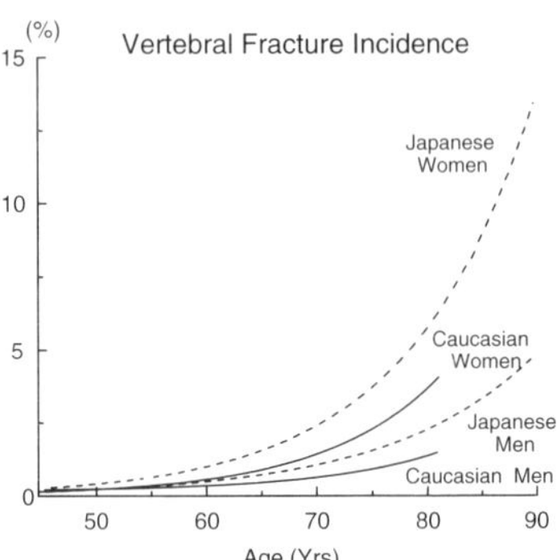

Figure 1. Left panel: the prevalence of vertebral fractures is similar in Chinese and European Caucasians in both sexes aged between 70 and 79 years. Right panel: the incidence of vertebral fracture is higher in Japanese than Caucasians in both sexes and higher in women than in men for each race. Adapted from Tsai et al [1], Lau et al [2], Xu et al [5], O'Neil et al [9], and Fujiwara et al [7] with permission.

## 2.2.	*Hip fracture*

Comparing races, almost all of the studies have consistently reported that the age-adjusted annual rate of hip fracture is lower in Asians than Caucasians [18-27]. Very low rates are reported in Korea and in Northern China [19-21,25]. Rates in the Japanese are about 50% lower than that in American Caucasians [24]. Intermediate rates of hip fracture were reported in Malaysia, Thailand and the Middle East [22, 26]. Lower rates have also been reported in Asian-Americans [27]. Earlier studies in Hong Kong and Singapore also showed a much lower rate of hip fracture in Chinese than Caucasians [23, 28], but recent studies suggest that rates are approaching Caucasians [22, 26]. However, rates are still around 20% lower than that in American Caucasians and much lower than the highest rates reported in Northern European countries [18] (**Figure 2**).

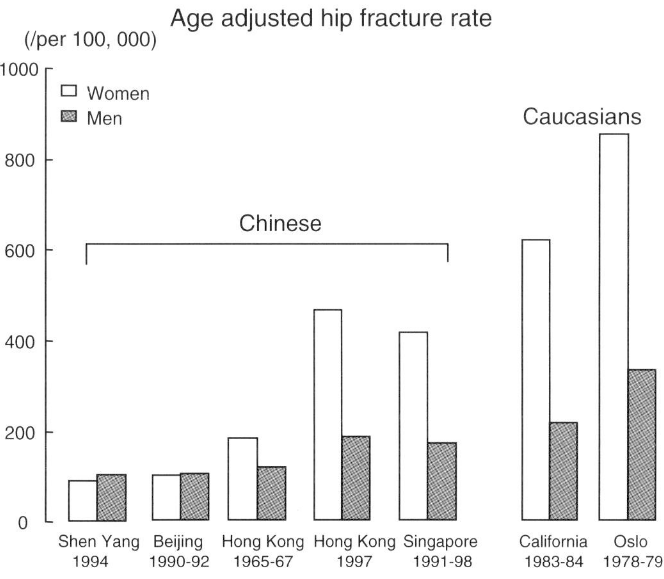

Figure 2 The age-standardised hip fracture rates aged 50 years and over are lower in Chinese than Caucasians but both sexes vary greatly in different regions. Adapted from Xu et al [19], Yan et al [20], Koh et al [22], Lau et al [26], and Villa et al [18] with permission.

The pattern of age-related increased hip fracture rates is similar in women and men, but incidence rates are two to three fold higher in Caucasian women than men [18]. In Asians, most, but not all studies, reported higher rates of hip fracture in women compared with men [19-26]. Even within the same ethnic group, rates of fracture varied greatly by sex and by geographical regions [19-26] (**Figure 2**). For example, between sexes, lower incidence of hip fracture in women than men has been reported in three studies from Northern China [19-21], while the two recent studies in Southern China and Singaporean Chinese show a much higher rate in women than men with a ratio of 2.5:1 [22, 26]. Within a geographic region, rates are also reported to be much lower in Northern than Southern Chinese in both women and men [19, 20, 26]. Xu et al [19] and Yan et al [20] each reported rates of 100 for men and 90 for women (per 100, 000) aged 50 years and over in Northern Chinese, while Lau et al [26] reported rates of 180 in men and 459 in women in Hong Kong, respectively. Most of these studies are based on retrospective data. Thus, methodological and ascertainment problems may partly explain these variable annual incidence rates between races and between sexes.

3. Reduced bone density and fracture risk

Patients with fractures have reduced areal bone mineral density (aBMD) and aBMD is a predictor of fracture [29]. Many studies have established the relationship between aBMD and the fracture risk in Caucasian women [30-33]. In general, a one standard deviation (SD) reduction of aBMD was associated with approximately 2- to 3-fold increase of risk for spine or hip fracture [33].

The relationship between aBMD and fracture risk in Asian women is less well defined but may be the same as that reported in Caucasians [5, 34-39] (**Figure 3**). For example, both Kung et al [34] and Xu et al [5] have reported that for each SD reduction in lumbar spinal aBMD there was an associated 2.4-fold increase in vertebral fracture risk in Chinese women. Huang et al [35] reported each one SD reduction in lumbar spinal aBMD was associated with a 2-fold increased risk of spine fracture in Japanese women living in Japan and America. Limited data

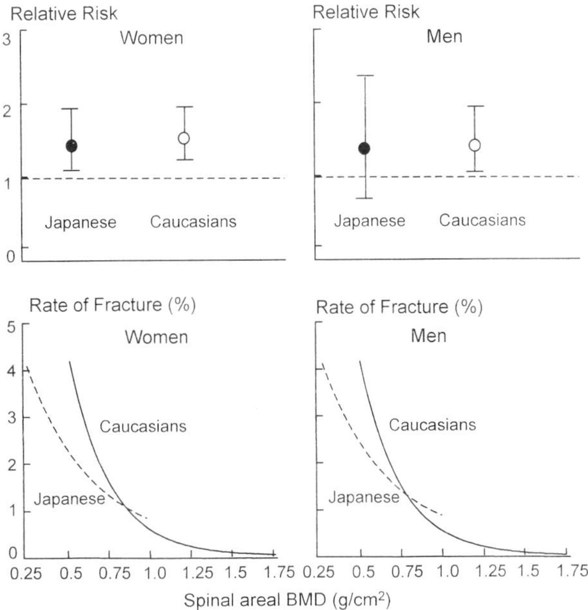

Figure 3. Upper panel, the relative risk of a one SD reduction in spinal aBMD (adjusted for age and prevalent vertebral fractures) is similar in Japanese and Caucasians for both women and men. Lower panel, at a given spinal aBMD for the same age, the absolute risk (incidence) of vertebral fractures is lower or similar in Japanese than Caucasians for both sexes. Adapted from O'Neil et al [16], and Fujiwara et al [7] with permission.

suggests that a one SD reduction in femoral neck aBMD predicts a similar hip fracture risk in Chinese/Japanese women compared to Caucasian women [7, 36].

It is less certain whether the rate of fracture (absolute risk) for a given aBMD level of the same age is the same in Asian and Caucasian women. In a recent prospective study conducted in Japan, the predicted rate of vertebral fracture at a given level of aBMD adjusted for age and baseline prevalent fracture appears to be lower in Japanese compared to Caucasians in both women and men [7] (**Figure 3**). However, the problem of comparing racial differences in fracture rate associated with aBMD is that Asians have lower aBMD than Caucasians, so a large proportion of the Asian population could not be matched with Caucasian population.

If the predictive value of a one SD reduction in aBMD is associated with a similar increase in fracture risk, and a given aBMD at the same age is associated with a lower or similar fracture rate between Asian and Caucasian women, then why do Asians have lower hip fracture rate but similar or higher vertebral fracture rates than Caucasians?

Bone fragility fractures attributable to low aBMD is only around 10-40% at different skeletal sites [30]. Only a small proportion of patients with fragility fractures have aBMD below the threshold value of –2.5 SD [40, 41]. In part, this is because measurement of aBMD only reflects one component of bone strength, the other material and structural properties of bone that contribute to bone fragility such as skeletal size, geometric distribution of bone mass, and architecture of trabecular and cortical bone are not captured by the aBMD measurement [42]. The loads imposed on bone during daily life are also not taken into account [43-46]. Thus, the smaller bone and lower aBMD in Asians than Caucasians may not necessary imply that Asians have a higher risk of fracture than Caucasians because their bone structure may be better preserved and their smaller bone is subjected to withstanding smaller loads, so the load per unit cross-sectional area (stress) may be the same compared to Caucasians.

4. Bone size and structural abnormalities in patients with fractures

Postmenopausal women with vertebral fractures have been reported to have smaller bone size at the vertebral body and other skeletal sites [47-51]. Using quantitative computed tomography (QCT), Gilsanz et al [47] reported that women with vertebral fractures had reduced vertebral body cross-sectional area compared to age-matched controls without fractures matched by volumetric BMD as well as height and weight. Smaller vertebral body width and volume in women with fractures has also been reported by other investigators [48-50]. In contrast, it has been found that women with vertebral fractures have increased vertebral body depth and spinal muscle moment arm [50, 52]. The increased vertebral body depth and moment arm may confer a biomechanical disadvantage because when bending forward, the spinal muscle contractions may produce a larger force/stress on the spine associated with the longer moment arm. At other skeletal sites such as iliac crest, the outer periosteal diameter was reduced in patients with vertebral fractures [53, 54]. Reduced bone diameter of the metacarpal was also reported in women with vertebral fractures [51].

Both trabecular and cortical bone structure are more severely destroyed in postmenopausal women with vertebral fractures. In the trabecular bone of iliac crest bone biopsies, the normal plate-shaped trabeculae are converted into rod-shaped trabeculae, and trabeculae are thinner and perforated. Many of the entire trabecular plates are completely removed, leading to the remaining trabeculae being more separated and less connected [53-59] (**Figure 4**). In the vertebral body, thinning, perforation and loss of trabecular numbers and connectivity are primarily confined to the horizontal trabeculae [60]. Vertebral body cortices are also thinner and more porous in postmenopausal women with vertebral fractures [61]. The reduction in cortical thickness is usually around 30-40% in patients with fracture compared to age matched controls [53, 54, 61]. Thus, both cortical thinning, increased porosity and trabecular structural disruption may all contribute greatly to the increased vertebral fragility with age.

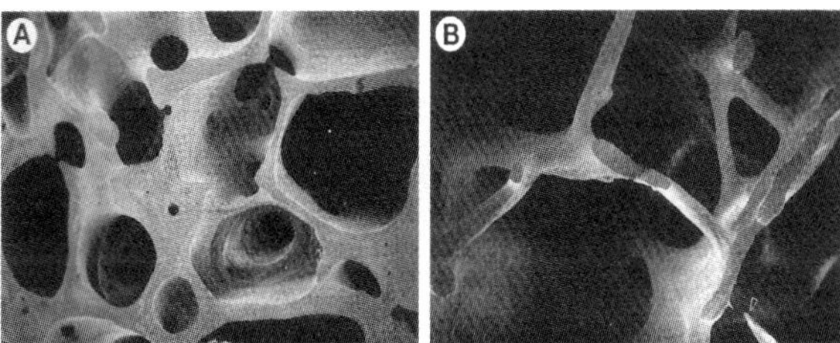

Figure 4. In normal cancellous bone (A) from an iliac crest bone biopsy, the cancellous bone is composed of curved plates interconnected by thicker bars; in osteoporotic bone (B) of women with vertebral fractures, the trabecular network is destroyed, being rod-like, perforated, more separated and loss of connectivity. Courtesy of Dempster et al [55].

In contrast to the smaller bone size and the more severe trabecular structural disruption in postmenopausal women with vertebral fracture, bone size at the femoral neck in patients with hip fracture has been variously reported to be smaller, normal or even increased [62-70]. Larger femoral neck periosteal diameter in elderly women with hip fractures has been reported in several studies [67-70]. It has been found that reduction in trabecular bone volume and loss of structural networks are less important in women with hip fracture [71]. In the femoral neck bone biopsies, elderly women with hip fractures were reported to have similar trabecular bone mass and structural disruption compared with age-matched controls [72-75]. Cortical thinning and increased cortical porosity in the femoral neck region are the major features of structural disruption in patients with hip fracture [71, 75]. It has been reported that the reduction in cortical thickness in elderly women with hip fracture is mainly confined to the inferior to anterior region of the femoral neck, a site withstanding the greatest stress during fall [75-77]. Larger femoral neck diameter with a very thin cortex may produce structural instability, predisposing to local buckling of the inner curvature of bone, therefore increasing hip fracture risk [78].

Accumulation of unrepaired microdamage may play an important role in the pathogenesis of bone fragility [71, 79]. Although direct evidence of the causal relationship between microcracks and fracture is lacking [82], several studies have shown that accumulation of microcracks increased with age at the femoral neck and the femoral shaft cortices [80, 81]. Because of lower bone remodelling indices and less structural disruption in the femoral neck than the vertebral body, it has been proposed that the accumulation of microdamage with age is more important for the bone fragility at the hip than the spine [71]. Decreased osteocyte number and density are associated with increased microcracks [82, 83]. A recent study indicates that osteocyte density is significantly reduced in women with vertebral fractures [83], and trabecular microcracks are present in human vertebral bodies [84], suggesting that microdamage may also play an important role in the pathogenesis of vertebral fractures.

These observations of macro- and micro-architectural abnormalities in patients with fractures are mainly derived from Caucasian women. The structural damage and disruption in patients with vertebral or hip fracture in Asian women and men are seldom reported in peer-reviewed international journals. In a small study of Japanese postmenopausal women with vertebral fractures, trabecular numbers were lower and trabecular separation were increased as measured by histomorphometry and microCT at the iliac crest bone biopsies, in cases compared to controls. Trabecular thickness did not differ between the two groups [85]. Thus, in both Asian and Caucasian women, the extent of structural disruption and the deficit in bone mass may be similar in patients with fragility fractures. However, whether the structural basis and the cellular mechanisms that lead to these structural abnormalities are similar in Asian and Caucasian women is largely unknown. Some of the issues are explored below.

5. Origins of bone fragility in Asian and Caucasian women

Riggs and colleagues have proposed a unifying model to explain the pathogenesis of bone fragility, Type I (postmenopausal) osteoporosis, postmenopausal bone loss characterised by early and rapid trabecular bone loss associated with vertebral fractures; and Type II (age-related) osteoporosis, characterised by the late slow phase of age-related bone loss mainly of cortical bone and associated with hip fractures [86]. The evidence to support this concept is largely based on the observations derived from the different patterns of fracture type, bone loss and the different pathophysiologic mechanisms that lead to bone loss [87]. This model failed to consider the role of peak bone mass in the pathogenesis of bone fragility in patients with fragility fractures [88].

5.1. Growth-related origin

Knowledge of growth-related factors to the contribution of understanding bone fragility in elderly women is largely based on studies in Caucasian women. There is insufficient data of Asian women. In Caucasian women, it has been suggested that reduced peak bone mass and subsequent bone loss after menopause contribute equally to the deficit in bone mass in older age [89]. Twin and family studies have shown important genetic effects on skeletal growth in bone mass, size and structure [90-92]. Family studies of mother-daughter pairs have also provided evidence of family bone trait resemblance and a tracking of bone mass and size during growth [93, 94]. Reduced peak bone mass in the premenopausal daughters of women with vertebral and hip fractures has been reported [95-100]. Family history of osteoporotic fractures is well documented as is the influence of genetic factors on fracture occurrence [91, 101, 102]. There is also some evidence to suggest that the sex-differences in bone fragility may originate in growth [68, 103]. Thus, although these are indirect inferences, these studies do suggest that there may be a casual linkage between growth and bone fragility.

It has been suggested that the higher bone mass and lower fracture risk in Blacks compared to Caucasians is growth-related because the pattern and amount of bone loss is similar in Black and Caucasian women after menopause [104]. It has also been reported that growth was associated with racial differences in several structural features of Asian and Caucasian children [105]. The question arising here is that if there are racial differences in fracture rates between Asians and Caucasians, is this due to racial differences in growth-related or age-related factors, or both? If it is largely growth-related, is this due to prepubertal growth or peripubertal growth? Answers to these questions are difficult to determine as most of the racial comparative studies between Asian and Caucasian girls and boys were performed using aBMD as the phenotype, in which aBMD is largely influenced by growth in bone size [42].

Limited data suggests that there appears to be no racial differences in total body length, total body area and total body bone mass in Asians and Caucasians before puberty [106], while the difference in timing (tempo) of the peak pubertal growth spurt has been reported between Asian and Caucasian girls and boys [107]. It has been reported that the timing, not the magnitude, of the peak bone mass accrual expressed as aBMD tended to occur earlier in Asian than Caucasian girls [107]. There is also some evidence to suggest that the age of onset of puberty and the age at menarche may be earlier in Asian than Caucasian girls [107-110]. Insights into the racial differences of skeletal growth can be partly gained by comparing racial differences of the peak growth velocity during puberty.

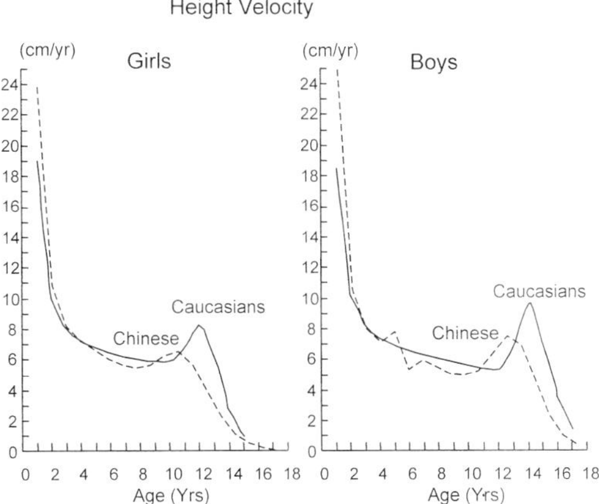

Figure 5. The peak height growth velocity during puberty is lower and occurs approximately one year earlier in Chinese than Caucasians of both sexes. Adapted from Parfitt [111] and Leung et al [112] with permission.

Based on indirect comparison from the published literature, the pattern of linear growth velocity of total body length is similar in Asian and Caucasian girls and boys [111-113]. However, the peak height growth velocity during puberty is lower and occurs approximately one year earlier in Asians than Caucasians (**Figure 5**).

Growth of length of the axial and appendicular skeleton is race specific. The shorter stature of Asians is predominantly due to the shorter leg length, the trunk length is very similar in Asians and Caucasians [113, 114]]. These racial differences in the upper body and lower body segment length can probably be attributed to the racial differences in the tempo, the duration and extent of the pubertal growth spurt between the two race groups. In both Asian and Caucasian girls and boys, before puberty, leg growth is faster than trunk growth. During puberty, trunk growth is accelerated while leg growth slows down [112, 115, 116]. Although a comparative study has never been reported between Asian and Caucasian children, there was some indirect comparisons that suggested that the peak pubertal growth spurt of trunk length is similar in Asian and Caucasian girls and boys [112, 115, 116].

Whether growth of bone width/diameter, structure and volumetric BMD (vBMD) of the axial and appendicular skeleton is race specific is uncertain. Whether the similar or higher vertebral fracture rate but lower hip fracture rates in Asian than Caucasian women is due to different racial effect of growth on axial and appendicular skeletons is also unknown. The region specific growth effect of race has been reported in Black and Caucasian children. For example, Gilsanz et al [117] reported that vertebral body trabecular vBMD, not cross-sectional area, measured by QCT, is higher in Black than Caucasian girls. In contrast, in the appendicular site of the mid-femur shaft, whole bone cross-sectional area, not cortical vBMD and cortical thickness, is higher in black than Caucasian girls [117]. Asian women achieve smaller vertebral size during growth than Caucasian women, however, it appears that peak vertebral trabecular vBMD measured by QCT is higher in Chinese than Caucasian women [118], but lower in Japanese than Caucasian women [119] (**Figure 6**). Asian women also have smaller appendicular skeletal diameter and thinner cortex [120]. Whether the long bone diameter and cortical thickness remained lower in Asians after adjustment for their shorter status, and whether cortical vBMD is the same in Asian and Caucasian women is unknown.

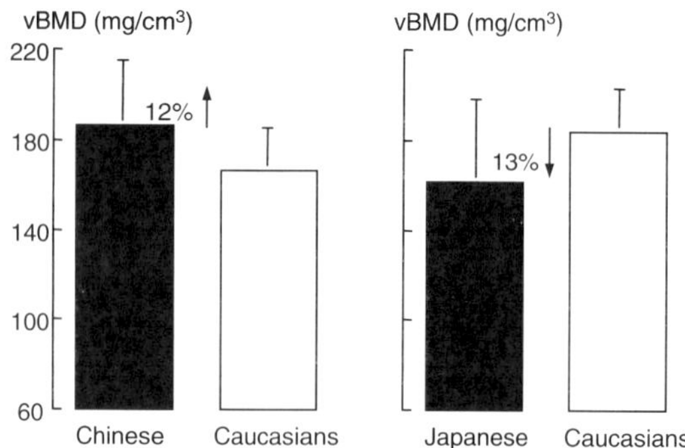

Figure 6. **The cross-calibrated peak vertebral body trabecular volumetric BMD (vBMD)** measured by QCT is higher in Chinese than Caucasian women, but lower in Japanese than Caucasian women. Adapted from Yu et al [118] and Ito et al [119] with permission.

5.2. *Menopause- and age-related origin*

Increased bone loss after menopause has been well documented as a major contributor to the increased bone fragility in both Asian and Caucasian women. The inference of bone loss has been largely derived from bone densitometry studies, which typically shows that menopause is associated with an early phase of accelerated decline in aBMD, and a late phase of slow decline in aBMD at the lumbar spine [86]. This pattern of postmenopausal bone loss is the same in Asian and Caucasian women [121]. However, as bone density is an integrated measurement of bone, it does not distinguish the surface specific changes of bone loss on the endosteal surfaces and bone gain on the periosteal surface [122]. Thus, neither the expression of aBMD nor vBMD is incorrect and is a misleading term when comparing racial differences in bone loss because these expressions are influenced by the amount of endosteal bone loss, the magnitude of periosteal bone gain and the increased bone size associated with periosteal expansion during aging.

Bone loss is a surface-based phenomenon. Menopause and aging associated bone loss only occur on the three subregions of endosteal surfaces (trabecular, endocortical and intracortical surfaces). There is no net bone loss on the periosteal surfaces [123]. In contrast, menopause/aging is associated with slow increased periosteal new bone apposition [124]. Thus, *net* bone loss during aging is a summation of bone loss on the endosteal surfaces and bone gain on the periosteal surface [50, 122] (**Figure 7**). *Net* bone loss is greater in Caucasian women than Caucasian men. This greater *net* bone loss in Caucasian women than men has been suggested to be due to the fact that women have lesser periosteal apposition because endosteal bone loss is similar in Caucasian women and men [50, 125-130]. *Net* bone loss is also greater in Asian women than Asian men [131-133], however, the relative contribution of periosteal apposition and endosteal bone loss to the sex differences in *net* bone loss in Asian women and men has not been reported.

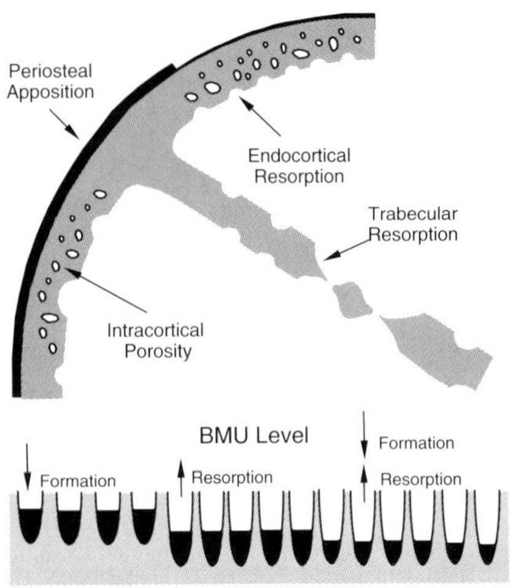

Figure 7. At the organ level (upper panel), *net* bone loss during aging is a summation of bone loss on the three subregions of endosteal (inner) surfaces and bone apposition on the periosteal (outer) surface. At the tissue level (lower panel), bone loss is determined by the numbers of negative BMUs activated. At the cellular level, bone loss is determined by the extent of each BMU imbalance, either due to reduced bone formation, increased bone resorption, or both. These processes are likely to be varied by race and sex. Adapted from Seeman [122] with permission.

A great deal of studies have been done to compare racial differences in aBMD. The lower aBMD in Asians compared to Caucasians is largely due to Asians have smaller bone size [105, 134-136]. Most of these studies suggested that the racial differences in aBMD disappeared after adjusting for bone size or body size [134-136]. However, as discussed above, inference regarding racial differences in bone loss should be made cautiously because the menopause and age-related changes on the periosteal surface and endosteal surface may be race specific. Hypothesis-driven studies comparing racial differences in the extent of bone modelling/remodelling on the periosteal and endosteal surfaces have never been done in Asian and Caucasian women. Whether the growth related racial differences in bone size, mass, and structural properties established during growth increase, decrease or remain the same with age, and whether these racial differences in menopause- and age-related changes account for racial differences in bone fragility fracture is unknown.

Whether race produces a different effect of menopause/aging on the axial skeleton and appendicular skeleton is also uncertain. If vertebral fracture rates are similar in Asian and Caucasian women, is this because menopause and aging are associated with similar structural disruption on endosteal surfaces in both Asian and Caucasian women? If hip fracture rates are lower in Asians than Caucasians, is this because Asians have lesser cortical thinning or lesser increased intracortical porosity with age than Caucasians? Do Asian women have lesser age-related increases in accumulation of unrepaired microdamage? If cortical thinning is less in Asians, is this due to Asians having greater periosteal apposition, slower endosteal bone resorption, or both?

6. Structural and biomechanical basis of bone fragility

6.1.   Vertebral skeleton

The structural basis for vertebral fragility in Caucasian women has been studied using histomorphometry and scanning electron microscopy [60, 61, 137-139]. The trabecular network of vertebral body consists of horizontal and vertical trabecular planes. The loss of trabecular bone is featured by structural disruption primarily of the horizontal trabeculae, with thinning, perforation and disappearance of horizontal structural plates, leading to the remaining vertical trabeculae being more separated and less connected, thereby increasing the structural instability [60, 139]. These trabecular structural disruptions have been suggested to be a major contributor to the increased vertebral body fragility in postmenopausal women. For example, disruption of trabecular networks, such as loss of connectivity has been documented to be a major feature of vertebral fracture independent of reduced bone mass [140-142].

The structural basis for vertebral fragility in Asian women is less well defined. Histomorphometric studies in Asians are rare. Using stereoscopic microscopy, Oda et al [143] studied the trabecular structure of lumbar vertebral body specimens from Japanese women and men.

Structural disruptions such as loss of trabecular number and increased trabecular separation were all observed in elderly women. Moreover, loss of structural elements was mainly confined to the anterior subregion of vertebral body, which is consistent with the view that anterior wedge vertebral fracture is more common in Japanese women [143] (**Figure 8**).

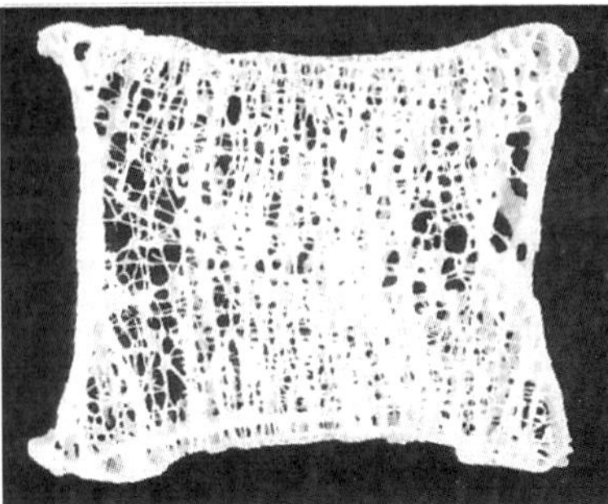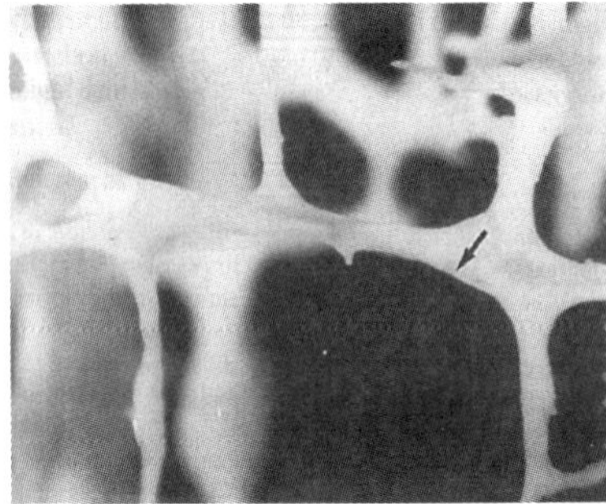

Figure 8. In postmenopausal Japanese women, trabecular structural disruption is more severe in the anterior region of vertebral body (left panel). Vertebral body trabecular thinning, loss of connectivity, and increased trabecular separation are present (right panel). Courtesy of Oda et al [143].

The cortical thickness of the vertebral body shell may also be important for vertebral strength. Decreased vertebral body cortical thickness and increased intracortical porosity with age have been documented in Caucasian women [137, 144]. Although not reported in all studies, several studies show the important contributions of vertebral body cortical thickness to the compressive strength of vertebral body in vitro [144, 145]. Thus, it remains to be defined as to what the role of trabecular structural disruption, cortical thinning and increased porosity have to the declined vertebral body strength and increased fragility with age in both Asian and Caucasian women.

The degree of thinning of the cortex during aging is determined by the endocortical resorption and a very slow process of periosteal apposition. The significant contribution of cortical thinning to increased vertebral fragility raises an important issue regarding the relative contribution of periosteal bone gain and endocortical resorption to the determinant of cortical thinning, and the role in establishing racial and sex differences in vertebral fragility. Although periosteal surface at the vertebral body has not been studied, vertebral body depth and cross-sectional area have been reported to be increased with age in Caucasian women [50, 146] and in Asian women [147]. Periosteal apposition has a protective effect on bone during aging because it partly compensates for endosteal bone loss and increases vertebral size, and therefore reduces the load falling on bone. For example, vertebral body bone mass is usually reported to be reduced by 30% in elderly Caucasian women, a study has shown that bone mass was reduced by 60% in elderly women after adjustment for the increased periosteal expansion [50].

Among Asian women, age-related decline in vertebral aBMD shows a similar pattern when compared to Caucasian women [118, 121]. Racial differences in age-related cortical thinning and declined cortical vBMD have not been documented. However, the amount of trabecular bone diminution has been variously reported to be similar or faster in Asian than Caucasian women. Fujii et al [147] reported that vertebral body trabecular vBMD measured by QCT declined with age similarly in Japanese and Caucasian women and in Japanese and Caucasian men. In contrast, using the same Caucasian reference database, both Ito et al [148] and Yu et al [118] reported that vertebral body trabecular vBMD measured by QCT declined faster in Japanese and Chinese women than Caucasian women (**Figure 9**).

Racial differences in the structural basis of trabecular and cortical bone loss have been studied in Black and Caucasian women [104]. The pattern and magnitude of bone loss on the endocortical and trabecular surfaces are similar, the structural disruption, such as trabecular thinning, loss of structural elements and the thinning of the cortex are all similar in Black and Caucasian women [104]. It is yet to be determined whether menopause is associated with racial differences in the structural changes on the periosteal and endosteal surfaces in Asian and Caucasian women. Comparative studies of these will give us a clue whether there are racial differences in vertebral fragility, and if so, what structural basis may explain the racial differences in vertebral fragility.

The vertebral body structural stability and compressive strength are also determined by the vertebral body cross-sectional area and the loads applied to spine. During normal daily activity, the loads on vertebral

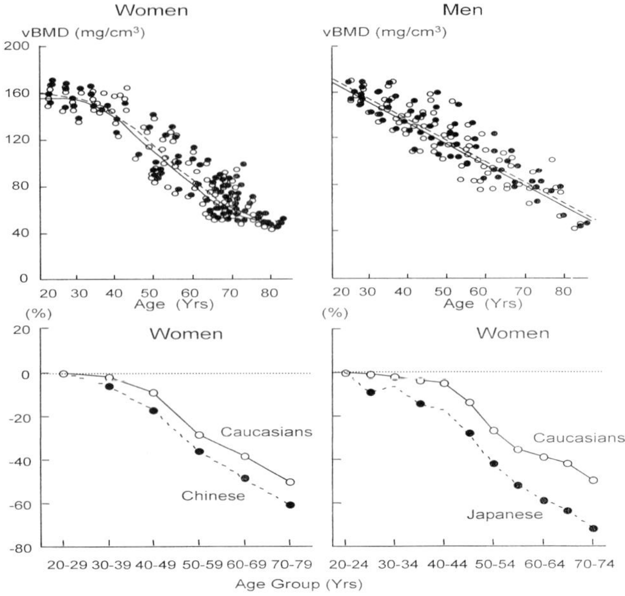

Figure 9. Upper panel, vertebral body trabecular volumetric bone mineral density (vBMD) measured by QCT declined with age similarly in Japanese (filled circles, dashed line) and Caucasians (open circles, solid line) in both sexes. Lower panel, the age-related diminution of vertebral body trabecular vBMD was faster in Chinese than Caucasian women and faster in Japanese women than Caucasian women. Adapted from Fujii et al [148], Yu et al [118] and Ito et al [119] with permission.

body are a function of upper body weight and extensor force caused by the spinal muscle contraction when bending forward [150]. The spinal muscle force contraction that occurs when bending forward generates considerable more stress on spine than the normal position of standing erect. Using static engineering principles, a study has shown that bending forward causes a 10-fold force increase on the spine than when standing erect [150]. The implication of these findings for racial comparison is that despite Asians having smaller vertebral body size than their Caucasian counterparts, Asians also have a lower body weight and a smaller muscle mass than Caucasians. This means that the loads falling on bone expressed as loads per unit cross-sectional area (stress) may be no different between the two racial groups. Unpublished data suggests that this is the case [147].

Vertebral fracture risk increases with age because vertebral body strength declines with age, while loads change little with age, so the ratio of load to strength increases with age dramatically. Thus, insights into racial differences in vertebral fragility and fracture rates may be gained by the application of biomechanical principles to the relationship between loads imposed on bone and the bone strength to resist that load. This concept of "factor of risk" has been proposed and applied to the study of vertebral fracture in different loading conditions [45, 46]. We have applied this model to study the biomechanical basis of sex differences in the vertebral body fragility fractures in Caucasian women and men [150]. Vertebral fracture risk index (FRI, stress/strength) increased with age, more in women than in men, and a greater proportion of elderly women than men (26% vs. 5%) have an FRI ≥ 1, a threshold value of fracture in both women and men. Thus, the higher incidence of vertebral fracture rates in women than in men is most likely due to more women than in men being placed in the higher risk group [150]. The similar vertebral fracture prevalence in Asian and Caucasian women may reflect a parellel load to strength relationship in the spine between the two groups. Preliminary data suggests that the proportion of elderly Asian and Caucasian women that have an FRI greater than unity is the same [147].

6.2. *Proximal femur*

The structural basis for bone fragility at the femoral neck is less well defined in Caucasian women. Available data suggests that the structural abnormalities that predispose an increase in femoral neck fragility are likely to be different from that of the vertebral body. There appears to be no accelerated bone loss at the femoral neck during the early phase of menopause as densitometry studies have shown that the femoral neck aBMD declines with age in a linear relationship [151, 152]. Structural disruption of femoral neck cortical bone, not trabecular bone, may play an important role in femoral neck fragility [72, 75]. Indeed, several studies have shown that menopause and aging are associated with a greater reduction in cortical thickness and an increase in cortical porosity in normal Caucasian postmenopausal women. These changes contribute largely to the reduction of femoral neck strength [76, 153, 154]. The biomechanical disadvantage of thinner and porous cortices is that they create an unstable structural condition associated with increased risk of local buckling, thereby increasing hip fracture risk [155].

The role of periosteal apposition in protecting against the age-related increase in femoral neck cortical thinning caused by endocortical resorption is unknown. It is believed that there is no periosteum at the femoral neck because it is surrounded by the capsule of the hip joint [156, 157]. However, recent studies using histomorphometry do demonstrate that periosteum is present at the femoral neck, and there is a non significant reduction of periosteal apposition in elderly Caucasian women with hip fractures compared to age-matched controls [156, 158]. In addition, most, but not all studies, reported that femoral neck periosteal diameter measured using x-ray technique increased with age in Caucasian women and men [68, 152, 155, 159-161]. It is likely periosteal apposition is important for Caucasian women as well as for men, to protect against the age-related increases in bone fragility by offsetting the endosteal bone loss and maintaining bending strength throughout life. Whether this is the reason why hip fracture occurs after vertebral fractures and usually occurs in old age remained to be answered.

There is very limited data on menopause- and age-related changes on the periosteal and endosteal surfaces of the femoral neck in Asian women and men. It has been reported that periosteal expansion at the femoral neck increases with age in Asian men but not in Asian women [131, 162]. Horikoshi et al [162] studied femoral neck geometric and structural properties in a small number of healthy Japanese women aged 23-81 years using peripheral quantitative computed tomography (pQCT). Femoral neck periosteal diameter did not increase with age. There was a small increase in endocortical diameter and a slight decline in cortical thickness. However, cortical vBMD declined significant with age, so the authors inferred that the declined cortical vBMD may be largely due to increased cortical porosity. Increased age-related femoral neck cortical porosity was documented in elderly Chinese women [163].

The age-related decline in femoral neck aBMD seems to be faster in Asian than Caucasian women and in Asian than Caucasian men [121, 164] (**Figure 10**). Similarly, as studies reported in Caucasians [165, 166], bone loss at the proximal femur is probably accelerated, rather than decelerated, in elderly Asian women and men [167, 168].

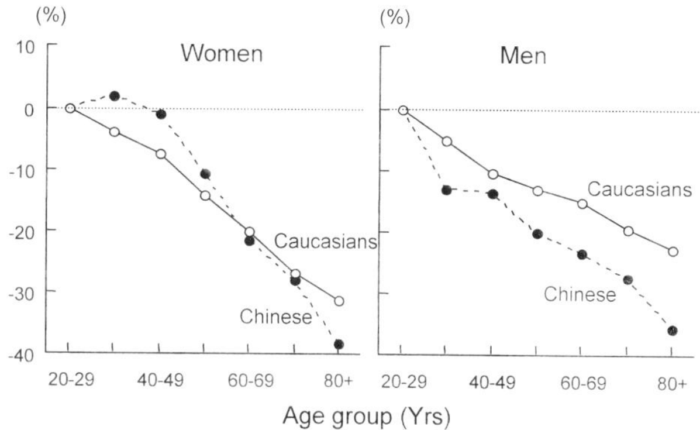

Figure 10. The age-related diminution of femoral neck aBMD relative to peak (% change) seems to be faster in Chinese than Caucasian women and in Chinese than Caucasian men. Adapted from Beck et al [152] and Liao et al [121], Duan et al [164] with permission.

In a 10-year follow up study in Japanese women and men, Yoshimura et al [167] reported that the annual decline rate of aBMD is faster in the elderly group (–1.2% in women and –1.2% in men) aged between 70 and 79 years compared to the younger group (range from –0.3 to –0.8%, respectively) of from 40 to 69 years. Ho et al [168] reported that compared to the age group of less than 75 years, femoral neck aBMD declined by 22% and 16% in very elderly Chinese women and men aged 85 years and over, respectively. These observations did not provide the information of the relative contribution of periosteal bone gain and endosteal bone loss to the net decline in bone loss. However, this data does suggest that bone remodelling, particularly on the endosteal surfaces is increased in elderly Asian women and men.

Asian women have smaller femoral neck diameter even after adjustment for their shorter status [169, 170]. The smaller femoral neck size in Asian women is associated with lower bending strength compared to Caucasian women because bending strength varies with the square distance of the radius of bone [171], therefore hip fracture rate would be expected to be higher in Asian women than Caucasian women. However, it is unknown whether bone structure, particularly in the cortical bone is better maintained during aging in Asian women than in Caucasian women. It remains to be determined whether Asian women are associated with lesser age-related reduction in femoral neck cortical thinning, increased cortical porosity and increased accumulation of unrepaired microdamge than Caucasian women. It also remains to be determined whether there are racial differences in age-related periosteal apposition and endocortical resorption since these surface changes determine the racial differences in the extent of cortical thinning and the distance of the cortex from neutral long axis of bone, which in turn determine the bending strength.

Shorter hip axis length (HAL) or shorter femoral neck axis length (FNAL) in Asian women compared to Caucasian women may be an additional important contributor to the lower hip fracture rates in Asian women [174, 175]. However, this is a controversial and an unresolved issue [172, 173]. Shorter femoral neck length is associated with increased resistance to bending and the contribution of shorter femoral neck length to bone strength has been reported [169]. Nakamura et al [169] reported that Japanese women have shorter stature, lower BMC, lower cross-sectional moment on inertia (a measure of bending strength) than in Caucasian women. However, when the femoral neck length and loading applied to bone were taken into account of, the safety factor, the bone's ability to resist the applied load, was about 50% higher for Japanese women than for Caucasian women [169]. The authors suggest that the shorter femoral neck length is a major contributor to the higher femoral neck safety factor in Asians. This explains why Japanese women have a lower hip fracture risk than Caucasian women [169]. However, in a recent study of Chinese women compared to Caucasian women, there was no difference in safety factors despite the fact of Chinese women have a shorter femoral neck axis length [170] **(Figure 11)**.

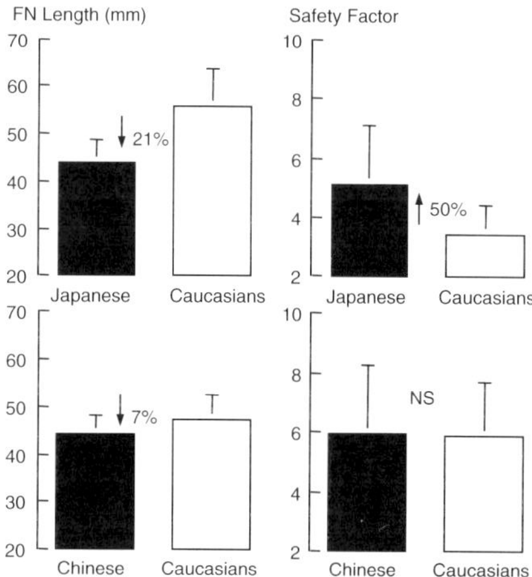

Figure 11. In both Japanese and Chinese women, femoral neck (FN) length is shorter. However, the safety factor is 50% higher in Japanese women than Caucasian women, but no different in Chinese women from Caucasian women. Adapted from Nakamura T et al [169] and Yan et al [170] with permission.

As discussed before, the shorter stature of Asian women relative to Caucasian women is primarily due to their shorter leg length, whilst the trunk length is very similar [113, 114]. Whether the lower ratio of leg length to trunk length in Asians is associated with better gait balance so produce less falls in Asian women than Caucasian women is uncertain. Whether this is the reason why Asians have less falls than Caucasians is also uncertain [6, 176]. When falls occur, the relative shorter distance of the proximal femur to the ground in Asian women than Caucasian women may be associated with lesser forces on the hip in Asian women compared to Caucasian women [6].

7. Pathophysiologic mechanism of bone fragility

7.1.   *Estrogen deficiency*

Estrogen deficiency after menopause is associated with an increased bone remodelling rate as reflected by increased bone turnover markers

[177-181].   In Asian women, biochemical markers of bone turnover increased significantly after menopause and maintained a higher level into old age [168-170]. The increased bone resorption makers seem to be associated with the number of years post menopause [168] **(Figure 12)**.

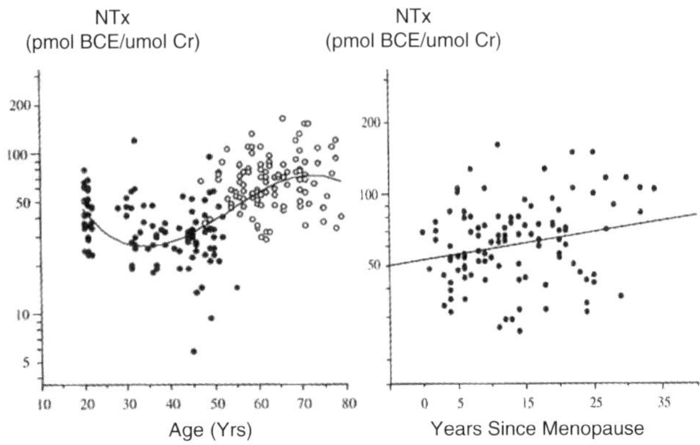

Figure 12. Bone resorption marker, urinary NTx, was increased after menopause in Japanese women (left panel), and there was a weaker positive association between increased NTx and years since menopause (right panel). Adapted from Sone et al [177] with permission.

Moreover, elderly Asian women with hip fracture have increased bone resorption markers than age-matched controls [180]. The results of these studies indicate that the bone remodelling rate at the entire skeletal level probably remains elevated, rather than decreasing with age in Asian women.

In both Asian and Caucasian women, the early phase of increased bone remodelling rate after menopause is probably confined to the trabecular bone because it has high surface-volume ratio, while cortical bone remodelling rate is probably slower due to its lower surface-volume ratio [71]. As age advances, trabecular bone loss is slow because trabecular bone surfaces available for bone remodelling are decreased due to irreversible loss of many trabecular plates and perforations. While bone remodelling rate on the endocortical and intracortical surfaces is increased, cortical bone becomes "trabecularized" particularly on its inner third surface [71, 182], so the cortical bone surface-volume ratio increases and bone loss is primarily on cortical bone in old age. Thus, the total bone surfaces for bone remodelling probably continues to increase rather than decrease with age, and this is why bone turnover markers remain elevated and bone loss continues into old age.

Racial differences of endogenous estrogen levels and bone turnover markers have been reported in Asian and Caucasian women. In pre- and early perimenopausal women, estrogen levels were lower in Asian women than Caucasian women and were associated with lower bone formation and resorption markers [183]. After menopause, residual estrogen levels were also lower in Asian women than Caucasian women [184]. However, the magnitude of menopause associated with increased bone resorption makers was similar in Asian women than Caucasian women, but lower in Asian than Caucasian men [179] (**Figure 13)**. As discussed earlier, menopause- and age-related bone loss seems to be faster in Asian women than Caucasian women [118]. These observations suggest that the lower endogenous estrogen levels in postmenopausal Asian women may enhance the skeletal responsiveness to estrogen deficiency than Caucasian women, resulting in faster bone loss in Asian than Caucasian women.

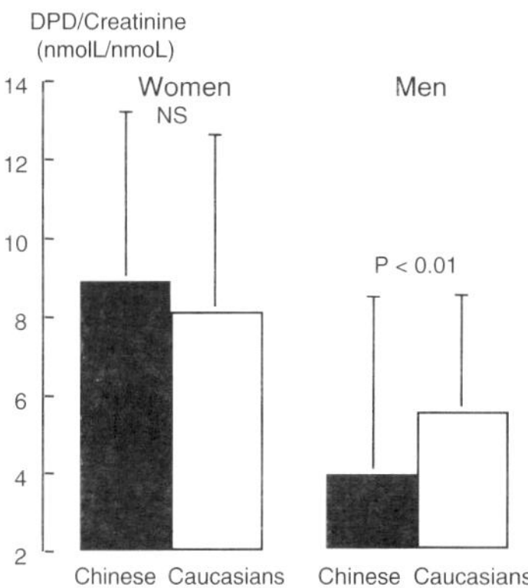

Figure 13. Bone resorption marker is similar in postmenopausal Chinese and Caucasian women, but is lower in Chinese than Caucasian men. Adapted from Yan et al [177] with permission.

At the cellular level, in Caucasian women, estrogen deficiency is associated with increased bone remodelling imbalance caused by increased bone resorption with reduced bone formation at basic multicellular unit (BMU) level [71, 185]. The cellular mechanism of estrogen deficiency associated with bone loss and structural damage in Asian postmenopausal women is less well defined. The observed trabecular disruption caused by estrogen deficiency, such as perforation and loss of structural elements in postmenopausal Asian women, suggests that the morphological basis for trabecular bone loss may be similar in Asian and Caucasian women, despite the relative contribution of increased bone resorption and reduced bone formation being unknown. In the cortical bone, using electron scanning microscopy, Chai et al [163] reported that the active osteoclast resorption was associated with age-related increases in expansion of osteonal diameter at the femoral neck cortex, resulting in increased cortical porosity in elderly Chinese women. However, whether this is due to estrogen deficiency alone or there is some interaction between estrogen deficiency and secondary hyperparathyroidism as reported in Caucasian women is unknown [87].

There are several studies exploring the racial differences in the structural basis and cellular mechanism of estrogen deficiency associated with bone loss and structural damage in Black and Caucasian women, in which the biological basis for bone remodelling imbalance after menopause is similar between the two groups [104, 186-188]. Comparative studies between Asian and Caucasian women have not been done. The question being asked here is what are the really fundamental differences in the bone remodelling imbalance at the tissue or cellular level between the two race groups? If there are biological differences, is this surface specific or skeletal site specific? Do Asian women have similar bone surface-volume ratio on trabecular, endocortical and intracortical surfaces as Caucasian women? Does the bone remodelling rate at the tissue level increase with age similarly in both Asian and Caucasian women? Does the extent of the negative BMU balance differ in Asian women from Caucasian women? What is the relative contribution of increased bone resorption and reduced bone formation to the negative BMU balance in Asian and Caucasian women? Answers to these questions are not yet available.

7.2. Secondary hyperparathyroidism

Many studies in Caucasians have suggested that secondary hyperparathyroidism may be largely responsible for the age-related increased bone loss and increased bone resorption markers in elderly women, therefore contributing to the pathogenesis of hip fracture [87, 189-191]. Patients with hip fracture usually reported to have increased serum concentration of parathyroid hormone (PTH) [189, 190]. The co-existing higher PTH and increased markers of bone resorption in patients with hip fracture is consistent with this notion [191]. Vitamin D deficiency associated with declining intestinal calcium absorption is a major contributing factor to the secondary hyperparathyroidism in the elderly [192].

There are also several studies in Asians that explore the role of vitamin D deficiency and increased PTH level in the pathogenesis of hip fracture [179, 193-195]. These results seem to be contradictory to the findings in Caucasian women. Yan et al [179] failed to detect an association between increased PTH and increased bone resorptions markers in elderly Chinese women and men. In a case control study in Hong Kong, MacDonald et al reported that serum 1,25-dihydrovitamin D and PTH were no different in elderly Chinese women with hip fracture compared to age matched controls [195]. Vitamin D deficiency is more common in the elderly Chinese living in the north, but not in the south of China. This is primarily due to the lesser sunshine exposure in the north than in the south Chinese [179, 193, 194, 196]. The paradox of this observation is that hip fracture rates are generally lower in the inhabitants of the north China [19, 20, 22, 26]. So the high hip fracture rates reported in Hong Kong or Singapore Chinese are unlikely to be explained by vitamin D deficiency and increased PTH level.

Whether the racial difference in hip fracture rate is attributed to the racial difference in secondary hyperparathyroidism is a question that remains unresolved. Racial differences in vitamin D-parathyroid hormone axis have been reported between Chinese and Caucasians [179]. It has been suggested but not proven that Chinese may be resistant to the skeletal effect of increased PTH [179]. Yan et al reported that vitamin D deficiency is associated with greater increases in serum PTH in elderly Chinese women than British Caucasian women [179]. However, there was no association between increased PTH and declining bone density or increased bone resorption markers in elderly Chinese women, but the association were detected in Caucasian women [179]. These observations led the authors to suggest that elderly Chinese may be resistant to PTH on the resorbing effect on bone [179]. However, the interpretation of this data should be treated cautiously because this is a cross-sectional study and the measurement of aBMD was blinded to the surface change on periosteal and endosteal envelope, in which increased PTH may have different effect on these surfaces.

Increased PTH is associated with increased age-related bone loss but PTH has different effect on bone – anabolic on trabecular bone and catabolic on cortical bone [196-199]. In postmenopausal women with primary hyperparathyroidism, trabecular bone mass and structure were better preserved while loss and thinning of cortical bone were the predominant features [196, 198, 200]. Increased levels of PTH with age may be associated with increased periosteal apposition on the outer surface of bone [200], but it is probably at the expense of increased endocortical bone resorption. So these surface specific effects of increased PTH are difficult to be detected by cross-sectional study and by densitometry. Studies are needed to determine whether the racial differences in the age-related changes on the periosteal and endocortical surfaces can be explained by the racial differences in the levels of increased PTH.

8. Summary and conclusion

Vertebral fracture incidence rates are higher in Caucasian women than in Caucasian men, and probably higher in Asian women than in Asian men. Whether vertebral fracture rates are lower, similar or higher in Asians compared to Caucasians is uncertain because there is insufficient epidemiological data in Asian countries and the methodology for defining vertebral fracture has not been resolved. The incidence of hip fracture is higher in women than in men in both Asian and Caucasian populations, while hip fracture rates appear to be lower in Asian women than Caucasian women and lower in Asian men than Caucasian men.

Patients with fractures have reduced aBMD and aBMD is an independent predictor of fracture risk. In both Asian and Caucasian women, the relative risk of each SD reduction in aBMD was associated with a similar increased risk of fracture. The absolute risk at a given aBMD level of the same age may be lower in Asians than Caucasians. However, the predictive value is limited by its sensitivity because aBMD only reflects one component of bone strength, the other structural and material properties of bone that contribute to increased bone fragility are not captured by aBMD. Moreover, the loading imposed on bone is not taken into account. This may be particularly important when comparing racial differences in fragility fractures because the extent and distribution of the load applied to bone may vary between the two race groups.

Structural abnormalities may be more important to the occurrence of fracture independent of reduced bone mass. The structural disruption in Caucasian postmenopausal women with vertebral fracture is different to that of hip fracture. Smaller bone size and structural disruption such as trabecular thinning, perforation and loss of connectivity as well as cortical thinning and intracortical porosity are all the major histological features of osteoporotic bone in postmenopausal women with vertebral fractures. In contrast, structural disruptions in postmenopausal women with hip fracture are mainly characterised by cortical thinning and increased intracortical porosity, while the trabecular perforation and loss of connectivity are less severe. The structural abnormalities in Asian women with fracture, particularly in patients with hip fracture require study.

Growth-related factors may contribute to the pathogenesis of bone fragility and to the racial differences in fracture rates. Available data suggest that there are racial differences in skeletal growth in Asian compared to Caucasian children, and these racial differences in skeletal growth are probably attributed to the racial differences in the tempo, duration and pubertal growth spurt between the two race groups.

Bone loss after menopause is a major contributor to the increased bone fragility in both Asian and Caucasian women. Bone densitometry studies show a similar pattern of postmenopausal bone loss in Asian and Caucasian women. The structural basis for postmenopausal bone loss in the trabecular and cortical bone is largely derived from Caucasian women. In Asian women, limited data suggest that trabecular bone loss occurs by a similar morphological basis as in Caucasian women. However, the pattern and magnitude of menopause and age-related cortical thinning and increased intracortical porosity in Asian women and men has not been documented.

Estrogen deficiency after menopause is associated with increased bone remodelling rate in Asian and Caucasian women. The bone remodelling rate as reflected by bone turnover markers increases after menopause and remains elevated. The magnitude of menopause/age associated with increased bone resorption markers appear to be similar in Asian and Caucasian women. At the cellular level, in Caucasian women, estrogen deficiency is associated with increased negative bone remodelling balance caused by increased bone resorption with reduced bone formation at the BMU level. The cellular mechanism of estrogen deficiency associated with bone loss and structural damage in Asian postmenopausal women is poorly defined. Moreover, the relative contribution of estrogen deficiency and secondary hyperparathyroidism to the pathophysiologic mechanism of bone fragility in Asian women is largely unknown.

There are no histological studies that compare the racial differences in menopause and age-related structural changes in the trabecular and cortical bone between Asians and Caucasians. There are few hypothesis-driven studies which compare the racial differences to the extent of periosteal and endosteal bone modelling and remodelling in Asian and Caucasians. This is a neglected area and studies are required to investigate the structural changes in the cortical and trabecular bone and on the periosteal and endosteal surfaces, and whether the racial differences in these surface specific changes account for the racial differences seen in fracture rates between the two populations.

Acronym and Symbol Definition

BMD	Bone mineral density
aBMD	Areal bone mineral density
vBMD	Volumetric bone mineral density
SD	Standard deviation
QCT	Quantitative computed tomography
PQCT	Peripheral quantitative computed tomography
FRI	Fracture risk index
HAL	Hip axis length
FNAL	Femoral neck axis length
BMU	Basic multicellular unit
PTH	Parathyroid hormone
Ntx	Type I collagen crosslinked N-telopeptides
DPD	Urinary free deoxypyridinoline
Cr	Creatinine

Acknowledgment

I would like to thank my supervisor Professor Ego Seeman for his helpful and critical comments on the paper and also Mrs Helen Patterson for reading and correcting the grammar errors of the draft.

REFERENCES

1. Tsai, K-S., Twu, S-J., Chieng, P-U., Yang, R-S., and Lee, T-K., Calcif. Tissue. Int., 249 (1996).
2. Lau, E.M.C., Woo, J., Chan, H., Chan, M.K.F., Griffith, J., and Chan, Y.H., Calcif. Tissue. Int., 1 (1998).
3. Nevitt, M., Bent, S., Lui, L., Zhang, Y., Yu, W., and Cummings, S., J. Bone. Miner. Res., Suppl.1:S170 (2001).
4. Lau, E.M.C., Chan, H.H.L., Woo, J., Lin, F., Black, D., and Nevitt. M., et al., J. Bone. Miner. Res., 1364 (1996).
5. Xu, L., Cummings, S.R., Qin, M., Zhao, X., Chen, X., and Nevitt, M., et al., J. Bone. Miner. Res., 2019 (2000).
6. Ross, P.D., Fujiwara, S., Huang, C., Davis, J.W., Epstein, R.S., and Wasnich, R.D., Int. J. Epidemiol., 1171 (1995).
7. Fujiwara, S., Kasagi, F., Masunari, N., Naito, K., Suzhki, G., and Fukunaga, M., J. Bone. Miner. Res., 1547 (2003).
8. Jones, G., Nguyen, T., Sambrook, P.N., Kelly, P.J., Gilbert, C., and Eisman, J.A., Osteoporos. Int., 277 (1994).
9. O'Neill, TW., Felsenberg, D., Varlow, J., Cooper, C., Kanis, J.A., and Silman, A.J., J. Bone. Miner. Res., 1010 (1996).
10. Jackson, S.A., Tenenhouse, A., Robertson, L., and the CaMos study group., Osteoporos. Int., 680 (2000).
11. Burger, H., van Daele, P.L.A., Grashuis, K., Hofman, A., Grobbee, D.E., and Schütte, H.E., et al., J. Bone. Miner. Res., 152 (1997).
12. Davies, K.M., Stegman, M.R., Heaney, R.P., and Recker, R.R., Osteoporos. Int., 160 (1996).
13. Cooper, C., Atkinson, E.J., O'Fallon, W.M., and Melton, III. L.J., J. Bone. Miner. Res., 22 (1992).
14. Sanders, K.M., Seeman, E., Ugoni, A.M., Pasco, J.A., Martin, T.J., and Skoric, B., et al., Osteoporosis. Int., 240 (1999).
15. Ross, P.D., Lombardi, A., and Freedholm, D., In: Osteoporosis in Men, Eds. Orwoll, E., (Academic Press, San Diego, California, 1999), p.505.
16. The European Prospective Osteoporosis Study (EPOS) Group., J. Bone. Miner. Res., 716 (2002).
17. van der Klift, M., De laet, C.E.D.H., McCloskey, E.V., Hofman, A., and Pols, H.A.P., J. Bone. Miner. Res., 1051 (2002).
18. Villa, M.L., Nelson, L., and Nelson, D., In: Osteoporosis, 2nd Ed., vol. 1. Eds, Marcus, R., Feldman, D., Kelsey, J., (Academic Press, San Diego CA, 2001), p.569.

19. Xu, L,, Lu, A., Zhao, X., Chen, X, and Cummings, S.R., et al., Am. J. Epidemiol., 901 (1996).

20. Yan, L., Zhou, B., Prentice, A., Wang, X., and Golden, M.H.N., Bone., 151 (1999).

21. Zhang, L., Cheng, A., Bai, Z., Lu, Y., Endo, N., and Dohmae, Y., J. Bone. Miner. Metab., 84 (2000).

22. Koh, L.K.H., Saw, S-M., Lee, J.J.M., Leong, K-H., and Lee, J., Osteoporos. Int., 311 (2001).

23. Wong, P.C., Clin. Orthop. RR., 55 (1966).

24. Ross, P.D., Norimatsu, H., Davis, J.W., Yano, K., Wasnich, R.D., and Fujiwara, S., et al, Am. J. Epidemiol., 801 (1991).

25. Rowe, S.M., Yoon, T.R., and Ryang, D.H., Int. Orthop., 139 (1993).

26. Lau, E.M.C., Lee, J.K., Suriwongpaisal, P., Saw, S.M., Das De, S., and Khir, A., et al., Osteoporos. Int., 239 (2001).

27. Lauderdale, D.S., Jacobsen, S.J., Furner, S.E., Levy, P.S., Brody, J.A., and Goldberg, J., Am. J. Epidemiol., 146 (1997).

28. Chalmers, T.J., Ho, S.C., J. Bone. Jt. Surg., 52B, 667 (1970).

29. Hui, S.L., Slemenda, C.W., Johnston, C.C.J., J. Clin. Invest., 1804 (1988).

30. Stone, K.L., Seeley, D.G., Lui, L-Y., Cauley, J.A., Ensrud, K., Browner, W.S., Nevitt, M.C., and Cummings, S.R., for the study of Osteoporotic Fracture Research Group., J. Bone. Miner. Res., 1947 (2003).

31. Kanis, J.A., Gluer, C.C., Osteoporos. Int., 192 (2000).

32. Orwoll, E., J. Bone. Miner. Res., 1867 (2000).

33. Marshall, D., Johnell, O., Wedel, H., BMJ., 1254 (1996).

34. Kung, A.W.C., Luk, K.D.K., Chu, L.W., Tang, G.W.K., Osteoporos. Int., 456 (1999).

35. Huang, C., Ross, P.D., Fujiwara, S., Davis, J.W., Epstein, R.S., Kodama, K., and Wasnich, R.D., Bone., 437 (1996).

36. Wei, T.S., Hu, C.H., Wang, S.H., and Hwang, K.L., Osteoporos. Int., 1050 (2001).

37. Siris, E.S., Chen, Y-T., Weiss, T.W., Brenneman, S.K., and Miller, P.D., Drug. Benefit. Trends., 36 (2003).

38. De Laet, C.E.D.H., van Hout, B.A., Burger, H., Hofman, A., and Pols, H.A., BMJ., 221 (1997).

39. Melton, III. L.J., Orwoll, E.S., and Wasnich, R.D., Osteoporos. Int., 707 (2001).

40. Schuit, S.C.E., van der Klift, M., Weel, A.E.A.M., de Laet, C.E.D.H., Burger, H., Seeman, E., Hofman, A., Uitterlinden, A.G., van Leeuwen, J.P.T.M., and Pols, H.A.P., Bone., 195 (2003).

41. Siris, E.S., Chen, Y-T., Abbott, T.A., Barrett-Connor, E., Miller, P.D., Wehren, L.E., and Berger, M.L., Arch. Intern. Med., 1108 (2004).

42. Seeman, E., J. Clin. Endocrinol. Metab., 4576 (2001).

43. Duan, Y., Seeman, E., and Turner, C.H., J. Bone. Miner. Res., 2276 (2001).

44. Peacock, M., Turner, C.H., Liu, G., Manatunga, A.K., Timmerman, L., and Johnston, C.C. Jr., Osteoporos. Int., 167 (1995).

45. Myers, E.R., Wilson, S.E., Spine., 25s (1997).

46. Bouxsein, M.L., In: Osteoporosis, 2nd Edition. Eds., Marcus, R., Feldman, D., and Kelsey, J., (Academic Press, San Diego CA USA, 2001), p.509.

47. Gilsanz, V., Loro, M.L., Roe, T.F., Sayre, J., Gilsanz, R., and Schulz, E.E., J. Clin. Invest., 2332 (1995).

48. Duan, Y., Parfitt, A.M., and Seeman, E., J. Bone. Miner. Res., 1796 (1999).

49. Krølner, B., Clin. Physiol., 139 (1982).

50. Duan, Y., Turner, C.H., Kim, B.T., and Seeman, E., J. Bone. Miner. Res., 2267 (2001).

51. Rico, H., Revilla, M., Fraile, E., Martin, F.J., Cardenas, J.L., and Villa, L.F., Bone., 303 (1994).

52. Ross, P.D., Huang, C., Davis., J.W., and Wasnich, R.D., Bone., 257S (1995).

53. Kimmel, D.B., Recker, R.R., Gallagher, J.C., Vaswani, A.S., and Aloia, J.F., Bone. Miner., 217 (1990).

54. Foldes, J., Parfitt, A.M., Shih, M-S., Rao, D.S., and Kleerekoper, M., J. Bone. Miner. Res., 759 (1991).

55. Dempster, D.W., Shane, E., and Lindsay, R., J. Bone. Miner. Res., 15 (1986).

56. Parfitt, A.M., Mathews, C.H.E., Villanueva, A.R., Kleerkoper, M., Frame, B., and Rao, D.S., J. Clin. Invest., 1396 (1983).

57. Arlot, M.E., Delmas, P.D., Chappard, D., and Meunier, P.J., Osteoporos. Int., 41 (1990).

58. Parfitt, A.M., Am. J. Med., 82 (suppl B), 68 (1987).

59. Recker, R.R., Calcif. Tissue. Int., S139 (1993).

60. Mosekilde, L., Bone. Miner., 13 (1990).

61. Ritzel, H., Amling, M., Posl, M., Hahn, M., and Delling, G., J. Bone. Miner. Res., 89 (1997).

62. Faulkner, K.G., Cummings, S.R., Black, D., Palermo, L., Glüer, C.C., and Genant, H.K., J. Bone. Miner. Res., 1211 (1993).

63. Partanen, J., Jamsa, T., and Jalovaara, P., J. Bone. Miner. Res., 1540 (2001).

64. Peacock, M., Turner, C.H., Liu, G., Manatunga, A.K., Timmerman, L., and Johnston, Jr. C.C., Osteoporos. Int., 167 (1995).

65. Boonen, S., Koutri, R., Dequeker, J., Aerssens, J., Lowet, G., Nijs, J., Verbeke, G., Lesaffre, E., and Geusens, P., J. Bone. Miner. Res., 1908 (1995).

66. Duboeuf, F., Hans, D., Schott, A.M., Kotzki, P.O., Favier, F., Marcelli, C., Meunier, P.J., and Delmas, P.D., J. Bone. Miner. Res., 1895 (1997).

67. Tabensky, A., Duan, Y., Edmonds, J., and Seeman, E., J. Bone. Miner. Res., 1101 (2001).

68. Duan, Y., Beck, T.J., Wang, X.F., and Seeman, E., J. Bone. Miner. Res., 1766 (2003).

69. Michelotti, J., and Clark, J., J. Bone. Miner. Res., 1714 (1999).

70. Karlsson, K.M., Sernbo, I., Obrant, K.J., Redlund-Johnell, I., and Johnell, O., Bone., 327 (1996).

71. Parfitt, A.M., In: Osteoporosis, 2nd Edition, Vol.1., Eds., Marcus. R., Feldman. D., and Kelsey. J., (Academic Press, San Diego, CA USA, 2001), p.433.

72. Johnston, C.C., Norton, J., Khairi, M.R.A., Kernek, C., Edouard, C., Arlot, M., and Meunier, P.J., J. Clin. Endocrinol. Metab., 551 (1985).

73. Uitewaal, P.J.M., Lips, P., and Netelenbos., J.C., Bone. Miner., 63 (1987).

74. Mori, S., Harruff., R., Ambrosius, W., and Burr, D.B., Bone., 521 (1997).

75. Bell, K.L., Loveridge, N., Power, J., Garrahan, N., Stanton, M., Lunt, M., Meggitt, B.F., and Reeve, J., J. Bone. Miner. Res., 111 (1999).

76. Bell, K.L., Loveridge, N., Power, J., Garrahan, N., Meggitt, B.F., and Reeve, J., Bone., 57 (1999).

77. Bell, K.L., Loveridge, N., Power, J., Rushton, N., and Reeve, J., Osteoporos. Int., 248 (1999).

78. Beck, T.J., Oreskovic, T.L., Stone, K.L., Ruff, C.B., Ensrud, K., Nevitt, M.C., Genant, H.K., and Cummings, S.R., J. Bone. Miner. Res., 1108 (2001).

79. Burr, D.B., Forwood, M.R., Fyhrie, D.P., Martin, R.B., Schaffler, M.B., and Turner, C.H., J. Bone. Miner. Res., 6 (1997).

80. Schaffler, M.B., Choi, K., and Milgrom, C., Bone., 521 (1995).

81. Norman, T.L., and Wang, Z., Bone., 375 (1997).

82. Qiu, S., Rao, D.S., Palnitkars, S., and Parfitt, A.M., Bone., 709 (2002).

83. Qiu, S., Rao, D.S., Palnitkar, S., and Parfitt, A.M., J. Bone. Miner. Res., 1657 (2003).

84. Wenzel, T.E., Schaffler, M.B., and Fyhrie, D.P., Bone., 89 (1996).

85. Ito, M., Nakamura, T., Matsumoto, T., Tsurusaki, K., and Hayashi, K., Bone., 163 (1998).

86. Riggs, B.L., and Melton, III. L.J., N. Engl. J. Med., 1676 (1986).

87. Riggs, B.L., Khosla, S., and Melton, III L.J., Endocri. Rev., 279 (2002).

88. Seeman, E., Osteoporos. Int., Suppl 1:S15 (1994).

89. Hui, S.L., Slemenda, C.W., and Johnston, Jr. C.C., Osteoporos. Int., 30 (1990).

90. Sambrook, P.N., Kelly, P.J., White, C.P., Morrison, N.A., and Eisman, J.A., In: Osteoporosis, Eds. Marcus, R., Feldman. D., and Kelsey, J., (Academic press, San Diego, CA USA,1996), p.477.

91. Peacock, M., Turner, C.H., Econs, M.J., and Foroud, T., Endocrine. Rev., 303 (2002).

92. Pocock, N.A., Eisman, J.A., Hopper, J.L., Yeates, M.G., Sambrook, P.N., and Eberl, S., J. Clin. Invest., 706 (1987).

93. Ferrari, S., Rizzoli, R., Slosman, D., and Bonjour, J.P., J. Clin. Endocrinol. Metab., 358 (1998).

94. Loro, M.L., Sayre, J., Roe, T.F., Goran, M.I., Kaufman, F.R., and Gilsanz, V., J. Clin. Endocrinol. Metab., 3908 (2000).

95. Seeman, E., Hopper, J.L., Bach, L., Cooper, M., McKay, J., and Jerums, G., N. Engl. J. Med., 554 (1989).

96. Seeman, E., Hopper, J.L., Tsalamandris, C., and Formica, C., J. Bone. Miner. Res., 739 (1994).

97. Danielson, M.E., Cauley, J.A., Baker, C.E., Newman, A.B., Dorman, J.S., Towers, J.D., and Kuller, L.H., J. Bone. Miner. Res., 102 (1999).

98.   Barthe, N., Basse-Cathalinat, B., Meunier, P.J., Ribot, C., Marchandise, X., Sabatier, J.P., Braillon, P., Thevenot, J., and Sutter, B., Osteoporos. Int., 379 (1998).

99.   Tabensky, A., Duan, Y., Edmonds, J., and Seeman, E., J. Bone. Miner. Res., 1101 (2001).

100.   Filardi, S., Zebaze, R.M.D., Duan, Y., Edmonds, J., Beck, T.J., and Seeman, E., Osteoporos. Int., 103 (2004).

101.   Cummings, S.R., Nevitt, M.C., Browner, W.S., Stone, K., Fox, K.M., Ensrud, K.E., Cauley, J., Black, D., and Vogt, T.M., N. Engl. J. Med., 767 (1995).

102.   Deng, H.W., Chen, W.M., Recker, S., Stegman, M.R., Li, J.L., Davies, K.M., Zhou, Y., Deng, H.Y., Heaney, R., and Recker, R.R., J. Bone. Miner. Res., 1243 (2000).

103.   Looker, A., Beck, T., and Orwoll, E., J. Bone. Miner. Res., 1291 (2001).

104.   Han, Z-H., Palnitkar, S., Rao, D.S., Nelson, D., and Parfitt, A.M., J. Bone. Miner. Res., 1967 (1996).

105.   Bhudhikanok, G.S., Wang, M-C., Eckert, K., Matkin, C., Marcus, R., and Bachrach, L.K., J. Bone. Miner. Res., 1545 (1996).

106.   Horlick, M., Thornton, J., Wang, J., Levine, L.S., Fedun, B., and Pierson, R.N., J. Bone. Miner. Res., 1393 (2000).

107.   Bachrach, L.K., Hastie, T., Wang, M-C., Narasimhan, B., and Marcus, R., J. Clin. Endocrinol. Metab., 4702 (1999).

108.   Huen, K.F., Leung, S.S.F., Lau, J.T.F., Cheung, A.Y.K., Leung, N.K., and Chiu, M.C., Acta. Pædiatr., 1121 (1997).

109.   Wong, G.W.K., Leung, S.S.F., Law, W.Y., Yeung, V.T.F., Lau, J.T.F., and Yeung, W.K.Y., Acta. Pædiatr., 620 (1996).

110.   Novotny, R., Davis, J., Ross, P.D., and Wasnich, R.D., J. Am. Diet. Assoc., 802 (1996).

111.   Parfitt, M.A., Osteoporos. Int., 382 (1994).

112.   Leung, S.S.F., Lau, J.T.F., Xu, Y.Y., Tse, L.Y., Huen, K.F., Wong, G.W.K., Law, W.Y., Yeung, V.T.F., Yeung, W.K.Y., and Leung, N.K., Ann. Hum. Biol., 297 (1996).

113.   Meredith, H.V., Growth., 37 (1978).

114.   Wang, X.W., Duan, Y., and Seeman, E., J. Bone. Miner. Res., 19 (suppl 1): abstract (2004),

115.   Bass, S., Delmas, P., Pearce, G., Hendrich, E., Tabensky, A., and Seeman, E., J. Clin. Invest., 795 (1999).

116.   Bradney, M., Karlsson, M.K., Duan, Y., Stuckey, S., Bass, S., and Seeman, E., J. Bone. Miner. Res., 1871 (2000).

117.   Gilsanz, V., Skaggs, D.L., Kovanlikaya, A., Sayre, J., Loro, M.L., Kaufman, F., and Korenman, S.G., J. Clin. Endocrinol. Metab., 1420 (1998).

118.   Yu, W., Qin, M., Xu, L., Van Kujk, C., Meng, X., Xing, X., Cao, J., and Genant, H.K., Osteoporos. Int., 468 (1999).

119.   Ito, M., Lang, T.F., Jergas, M., Ohki, M., Takada, M., Nakamura, T., Hayashi, K., and Genant, H.K., Calcif. Tissue. Int., 123 (1997).

120.   Garn, S.M., Pao, E.M., and Rihl, M.E., Science., 1439 (1964).

121.   Liao. E-Y., Wu, X-P., Deng, X-G., Huang, G., Zhu, X-P., Long, Z-F., Wang, W-B., Tang, W-L., and Zhang, H., Osteoporos. Int., 669 (2002).
122.   Seeman, E., Osteoporosis. Int., 14 (Suppl3):S2 (2003).
123.   Parfitt, A.M., J. Bone. Miner. Res., 1213 (1998).
124.   Balena, R., Shih, M-S., and Parfitt, A.M., J. Bone. Miner. Res., 1475 (1992).
125.   Mosekilde, L., and Mosekilde, L., Bone., 67 (1990).
126.   Ebbesen, E.N., Thomsen, J.S., Beck-Nielsen, H., Nepper-Rasmussen, H.J., and Mosekilde, L., J. Bone. Miner. Res., 1394 (1999).
127.   Ruff, C.B., and Hayes, W.C., J. Orthop. Res., 886 (1988).
128.   Kalender, W.A., Felsenberg, D., Louis, O., Lopez, P., Klotz, E., Osteaux, M., and Fraga, J., Europ. J. Radiol., 75 (1989).
129.   Genant, H.K., Ettinger, B., Harris, S.T., Block, J.E., and Steiger, P., In: Osteoporosis: aetiology, diagnosis and management., Eds. Riggs, B.L., Melton, L.J. III. (Raven Press, New York, 1988), p.221.
130.   Aaron, J.E., Makins, N.B., and Sagreiy, K., Clin. Orth. RR., 260 (1987).
131.   Tsai, K.S., Cheng, W.C., Sanchez, T.V., Chen, C.K., Chieng, P.U., and Yang, R.S., Bone., 365 (1997).
132.   Tsai, K.S., Cheng, W.C., Chen, C.K., Sanchez, T.V., Su, C.T., and Chieng, P.U., et al., Bone., 547 (1997).
133.   Cheng, W-C., Yang, R-S., Hsu, S.H.J., Chieng, P-U., and Tsai, K-S., Spine., 964 (2001).
134.   Ross, P.D., He, Y-F., Yates, A.J., Couland, C., Ravn, P., McClung, M., Thompson, D., and Wasnich, R.D., for the EPIC Study Group., Calcif. Tissue. Int., 339 (1996).
135.   Russell-Aulet, M., Wang, J., Thornton, J.C., Colt, E.W.D., and Pierson, R.N. Jr., J. Bone. Miner. Res., 1109 (1991).
136.   Cundy, T., Cornish, J., Evans, M.C., Gamble, G., Stapleton, J., and Reid, I.R., J. Bone. Miner. Res., 368 (1995).
137.   Edwards, W.T., Zheng, Y., Ferrara, L.A., and Yuan, H.A., Spine., 218 (2001).
138.   Banse, X., Devogelaer, J.P., Munting, E., Delloye, C., Cornu, O., and Grynpas, M., Bone., 563 (2001).
139.   Thomsen, J.S., Ebbesen, E.N., and Mosekilde, L., Bone., 664 (2002).
140.   Kleerekoper, M., Villanueva, A.R., Stanciu, J., Sudhaker Rao, D., and Parfitt, A.M., Calcif. Tissue. Int., 594 (1985).
141.   Aaron, J.E., Shore, P.A., Shore, R.C., Beneton, M., and Kanis, J.A., Bone., 277 (2000).
142.   Oleksik, A., Ott, S.M., Vedi, S., Bravenboer, N., Compston, J., and Lips, P., J. Bone. Miner. Res., 1368 (2000).
143.   Oda, K., Shibayama, Y., Abe, M., and Onomura, T., Spine., 1050 (1998).
144.   Vesterby, A., Mosekilde, L., Gundersen, H.J.G., Melsen, F., Mosekilde, L., Holme, K., and Sorensen, S., Bone., 219 (1991).
145.   McBroom, R.J., Hayes, W.C., Edwards, W.T., Goldberg, R.P., and White, III A.A., J. Bone. & Joint. Surg. (Am)., 67A:1206 (1985).
146.   Israel, H., Age. Ageing., 71 (1973).
147.   Duan, Y., Wang, X-F., Evans, A., and Seeman, E., Bone., 2004 submitted.

148. Fujii, Y., Tsutsumi, M., Tsunenari, T., Fukase, M., Yoshimoto, Y., Fujita, T., and Genant, H.K., Bone. Miner., 87 (1989).

149. Ito, M., Lang, T.F., Jergas, M., Ohki, M., Takada, M., Nakamura, T., Hayashi, K., and Genant, H.K., Calcif. Tissue. Int., 123 (1997).

150. Duan, Y., Seeman, E., and Turner, C.H., J. Bone. Miner. Res., 2276 (2001).

151. Riggs, B.L., Wahner, H.W., Seeman, E., Offord, K.P., Dunn, W.L., Mazess, R.B., Johnson, K.A., and Melton, L.J. III., J. Clin. Invest., 716 (1982).

152. Beck, T.J., Looker, A.C., Ruff, C.B., Sievanen, H., and Wahner, H.W., J. Bone. Miner. Res., 2297 (2000).

153. Bousson, V., Meunier, A., Bergot, C., Vicaut, E., Rocha, M.A., Morais, M.H., Laval-Jeantet, A-M., Laredo, J-D., J. Bone. Miner. Res., 1308 (2001).

154. Bousson, V., Bergot, C., Meunier, A., Vicaut, E., Barbot, F., Parlier-Cuau, C., Laval-Jeantet, A-M., and Laredo, J-D., Radiology., 179 (2000).

155. Beck, T.J., Oreskovic, T.L., Stone, K.L, Ruff, C.B., Ensrud, K., Nevitt, M.C., Genant, H.K., and Cummings, S.R., J. Bone. Miner. Res., 1108 (2001).

156. Orwoll, E.S., J. Bone. Miner. Res., 949 (2003).

157. Pankovich, A.M., Arch. Surg., 20 (1975).

158. Power, J., Loveridge, N., Rushton, N., Parker, M., and Reeve, J., Osteoporos. Int., 141 (2003).

159. Crabtree, N., Lunt, M., Holt, G., Kröger, H., Burger, H., Grazio, S., Khaw, K-T., Lorenc, R.S., Nijs, J., Stepan, J., Falch, J.A., Miazgowski, T., Raptou, P., Pols, H.A.P., Dequeker, J., Havelka, S., Hoszowski, K., Jajic, I., Czekalski, S., Lyritis, G., Silman, A.J., and Reeve, J., Bone., 151 (2000).

160. Heaney, R.P., Barger-Lux, M.J., Davies, K.M., Ryan, R.A., Johnson, M.L., and Gong, G., Osteoporos. Int., 426 (1997).

161. Kaptoge, S., Dalzell, N., Loveridge, N., Beck, T.J., Khaw, K-T., and Reeve, J., Bone., 561 (2003).

162. Horikoshi, T., Endo, N., Uchiyama, T., Tanizawa, T., and Takahashi, H.E., Calcif. Tissue. Int., 447 (1999).

163. Chai, B., Tang, X., Chin. Med. J. (Engl)., 705 (1996).

164. Duan, Y., and Seeman, E., Ann. Acad. Med. Singapore., 54 (2002).

165. Ensrud, K.E., Palermo, L., Black, D.M., Cauley, J., Jergas, M., Orwoll, E.S., Nevitt, M.C., Fox, K.M., and Cummings, S.R., J. Bone. Miner. Res., 1778 (1995).

166. Jones, G., Nguyen, T., Sambrook, P., Kelly, P.J., and Eisman, J.A., B.M.J., 691 (1994).

167. Yoshimura, N., Kinoshita, H., Danjoh, S., Takijiri, T., Morioka, S., Kasamatsu, T., Sakata, K., and Hashimoto, T., Osteoporos. Int., 803 (2002).

168. Ho, S.C., Chan, S.S.G., Woo, J., Leung, P.C., and Lau, J., Osteoporos. Int., 161 (1995).

169. Nakamura, T., Turner, C.H., Yoshikawa, T., Slemenda, C.W., Peacock, M., Burr, D.B., Mizuno, Y., Orimo, H., Ouchi, Y., and Johnston, Jr. C.C., J. Bone. Miner. Res., 1071 (1994).

170. Yan, L., Crabtree, N.J., Reeve, J., Zhou, B., Dequeker, J., Nijs, J., Falch, J.A., and Prentice, A., Bone., 584 (2004).

171. Turner, C.H., Osteoporos. Int., 12 (1991).
172. Cummings, S.R., Cauley, J.A., Palermo, L., Ross, P.D., Wasnich, R.D., Black, D.M., and Faulkner, K.G., Osteoporos. Int., 226 (1994).
173. Chin, K., Evans, M.C., Cornish, J., Cundy, T., and Reid, I.R., Osteoporos. Int., 344 (1997).
174. Greendale, G.A.,Young, J.T., Huang, M-H., Bucur, A., Wang, Y., and Seeman, T., Osteoporos. Int., 320 (2003).
175. Wang, M-C., Aguirre, M., Bhudhikanok, G.S., Kendall, C.G., Kirsch, S., Marcus, R., and Bachrach, L.K., J. Bone. Miner. Res., 1922 (1997).
176. Aoyagi, K., Ross, P.D., Davis, J.W., Wasnich, R.D., Hayashi, T., Takemoto, T-I., J. Bone. Miner. Res., 1468 (1998).
177. Sone, T., Miyake, M., Takeda, N., and Fukunaga, M., Bone., 335 (1995).
178. Tsai, K.S., Pan, W.H., Hsu, S.H.J., Cheng, W.C., Chen, C.K., Chieng, P.U., Yang, R.S., and Twu, S.T., Calcif. Tissue. Int., 454 (1996).
179. Yan, L., Zhou, B., Wang, X., D'Ath, S., Laidlaw, A., Laskey, M.A., and Prentice, A., Bone., 620 (2003).
180. Hoshino, H., Takahashi, M., Kushida, K., Ohishi, T., and Inoue, T., Calcif. Tissue. Int., 36 (1998).
181. Yoshimura, N., Hashimoto, T., Sakata, K., Morioka, S., Kasamatsu, T., and Cooper, C., Calcif. Tissue. Int., 198 (1999).
182. Recker, R.R., Barger-Lux, M.J., In: Osteoporosis 2nd Edition, Vol.2., Eds., Marcus, R., Feldman, D., Kelsey, J., (Academic Press, San Diego, CA USA, 2001). p.59.
183. Randolph, J.F., Sowers, J.R., Gold, M.F., Mohr, E.B., Luborsky, B.A., Santoro, J., McConnel, N., Finkelstein, J.S., Korenman, S.G., Matthews, K.A., Sternfeld, B., Lasley, B.L., J. Clin. Endocrinol. Metab., 1516 (2003).
184. Key, T.J.A., Chen, J., Wang, D.Y., Pike, M.C., and Boreham, J., Br. J. Cancer., 631 (1990).
185. Eriksen, E.F., Hodgson, S.F., Eastell, R., Cedel, S.L., O'Fallon, W.M., and Riggs, B.L., J. Bone. Miner. Res., 311 (1990).
186. Han, Z.H., Palnitkar, S., Rao, D., Sudhaker, S., Nelson, D., and Parfitt, A.M., J. Bone. Miner. Res., 498 (1997).
187. Parisien, M., Cosman, F., Morgan, D., Schnitzer, M., Liang, X., Nieves, J., Forese, L., Luckey, M., Meier, D., Shen, V., Lindsay, R., and Dempster, D.W., J. Bone. Miner. Res., 948 (1997).
188. Parfitt, A.M., Han, Z-H., Palnitkar, S., Rao, D.S., Shih, M-S., and Nelson, D., J. Bone. Miner. Res., 1864 (1997).
189. Meunier, P. J., Chapuy, M. C., Arlot, M. E., Delmas, P. D. and Duboeuf, F., Osteoporos. Int., (Suppl 1), S71 (1994).
190. Lips, P., Endocri. Rev., 477 (2001).
191. Boonen, S., Vanderschueren, D., Cheng, X. G., Verbeke, G., Dequeker, J., Geusens, P., Broos, P., and Bouillon, R., J. Bone. Miner. Res., 2119 (1997).
192. Chapuy, M. C., Schott, A. M., Garnero, P., Hans, D., Delmas, P. D., and Meunier, P. J., J. Clin. Endocrinol. Metab., 1129 (1996).
193. Tsai, K.S., Hsu, S.H.J., Cheng, J.P., and Yang, R.S., Bone., 371 (1997).

194.   Chan, E.L.P., Lau, E., Shek, C.C., MacDonald, D., Woo, J., Leung, P.C., and Swaminathan, R., Clin. Endocrinol., 375 (1992).
195.   MacDonald, D., Lau, E., Chan, E.L.P., Mak, T., Woo, J., Leung, P.C., and Swaminathan, R., Calcif. Tissue. Int., 412 (1992).
196.   Bilezikian, J.P., and Silverberg, S.J., In: Osteoporosis, 2nd Edition., Vol.2., Eds., Marcus, R., Feldman, D., and Kelsey, J., (Academic Press, San Diego CA USA 2001). p.71.
197.   Dempster, D. W., Cosman, F., Parisien, M., Shen, V., and Lindsay, R., Endocr. Rev., 690 (1993).
198.   Parisien, M. V., Silverberg, S. J., Shane, E., de la Cruz, L., Lindsay, R., Bilezikian, J. P., and Dempster, D. W., J. Clin. Endocrinol. Metab., 930 (1990).
199.   Duan, Y., DeLuca, V., and Seeman, E., J. Clin. Endocrinol. Metab., 718 (1999).
200.   Parfitt, A.M., J. Bone. Miner. Res., 1741 (2002).

CHAPTER 4

NUTRITION AND OSTEOPOROSIS

Robert P. Heaney, M.D.

John A. Creighton University Professor
Creighton University Medical Center
601 North 30th Street – Suite 4841,Omaha, Nebraska 68131, USA
Phone: (402) 280-4029 Fax: (402) 280-4751 E-mail: rheaney@creighton.edu

OUTLINE

INTRODUCTION – THE CAUSES OF OSTEOPOROTIC FRAGILITY

Decreased Intrinsic Bone Strength

Decreased Bone Mass

Defective Bone Architecture

Impaired Bony Material Quality

Increased Propensity for Injury

CALCIUM

The Skeleton as the Calcium Nutrient Reserve

The Calcium Requirement and the Consequences of Suboptimal Intake

Defining the Requirement for Calcium

Nutrient-Nutrient Interactions: Factors that Influence the Calcium Requirement

Influences on Intestinal Absorption

Fiber

Caffeine

Influences on Renal Conservation

1. Introduction: The Causes of Osteoporotic Fragility

Osteoporosis can be defined as a condition of skeletal fragility associated with decreased bone mass and with microarchitectural deterioration of bone tissue, with a consequent increase in risk of fractures. All bone will fracture when exposed to a greater load than it is designed to resist. Hence the fractures of osteoporosis are frequently distinguished from fractures generally by designating them "low trauma fractures", or "fragility fractures". In brief, the fractures of osteoporosis can be characterized as those that occur because the skeleton does not have the strength called for in the individual's genetic program. Fractures may come about either because the bone itself does not have the requisite strength, or because it is, for other reasons, subjected to unusual forces occasioned by, for example, an increased propensity for injury.

Fig. 1 sets forth, schematically, some of the factors contributing to what is probably the most serious of the osteoporotic fractures, i.e., fracture of the proximal femur. The factors for which there is evidence of a nutritional influence are indicated by stars, and will be discussed at length in what follows. Good nutrition is essential for the optimal functioning of all body tissues and systems, and bone is no exception. Hence it is not surprising that nutrition enters into the osteoporotic fracture context at many different levels.

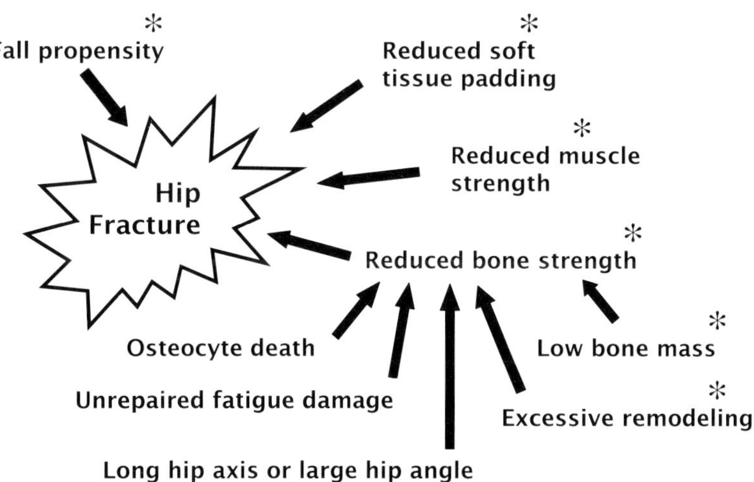

Fig. 1. Interplay of various factors contributing to risk of hip fracture, illustrating both the multifactorial character of osteoporotic fracture and the points at which nutrition influences fracture risk. Those factors for which there is an established role of inadequate nutrition are indicated by *. (Copyright, Robert P. Heaney, 2004. Used with permission.)

                    R. P. Heaney

Decreased Intrinsic Bone Strength

Strength in bone as in any structure, is a function of its massiveness, its architectural arrangement in space, and the physical properties of the component materials.

Decreased Bone Mass. The decrease in bone massiveness which is commonly a part of the physical manifestations of osteoporosis has, in fact, given the disease its name. Typically, osteoporotic bone will be characterized by thin cortices, thin and/or sparse trabeculae, severed trabecular cross-braces, and increased cortical porosity. It is intuitively clear why such a diminution in mass would cause an increase in fragility. However, not all individuals with the same bone mass will have the same degree of fragility, and it is necessary to recognize the role of other factors.

Defective Bone Architecture. Natural selective forces have led to the development of skeletons in all mammals that are compromises between strength and massiveness. Overly massive skeletons will, of course, be very strong (other things being equal), but much of the mass can be dispensed with if the architecture is optimized. Thus, for the same cross-sectional area (and hence the same quantity of material), a thin walled tube will be stiffer (and hence better able to resist bending forces) than will a solid rod of exactly the same mass (Fig. 2).

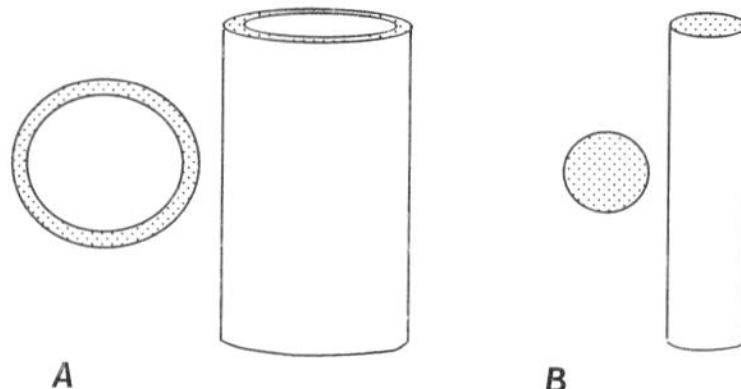

Fig. 2. Two cylindrical elements containing the same mass, but arranged in different spatial distributions. **B** is a solid rod, while **A** is a hollow cylinder. The true density of **A** is ~0.45, while the density of **B** is ~1.02 (arbitrary units). Despite the substantially lower density, **A** is stiffer and hence more resistant to bending than **B**, *i.e.*, it is structurally stronger. (Copyright, Robert P. Heaney, 2004. Used with permission.)

Similarly, in cancellous bone, horizontal cross-bracing trabeculae are important because they provide stiffness, protecting the vertical, load-bearing trabeculae from excessive bowing (and therefore snapping). In these ways architecture affects bone strength independently of bone mass.

Impaired Bone Material Quality. Bone is a two-phase material consisting of mineral crystals embedded in a dense protein matrix. Most of the mass of bone (approximately 98%) is extracellular and is laid down by bone-forming cells during the process of bone formation. In the past it has generally been considered that bony material did not vary appreciably from person to person or disease to disease (with the notable exception of osteomalacia, in which there is a failure of adequate mineralization of the protein matrix). However, this presumed constancy is an over-simplification. All structural materials, when repeatedly loaded, develop fatigue damage, which alters their material properties and increases the propensity to structural failure. Additionally, collagen cross-links are important for the tensile strength of bone. There is at least one report [1] of reduced cross-links in osteoporotic bone, pointing to a qualitative defect in bony material in at least some cases of osteoporosis.

In many mammals the bone contains a repair apparatus which detects fatigue-damaged bony volumes and replaces them. This process helps to keep the bony material at optimal strength despite ongoing damage, and represents an evolutionary compromise that avoids the need for excessively massive structures. By contrast human engineering constructions are commonly "over engineered", i.e., they are made many times more massive than would be necessary to resist the maximum estimated load to which the structure would be exposed. Bone, by contrast, has much less structural reserve and depends upon repair of fatigue damage to maintain its structures at the peak strength possible for their mass and architecture.

Thus, in brief, bone will sustain fragility fractures if it experiences either a significant decrease in bone mass, a deterioration in bone architecture, or an impairment of bone material quality that is not suitably repaired.

Increased Propensity for Injury

Even fragile bones will not necessarily result in fracture if they are not subjected to excessive force, such as would come about from falls from standing height. Individuals subject to frequent falling, whether from age-related declines in central nervous functioning, inappropriate postural reflexes, alterations in gait pattern, the use of drugs that influence balance and blood pressure, or many other forces, will expose their skeletons to forces that may be greater than the intrinsic bony strength can sustain. Sometimes these forces are sufficient to break even fully normal bones, e.g., a fall to the side, striking the lateral surface of the upper femur, will often produce a typical hip fracture even in young individuals. In brief, a significant portion of the fracture risk associated with osteoporosis resides in the fragile person, rather than in his/her fragile bones.

2. Calcium

The Skeleton as the Calcium Nutrient Reserve

Throughout the course of vertebrate evolution, bone developed several times and has served many functions, such as dermal armor and internal stiffening [2]. Evidence from a variety of lines suggests that the most primitive function of the skeleton is actually to buffer the internal milieu for several essential minerals, notably calcium and phosphorus [3]. For both nutrients, the skeleton serves both as a source and as a sink, that is, as a reserve to offset shortages and, to a limited extent, as a place for safely storing surpluses.

We see this reserve feature of skeletal function expressed in diverse ways. For example, laboratory animals such as cats, rats, and dogs will reduce bone mass as needed to maintain near constancy of calcium levels in the extracellular fluid [4–6]. This activity is mediated by PTH and involves actual bone destruction, not leaching of calcium from bone. When calcium-deprived animals are parathyroidectomized, bone is spared, but severe hypocalcemia develops [7]. More physiologically, perhaps, deer temporarily increase bone resorption each year to meet the calcium and phosphorus demands of annual antler formation (which exceed the nutrient supply of late winter and spring foliage) [8]. Finally, we see the opposite side of the same function expressed in the now well established fact that augmented calcium intake will slow or reduce age-related bone loss in humans (see below).

While retaining its primitive, reserve function, bone in the higher, terrestrial vertebrates acquired a second role, namely internal stiffening and rigidity – what is today the most apparent feature of the skeleton. As such, calcium (or phosphorus) is the only nutrient with a reserve that possesses such a secondary function (with the possible exception of the thermal insulation provided by energy reserves). For typical nutrients, the reserve is first depleted, without detectable impact upon the health or functioning of the organism. Then, after the reserve is exhausted and the metabolic pool begins to be depleted, clinical disease expresses itself. For some nutrients (e.g., vitamin A or energy), the reserve can be quite large, and the latent period may last many months (or even years). But for others (e.g., the water-soluble vitamins), the reserve may be very small and detectable dysfunction develops soon after intake drops.

With calcium, the reserve is vast relative to the cellular and extracellular metabolic pools of calcium. As a result, dietary insufficiency virtually never impairs biochemical functions that are dependent upon calcium, at least in ways we can now recognize. However, since bone strength is a function of bone mass, it follows inexorably that any decrease whatsoever in the size of the calcium reserve – any decrease in bone mass – will produce a corresponding decrease in bone strength. We literally walk about on our calcium reserve. It is this unique relationship which is both the basis for the linkage of calcium nutriture with bone status and the explanation why reduction in the size of the reserve is a principal defining characteristic of the major human calcium deficiency syndrome.

At the same time it must be stressed that the mass of the skeleton, i.e., the size of the calcium nutrient reserve, can be depleted for non-nutritional reasons, and such depletion cannot be prevented by nutritional means, i.e., by increasing calcium intake. Examples are the bone loss that occurs with immobilization or disuse, the bone loss that occurs following estrogen withdrawal in human females at menopause (or following ovariectomy at an earlier age), and the bone loss that occurs during lactation in most mammalian species. This fact underscores the difficulty of interpreting bone mass in individuals. The bone mass may be low because of heredity, because of reduced physical activity, because of stunted growth in childhood, because of normal physiological processes, as well as because of inadequate calcium intake. Ensuring an adequate calcium intake will prevent or reverse only the bone loss associated with the latter mechanism. The goal of an adequate calcium intake, therefore, is not so much to ensure optimal bone status (which is a multifactorial project), but to ensure that inadequate calcium intake is not the limiting factor in determining current bone status.

The Calcium Requirement and the Consequences of Suboptimal Calcium Intake

The requirement for calcium may be notionally defined as the intake necessary to achieve and sustain the skeletal mass called for in the genetic program, as modified by current mechanical loading patterns. Because the calcium nutrient density of the diets of the high primates and human hunter-gatherers prior to the agricultural revolution, was high, humans, and indeed most mammals, do not have efficient mechanisms for utilizing or conserving food calcium. Absorption efficiency is low (net absorption from the intestine averaging between 10 and 15%), and cutaneous and obligatory excretory losses high. This behavior can be contrasted with that of sodium, which was a trace nutrient in the primitive terrestrial environment. With sodium, intestinal absorption efficiency approaches 100%, and both renal and cutaneous losses can be reduced to extremely low levels in response to extracellular fluid (ECF) volume depletion (which would, of course, occur with excessive sodium losses).

Intestinal absorption efficiency rises during the most rapid of the growth phases (infancy, adolescence, and pregnancy), resulting in substantially greater extraction of calcium from the diet, but for most other life stages calcium utilization efficiency is very poor. For example, when an individual ingests a calcium-rich food, such as milk, containing typically 300 mg of calcium, net absorption will average only 10% of that figure, or 30 mg; and urinary wastage (from the mild absorptive calcemia following absorption), will spill approximately 15 mg of that total, leaving only 15 mg from that 300 mg serving to offset cutaneous losses and/or support bone growth or maintenance.

Bone is continuously being torn down and replaced, in a process known collectively as "remodeling", and in a typical healthy adult the fluxes of calcium into and out of bone through the processes of bone formation and bone resorption are as large or larger than all of the other fluxes into or out of the extracellular fluid calcium compartment combined. The calcium "traffic" involved in bone remodeling thus constitutes a system that can be modulated either to store calcium that may be entering the body in excess of current excretory losses, or to release calcium when excretory losses exceed intake. This modulation comes about principally by increasing or decreasing the rate of bone resorption, which in turn is controlled by the action of parathyroid hormone (PTH), which is exquisitely responsive to the concentration of calcium ions in the extracellular fluid. It is important to note that the net release of calcium from bone actually involves a net loss of bone tissue. Calcium is never taken out of bone. Rather, small quantities of bone are torn down, and the calcium released thereby is scavenged by the system to meet the needs for maintenance of ECF calcium ion concentration

Defining the Requirement for Calcium. Unlike other nutrients, the requirement for calcium relates solely to calcium's secondary function, i.e., to the size of the calcium reserve, in other words, to total skeletal and regional bone mass. However, unlike energy, which can be stored as fat without practical limit, the size of the calcium reserve is limited, even in the face of dietary surfeit, by genetic and mechanical factors. As a result, calcium functions as a threshold nutrient, much as does iron. This means that, below some critical value, the effect (bone mass for calcium or hemoglobin mass for iron) will be limited by available supplies, while above that value, i.e., the "threshold", no further benefit will accrue from additional intake. This biphasic relationship is depicted schematically in Fig. 3, in which the intake-effect relationship is depicted first schematically (A), and then (B) as exemplified by data derived from a growing animal model. In panel B the effect of the nutrient is expressed directly as the amount of bone calcium an animal is able to accumulate from any given intake.

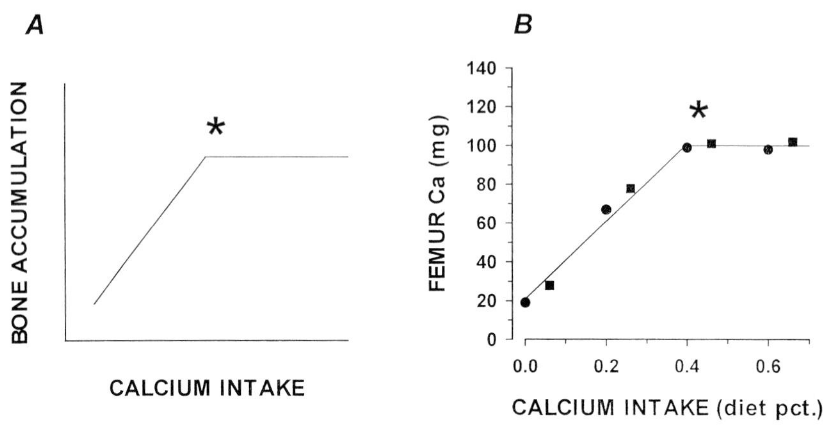

Fig. 3. Schematic illustration of the relationship between health status and body depletion of a nutrient. In A. is depicted the depletion of body stores of a typical nutrient after placing the organism on a deficient intake. In B. (the pattern exhibited by calcium), the reserve is very large relative to the metabolic pool, but health, as reflected in skeletal strength, declines steadily as the reserve itself is depleted. The data of panel B have been redrawn from Forbes et al. [9]. (Copyright, Robert P. Heaney, 1995, 2004. Reproduced with permission.)

However, if the notion of "effect" is taken to mean "any change whatsoever", then the diagram fits all life stages, even when bone may be undergoing some degree of involution. This generalized form of the threshold diagram is set forth in Fig. 4, which shows schematically what the intake/retention curves look like during growth, maturity, and involution (senescence). In brief, the plateau occurs at a positive value during growth, at zero retention in the mature individual, and sometimes at a negative value in the elderly. (Available evidence suggests that there are probably several involutional curves, with the plateau during involution at a negative value in the first 3–5 years after menopause, at zero for the next ~10 years, and then at increasingly negative values with advancing age.)

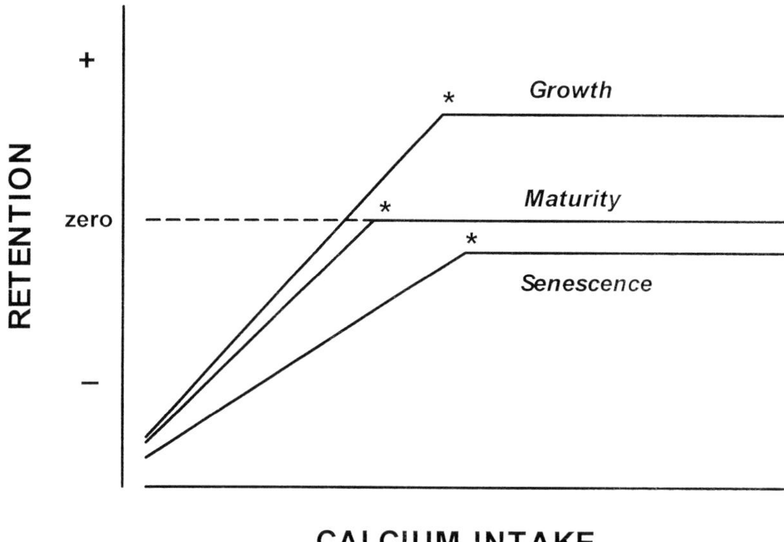

Fig. 4. Threshold curves for calcium retention as a function of calcium intake at three life stages. Increasing intakes up to the threshold values (indicated by *) improves retention; whereas increasing intakes beyond the threshold value produces no further change in retention. At subthreshold intakes, retention will be less than optimal (or even negative). During growth, suprathreshold intakes produce net calcium retention (i.e., augmentation of skeletal reserves); during maturity, zero balance (i.e., maintenance of skeletal reserves); and during senescence, either zero balance or slight negative balance (depending upon other involutional forces acting upon the aging individual). (Copyright, Robert P. Heaney, 1998, 2004. Used with permission.)

The functional indicator of nutritional adequacy for such a threshold nutrient is termed "maximal retention" and can be located in Figs. 4 and 5 at the asterisks above the curves. The intake corresponding to this point represents the minimum daily requirement. Calcium retention in this sense is "maximal" only in that further intake of calcium will produce no further retention. (This is in contrast to treatment with hormones or drugs, which can sometimes produce further calcium retention.) This approach was used by the Food and Nutrition Board of the National Academy of Sciences of the U.S. in its development of recommended intakes for calcium in 1997 [10].

There has been much uncertainty and confusion in recent years about what the threshold intake may be for various ages and physiological states. With the 1994 Consensus Development Conference on Optimal Calcium Intake [11] and the report of the Panel on Calcium and Related Nutrients [10], the bulk of that confusion has been resolved. The evidence for the intakes recommended by the consensus panel is summarized both in the Conference and Panel reports and in recent reviews of the relationship of nutrition and osteoporosis [12,13], and will be summarized briefly in ensuing sections of this chapter.

The most persuasive of the evidence supporting the conclusion that raising calcium intake will reduce fracture risk came in the form of several randomized controlled trials showing both reduction in age-related bone loss and reduction in fractures following augmentation of prevailing calcium intakes [14–23].

These studies are reviewed briefly in the following paragraphs. However, as already noted, the effects of inadequate calcium intake are most evident at the two extremes of life. During growth that is because the skeletal mass must increase from approximately 25 g calcium at birth to approximately 1000 g calcium at age 30, with the largest percentage gains occurring during infancy and at the adolescent growth spurt. And during senescence mechanisms for conserving calcium tend to deteriorate, just as do the reserve capacities of most other body systems. As a result, the ability of elderly individuals to adapt to insufficient calcium intakes deteriorates, and bone much more clearly expresses the effects of diet. Figures 5 and 6 show this skeletal vulnerability, first for children and then for octogenarians when calcium intakes are far short of what is needed to protect the skeletons.

Fig. 5 shows the relative risk of sustaining any prepubertal fracture in children who are milk avoiders [24]. Such risk is increased approximately 2.5-fold over what would be expected for age–matched, community controls. Although the term "osteoporosis" is usually confined to older individuals, or to individuals with a demonstrable decrease in bone mass, the fractures occurring in these children are in no essential way different from the fractures occurring in older individuals in whom the diagnosis might be more readily applied. The definition of osteoporosis set forth earlier in this chapter is broad enough to include these childhood fractures as truly osteoporotic.

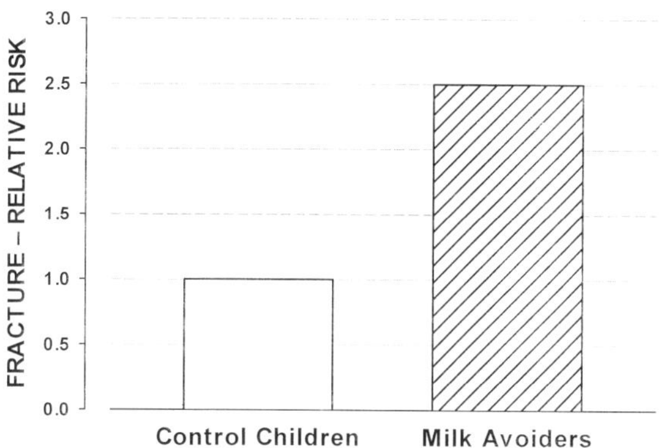

Fig. 5. Relative risk of prepubertal fracture in 50 New Zealand children, aged 3–13, who had been habitual milk avoiders from age ~1. (Plotted from data of Goulding et al. [24].) (Copyright, Robert P. Heaney, 2004. Used with permission.)

Fig. 6, by contrast, is derived from a study of elderly French women who were randomized to receive either a calcium and vitamin D supplement or placebo [14]. The supplemental calcium elevated their dietary intakes from 500 to 1700 mg/d, and the supplemental vitamin D, at least in part, served to ensure that the ingested calcium would be absorbed efficiently (see also below, vitamin D). As Fig. 6 shows, hip fracture risk was decreased by approximately 30% within 18 months of starting supplementation. At the same time the Figure shows that the bone loss occurring in the unsupplemented individuals was completely stopped in the supplemented group. In fact, the measured bone loss in the placebo-treated individuals averaged better than 3%/year while there was, by contrast, a small gain in bone in the calcium-supplemented individuals. Fig. 7 depicts the threshold diagram for calcium for the elderly, as set forth earlier in Fig. 4. It allows the tentative placement of the two treated groups in the French trial. From the bone loss that the placebo-treated individuals were sustaining, it is clear that they were located somewhere on the ascending limb of the calcium threshold diagram (point B); while the supplemented individuals clearly had intakes at or above the threshold (point A). The goal of all calcium regimens must be to achieve a calcium intake that is above the threshold point of the diagram. As Fig. 7 shows, however, even a supra-threshold intake may not be sufficient to ensure calcium retention in all individuals, simply because other age-related factors may be leading to a decline in bone mass.

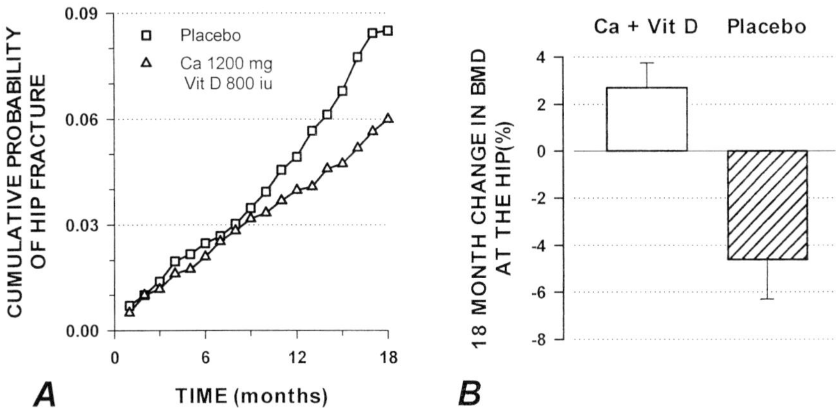

Fig. 6. Risk of incident hip fracture and change in hip bone mass in a randomized, placebo-controlled trial of 1847 elderly French women. (Redrawn from Chapuy et al. [14]. Hip fracture incidence was reduced by more than 30% in the supplemented individuals. The placebo-treated women were losing bone at a rate greater than 3%/yr, while the supplemented women actually experienced a small bone gain. (Copyright, Robert P. Heaney, 1992, 2004. Used with permission.)

Table 1 sets forth recent recommendations for the calcium requirement. As can be seen, while the 1994 NIH recommendations are, for most ages, substantially higher than the 1989 RDAs, they are actually quite close both to values derivable both from available balance studies and to the 1997 recommendations of the Food and Nutrition Board.

Table 1. Various estimates of the calcium requirement in North American women

Age	1989 RDA[a]	NIH[b]	1997 RDI[c]
1–5	800	800	--
6–10	800	800–1200	960
11–24	1200	1200–1500	1560
Pregnancy/lactation	1200	1200–1500	1200–1560
24–50/65	800	1000	1200
65–	800	1500	1440

[a]Reference 25
[b]Recommendations for women as proposed by the Consensus Development Conference on Optimal Calcium Intake [11].
[c]The so-called "adequate intakes" of the new RDI values, multiplied by a factor of 1.2× to convert them into RDA format [10].

As noted earlier, the calcium requirement is related to a bone mass endpoint, but recent evidence indicates that calcium may be affecting bone in other ways entirely, ways that may be even more important that its effect on bone massiveness [26]. When calcium intake is inadequate, the level of secretion of parathyroid hormone rises, and if the intake remains low, then the production of PTH remains high. This leads to a chronic increase in bone remodeling rate. Recker et al. [27], for example, have shown that remodeling rate doubles across menopause, and then reaches nearly 3× premenopausal levels by age 65. That increase in remodeling rate is responsible for much of the enhanced fragility of the postmenopausal period in women. Agents which reduce remodeling to the premenopausal level reduce fracture risk as well. Gonadal hormones during the reproductive years are responsible for a quasi-physiological antagonism of PTH-mediated bone remodeling. The release of this tonic inhibition is at least a major part of the explanation for the postmenopausal rise in remodeling. While high calcium intakes do stop the bone loss of the late postmenopausal period (as shown in Fig. 6), their effect on fracture rate is virtually immediate, indicating that the fracture reduction is not due to an effect on bone mass. By contrast, remodeling rate drops immediately when calcium intake is elevated substantially.

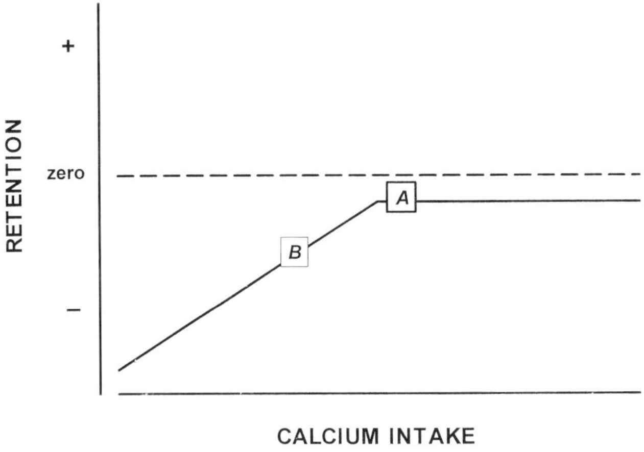

Fig. 7. Calcium threshold curve for elderly individuals from Fig. 4. *B* represents the intake typical of most older persons, and is associated with negative retention, i.e., bone loss. *A* represents the threshold value, i.e., an intake sufficient to protect the skeletal reserves. The control group in the study depicted in Fig. 6 had intakes in the region of point *B*, while the calcium-supplemented individuals had intakes in the region of point *A*. (Copyright, Robert P. Heaney, 1998. Used with permission.)

While, theoretically, high calcium intake is important for bone health at all stages of life, in the practical order the largest measurable effects are seen during growth and senescence. This is partly because the gonadal hormones that are produced during the reproductive years and much of the mature life of individuals protect the skeleton by a physiological partial antagonism of the resorptive effects of parathyroid hormone. As a consequence, individuals with low calcium intakes may be only marginally disadvantaged, so long as they are otherwise well nourished and have normal hormonal status.

Nutrient-Nutrient Interactions: Factors that Influence the Calcium Requirement

There are several nutritional factors which influence or have been proposed to influence the calcium requirement. These are probably less important than once thought, since at calcium intakes in the ranges currently recommended, interactions tend to have negligible impact on the calcium economy. Nevertheless, the issue of interactions continues to arise, and so will be addressed briefly here.

The principal interacting nutrients are sodium, protein, caffeine, and fiber. Fiber and caffeine influence calcium absorption [28–31] and typically exert relatively minor effects, while sodium and protein influence urinary excretion of calcium, [31,32] and can be of much greater significance for the calcium economy when calcium intakes are low. The net effects of phosphorus and fat in humans are minor to non-existent.

Absorption efficiency and excretory loss are at least as important as actual calcium intake. In 560 balances in healthy middle-aged women consuming typical intakes performed in the author's laboratory, only 11% of the variance in balance among these women was explained by differences in their actual calcium intakes. By contrast, absorption efficiency explains about 15%, while urinary losses explained about half.

Influences on Intestinal Absorption of Calcium. *Fiber.* The effect of fiber is variable, and generally small. Many kinds of fiber have no influence at all on absorption, such as the fiber in green, leafy vegetables [33,34]. The fiber in wheat bran, by contrast, reduces absorption of co-ingested calcium, although except for extremes of fiber intake [35], the overall effect is generally relatively small. Often lumped together with fiber are associated plant food constituents such as phytate and oxalate. Both can reduce the availability of any calcium contained in the same food, but, unlike bran, generally do not affect co-ingested calcium from other foods. For example, for equal ingested loads, the calcium of beans is only about half as available as the calcium of milk [36], while the calcium of spinach and rhubarb is nearly totally unavailable [37]. For spinach and rhubarb, the inhibition is mostly due to oxalate. For common beans, phytate is responsible for about half the interference, and oxalate, the other half. Even so, the effects of phytate and oxalate are highly variable from food to food. There is a sufficient quantity of both anti-absorbers in beans to complex all the calcium also present, and yet absorptive interference is only half what might be expected.

Caffeine. Often considered to have a deleterious effect on the calcium economy, caffeine actually has the smallest effect of the known interacting nutrients [29]. A single cup of brewed coffee causes deterioration in calcium balance of ~3 mg [30,31,38], mainly by reducing absorption of calcium [30]. The effect is probably on active transport, although this is not known for certain. This small effect is more than adequately offset by a tablespoon or two of milk [30,38].

Influences on Renal Conservation of Calcium. Protein and Sodium. As noted, the effects of protein and of sodium can be substantial [31,39,40]. Both nutrients can increase urinary calcium loss across the full range of their own intakes, from very low to very high – so it is not a question of harmful effects of an *excess* of these nutrients. Sodium and calcium share the same transport system in the proximal tubule, and every 2300 mg sodium excreted by the kidney pulls 20–60 mg of calcium out with it. And every gram of typical protein (whether from animal or vegetable sources) metabolized in adults causes an increment in urine calcium loss of about 1 mg. This latter effect is probably due to excretion of the sulfate load produced in the metabolism of sulfur-containing amino acids (and is thus a kind of endogenous analog of acid-rain).

Although much of the literature in this field stresses the role of sodium, as such, it is important to recognize that most dietary sodium is in the form of table salt, sodium chloride, and that the often ignored anion plays an important role in these interactions. This issue is too complex for exhaustive treatment here, and it will be sufficient only to note that sodium bicarbonate does not have the same hypercalciuric effect as sodium chloride [41], and that potassium bicarbonate completely obliterates the calciuria of a high sodium chloride intake [42].

At low salt and protein intakes, the minimum calcium requirement to maintain calcium balance for an adult premenopausal female may be as little as 450 mg/d, whereas if her intake of both nutrients is high, she may require as much as 2000 mg/d. A forceful illustration of the importance of sodium intake is provided by the report of Matkovic et al. [43], showing that urine calcium remains high in adolescent girls on calcium intakes too low to permit bone gain. The principal determinant of urinary calcium in such young women is sodium intake [44], not calcium intake.

Differences in protein and sodium intake from one national group to another are perhaps part of the explanation why studies in different countries have shown sometimes strikingly different calcium requirements. At the same time, one usually finds a positive correlation between calcium intake and bone mass within each national range of intakes [45]. Hence although sodium (and protein) intake differences between cultures obscure the calcium effect, they do not obliterate it.

For diets high in calcium, as would have been the case for our hunter-gatherer ancestors, high protein and possibly high sodium intakes could have been handled by the body perfectly well. At the low intakes that prevail today, an individual's absorptive performance is close to maximal. Augmented loss from increased sodium or protein intake cannot be offset by increasing extraction from the diet, both because there is less there to extract, and because extraction efficiency is already at the upper end of its possible range. By contrast, at intake levels typical of those that prevailed during hominid evolution, intestinal absorption is predominantly passive, and the full range of absorptive adaptation is available to offset increased excretory or cutaneous losses. In brief, these nutrients create problems for the calcium economy of contemporary adult humans mainly because we typically have calcium intakes that are low relative to those of pre-agricultural humans, and sodium intakes that are high.

Acid Ash Residue. The acid/alkaline ash characteristic of the diet may also be important, although the quantitative relationship of this diet feature to the calcium requirement has been less fully explored to date. Nevertheless, it has clearly been shown that substitution of metabolizable

                                    R. P. Heaney

anions (e.g., bicarbonate or acetate) for fixed anions (e.g., chloride) in various test diets will lower obligatory urinary calcium loss substantially [46,47]. This suggests that primarily vegetarian diets create a lower calcium requirement, and provides a further explanation for the seemingly lower requirement in many non-industrialized populations. However, it is not yet clear whether, within a population, vegetarians have higher bone mass values than omnivores, and some data suggest they may actually have less dense skeletons, possibly because of the often very low calcium levels of such diets [48,49].

Calcium Requirement and Body Size

The calcium requirements established by the joint U.S.-Canadian Task Force [10] are predicated on typical North American body size. The correct size adjuster (height, weight, or surface area) is not known. Nevertheless, it is likely that the minimum daily calcium requirement for bone health is a function of body size. Taking, for example, weight as the adjustment variable, a population whose women average 50 kilo would get the same protective effect from a diet containing 700–750 mg/d as would a North American woman from a diet containing 1000 mg/d. However, it should be noted that, as nutrition improves in many nations that formerly had high levels of poverty, body size tends to increase, as well, and simply because older individuals today are smaller (and hence can probably get by on less dietary calcium), it does not necessarily follow that future age cohorts would need less calcium than North Americans.

Calcium Sources

In Western nations individuals with low calcium intakes have diets that typically are deficient in four or more other nutrients, as well [50]. It follows that the preferred way to address such deficiency is from food sources that contain more than a single nutrient. Thus, while medicinal calcium supplements may be indicated, and certainly have a place in co-therapy of osteoporosis along with bone active agents, primary prevention should be focused on total nutritional quality of the diet, i.e., using food sources of calcium. Such sources include most dairy products, green leafy vegetables, particularly of the Brassica species, calcium-set tofu, small bony fish, and a few shell fish and nuts. By contrast, seed foods such as corn, rice, wheat, and millet, and most meats, tend to be poor calcium sources.

Among the vegetable sources there is great variability in the bioavailability of their calcium. For example, the calcium of high oxalate vegetables (such as spinach and rhubarb) is almost completely unavailable. Fig. 8 displays the *available* calcium in a variety of foods. "Available" represents the product of the fractional absorbability of the calcium in a food and its total calcium content. It is thus the actual, gross[*] amount of calcium a particular food delivers into the blood of the absorbing subject.

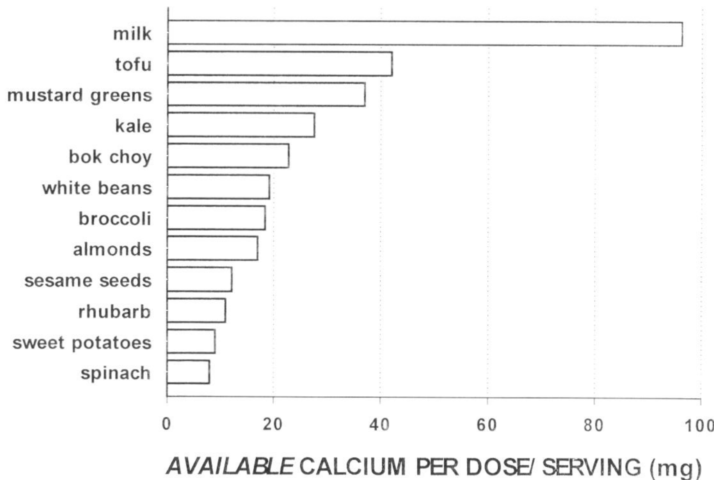

Fig. 8. Available calcium per serving of a variety of food sources. "Available" represents the product of the calcium content of the food and its fractional absorption, and thus represents gross absorption. Calcium contents of the various foods have been derived from standard food databases. (Copyright, Robert P. Heaney, 1998, 2004. Used with permission.)

---

[*] In the process of digestion substantial quantities of calcium enter the gut in the form of digestive secretions and sloughed mucosa. For this reason, net absorption is always less than gross.

If calcium supplements are used to make up for what cannot be realistically provided in the diet, it should be noted that, mimicking food, supplements should be taken with meals. Divided doses enhance absorption from any source – supplement or food – since absorption fraction is an inverse function of load size [51]. Various calcium salts (e.g., calcium carbonate, calcium citrate, calcium phosphate) are absorbed with approximately equal efficiency, other things being equal [52,53]. Pharmaceutical formulation, however, may have a large effect on absorbability. Different tablets of the same salt (e.g., calcium carbonate) may exhibit a two-fold range in absorbability, depending upon other materials added in the tableting process. In all instances reliance should be had only on products that have established their bioavailability by formal testing in humans.

All calcium sources (including food) interfere with iron absorption when the two nutrients are ingested at the same meal. However, single-meal studies miss the body's up-regulation of iron absorption in the face of need, and chronic feeding studies have revealed no deterioration of iron status in subjects consuming high calcium diets. Perhaps of greater relevance, Matkovic and his colleagues have convincingly shown that

adolescent girls are able to increase total body iron stores normally in the presence of 1600 mg calcium intakes [54]. This is a particularly reassuring finding since females in this age group are among the most vulnerable to iron deficiency. However, if an adult is iron-deficient (e.g., as a result of severe blood loss) and is taking an iron supplement, it may be best if the meal at which the iron is taken not contain a large amount of calcium (food or supplement).

3. Vitamin D

The Functioning of Vitamin D in the Calcium Economy

It has long been recognized that vitamin D is important for absorption of calcium from the diet. Its role in that regard lies in facilitating active transport, mainly by inducing the formation of a calcium-binding transport protein in intestinal mucosal cells. This function is particularly important for adaptation to low intakes. This effect is produced mainly by $1,25(OH)_2D$ (calcitriol), the metabolically most active form of the vitamin. $1,25(OH)_2D$ is produced in the kidney in response to PTH stimulation, and circulates to the intestine where it binds to the vitamin D receptor of the mucosal cells. There is also, apparently, a second, more rapidly acting vitamin D-related absorption mechanism [55], which is non-genomic in nature but nevertheless requires occupancy of the classical vitamin D receptor by $1,25(OH)_2D$. Finally absorption also occurs passively, probably mainly by way of paracellular diffusion. This route is not dependent upon vitamin D, and is not as well studied. The proportion of absorption by the three mechanisms varies with intake and is not well characterized in humans; at high calcium intakes (above 2000 mg/day) absorption fraction approaches that observed in anephric individuals (ca. 10–15 percent of intake). Under these circumstances it is likely that active transport contributes relatively little to the total absorbed load. Nevertheless, it is clear, at prevailing calcium intakes, that vitamin D status influences absorptive performance and that it thereby influences the minimum calcium requirement.

A simple calculation suffices to establish the magnitude of this influence. Assume an intake of 1000 mg Ca/d. To that is added about 150 mg in the form of digestive secretions and sloughed off mucosa. If passive absorption is at a level of 12.5 percent of intake, gross absorption would amount to 144 mg, leaving the individual with a net absorption of –6 mg/d, or *negative* balance across the gut (and, of course, providing no calcium gain for the body to offset renal and dermal losses). If, however, vitamin D-mediated, active transport is operating, so that, for example, gross absorption efficiency is 27.5 percent, net absorption becomes +109 mg from the same intake. The relationship of active transport to net absorption is shown graphically, for various intakes, in Fig. 9. The Figure makes clear that meeting physiological demands for calcium would require very high calcium intakes in the absence of vitamin D. (That situation is depicted by the bottom line in the figure, which is the net absorption contour for zero active absorption, as well as by the other lines depicting lower levels of active transport, reflecting, in turn, varying degrees of vitamin D insufficiency.)

A principal storage form of the vitamin is 25-hydroxyvitamin D (25OHD), and its plasma level is generally regarded as the best clinical indicator of vitamin D status. Although usually considered to be about three orders of magnitude less potent than calcitriol in promoting active transport in animal receptor assays, there is growing evidence that it may possess physiological functions in its own right [55–61], and in the only human dose-response studies performed to date, 25OHD was found to have a molar potency in the range of 1/125 to 1/400 that of $1,25(OH)_2D_3$ [60–62], not the 1/2000 figure usually considered to reflect relative 25OHD activity.

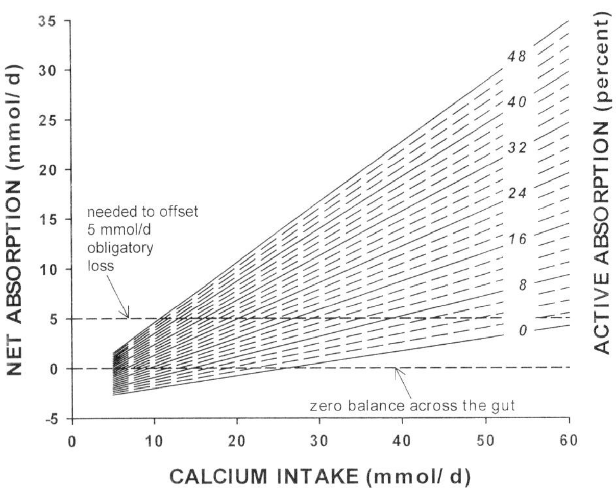

Fig. 9. Relationship of vitamin D-mediated, active calcium absorption, calcium intake, and net calcium gain across the gut. Each of the contours represents a different level of active absorption above a baseline passive absorption of 12.5%. (The values along each contour represent the sum total of passive and variable active absorption.) The horizontal and dashed lines indicate 0 and 5 mmol/d net absorption, respectively. The former is the value at which the gut switches from a net excretory to a net absorptive mode, and the latter is the value needed to offset typical urinary and cutaneous losses in mature adults. (To convert mmol to mg, multiply by 40.) (Copyright, Robert P. Heaney, 1999. Used with permission.)

Vitamin D status commonly deteriorates in the elderly, whose plasma 25OHD levels are generally lower than in young adults [63,64]. These elderly persons, without histological or biochemical evidence of osteomalacia, nevertheless exhibit high PTH levels, high serum alkaline phosphatase levels, and low absorptive performance, all of which move to or toward normal with physiological amounts of supplemental vitamin D [63–66].Bone mass is·directly correlated with serum 25OHD in the NHANES-III database [67], and the rate of age-related loss of bone has been found to be inversely correlated to dietary vitamin D [68]. Low dosage vitamin D supplementation of ostensibly healthy postmenopausal women significantly slows wintertime bone loss and reduces the annual parathyroid-mediated activation of the bone remodeling system that occurs in winter through late spring [64]. These data all suggest that relative vitamin D insufficiency is common. This conclusion is confirmed in several population studies. For example, Thomas et al. [69] reported that 57 percent of patients admitted to a general medicine service had serum 25OHD values below the lower end of the reference range. With recent evidence that the laboratory reference range is itself suboptimal [70–72], it is likely that better than 80 percent of these patients had subnormal vitamin D status.

Low serum 25OHD levels in the elderly are partly due to decreased solar exposure and partly to decreased efficiency of skin vitamin D synthesis. In North America decreased intake of milk, the principal dietary source of the vitamin also plays a role. Moreover, the elderly exhibit other abnormalities of the vitamin D endocrine system which may further impair their ability to adapt to reduced calcium intake. These include decreased responsiveness of the renal 1-α-hydroxylase to parathyroid hormone [73] and possibly, also, decreased mucosal responsiveness to calcitriol [74] (although available data do not permit distinguishing a decrease in mucosal responsiveness from a simple decrease in mucosal mass).

For all these reasons there is a growing body of opinion that the requirement for vitamin D rises with age [72,75–79], and a body of data which strongly suggests that relative vitamin D deficiency plays a role in several components of the osteoporosis syndrome. For example, calcium absorption efficiency falls as serum 25OHD decreases within the range of serum values from 80 to 50 nmol/L (both well within the reference range), and fracture risk is reduced by vitamin D supplementation at 800 IU/d [71,72], involving serum 25OHD levels in exactly the same range. Lips et al. on the other hand, found no benefit from a smaller supplemental dose (400 IU) in a Dutch population [80].

The foregoing studies (as well as others) lead inexorably to the conclusion that vitamin D insufficiency is prevalent in the middle-aged and elderly of Northern Europe and North America (and undoubtedly northern Asia as well). Moreover, in virtually none of the studies showing a benefit of supplemental vitamin D was clinically evident osteomalacia a significant feature of the problem. Hence, as discussed above, this criterion for true vitamin D deficiency is much too strict to be clinically useful today. How the vitamin D requirement ought to be defined is another matter. Holick [79] and Heaney et al. [70,81] have presented data showing that it takes an intake of at least 600–1000 IU/day, from all sources, to sustain serum 25(OH)D levels in healthy young males, and the doses of vitamin D used in the studies summarized above also suggest that an intake of at least 500–800 IU/day is required for full expression of the known effects of vitamin D in adults. Available evidence indicates that daily utilization of vitamin D approximates 4000 IU, most of which must be derived from cutaneous synthesis in response to solar UV-B radiation [81].

What is not clear from the above is how much of the effect of vitamin D in studies such as the fracture prevention trial of Heikinheimo et al. [82] is due to facilitating gut adaptation to marginal calcium intakes [70], and how much may represent an extra-intestinal effect of the vitamin in its own right. In addition to its calcium-related functions, vitamin D is an important determinant of neuromuscular function. Short-term treatment with vitamin D reduces fall frequency substantially [83], and lower extremity muscle function has been shown to be a linear function of serum 25(OH)D level throughout the entire range usually encountered in persons living at mid to high latitudes [84]. Both effects could explain a reduction in osteoporotic fracture risk. Calcitriol receptors are widely distributed in many tissues, and calcitriol enhances PTH-mediated bone resorption and exhibits autocrine action in cell differentiation and in immune modulation. Additionally, elevating serum 25OHD levels in the elderly improves the often incomplete gamma carboxylation of osteocalcin (see below – Vitamin K).

Sources of Vitamin D

Vitamin D is not a normal constituent of most foods. It is added in some nations as a fortificant to products such as milk. The principal source of vitamin D for most populations is exposure of the skin to the sun. However, the amount of vitamin D that can be acquired in this way depends upon latitude, season, skin pigmentation (both constitutive and tanning), and air quality. Thus, at mid to high latitudes (greater than 37°), vitamin D synthesis in the skin in winter months is negligible [85]. The rate of utilization of vitamin D is sufficiently high that even generous summer sun exposure will usually not be enough to provide sufficient vitamin D to ensure vitamin D adequacy throughout the winter and spring months [86]. As evidence accumulates pointing toward a higher vitamin D requirement than that needed to prevent rickets or osteomalacia, it will be necessary for various nations to develop and implement national fortification and/or supplementation strategies.

4. Protein

The importance of protein for bone is at least two-fold. First, protein is a bulk constituent of bone, comprising roughly half its volume. Because of extensive post-translational modification of the collagen molecule (e.g., cross-linking, hydroxylation, etc.) many of the amino acids released in bone resorption cannot be recycled. Hence, bone turnover requires a continuing supply of fresh dietary protein. Second, protein elevates serum IGF-1 [87,88], which is trophic for bone.

In various clinical and metabolic studies, protein exerts two seemingly contradictory effects with respect to bone: 1) protein increases urinary calcium loss [89]; and 2) protein aids recovery from hip fracture [90,91] and slows age-related bone loss [91,92]. For the most part, the studies establishing these diverse and to some extent contradictory effects have been performed by varying only the nutrient concerned. For example, the calciuric effects of protein have been demonstrated most clearly in studies in which purified protein or protein hydrolysates were used, with each gram of protein resulting in an approximate rise in urinary calcium excretion of 1 mg. Spencer, however, observed that, when the protein was fed as ground beef, urinary calcium did not rise, with the difference in response being due, presumably, to the fact that the meat contained substantial quantities of phosphorus [93]. Similarly, in multiple regression models adjusting for calcium intake, estrogen status, body size, and phosphorus intake, and involving data from 644 balance studies in middle-aged women, we were unable to find an effect of protein on urine calcium [94].

Kerstetter et al. [95] have reported that high protein intakes enhance calcium absorption, an effect which would counter a calciuric effect (were there to be one). Not everyone has been able to reproduce this finding in chronic feeding studies [96], and it may be, to the extent that the phenomenon is operative, that it applies only acutely. Very recently Roughead et al. [97] in a controlled feeding study have reported no effect of high and low protein intakes from meat (117 g/d vs. 68 g/d) either on calcium balance or on urinary calcium excretion, a finding consistent with that of Spencer et al. [93] and Heaney [96], but at odds with that of Kerstetter [95].

The generally very reproducible calciuric effect of pure protein or amino acids had led, several years ago, to the tentative conclusion that high protein intakes might be deleterious for the skeleton. However, not only do the studies involving food sources of protein, such as those just cited, not support that conclusion, but epidemiological studies, such as those from the Framingham osteoporosis cohort [92] indicate instead that age-related bone loss in postmenopausal women is *inversely* related to protein intake, not *directly*, as might have been predicted from the calciuric effect. Further, there is one population-based study [98] that indicates reduced hip fracture risk with high protein intake.

In their randomized controlled trial of calcium supplementation, Dawson-Hughes and colleagues [99] showed that the bone gain associated with calcium supplementation was confined to individuals in the highest tertile of protein intake, while in the placebo group there was a nonsignificant trend toward worsening bone status as protein intake rose. This latter effect is what would be predicted if there were some degree of protein-induced calciuria without an offsetting increase in absorbed calcium. Protein intake in this study spanned only a relatively narrow range, and was not randomly assigned to the subjects, and so these results cannot be considered final. Nevertheless they do exhibit two interesting features: 1) high protein intake clearly did not block the positive effect of calcium; and 2) most of the protein was from animal sources (as was true for the Framingham osteoporosis cohort, as well). This latter point provides no support for the hypothesis that animal foods (as contrasted with vegetable protein sources), by increasing urinary calcium loss, artificially elevate the calcium requirement.

The IGF-1 response is of particular interest. IGF-1 rises with protein intake, but above certain protein intakes, no further increase in IGF-1 can be produced. This effect is analogous to calcium retention, which rises at suboptimal calcium intakes, but which plateaus at or above the individual's calcium intake requirement. For both nutrients a rise in retention (for calcium) or a rise in IGF-1 (for protein) can be taken as evidence that the pre-supplement intake of the corresponding nutrient was suboptimal. The fact that IGF-1 has not reached its plateau at intakes in the range of current RDAs, have led some to conclude that the current RDA for protein is set too low, particularly for the elderly. In any case, it is important to understand this relationship of nutrient intakes in various studies to the respective plateaus. Different studies would be expected to show more or less of a beneficial effect of increasing one or both nutrient intakes depending upon whether the pre-supplement intake were below or above the respective threshold level.

5. Phosphorus

Bone mineral is typically considered to be in the form of hydroxyapatite, i.e., $Ca_{10}(OH)_2(PO_4)_6$. The phosphate anion accounts for nearly 60 percent of the mass of the mineral, and calcium and phosphorus exist in bone at a molar ratio of 10:6. Clearly, therefore, adequate dietary phosphorus is essential for bone health.

Fortunately phosphorus intake is generally above the applicable RDA in individuals consuming adequate amounts of protein; hence dietary phosphorus deficiency is not common, and an isolated phosphorus deficiency essentially never occurs. (There has even been some concern expressed that there is too much phosphorus in contemporary diets. That is probably not correct.) However, low phosphorus intakes are relatively common among the elderly (i.e., 10–15% of women over 60 in the U.S. ingest under two thirds of the RDA). Whether such low intakes directly contribute to the problem of osteoporosis is not known, but unlikely. When serum inorganic phosphorus (P_i) levels are low, bone mineralization will be limited by phosphate depletion in the micro-environment of the mineralizing front. Depending upon serum P_i, this may occur before calcium is locally depleted. It is probable that osteoblast function is compromised by such low ambient phosphate concentrations. This relationship may become important when patients with low phosphorus intakes are given large calcium supplements and placed on anabolic agents (such as teriparatide or fluoride). Calcium supplements, if given as the carbonate or citrate salts (e.g.), will bind most or all of the ingested food phosphorus [100], thereby limiting the bone gain potentially achievable with anabolic agents.

Phosphorus is commonly believed to reduce calcium absorption, but the evidence for that effect is scant to non-existent, and there is much contrary evidence. In analysis of 567 metabolic balances performed in healthy middle-aged women studied on their usual diets, variation in phosphorus intake over a nearly 6-fold range had no detectable effect on calcium absorption efficiency [96]. And in a controlled metabolic study, Spencer found no effect of even large increments in phosphate intake on overall calcium balance at low, normal, and high intakes of calcium [101]. In adults, Ca:P ratios ranging from 0.2 to above 2.0 are without effect on calcium balance, at least so long as adjustments are made for calcium intake [31,96].

What phosphorus does is depress urinary calcium loss and elevate digestive juice secretion of calcium, by approximately equal amounts, with little or no net effect on balance [102]. While it is true that stoichiometric excesses of phosphate will tend to form complexes with calcium in the chyme, various calcium phosphate salts have been shown to exhibit absorbability similar to other calcium salts, and phosphate is, of course, a principal anion of the major food source of calcium (dairy products). In any case, phosphate itself is more readily absorbed than calcium (by a factor of 2–5×), and at intakes of both nutrients in the range of their respective RDAs, absorption will leave a stoichiometric excess of calcium in the ileum, not the other way about. This explains the seeming paradox that high calcium intakes can block phosphate absorption (as in management of end-stage renal disease), while achievably high phosphate intakes have little or no effect on calcium absorption.

6. Minerals and Trace Nutrients

Trace Minerals

Several minerals in addition to calcium and phosphorus may be involved in bone status. These include the bulk minerals, potassium and magnesium, and the trace minerals notably zinc, manganese, and copper. The latter are essential metallic co-factors for enzymes involved in synthesis of various bone matrix constituents [103]. In growing animals, diets deficient in these nutrients produce definite skeletal abnormalities [104]. Additionally, zinc deficiency is well known to produce growth retardation and other abnormalities in humans. But it is not known with certainty whether significant deficiencies of these elements develop in previously healthy adults, or at least, if they do, whether such deficiencies contribute detectably to the osteoporosis problem. Finally, bone mineral contains large quantities of magnesium, which can become deficient in adults. But, as with the trace elements, the impact of such deficiency on osteoporosis is unclear.

Copper. Copper is of particular interest. The principal sources of copper in the diet are shellfish, nuts, legumes, whole grain cereals, and organ meats. True dietary copper deficiency is considered to be rare and to be confined to special circumstances, such as with total parenteral nutrition or infants recovering from malnutrition. Recognized manifestations in humans have usually centered on disorders of hemopoiesis, mainly as an iron-refractory, hypochromic anemia and leukopenia. Osteoporosis or fragility fractures have not been generally considered to be a part of the syndrome. However, copper-deficient premature infants have underdeveloped, weak bones that fracture easily and respond to copper supplementation [105], and in one human with copper deficiency due to a copper transport defect, the patient's morbidity included osteoporosis [106].

Copper is a necessary co-factor for lysyl oxidase, one of the principal enzymes involved in collagen cross-linking. These cross-links are important for connective tissue strength, both in tension and in compression, as they prevent the fibrils from sliding along one another's length. Bone formed under conditions of lysyl oxidase inhibition is mechanically weak, independent of mass. Copper deficiency is reported to be associated with osteoporotic lesions in sheep, cattle, and rats [103,107]. Copper has not been much studied in connection with human osteoporosis, but in one study in which serum copper was measured, levels were negatively correlated with lumbar spine BMD, even after adjusting for body weight and dietary calcium intake [108]. In another [106] postmortem specimens of bone from osteoporotic individuals were reported to contain fewer cross-links than bone from age-matched controls.

Zinc. Zinc is a known constituent of about 300 enzymes, including alkaline phosphatase, and it plays a role with other proteins, such as the estrogen receptor molecule. Its principal sources in the human diet are red meat, whole grain cereals, shellfish, and legumes. A 70 kg adult body contains 2–3 g zinc, about half in bone. Most of this bony zinc is located on the surfaces of the calcium phosphate crystals and probably has no metabolic significance. (Many cations present in the mineralizing environment adsorb to the oxygen-rich phosphate groups on crystal surfaces and get stuck there as free water is displaced by new mineral deposition.) A fortuitous consequence of this situation is that urine zinc reflects bone resorption. Thus Herzberg *et al.* [109] have shown that urine zinc rises with age, is higher in patients with osteoporosis, and is reduced when postmenopausal women are given estrogen [110]. While some etiologic connection between zinc and osteoporosis cannot be ruled out, these observations are most easily explained as reflections of the enhanced bone resorption found in many patients with osteoporosis, the elevated resorption of the estrogen-deprived, postmenopausal state, and the well known antiresorptive effect of estrogen. Urinary zinc excretion probably functions as a marker for bone resorption, rather than as a reflection of the underlying disease mechanisms.

On the other hand, of known nutrients, zinc is the one most strongly related to serum IGF-1 [111], a growth factor known to be osteotrophic even in adults. In this connection, Schürch *et al.* [112] have shown the importance of IGF-1 in recovery from hip fracture. In an observational study from Sweden, fracture risk was higher in individuals with low zinc intakes [113], and, after adjusting for other nutrients, the risk gradient showed the expected dose-response relationship. New et al. [114] in a dietary survey of nearly 1,000 British premenopausal women found high zinc intakes to be associated with higher bone density values at both spine and hip.

Manganese. While manganese is also recognized as an essential nutrient, its precise role in nutrition is much less well characterized than that of copper and zinc. Although manganese deficiency is well recognized in both laboratory and farm animals, there is no generally recognized manganese deficiency syndrome in humans. Manganese is widely distributed in foods and is especially rich in tea.

Bone manganese content is, like that of copper and zinc, a reflection mainly of serum levels prevailing at the time bone is formed, and thus a reflection of dietary manganese. Bone manganese probably has no other metabolic significance, per se. Manganese is capable of activating many enzymes, but for most the effect is nonspecific. Manganese is, however, believed to be the preferred metal ion for certain glycosylation reactions involved in mucopolysaccharide synthesis. In this connection, manganese deficiency could interfere with both cartilage and bone matrix formation.

Animals reared on manganese-deficient diets exhibit general growth retardation, but careful measurements indicate that long bone growth is disproportionately affected [115], possibly reflecting a specific problem with endochondral bone formation. There is also indication of delayed skeletal maturation, suggesting a role of manganese in chondrogenesis. Strause et al. [116] showed this quite nicely in a rat model in which demineralized bone powder is implanted subcutaneously. In control animals cartilage forms around the powder implant, then osteogenesis occurs. In manganese-deficient animals neither development took place. In further work, Strause et al. [117] showed that manganese-deficient rats had both disordered regulation of calcium homeostasis and decreased bone mineral density. Because histology was not performed, it is not possible to say whether this represented impaired mineralization or osteoporosis. Finally, Reginster et al. [118] found low serum manganese in a group of 10 women with osteoporosis. What significance any of these findings may have for the bulk of human osteoporosis is uncertain.

In one four-way, randomized intervention trial, a trace mineral cocktail including copper, zinc, and manganese slowed bone mineral loss in postmenopausal women, when given either with or without supplemental calcium [119]. There appeared to be a small additional benefit from the extra trace minerals; however, the only statistically significant effect in this study was associated with the calcium supplement. This could mean that trace mineral deficiency plays no role in osteoporosis, but it could also mean that not all of the women treated suffered from such deficiency. In fact, since both osteoporotic and age-related bone loss are multifactorial, one would presume that only some of the subjects in such a study would be deficient, since there is no known way to select subjects for inclusion on the basis of presumed trace mineral need. Thus the suggestive findings of this study have to be considered grounds for further exploration of this issue.

Magnesium. The adult female RDA for magnesium was 280 mg/d in the 1989 RDAs and revised upwards to 320 mg/d in the 1997 DRIs [10]. Only about 25% of adult North American females achieve this level of intake on any given day. Average intakes tend to be in the range of 70–80% of the RDA. While severe magnesium deficiency is a well-described syndrome, interfering both with PTH secretion and PTH action on bone, it is uncertain whether mild departures from the RDA have any adverse effect, or even whether the RDA needs to be as high as it is now set, at least for bone. There is, as well, a widespread popular belief that magnesium is necessary for optimal calcium absorption. However, the many studies establishing the benefit of supplemental calcium described earlier achieved their effect without adding magnesium to the diets of their subjects. Furthermore, Spencer, in a series of careful metabolic studies, showed that a tripling of magnesium intake had no effect on absorption efficiency for calcium [120]. Thus there is no known justification for supplemental magnesium in prevention or treatment of osteoporosis. Moreover, magnesium salts, when used as a component of a combined supplement tablet (e.g., as in dolomite), displace calcium and make it more difficult (i.e., more pills are required) to get sufficient calcium by this route.

However, an unknown, but probably small, proportion of patients with osteoporosis have silent celiac disease as a contributory factor in their disease. These individuals commonly have some degree of magnesium deficiency. Since the underlying problem in such cases is asymptomatic, it is usually unrecognized, and hence untreated. For that reason, there may well be a small group of osteoporotic patients who would benefit from supplemental magnesium (as well as from calcium and vitamin D).

Potassium. Potassium is a largely intracellular cation. Bone mineral contains mainly that amount which is trapped when calcium phosphate is precipitated out of an extracellular fluid phase that happens to contain some potassium. There are no recognized abnormalities of bone or bone cellular function associated with values of serum potassium in the range of concentrations typically encountered.

The principal importance of potassium lies in the effects it may exert on the processes that maintain calcium homeostasis, particularly urinary calcium conservation and excretion. Low potassium intakes increase urinary calcium loss and high potassium diets reduce it [121–124]. Such observations, by themselves, could mean simply that diet potassium is a marker for other food constituents responsible for the effect. This, in fact, is partly correct (see below). But pure potassium salts – typically the bicarbonate or citrate salts – exhibit the same inverse relationship to urine calcium, pointing to a role specifically for potassium itself.

Perhaps most striking of potassium's effects is the fact that potassium (as the citrate) completely blocks the calciuria of a large sodium chloride load [125]. It is believed that both the potassium cation and the bicarbonate anion (to which citrate is metabolized) work in the distal renal tubule facilitating reabsorption of the extra calcium not reclaimed in the proximal tubule because of competition with sodium for the transport mechanism.

However, just as the undoubted effects of sodium on urine calcium have not yet been unambiguously shown to have corresponding effects on bone, so, therefore, amelioration of those effects by potassium has not been clearly shown to confer a skeletal benefit, although, in short-term metabolic experiments, potassium bicarbonate does produce a positive calcium balance shift [124,126].

New et al. [127,128] showed in observational studies a significant inverse relationship between potassium intake and bone mineral density (BMD) at both hip and spine, but it cannot be determined whether the effect is due solely to the higher potassium content or whether potassium instead is a marker for other food constituents. Potassium is ubiquitous in the diet, but is found most abundantly in green and root vegetables, followed closely by fruits, then by legumes and milk (or yogurt). A diet high in potassium will necessarily be high in vegetables. In addition to their potassium content, such foods have an alkaline/ash characteristic and thus, effectively, the anion associated with potassium in such foods will be bicarbonate. By contrast, wheat, rice, corn, and other cereal grains have very low potassium contents and generally exhibit an acid ash characteristic (because of their high content of sulfur-containing amino acids). Thus, in brief, foods high in potassium generally have an alkaline ash characteristic, and alkaline ash foods will generally be good sources of potassium.

New et al. [129,130] have also shown a significant inverse relationship in free-living subjects between net endogenous acid production (NEAP) from ingested foods and lumbar spine bone mineral density. The effect was small (less than 2.5% difference in BMD between upper and lower quartiles of NEAP), but consistent with studies by others showing a calciuric effect of food-based acid production [121,122]. New has also shown significantly higher excretion of bone remodeling biomarkers at the highest quartile of NEAP, and she also reports a small, but significant difference in NEAP between postmenopausal women with and without fracture.

On the other hand, Rafferty et al., in a large series of balance studies, showed no effect of potassium intake on calcium balance [94]. While these investigators found the same effect on urine calcium as reported by others, they also found a significant negative effect of potassium on intestinal calcium absorption. Effectively, what was gained at the kidney was lost at the gut. Theirs is the only study of potassium effects in which calcium absorption was evaluated.

Another approach may be to contrast bone status data in individuals with vegan and omnivore diets, which represent quasi-extremes of food intake patterns. Studies using contemporary bone assessment technologies [131–133], indicate that, in general, not only do the vegans not have denser bones, but they tend actually to have somewhat lower BMD, despite the fact that they have higher potassium intakes than do omnivores. While the vegetable intake of vegans will usually be higher than that of omnivores, their intake of cereal grain products will usually be higher as well. Cereals, as already noted, are very poor sources of potassium and generally produce an acid-ash residue as well (i.e., high NEAP). Hence any switch between vegan and omnivore diets involves trade-offs. Clearly the mere substitution of vegetable for animal protein sources does not seem to confer a skeletal advantage, and may, in fact, do the opposite. One may note, in passing, that the primitive human diet was omnivorous.

Aluminum. Although not in any proper sense a nutrient, aluminum, in the form of Al-containing antacids, also exerts significant effects on obligatory calcium loss in the urine [134]. By binding phosphate in the gut, these substances reduce phosphate absorption, lower integrated 24-hr serum phosphate levels, and thereby elevate urinary calcium loss. (This is the opposite of the more familiar hypocalciuric effect of oral phosphate supplements.) Therapeutic doses of Al-containing antacids can elevate urine calcium by 50 mg/d or more.

Other Vitamins

Folic Acid. Folic acid may also play a role in the pathogenesis of osteoporosis. High levels of folate are required for the maximal conversion of homocysteine to methionine, and in the absence of adequate folate, serum homocysteine levels rise. Homocystinuria, an inherited disorder of folate metabolism, has as one of its cardinal features osteoporosis, developing early in life; and some nutritionists have hypothesized that the high blood levels of homocysteine are responsible for the skeletal effect [135]. Recently it has been reported that patients with hip fracture have higher homocysteine levels than normal controls and that high serum homocysteine may be a risk factor for osteoporotic fracture [136]. It is not known for certain how homocysteine may act in this context, but homocysteine is known to be an extremely active compound, binding irreversibly to sulfhydryl groups and other polar side chain elements in structural proteins. It is speculated that homocysteine may thus disrupt the cross-linking of collagen which is essential for the tensile strength of bone. At the same time, it must be acknowledged that high serum homocysteine levels are a marker for poor nutrition generally (since homocysteine reflects current intake of folate). Thus the association of high homocysteine with hip fracture may be simply an indicator (as with vitamin K) of the poor nutritional status that is common among hip fracture patients.

Vitamin K. The chemistry and physiology of Vitamin K have been extensively reviewed elsewhere [137,138]. In brief, Vitamin K is necessary for the gamma-carboxylation of glutamic acid residues in a large number of proteins. Most familiar are those related to coagulation, in which seven vitamin K dependent proteins are involved in one way or another. The gamma-carboxyglutamic acid residues in the peptide chain bind calcium, either free or on the surface layers of crystals, and have been thought to function in varying ways including catalysis of the coagulation cascade, inhibition of mineralization (as in urine), and generation of osteoclast chemotactic signals.

Three vitamin K-dependent proteins are found in bone matrix: osteocalcin (bone gla protein – BGP), matrix gla-protein, and protein S. Only BGP is unique to bone. There is also a kidney gla protein (nephrocalcin), which may be involved in renal reabsorption of calcium. BGP binds avidly to hydroxyapatite and is chemotactic for bone-resorbing cells. Roughly 30% of the synthesized BGP is not incorporated into matrix, but is released instead into the circulation, where, like alkaline phosphatase, it can be measured and used as an indicator of bone turnover. In vitamin K deficiency, such as would occur with coumarin anticoagulants, serum BGP levels decline, and the degree of carboxylation of the circulating BGP falls dramatically. While it would seem therefore that vitamin K deficiency would have detectable skeletal effects, they have been very hard to find. Rats reared and sustained to adult life under near total suppression of BGP gamma-carboxylation show only minor skeletal defects, mostly related to abnormalities in the growth apparatus [137]. In aging humans, the problem of detecting skeletal abnormalities is compounded by the fact that the bulk of the skeleton was formed prior to the onset of any deficiency, and thus bone tends to be an insensitive indicator of current nutritional stresses.

Various vitamin K-related abnormalities have been described in association with osteoporosis, but their significance to skeletal status remains unclear. Women with low dietary vitamin K intakes have significantly lower values for BMD at hip and spine than do those with higher intakes [139], and greater risk for hip fracture [140]. Circulating vitamin K and menaquinone levels are low in hip fracture patients [141]. BGP is under-carboxylated in osteoporotics, and this defect responds to relatively small doses of vitamin K. However, maximal suppression of undercarboxylation has been reported to require in excess of 1000 µg of vitamin K per day [142]. Finally, urine calcium has been reported to be high in osteoporotics and to fall on administering vitamin K [143].

Whether or not vitamin K is important for bone health, serum vitamin K levels are indicators of general nutritional status, and it may simply be that the observation of low vitamin K levels in osteoporotics, especially in those with hip fracture, is mainly a reflection of the often poor nutrition of these individuals.

Ascorbic Acid (Vitamin C). Although vitamin C deficiency was, in a sense, the first nutritional deficiency to be recognized and its cure or prevention identified, the full function of ascorbic acid in the body remains unclear. Vitamin C deficiency, when extreme, produces a syndrome known as "scurvy", characterized by capillary permeability, bleeding and bruising, muscle weakness, fatigue, and general disability.

In addition to functioning as an aqueous antioxidant, vitamin C is necessary for the synthesis, cross-linking, and aggregation of collagen fibrils in all connective tissues. During growth, vitamin C deficiency results in severe disruption of the growth apparatus of all bones and can produce a clinical picture somewhat like that of rickets. The amount of vitamin C required to prevent both these bony abnormalities during growth, and the hemorrhagic tendencies at all life stages, is only 60–100 mg/d, an amount relatively easily obtained from a diet containing fruits and vegetables. However, there is no consensus as to whether there may be less obvious manifestation of vitamin C deficiency at intakes that are substantially higher. Most mammals, including many primates, are able to synthesize vitamin C from glucose, and where it has been measured, this production far exceeds the amount required to prevent or treat scurvy, suggesting that the vitamin is exerting less obvious effects.

Some degree of vitamin C deficiency occurs relatively often in elderly individuals living alone, particularly when combined with alcoholism. Because body stores of ascorbic acid are limited and its body half-life short, it is easily possible for low vitamin C intakes to impair new bone formation and hence contribute to the osteoporosis problem.

Skeletal and urinary deoxypyridinoline cross-links vary directly with vitamin C intake [144,145], and individuals with low intakes have more rapid bone loss [146] and lower bone mass and fewer fractures [147] than suitable control individuals. Interestingly, individuals taking a combination of vitamin C supplements, estrogen, and calcium had significantly better bone mass than controls, with each component seeming to augment the difference [148].

At the same time it must be stressed that low vitamin C status, as with vitamin K and folate, is a marker for poor global nutrition, which is itself common in many elderly populations. Hence a causal connection between low vitamin C status and skeletal impairment must remain uncertain.

7. Conclusion

Nutritional forces influence osteoporotic fragility by virtue of affecting bone strength and altering the propensity for injury. The nutrients known with certainty to be important are calcium, vitamin D and protein. Phosphorus, certain trace minerals (manganese, copper, and zinc), and vitamins C and K, while involved in bone health generally, are less certainly involved in osteoporosis. Bone cells, of course, are as dependent on total nutrition – including all the vitamins and trace minerals – as are all other cells and tissues. However, current bone mass and bone strength are dependent on cell activity extending back in time over a many year period. Hence acute nutrient deficiencies, while undoubtedly impairing current cellular competence, tend to have less effect on overall bone strength, which is the concern in this primer. The major exceptions to this generalization are the nutrients, calcium, vitamin D, and protein.

Specifically bone mass is dependent upon the quantity of calcium in the diet, together with the amount of protein available for synthesis of the bone matrix. Calcium availability, in turn, is dependent upon vitamin D status, and calcium absorption will be less than optimal when vitamin D status is subnormal. Vitamin D is also important for maintenance of neuromuscular function. Low vitamin D status is associated with poor muscular strength, and impaired reflexes, resulting in excessive falling. Potassium and sodium intakes may also influence bone mass, primarily through their effect on the calcium economy, and hence will exert their influence mainly under conditions when calcium intake is marginal or inadequate.

Low calcium intake or low vitamin D status have an additional effect on bone architecture in that they lead to excessive remodeling. During the several months between initiation of a remodeling locus and its completion, bone mass is locally compromised (and hence weakened). In brief, while remodeling ultimately strengthens bone, any remodeling in excess of mechanical need contributes only structural weakness. Calcium and vitamin D deficiency lead to excessive remodeling by virtue of the fact that insufficient calcium intake is the principal stimulus for secretion of parathyroid hormone, which in turn is the principal regulator of the quantity of bone remodeling in the total skeleton.

Protein contributes to bone strength by enhancing IGF-1 levels, which are trophic for bone, and by providing the raw material needed for synthesis of new bone matrix. Typical diets, particularly for the elderly, in most modern societies will be deficient in one or all of these nutrients, and special attention should be paid to ensuring adequate intake, both for prevention of osteoporosis, and for the support of anti-osteoporosis pharmacotherapy.

Phosphorus is important for bone strength since it constitutes the principal anion of bone mineral, but phosphorus is less likely to be deficient in contemporary diets. It may become rate-limiting in situations in which anti-osteoporosis therapy is accompanied by high doses of calcium supplements (which will bind dietary phosphorus and limit its absorption).

Trace nutrients such as vitamin K, manganese, copper, and zinc are important for bony integrity, but their roles in pathogenesis or treatment of osteoporosis remain unclear

REFERENCES

1. Oxlund H, Mosekilde L, Ørtoft G. Reduced concentration of collagen reducible cross-links in human trabecular bone with respect to age and osteoporosis. Bone 19:479-484, 1996.
2. Urist MR. The origin of bone. Discovery 25:13-19, 1964.
3. Urist MR. The bone-body fluid continuum. Perspect Biol Med 6:75-115, 1962.
4. Bauer W, Aub JC, Albright F. Studies of calcium and phosphorus metabolism. J Exper Med 49:145- ,1929.
5. Gershon-Cohen J, Jowsey J. The relationship of dietary calcium to osteoporosis. Metabolism 13:221- ,1964.
6. Bodansky M, Duff VB. Regulation of the level of calcium in the serum during pregnancy. JAMA 112:223-229, 1939.
7. Jowsey J, Raisz LG. Experimental osteoporosis and parathyroid activity. Endocrinol 82:384-396, 1968.
8. Banks WJ Jr., Epling GP, Kainer RA, Davis RW. Antler growth and osteoporosis. Anat Rec 162:387-398, 1968.
9. Forbes RM, Weingartner KE, Parker HM, Bell RR, Erdman JW Jr. Bioavailability to rats of zinc, magnesium and calcium in casein-, egg- and soy protein-containing diets. J Nutr 109:1652-1660, 1979
10. Dietary Reference Intakes for Calcium, Magnesium, Phosphorus, Vitamin D, and Fluoride. Food and Nutrition Board, Institute of Medicine. National Academy Press, Washington, DC, 1997.
11. NIH Consensus Conference: Optimal Calcium Intake. JAMA 272:1942-1948, 1994.

12. Heaney RP. Nutritional factors in osteoporosis. Ann Rev Nutr 13:287-316, 1993.

13. Heaney RP. Calcium, dairy products, and osteoporosis. J Am Coll Nutr 19(2):83S-99S, 2000.

14. Chapuy MC, Arlot ME, Duboeuf F, et al. Vitamin D_3 and calcium to prevent hip fractures in elderly women. N Engl J Med 327:1637-1642, 1992.

15. Dawson-Hughes B, Dallal GE, Krall EA, Sadowski L, Sahyoun N, Tannenbaum S. A controlled trial of the effect of calcium supplementation on bone density in postmenopausal women. N Engl J Med 323:878-883, 1990.

16. Reid IR, Ames RW, Evans MC, Gamble GD, Sharpe SJ. Effect of calcium supplementation on bone loss in postmenopausal women. N Engl J Med 328:460-464, 1993.

17. Johnston CC Jr., Miller JZ, Slemenda CW, Reister TK, Hui S, Christian JC, Peacock M. Calcium supplementation and increases in bone mineral density in children. N Engl J Med 327:82-87, 1992.

18. Lloyd T, Andon MB, Rollings N, Martel JK, Landis JR, Demers LM, Eggli DF, Kieselhorst K, Kulin HE. Calcium supplementation and bone mineral density in adolescent girls. JAMA 270:841-844, 1993.

19. Chevalley T, Rizzoli R, Nydegger V, Slosman D, Rapin C-H, Michel J-P, Vasey H, Bonjour J-P. Effects of calcium supplements on femoral bone mineral density and vertebral fracture rate in vitamin D-replete elderly patients. Osteoporos Int 4:245-252, 1994.

20. Recker RR, Hinders S, Davies KM, Heaney RP, Stegman MR, Kimmel DB, Lappe JM. Correcting calcium nutritional deficiency prevents spine fractures in elderly women. J Bone Miner Res 11:1961-1966, 1996.

21. Dawson-Hughes B, Harris SS, Krall EA, Dallal GE. Effect of calcium and vitamin D supplementation on bone density in men and women 65 years of age or older. N Engl J Med 337:670-676, 1997.

22. Reid IR, Ames RW, Evans MC, Sharpe SJ, Gamble GD. Determinants of the rate of bone loss in normal postmenopausal women. J Clin Endocrinol Metab 79:950-954, 1994.

23. Aloia JF, Vaswani A, Yeh JK, Ross PL, Flaster E, Dilmanian FA. Calcium supplementation with and without hormone replacement therapy to prevent postmenopausal bone loss. Ann Intern Med 120:97-103, 1994.

24. Goulding A, Rockell JE, Black RE, Grant AM, Jones IE, Williams SE. Children who avoid drinking cow's milk are at increased risk for prepubertal bone fractures. J Am Diet Assoc 104:250-253, 2004.

25. Recommended Dietary Allowances, 10th edition. National Acad. Press, Washington, DC, 1989.

26. Heaney RP. Is the paradigm shifting? Bone 33:457-465, 2003.

27. Recker RR, Lappe JM, Davies KM, Heaney RP. Bone remodeling increases substantially in the years following menopause and remains increased in older osteoporosis patients. J Bone Miner Res (in press) 2004.

28. Pilch SM (editor). Physiological effects and health consequences of dietary fiber. Prepared for the Center for Food Safety and Applied Nutrition, Food and

Drug Administration under Contract No. FDA 223-84-2059 by the Life Sciences Research Office, Federation of American Societies for Experimental Biology. 1987. Available from FASEB Special Publications Office, Bethesda, MD.

29.   Heaney RP. Effects of caffeine on bone and the calcium economy. Food Chem Toxicol 40:1263-1270, 2002.

30.   Barger-Lux MJ, Heaney RP. Caffeine and the calcium economy revisited. Osteoporos Int 5:97-102, 1995.

31.   Heaney RP, Recker RR. Effects of nitrogen, phosphorus, and caffeine on calcium balance in women. J Lab Clin Med 99:46-55, 1982.

32.   Nordin BEC, Need AG, Morris HA, Horowitz M. The nature and significance of the relationship between urinary sodium and urinary calcium in women. J Nutr 123:1615-1622, 1993.

33.   Heaney RP, Weaver CM, Hinders SM, Martin B, Packard P. Absorbability of calcium from Brassica vegetables. J Food Sci 58:1378-1380, 1993.

34.   Weaver CM, Heaney RP, Nickel KP, Packard PT. Calcium bioavailability from high oxalate vegetables: Chinese vegetables, sweet potatoes, and rhubarb. J Food Sci 62:524-525, 1997.

35.   Weaver CM, Heaney RP, Martin BR, Fitzsimmons ML. Human calcium absorption from whole wheat products. J Nutr 121:1769-1775, 1991.

36.   Weaver CM, Heaney RP, Proulx WR, Hinders SM, Packard PT. Absorbability of calcium from common beans. J Food Sci 58:1401-1403, 1993.

37.   Heaney RP, Weaver CM, Recker RR. Calcium absorbability from spinach. Am J Clin Nutr 47(4):707-709, 1988.

38.   Barrett-Connor E, Chang JC, Edelstein SL. Coffee-associated osteoporosis offset by daily milk consumption. JAMA 271:280-283, 1994.

39.   Nordin BEC, Polley KJ, Need AG, Morris HA, Marshall D. The problem of calcium requirement. Am J Clin Nutr 45:1295-1304, 1987.

40.   Nordin BEC, Need AG, Morris HA, Horowitz M. Sodium, calcium and osteoporosis In: Burckhardt P, Heaney RP, eds. Nutritional Aspects of Osteoporosis, 85:279-295. Raven Press, New York, 1991:

41.   Morris RC Jr, Frassetto LA, Schmidlin O, Forman A, Sebastian A. Expression of osteoporosis as determined by diet-disordered electrolyte and acid-base metabolism. In: Nutritional Aspects of Osteoporosis, pp. 357-378. Burckhardt P, Dawson-Hughes B, Heaney RP, eds. Academic Press, New York, 2001

42.   Sellmeyer DE, Schloetter M, Sebastian A. Potassium citrate prevents increased urine calcium excretion and bone resorption induced by a high sodium chloride diet. J Clin Endocrinol Metab 87:2008-2012, 2002.

43.   Matkovic V, Fontana D, Tominac C, Goel P, Chesnut CH III. Factors that influence peak bone mass formation: a study of calcium balance and the inheritance of bone mass in adolescent females. Am J Clin Nutr 52:878-888, 1990.

44.   Matkovic V, Ilich JZ, Andon MB, et al. Urinary calcium, sodium, and bone mass of young females. Am J Clin Nutr 62:417-425, 1995.

45. Lau EMC, Cooper C, Woo J. Calcium deficiency – a major cause of osteoporosis in Hong Kong Chinese. In: Burckhardt P, Heaney RP, eds. Nutritional Aspects of Osteoporosis. New York: Raven Press, 1991;85:175-180.

46. Berkelhammer CH, Wood RJ, Sitrin MD. Acetate and hypercalciuria during total parenteral nutrition. Am J Clin Nutr 48:1482-1489, 1988.

47. Sebastian A, Harris ST, Ottaway JH, et al. Improved mineral balance and skeletal metabolism in postmenopausal women treated with potassium bicarbonate. N Engl J Med 330:1776-1781, 1994.

48. Barr SI, Prior JC, Janelle KC, Lentle BC. Spinal bone mineral density in premenopausal vegetarian and nonvegetarian women: cross-sectional and prospective comparisons. J Am Diet Assoc 98:760-765, 1998.

49. Chiu J-F, Lan S-J, Yang C-Y, Wang P-W, Yao W-J, Su I-H, Hsieh C-C. Long-term vegetarian diet and bone mineral density in postmenopausal Taiwanese women. Calcif Tissue Int 60:245-249, 1997.

50. Barger-Lux MJ, Heaney RP, Packard P, Lappe JM, Recker RR. Nutritional correlates of low calcium intake. Clinics in Applied Nutrition 2:39-44, 1992.

51. Heaney RP, Weaver CM, Fitzsimmons ML. The influence of calcium load on absorption fraction. J Bone Miner Res 11(5):1135-1138, 1990.

52. Heaney RP, Recker RR, Weaver CM. Absorbability of calcium sources: the limited role of solubility. Calcif Tissue Int 46:300-304, 1990.

53. Heaney RP, Dowell MS, Barger-Lux MJ. Absorption of calcium as the carbonate and citrate salts, with some observations on method. Osteoporos Int 9:19-23, 1999.

54. Ilich-Ernst JZ, McKenna AA, Badenhop NE, Clairmont AC, Andon MB, Nahhas, RW, Goel P, Matkovic V. Iron status, menarche, and calcium supplementation in adolescent girls. Am J Clin Nutr 68:880-887, 1998.

55. Norman AW. Intestinal calcium absorption: a vitamin-D hormone-mediated adaptive response. Am J Clin Nutr 51:290-300, 1990.

56. Bell NH, Epstein S, Shary J, Greene V, Oexmann MJ, Shaw S. Evidence of a probable role for 25-hydroxyvitamin D in the regulation of calcium metabolism. J Bone Miner Res 3:489-495, 1988.

57. Barger-Lux MJ, Heaney RP, Lanspa SJ, Healy JC, DeLuca HF. An investigation of sources of variation in calcium absorption physiology. J Clin Endocrinol Metab 80:406-411, 1995.

58. Francis RM, Peacock M, Storer JH, Davies AEJ, Brown WB, Nordin BEC. Calcium malabsorption in the elderly: the effect of treatment with oral 25-hydroxyvitamin D_3. Eur J Clin Invest 13:391-396, 1983.

59. Reasner CA, Dunn JF, Fetchick D, et al., Alteration of vitamin D metabolism in Mexican-Americans (letter to editor). J Bone Miner Res 5:793-794, 1990.

60. Colodro IH, Brickman AS, Coburn JW, Osborn TW, Norman AW. Effect of 25-hydroxy-vitamin D_3 on intestinal absorption of calcium in normal man and patients with renal failure. Metabolism 27:745-753, 1978.

61. Devine A, Dick IM, Wilson W, Prince RL. Vitamin D status is unrelated to bone density or turnover in elderly postmenopausal women: a cross-sectional

and longitudinal vitamin D intervention study. J Bone Miner Res 14:S382, 1999.

62.   Heaney RP, Barger-Lux MJ, Dowell MS, Chen TC, Holick MF. Calcium absorptive effects of vitamin D and its major metabolites. J Clin Endocrinol Metab 82:4111-4116, 1997.

63.   McKenna JM, Freaney R, Meade A, Muldowney FP. Hypovitaminosis D and elevated serum alkaline phosphatase in elderly Irish people. Am J Clin Nutr 41:101-109, 1985.

64.   Dawson-Hughes B, Dallal GE, Krall EA, Harris S, Sokoll LJ, Falconer G. Effect of vitamin D supplementation on wintertime and overall bone loss in healthy postmenopausal women. Ann Int Med 115:505-512, 1991.

65.   Heaney RP. Calcium, bone health, and osteoporosis. In: Bone and Mineral Research, Annual IV, W. A. Peck, ed. Elsevier Science Publishers, Amsterdam, pp. 255-301, 1986.

66.   Krall EA, Sahyoun N, Tannenbaum S, Dallal GE, Dawson-Hughes B. Effect of vitamin D intake on seasonal variations in parathyroid hormone secretion in postmenopausal women. N Engl J Med 321:1777-1783, 1989.

67.   Bischoff--Ferrari HA, Dietrich T, Orav EJ, Dawson-Hughes B. Positive association between 25-hydroxy vitamin D levels and bone mineral density: a population-based study of younger and older adults. Am J Med 116:634-639, 2004.

68.   Lukert B, Higgins J, Stoskopf M. Menopausal bone loss is partially regulated by dietary intake of vitamin D. Calcif Tissue Int 51:173-179, 1992.

69.   Thomas MK, Lloyd-Jones DM, Thadhani RI, Shaw AC, Deraska DJ, Kitch BT, Vamvakas EC, Dick IM, Prince RL, Finkelstein JS. Hypovitaminosis D in medical inpatients. N. Engl. J. Med. 338:777-783, 1998.

70.   Heaney RP, Dowell MS, Hale CA, Bendich A. Calcium absorption varies within the reference range for serum 25-hydroxyvitamin D. J Am Coll Nutr 22(2):142-146, 2003.

71.   Trivedi DP, Doll R, Khaw KT. Effect of four monthly oral vitamin D3 (cholecalciferol) supplementation on fractures and mortality in men and women living in the community: randomised double blind controlled trial. BMJ 326:469-474, 2003.

72.   Lips P, Holick MF, Heaney RP, Meunier PJ, Vieth R, Dawson-Hughes B. Vitamin D Round Table. In: Nutritional Aspects of Osteoporosis, 2nd Edition. Burckhardt P, Dawson-Hughes B, Heaney RP, eds. Elsevier Inc., San Diego, CA (in press 2004).

73.   Slovik DM, Adams JS, Neer RM, Holick MF, Potts JT, Jr., Deficient production of 1,25-dihydroxyvitamin D in elderly osteoporotic patients. N Engl J Med 305:372-374 1981.

74.   Francis RM, Peacock M, Taylor GA, Storer JH, Nordin BEC. Calcium malabsorption in elderly women with vertebral fractures: evidence for resistance to the action of vitamin D metabolites on the bowel. Clin Sci 66:103-107, 1984.

75. Vieth R. Vitamin D supplementation, 25-hydroxyvitamin D concentrations, and safety. Am J Clin Nutr 69:842-856, 1999.

76. Gloth FM III, Tobin JD, Sherman SS, Hollis BW. Is the recommended daily allowance for vitamin D too low for the homebound elderly? J Am Geriatr Soc 39:137-141, 1991.

77. Parfitt AM, Gallagher JC, Heaney RP, Johnston CC Jr, Neer R, Whedon GD. Vitamin D and bone health in the elderly. Am J Clin Nutr 36:1014-1031, 1982.

78. Suter PM, Russell RM. Vitamin requirements of the elderly. Am J Clin Nutr 45:501-512, 1987.

79. Holick MF. Sources of vitamin D: diet and sunlight. In: P. Burckhardt, R. P. Heaney, eds. Nutritional Aspects of Osteoporosis, (Proceedings of 2nd International Symposium on Osteoporosis, Lausanne, May 1994). Challenges in Modern Medicine 7, 289-309, 1995. Ares-Serono Symposia Publications, Rome, Italy.

80. Lips P, Graafmans WC, Ooms ME, Bezemer PD, Bouter LM. Vitamin D supplementation and fracture incidence in elderly persons. Ann Intern Med 124:400-406, 1996.

81. Heaney RP, Davies KM, Chen TC, Holick MF, Barger-Lux MJ. Human serum 25-hydroxy-cholecalciferol response to extended oral dosing with cholecalciferol. Am J Clin Nutr 77:204-210, 2003.

82. Heikinheimo RJ, Inkovaara JA, Harju EJ, Haavisto MV, Kaarela RH, et al. Annual injection of vitamin D and fractures of aged bones. Calcif Tissue Int 51:105-110, 1992.

83. Bischoff-Ferrari HA, Dawson-Hughes B, Willett WC, Staehelin HB, Bazemore MG, Zee RY, Wong JB. Effect of vitamin D on falls. JAMA 291:1999-2006, 2004.

84. Bischoff HA, Dietrich T, Orav EJ, Zhang Y, Karlson EW, Dawson-Hughes B. Higher 25-hydroxyvitamin D levels are associated with better lower extremity function in active and inactive ambulatory elderly in the US. (Abstract #1203) J Bone Miner Res 18(Suppl 2):S52, 2003.

85. Webb AR, Kline L, Holick MF. Influence of season and latitude on the cutaneous synthesis of vitamin D3: Exposure to winter sunlight in Boston and Edmonton will not promote vitamin D3 synthesis in human skin. J Clin Endocrinol Metab 67:373-378, 1988.

86. Barger-Lux MJ, Heaney RP. Effects of above average summer sun exposure on serum 25-hydroxyvitamin D and calcium absorption. J Clin Endocrinol Metab 87(11):4952-4956, 2002.

87. Heaney RP, McCarron DA, Dawson-Hughes B, Oparil S, Berga SL, Stern JS, Barr SI, Rosen CJ. Dietary changes favorably affect bone remodeling in older adults. J Am Diet Assoc 99:1228-1233, 1999.

88. Bonjour JP, Schürch MA, Chevalley T, Ammann P, Rizzoli R. Protein intake, IGF-1 and osteoporosis. Osteoporos Int 7(Suppl 3):S36-S42, 1997.

89. Johnson NE, Alcantara EN, Linkswiler HM. Effect of protein intake on urinary and fecal calcium and calcium retention of young adult males. J Nutr 100:1425-1430, 1970.

90.   Delmi M, Rapin C-H, Bengoa J-M, Delmas PD, Vasey H, Bonjour J-P. Dietary supplementation in elderly patients with fractured neck of the femur. Lancet 335:1013-1016, 1990.

91.   Schürch M-A, Rizzoli R, Slosman D, Vadas L, Vergnaud P, Bonjour J-P. Protein supplements increase serum insulin-like growth factor-I levels and attenuate proximal femur bone loss in patients with recent hip fracture. Ann Intern Med 128:801-809, 1998.

92.   Hannan MT, Tucker KL, Dawson-Hughes B, Cupples LA, Felson DT, Kiel DP. Effect of dietary protein on bone loss in elderly men and women: The Framingham Osteoporosis Study. J Bone Miner Res 15:2504-2512, 2000.

93.   Spencer H, Kramer L, Osis D. Effect of a high protein (meat) intake on calcium metabolism in man. Am J Clin Nutr 31:2167-2180, 1978.

94.   Rafferty K, Davies KM, Heaney RP. Potassium intake and the calcium economy. J Am Coll Nutr (in press) 2004.

95.   Kerstetter JE, O'Brien KO, Insogna KL. Dietary protein affects intestinal calcium absorption. Am J Clin Nutr 68:859-865, 1998.

96.   Heaney RP. Dietary protein and phosphorus do not affect calcium absorption. Am J Clin Nutr 72:758-761, 2000.

97.   Roughead ZK, Johnson LK, Lykken GI, Hunt JR. Controlled high meat diets do not affect calcium retention of bone status in healthy postmenopausal women. J Nutr 133:1020-1026, 2003.

98.   Wengreen HJ, Munger RG, West NA, Cutler DR, Corcoran CD, Zhang J, Sassano NE. Dietary protein intake and risk of osteoporotic hip fracture in elderly residents of Utah. J Bone Miner Res 19(4):537-545, 2004.

99.   Dawson-Hughes B, Harris SS. Calcium intake influences the association of protein intake with rates of bone loss in elderly men and women. Am J Clin Nutr 75:773-779, 2002.

100.   Heaney RP, Nordin BEC. Calcium effects on phosphorus absorption: implications for the prevention and co-therapy of osteoporosis. J Am Coll Nutr 21(3):239-244, 2002.

101.   Spencer H, Kramer L, Osis D, Norris C. Effect of phosphorus on the absorption of calcium and on the calcium balance in man. J Nutr 108:447-457, 1978.

102.   Heaney RP, Recker RR. Determinants of endogenous fecal calcium in healthy women. J Bone Miner Res 9:1621-1627, 1994.

103.   Davis GK, Mertz W. Copper. In: Mertz W, ed. Trace Elements in Human and Animal Nutrition-Fifth Edition, Vol. I. Academic Press, San Diego, CA, 1987; 301-364.

104.   Mertz W (editor). Trace elements in human and animal nutrition, 5th edition, (1987). Academic Press, Inc., San Diego, CA.

105.   Schmidt H, Herwig J, Greinacher I. The skeletal changes in premature infants with copper deficiency. Rofo. Fortschritte aud dem Gebiete der Rontgenstrahlen und der Neuen Bildgebenden Verfahren 155:38-42, 1991.

106.   Buchman AL, Keen CL, Vinters HV, Harris E, Chugani HT, et al, Copper deficiency secondary to a copper transport defect: a new copper metabolic disturbance. Metabolism 43:1462-1469, 1994.

107. Strain JJ. A reassessment of diet and osteoporosis – possible role for copper. Med Hypotheses 27:333-338, 1988.

108. Howard G, Andon M, Bracker M, Saltman P, Strause L. Low serum copper, a risk factor additional to low dietary calcium in postmenopausal bone loss. J Trace Elements Experimental Med 5:23-31, 1992.

109. Herzberg M, Foldes J, Steinberg R, Menczel J. Zinc excretion in osteoporotic women. J Bone Miner Res 5:251-257, 1990.

110. Herzberg M, Lusky A, Blonder J, Frenkel Y. The effect of estrogen replacement on zinc in serum and urine. Obstet Gynecol 87:1035-1040, 1996.

111. Devine A, Rosen C, Mohan S, Baylink DJ, Prince RL. Effects of zinc and other nutritional factors on IGF-1 and IGF binding proteins in postmenopausal women. Am J Clin Nutr 68:200-206, 1998.

112. Schürch M-A, Rizzoli R, Slosman D, Bonjour J-P. Protein supplements increase serum IGF-1 and decrease proximal femur bone loss in patients with a recent hip fracture. In: S. E. Papapoulos, P. Lips, H. A. P. Pols, C. C. Johnston, P. D. Delmas, eds. Osteoporosis 1996, Elsevier Science B.V., Amsterdam, The Netherlands, 1996; 327-329.

113. Elmstahl S, Gullberg B, Janzon L, Johnell O, Elmstahl B. Increased incidence of fractures in middle-aged and elderly men with low intakes of phosphorus and zinc. Osteoporos Int 8:333-340, 1998.

114. New SA, Bolton-Smith C, Grubb DA, Reid DM. Nutritional influences on bone mineral density: a cross-sectional study in premenopausal women. Am J Clin Nutr 65:1831-1839, 1997.

115. Asling CW, Hurley LW. The influence of trace elements on the skeleton. Clin Orthop 27:213-264, 1963.

116. Strause L, Saltman P, Glowacki J. The effect of deficiencies of manganese and copper on osteoinduction and on resorption of bone particles in rats. Calcif Tissue Int 41:145-150, 1987.

117. Strause LG, Hegenauer J, Saltman P, Cone R, Resnick E. Effects of long-term dietary manganese and copper deficiency on rat skeleton. J Nutr 116:135-141, 1986.

118. Reginster JY, Strause LG, Saltman P, Franchimont P. Trace elements and postmenopausal osteoporosis: a preliminary study of decreased serum manganese. Med Sci Res 16:337-338, 1988.

119. Strause L, Saltman P, Smith KT, Bracker M, Andon MB. Spinal bone loss in postmenopausal women supplemented with calcium and trace minerals. J Nutr 124:1060-1064, 1994.

120. Spencer H, Fuller H, Norris C, Williams D Effect of magnesium on the intestinal absorption of calcium in man. J Am College Nutr 1994;13:485-492.

121. Morris RC Jr, Frassetto LA, Schmidlin O, Forman A, Sebastian A. Expression of osteoporosis as determined by diet-disordered electrolyte and acid-base metabolism. In: Nutritional Aspects of Osteoporosis, pp. 357-378. Burckhardt P, Dawson-Hughes B, Heaney RP, eds. Academic Press, New York, 2001.

122.   Buclin T, Cosma M, Appenzeller M, Jacquet AF, Décosterd LA, Biollaz J, Burckhardt P. Diet acids and alkalis influence calcium retention in bone. Osteoporos Int 2001:12:493-499.

123.   Lemann J Jr, Pleuss JA, Gray RW, Hoffmann RG. Potassium administration reduces and potassium deprivation increases urinary calcium excretion in healthy adults. Kidney Int 1991;39:973-983.

124.   Lemann J Jr, Pleuss JA, Gray RW. Potassium causes calcium retention in healthy adults. J Nutr 1993;123:1623-1626.

125.   Sellmeyer DE, Schloetter M, Sebastian A. Potassium citrate prevents increased urine calcium excretion and bone resorption induced by a high sodium chloride diet. J Clin Endocrinol Metab 2002;87:2008-2012.

126.   Sebastian A, Harris ST, Ottaway JH, Todd KM, Morris RC Jr. Improved mineral balance and skeletal metabolism in postmenopausal women treated with potassium bicarbonate. N Engl J Med 1994;330:1776-1781.

127.   New SA, Bolton-Smith C, Grubb DA, Reid DM. Nutritional influences on bone mineral density: a cross-sectional study in premenopausal women. Am J Clin Nutr 1997;65:1831-1839.

128.   New SA, Robins SP, Campbell MK, Martin JC, Garton MJ, Bolton-Smith C, Grubb DA, Lee SJ, Reid DM. Dietary influences on bone mass and bone metabolism: further evidence of a positive link between fruit and vegetable consumption and bone health. Am J Clin Nutr 2000;71:142-151.

129.   New SA. The role of the skeleton in acid-base homeostasis. Proceedings Nutr Society 2002;61:151-164.

130.   New SA. Impact of food clusters on bone. In: Nutritional Aspects of Osteoporosis, pp. 379-397. Burckhardt P, Dawson-Hughes B, Heaney RP, eds. Academic Press, New York, 2001.

131.   Barr SI, J. Prior C, Janelle KC, Lentle BC. Spinal bone mineral density in premenopausal vegetarian and nonvegetarian women: cross-sectional and prospective comparisons. J Am Diet Assoc 1998;98:760-765.

132.   Chiu JF, Lan SJ, Yang CY, Wang PW, Yao WJ, Su IH, Hsieh CC. Long-term vegetarian diet and bone mineral density in postmenopausal Taiwanese women. Calcif Tissue Int 1997;60:245-249.

133.   Lau EMC, Kwok T, Woo J, Ho SC. Bone mineral density in Chinese elderly female vegetarians, vegans, lacto-vegetarians and omnivores. European J Clin Nutr 1998;52:60-64.

134.   Spencer H, Kramer L, Norris C, Osis D. Effect of small doses of aluminum-containing antacids on calcium and phosphorus metabolism. Am J Clin Nutr 36:32-40, 1982.

135.   Krumdieck CL, Prince CW. Mechanisms of homocysteine toxicity on connective tissues: implications for the morbidity of aging. J Nutr 130:365S-368S, 2000.

136.   McLean RR, Jacques PF, Selhub J, Tucker KL, Samelson EJ, Broe KE, Hannan MT, Cupples LA, Kiel DP. Homocysteine as a predictive factor for hip fracture in older persons. N Engl J Med 350:2042-2049, 2004.

137. Price PA. Role of vitamin-K-dependent proteins in bone metabolism. Ann Rev Nutr 8:565-583, 1988.

138. Szulc P, Delmas PD. Is there a role for vitamin K deficiency in osteoporosis? In: Burckhardt P, Heaney RP, eds. Challenges of Modern Medicine, Nutritional Aspects of Osteoporosis, (Proceedings of 2nd International Symposium on Osteoporosis, Lausanne, May 1994). Ares-Serono Publications, Rome, Italy, 1995;7:357-366.

139. Booth SL, Broe KE, Gagnon DR, Tucker KL, Hannan MT, McLean RR, Dawson-Hughes B, Wilson PWF, Cupples LA, Kiel DP. Vitamin K intake and bone mineral density in women and men. Am J Clin Nutr 77:512-516, 2003.

140. Feskanich D, Weber P, Willett WC, Rockett H, Booth SL, Colditz GA. Vitamin K intake and hip fractures in women: a prospective study. Am J Clin Nutr 69:74-79, 1999.

141. Hodges SJ, Pilkington MJ, Stamp TCB, et al. Depressed levels of circulating menaquinones in patients with osteoporotic fractures of the spine and femoral neck. Bone 12:387-389, 1991.

142. Binkley NC, Krueger DC, Kawahara TN, Engelke JA, Chappell RJ, Suttie JW. A high phylloquinone intake is required to achieve maximal osteocalcin γ-carboxylation. Am J Clin Nutr 76:1055-1060, 2002.

143. Knapen MHJ, Hamulyak K, Vermeer C. The effect of vitamin K supplementation on circulating osteocalcin (bone gla protein) and urinary calcium excretion. Annals Int Med 111:1001-1005, 1989.

144. Munday K. Vitamin C and bone markers: investigations in a Gambian population. Proc Nutr Soc 62(2):429-436, 2003.

145. Bates CJ, Tsuchiya H. Comparison of vitamin C deficiency with food restriction on collagen cross-link ratios in bone, urine and skin of weanling guinea-pigs. Br J Nutr 89(3):303-310, 2003.

146. Kaptoge S, Welch A, McTaggart A, Mulligan A, Dalzell N, Day NE, Bingham S, Khaw KT, Reeve J. Effects of dietary nutrients and food groups on bone loss from the proximal femur in men and women in the 7th and 8th decades of age. Osteoporos Int 14(5):418-428, 2003.

147. Simon JA, Hudes ES. Relation of ascorbic acid to bone mineral density and self-reported fractures among US adults. Am J Epidemiol 154(5):427-433, 2001.

148. Morton DJ, Barrett-Connor EL, Schneider DL. Vitamin C supplement use and bone mineral density in postmenopausal women. J Bone Miner Res 16(1):135-140, 2001.

CHAPTER 5

BONE ADAPTATION TO MECHANICAL LOADING: HOW DOES BONE SENSE THE NEED FOR CHANGE TO LOADING FROM EXERCISE?

K. Shawn Davison, C. J. R. Blimkie , R. A. Faulkner, L. Giangregorio

Depts. of Medicine, McMaster University and University of Laval
212-9th S,t E Saskatoon, SK, Canada S7N 0A4
Phone: 306.652.1734 Fax: 306.652.1768

The strength of a bone is directly related to its ability to resist fracture in a given loading environment. Bone strength is dependent on a number of factors that can be grouped broadly into three categories: material properties (i.e. mean levels of mineralization, organic properties), bone architecture (i.e. cortical thickness, distribution, porosity; trabecular thickness, connectivity, perforations) and bone mass (i.e. more massive bone is stronger).

Wolff's Law and the Mechanostat

Julius Wolff conceptualized the theory that bone mass and architecture can be remodeled to maintain a certain homeostatic load per unit area, so that changes in the function of a bone will be followed by proportional changes in bone mass and area (1). Frost expanded these concepts, suggesting that mechanisms exist in bone where typical mechanical usage is monitored and the mass and structure of bone are adapted to meet mechanical needs. Bone modeling/remodeling can be turned "on" or "off" depending on the level of mechanical strain the "mechanostat" detects (2). According to the mechanostat theory, mechanical loading-driven bone modeling and remodeling will adapt bone strength, in the form of bone mass and architecture, to keep the level of strain on bone within an operational range. The physiological loading zone, suggested to be at or below 1000 microstrain, but above 50-100 microstrain (3), is where the amounts of bone resorbed and subsequently formed are relatively balanced. Bone mass and strength will be increased via modeling if the peak strains on bone exceed the upper threshold, called a modeling threshold. When the typical level of strain is consistently below the lower (remodeling) threshold, the amount of loading is not producing strains sufficient to maintain bone in its current state. Disuse-mode remodeling is enhanced below the remodeling threshold and bone tissue is lost until a new, lower bone strength equilibrium is established. Increased mechanical usage above the modeling threshold and in the area of 3000 microstrain is proposed to result in the accumulation of microdamage, which can reduce the overall strength of the bone (for more information on the mechanostat theory, please see the chapter by Harold Frost in this book).

Characteristics of an Osteogenic Strain Stimulus

Animal studies have shown that mechanical loading can increase bone mass (4-7). The nature of the mechanical strain stimulus capable of driving bone adaptation has been explored in recent years, and has been the subject of several reviews (8-11). Early research emphasized the importance of the magnitude of imposed strain; using an isolated avian model, Rubin and Lanyon demonstrated a graded, dose-response relationship between the magnitude of the peak strain within bone tissue and the change in bone mass (12). More recent research (13;14) has also pointed to loading frequency as a critical factor mediating the skeletal adaptive response. Loading frequency and strain rate have been implicated as important determinants of bone adaptation, and like strain magnitude, also appear to have a direct influence on the bone formation response (15;16). As well, dynamic loading conditions, far more so than static loading, appear to elicit greater bone adaptation (7).

A dynamic mechanical loading stimulus of sufficient magnitude need only be applied for a short period of time to be osteogenic. Rubin and Lanyon demonstrated that as little as 36 loading cycles per day was sufficient to stimulate increased bone mineral content in avian ulnae, and that bones subjected to 360 or 1800 loading cycles per day under the same strain magnitude did not result in greater increases in the amount of bone formed (7). Recent research by Robling and collegues (17) suggests that bone can become desensitized to loading fairly quickly, but that its mechanosensitivity may be recovered several hours later, so only a short duration of loading is required for a stimulus to be osteogenic. Recovery between loading sessions and/or between loading cycles can improve the bone adaptive response to mechanical loading by allowing for recovery of mechanosensation (9). Furthermore, bone cells may become less responsive to routine signals; therefore, bone adaptation may be governed by bone strains that are unusual (18). Mathematical formulae incorporating available data on the nature of osteogenic mechanical stimuli have been proposed that predict bone adaptation to mechanical loading (18). In practical terms, when designing exercise programs for bone health, it is important to consider the frequency and timing of exercise bouts, the adequacy of strain rates and magnitudes, and the novelty of the exercise conditions to optimize skeletal adaptation. These considerations are based, however, mostly on findings from animal studies, and need to be verified in humans at different stages of the life cycle.

Muscle-Bone Interactions

The Utah Paradigm, proposed by Harold Frost, highlights the importance of muscle contractions in providing the largest loading stimulus for bone adaptation (2;19;20). It is proposed that muscle and bone form a unit, whereby changes in muscle strength will have a corresponding effect on bone strength (21). Comparisons of bone strength among different types of activity provide support for this theory; for example, long distance runners typically have smaller, weaker muscles than weight lifters, and correspondingly have less bone mass and bone strength than weight lifters (3). During growth, muscles increase in size and strength; bone modeling should therefore modify bone mass and size to meet the need for more bone strength. Exercise would further increase the applied loads to bone during this period of active modeling, allowing for further increases in bone mass and size (3). In a recent investigation by Rauch et al. (22), the peak velocity of lean mass accrual during growth (surrogate of muscle mass) preceded the peak velocity in bone mass by an average of 0.51 years in girls and by 0.36 in boys, demonstrating the importance of muscle development on bone mass. In young adulthood, muscle and bone strength plateau at a levels corresponding with the level of mechanical loading. Therefore, modeling ceases and conservation-mode bone remodeling ensues. The ability of exercise to increase bone mass and strength when modeling is no longer active is subsequently reduced. Further, as adults age, muscle mass and strength decrease and the level of muscle induced strain on bone is reduced, resulting in slow bone loss (3). As muscles become weaker, the ability of exercise to initiate modeling is diminished. This may explain why many exercise interventions in older adults often prevent bone loss, but usually result in only small gains, if any, in bone mass (23-25).

Schoenau and colleagues have demonstrated that a linear relationship exists between muscle CSA and BMC at the radial diaphysis in healthy children and adolescents, and suggest that deviations from this established "normal" bone-muscle relationship may be used as a diagnostic criterion for bone disease (26). A functional relationship between mechanical forces and bone development is supported by both clinical observations and studies of athletes. Clinical observations of individuals with disease processes that interfere with muscle development (i.e. muscle dystrophy, spina bifida) invariably demonstrate a negative effect on bone development (27;28). Side-to-side differences in muscle area attributed to tennis-playing in growing children and adolescents were associated with corresponding differences in bone mass, size and strength (29). Heinonen and collegues (30) also demonstrated significant correlations between tibial muscle cross-sectional area and cortical bone area in pre- and early pubertal girls. However, when the cortical cross-section was divided into three compartments, only the bone area lateral cortices (those under the highest muscle-generated strain) remained significantly correlated with muscle area, suggesting a localized effect of muscle on bone structure.

The hypothesis that exercise-related muscle adaptations result in corresponding adaptations in bone has been criticized, in that it does not consider other factors that may account for bone adaptation, such as genetics, hormones and nutrition (29). Mutations of the myostatin (suppresses muscle growth) gene produce mice with muscle mass that is three times that of control mice, yet there is no demonstrable difference in femoral shaft size or shape (31). In this example, genetics rather than the force producing capacity of the muscle appeared to regulate bone development. It is important to note that although the myostatin-null mice had more muscle mass, the amount of activity the mice engaged in was likely comparable to that of wild type mice. The larger muscles may not have a beneficial effect on bone if they are not required to produce greater forces. Additional research using the myostatin-null mouse model confirmed that the skeletal effects of increased muscle in these mice were limited to muscle attachment sites (i.e. femoral trochanter or deltoid crest), and were more likely to be manifested as site-specific increases in bone area rather than changes in BMD or mid-shaft bone strength (32).

Direct evidence supporting the link between increases in muscle mass and/or strength and corresponding bone adaptation as a result of exercise in humans is lacking. Side-to-side differences in muscle area associated with tennis playing during growth explained only 12-16% of the variance in the side-to-side differences in BMC, bone area, cortical area and polar moment of inertia (29). Muscle strength gains achieved during exercise interventions are not always accompanied by increases in bone mass (33). Future research in this area should aim to clarify the importance of muscle mass and/or strength in the growth and maintenance of skeletal mass and strength. As well, it remains to be determined if increasing or maintaining muscle mass and strength throughout the lifespan will have a meaningful impact on skeletal health and fracture risk.

Bone Adaptation: Mechanisms

The way in which bone cells detect mechanical signals and convert them into a bone adaptive response is still unclear, and has been the subject of several reviews (8;11;18). The network of lacunae and canaliculi in bone, containing osteocytes and matrix, has been proposed as the structure responsible for the sensation and transduction of mechanical signals (8). Osteocytes have been pinpointed as the primary mechanosensory cells in bone because they are ideally situated throughout the lacuno-canalicular network and have been demonstrated to be responsive to mechanical signals. Osteocytes maintain contact with cells on the bone surface and neighbouring osteocytes via gap junctions, and they respond to mechanical loading with increased metabolism, gene activation and the production of growth factors and matrix (8;11). Osteocytes deprived of mechanical loading became hypoxic after 24 hours of disuse, indicating that mechanical loading may be essential to sustain nutrient supply, waste removal and cell population viability (34). A brief (< 4 minutes) loading protocol prevented osteocyte hypoxia from occurring. Osteocyte apoptosis and/or the removal of osteoclast-inhibiting signals as a result of understimulation of osteocytes have been proposed as mechanisms for the recruitment of osteoclasts to resorb bone tissue (8).

Although bone strain can directly activate bone cells, it has been suggested that mechanical strain on bones indirectly activates bone cells via fluid flow through the canalicular spaces (18). Mechanical loading of bone causes movement of extracellular fluid through the network of lacunae and canaliculi, which can stimulate bone cells via the creation of streaming potentials and/or the generation of shear stress on the osteocyte cell membrane (8;11). The production of signaling intermediaries important in the response of bone to loading has been demonstrated to be shear stress-dependent (35). Mathematical modeling of these cellular mechanisms revealed that neither a fluid shear stress model nor a stress-generating electrical potential model could predict the impact of variation in frequency of loading on the osteogenic response (14). Loading frequency modulates the proportional relationship between mechanical strain and bone formation, such that formation is increased at higher frequencies. However, a third model suggested that fluid shear stress is osteogenic, but the mechanosensitivity of bone cells depends on interactions between fluid forces and the viscoelasticity of the cell and/or matrix (14).

The transformation of a mechanical signal to a biochemical signal is most likely the result of multiple signal transduction pathways, activated at the level of the bone cell membrane or cytoskeleton (36). Shear-stress activation of a G-protein-linked mechanoreceptor causes increased levels of intracellular calcium, prostaglandins and nitric oxide. As well, fluid flow may induce cytoskeletal reorganization in bone cells, which may affect gene expression via a direct linkage between the actin cytoskeleton and the bone cell nucleus (18). Nitric oxide and prostaglandins (i.e. prostacylcin and prostaglandin E_2) have been implicated as signaling intermediaries in the transduction of mechanical strain into osteoblast proliferation and differentiation, and increased bone formation (36). The activation of these signal transduction pathways ultimately leads to changes in bone formation that aim to alter bone structure to meet the mechanical demands placed on it.

Physical Activity and Bone

Immobilization

The importance of regular loading for the maintenance of skeletal integrity is most dramatically revealed in situations of extreme disuse. Reductions in weight-bearing, such as bed rest, spinal cord injury, and space travel all generate a skeletal adaptive response, resulting in the loss of bone mineral (37). Similar to exercise effects on bone, the skeletal response to immobilization or reduced loading is site-specific. For example, following 17 weeks of bed rest in healthy humans, significant losses of bone mineral were noted at weight-bearing sites, with no significant changes in the upper limbs and an increase in bone mineral at the skull (38). Increases in BMD in the skull and decreases in weight-bearing bones have also been reported after reduced activity due to hip fracture (39).

When comparing models of reduced loading, the degree to which bone mineral is lost appears to be related to the magnitude of the relative reduction in loading (37). After a spinal cord injury, the amount of bone lost has been associated with the degree of post-trauma immobilization and the duration post-injury (40). Individuals with incomplete lesions tend to lose less bone than those with complete lesions, and early mobilization after the injury may reduce bone loss (41;42). As well, re-establishing regular weight bearing may not result in a complete restoration of lost bone mass (43).

What Types of Exercises are Osteogenic?

Cross-sectional studies suggest that activities involving high forces, such as strength and power training, or high-impacts, such as basketball, racquet sports or gymnastics result in higher bone densities (2;44-47). Studies of retired gymnasts demonstrate that areal BMD at several sites, excluding the skull, are 0.7-1.4 standard deviations greater than controls, suggesting that gymnastics training during growth results in bone adaptations that result in a sufficient bone mineral surfeit to have a favorable impact on fracture risk (48). The influence of moderate-impact exercise, such as running or walking, on skeletal health, is less clear. A recent meta-analysis suggested that moderate-impact exercise interventions are sufficient to prevent bone loss and/or result in small bone gains (24). However, when comparing competitive female athletes, runners had significantly lower BMD at the whole body, lumbar spine and femoral neck than gymnasts and controls, despite a similar prevalence of menstrual dysfunction between the athlete groups (46). It is possible that the high impact loading experienced in gymnastics counteracted the detrimental effects of high training volumes in competitive gymnasts, but in runners, the nature (low impact) and or magnitude of loading strains were not sufficient to prevent bone loss at high training volumes. In adolescent males, badminton players had significantly higher BMDs at weight-bearing sites than hockey players, despite a lower average training volume (49). This reinforces the importance of higher impact loads in unusual directions as an important condition for augmenting bone at weight-bearing sites.

Effects of Physical Activity During Growth

The transition between childhood and adolescence is a crucial period for bone mineral accrual. It has been estimated that 26% of adult bone mineral is accrued during the two years around peak bone mineral content velocity (PBMCV), which corresponds with ages 11.5 to 13.5 for girls and 13.1 to 15.1 for boys (50). Cross-sectional studies support an association between physical activity during growth and increased bone mass, and these findings have been summarized previously (23;51-53).

A longitudinal study of six years duration demonstrated that bone mineral accumulation and peak bone mineral accrual rate were significantly greater in highly active children than in their inactive counterparts during the two years around PBMCV (50). Active boys and girls had total body bone mineral content values that were 9% and 17% greater, respectively, than those of inactive boys and girls.

The possibility of an optimal time to augment bone mineral accrual via exercise is an appealing concept for researchers and clinicians, particularly if the gains are maintained beyond childhood , even if activity levels decrease during adulthood. Regular exercise may have a greater osteogenic potential if initiated before puberty or in early puberty, due to possible synergistic effects with high levels of bone mineral accretion during that time. Cross-sectional data comparing the femoral shaft bone mineral content and cortical area in the playing and non-playing arms in female racquet sport players support the concept that exercise has a greater impact on the skeleton during growth, in that side-to-side differences were substantially greater in players who had begun their training before menarche (54;55). Similarly, activity-related bone gain in junior tennis players was heightened during the period of rapid growth just before menarche (56). A three-year longitudinal study demonstrated that gymnasts had higher bone mass throughout puberty when compared to controls, and the differences in the majority of bone variables were most apparent during the adolescent growth spurt (57). Another longitudinal study revealed that the increase in total body, spine and leg areal BMD (g/cm^2 per year) over one year was 30-85% greater in prepubertal gymnasts than in bone-age matched controls (48). Greater rates of bone mineral accrual were also noted in a three-year prospective study of adolescent gymnasts approaching puberty (58).

To address the question of whether a "window of opportunity" for bone response exists, MacKelvie et al. (59) conducted a systematic review of exercise intervention studies conducted in children and adolescents, separating the studies according to maturational age of the participants (prepubertal, early pubertal and post-pubertal). Support for the ability of intensive, aggressive exercise programs to engender a bone response in the **prepubertal** skeleton was provided by two studies, such that the difference in eight month bone mineral gain was 1.2% to 5.6%

depending on the skeletal site. Similar increases were noted more recently in Asian and white prepubertal boys (59). A less intense exercise program cited in the systematic review demonstrated a significant bone response in favour of the intervention only at the femoral trochanter (60).

In **early pubertal** girls (all premenarchal), the implementation of an extra-curricular exercise program resulted in significantly greater gains in bone mineral at the total body, lumbar spine and proximal femur in the intervention group than in controls (61). MacKelvie and collegues (62) conducted a seven-month study of jumping exercise in both prepubertal and early pubertal girls, and found that early pubertal girls experienced greater bone changes at the femoral neck and lumbar spine, as well as greater changes in femoral neck cross-sectional area and reduced endosteal expansion when compared to controls matched for maturity. In prepubertal girls, however, the bone changes observed did not differ between the intervention group and controls. After participating in the same exercise intervention for an additional 13 months, early pubertal and peri-pubertal girls experienced a 2% greater bone mineral accrual at two bone sites each year, for an overall bone benefit of 5% when compared to controls (63). A more recent study of exercise and calcium supplementation in pre-pubertal and early pubertal girls demonstrated increased bone mass at the femur and tibia-fibula, and a calcium-exercise interaction was reported at the femur (64).

In **postmenarcheal** girls, two studies reported in the systematic review failed to provide support for the ability of exercise to increase bone mass (59). Similarly, an intense jumping program performed twice per week for 9 months resulted in 3-4% higher BMC changes in premenarcheal girls when compared to controls, but the increase in BMC in postmenarcheal girls after the intervention was not significantly different from controls (65). Taken together, the results of the systematic review and more recent studies suggest that vigorous exercise can enhance bone adaptation in children if initiated before menarche. It remains to be determined if exercise-induced bone adaptation is greater during the prepubertal or early pubertal years. As well, the majority of studies are conducted in females. Whether similar conclusions can be inferred about males is uncertain given the differing endocrine changes between sexes during the transition from childhood to adulthood.

An important consideration is whether or not exercise-induced bone adaptations achieved during growth can be maintained into adulthood, especially if activity levels decrease. Several retrospective cross-sectional studies suggest that at least some of the bone mass gained as a result of exercise during growth is maintained; however, these studies may be limited by selection bias and other confounding factors (55;66). Longitudinal investigations are now starting to report that the gains made in childhood and adolescence bone typically result in greater amounts of bone during early adulthood (67). There are few prospective studies evaluating whether exercise-related bone adaptations can be maintained. Seven months of jumping exercise in prepubertal children produced 4.5% and 3.1% greater BMC gains at the femoral neck and lumbar spine, respectively, in the exercise group than in controls, but 7 months after training these earlier gains had regressed; a BMC gain of 4% was maintained at the femoral neck, but differences did not persist at the lumbar spine (68). A prospective 5-year follow up study of female racquet-sport players demonstrated that even with a reduction in training, there was maintenance of exercise-related bone gain independent of starting age of training (69). Intercollegiate gymnasts (mean age of 18.6 years) experienced increases in bone density at the lumbar spine, hip and proximal femur during competitive training seasons that were followed by declines in bone density during the "off seasons", but over a period of 24 months, significant overall increases of 2% and 4.3% were noted at the whole body and lumbar spine, respectively (70). However, a six-year longitudinal study of adolescent ice-hockey players demonstrated bone loss at the femoral neck in individuals who ceased regular training, and gains in bone mass in those that continued training (71). Additional research is required to ascertain whether exercise-induced bone adaptations achieved during growth can be maintained in adulthood if activity levels are not maintained.

Effects of Physical Activity in Adults

The ability of exercise to increase mechanical strain and subsequently enhance bone mineral apposition in adult humans has been explored and debated in recent years. An often-cited study is that of Jones et al. (72), where the humerus of the dominant arm in adult tennis players, had a greater cortical thickness than the non-dominant arm. Cross-sectional studies of athletes have demonstrated that physical activity has a positive impact on bone mass. (73-75). Although athletic studies provide promising evidence that physical activity confers an osteogenic benefit, selection bias may contribute to apparent differences in bone mass between athletic and non-athletic populations.

Both cross-sectional and longitudinal studies point toward a positive effect of progressive resistance training on bone mineral density in adults, and that the effects are specific to the bone sites associated with the active musculature (45). Meta-analyses of the skeletal effects of exercise in pre- and post-menopausal women reveal that although exercise has a positive effect on the skeleton, it is generally manifested in a prevention of bone loss rather than bone gain (24;76;77). Strenuous aerobic exercise in post-menopausal women had overall beneficial treatment effects at the lumbar spine and femoral neck of 0.96% and 0.90% per year, respectively (76). Both impact exercises (walking, running, aerobics) and non-impact (resistance or strength training, weightlifting) exercises had a positive impact on bone in **post-menopausal** women at the lumbar spine and femoral neck, and in **pre-menopausal** women at the lumbar spine. Effects of exercise on bone mass at the femoral neck in pre-menopausal women were not significant for impact exercise, and there was insufficient data for meta-analysis of the effects of non-impact exercise (24). Randomized controlled trials of exercise training demonstrated an overall prevention or reversal of bone loss of 1% per year in exercisers compared to controls. Overall treatment effects in non-randomized trials were almost twice as high, indicating that non-random allocation of subjects introduces confounding factors resulting in an overestimation of the effects of exercise on bone (76). The changes observed in bone mass with exercise in **men** is similar to that seen in women (78;79).

The large variability across studies with respect to the type of exercises employed, the duration and intensity of exercise protocols, participant compliance and drop out rates, and differences in measurement techniques make summarizing the effects of exercise on bone via meta- analysis difficult. In one meta-analysis, studies that demonstrated the largest bone gains at the lumbar spine and femoral neck were also those with the best compliance and highest intensity activities (80;81). Based on the existing data, it appears that mechanical loading through exercise has its greatest potential to affect bone mass in the growing skeleton compared to the mature skeleton. In adults, exercise can prevent age-related bone loss, but may not increase bone mass to a great extent, if at all (82).

Changes in Bone Size and Shape

Many studies have investigated the ability of exercise to improve bone mass at various skeletal sites, but bone structure is also an important component of bone strength. Physical activity may have an impact on bone structure that is not revealed by simply measuring BMD with densitometry. Mechanical loading may augment the changes in bone structure that occur during growth, but the effects may depend on the timing of exposure, the location (proximal, central or distal) along the limb, the bone surface (periosteal or endosteal), or the type of loading conditions (torsion, bending or axial compression) (73;83). Prepubertal tennis players had a 7-11% greater cortical area in the loaded arm compared to the unloaded arm, and the adaptations varied according to site; at the distal humerus, differences were due to greater periosteal expansion alone, at the mid-humerus they were a result of a greater periosteal than medullary expansion. In female racquet sport players, side-to-side differences in humeral shaft bone structure were manifested as a periosteal expansion of the cortex, but at the distal radius, the same adaptation was not as evident, and differences in trabecular density were more prominent (55). It has been suggested that sites that experience axial compressive loading, such as the ends of long bones, are more likely to adapt with increases in bone density, while sites that are subjected to bending loads, such as the shafts of long bones, adapt by increasing in size (73).

The importance of timing of exposure and site-specificity with respect to exercise-related changes in bone structure was demonstrated after a jumping intervention in young girls (84). Significant increases in areal BMD, bone cross-sectional area, cortical thickness and section modulus (a surrogate for bending strength) occurred at the femoral neck in early pubertal girls, but at the intertrochanteric region, the increases were noted only in areal BMD. Similar adaptations were not observed at any site in prepubertal girls, and no exercise-related adaptations were apparent at the femoral shaft in either group (84). An 8-month exercise intervention in prepubertal boys (consisting of a variety of weight-bearing activities) increased femoral midshaft BMD as a result of increased endosteal apposition, and therefore increased cortical thickness; however, the section modulus was not significantly increased (85).

Similar trends with respect to changes in bone size and shape in response to exercise have been observed in adults. Exercise-related gains in mechanical competence without corresponding improvement in bone mass have been demonstrated experimentally in both mature animals and adult humans (86;87). Cast immobilization in adults caused a reduction in bone mass and area at the radius, with no change in BMD (88). Site-specificity with respect to exercise-induced changes in bone structure also has been reported in a cross-sectional study of weight lifters (73). Declining BMD is a common consequence of aging, however, compensatory changes in bone structure have been demonstrated to occur which may maintain bending strength. A longitudinal study of 4187 elderly women demonstrated that bone loss at the femoral neck was accompanied by small increases in an index of bending strength (section modulus) (33). Women who had lost weight over a 3.5-year period experienced significant reductions in both BMD and section modulus. Little change in BMD and small increases in section modulus were observed in women who had gained weight, demonstrating that the adaptive response to altered mechanical loading may be better represented by indices of bone geometry (33).

It is difficult to describe the effects of physical activity on bone structure given the tremendous variability that exists among bone sites, surfaces and regions, among loading types and intensities, and among age and/or maturity level of study participants, since these factors may determine whether or not exercise-related changes in bone structure will occur. Exercise interventions may have an impact on bone structure that are independent of bone mass changes. If so, it may be necessary to re-evaluate the tools used to assess the strength of the skeleton. As well, future research should delineate the factors that have the greatest potential for modifying the mass and structure of bone for the reduction of fracture risk in later years.

Factors that May Influence the Skeletal Response to Exercise

Calcium

Calcium supplementation studies have reported greater gains in bone during growth, prevention of bone loss with aging, and even reduction in fracture risk in the elderly (89). Calcium intake may also modulate the osteogenic potential of exercise. Evidence from several studies(90-92) supports the concept that during childhood and/or adolescence a threshold intake of calcium optimizes the effect of physical activity on adult bone status (90-92). Greater gains in bone mass at the femur, but not the tibia-fibula, were achieved with moderate exercise and additional calcium (~ 440 mg/d to a diet containing ~ 700 mg/d) in prepubescent girls; at the latter site, there was a significant effect of exercise only (64). Adequate calcium intake and regular physical activity are required for optimizing the genetic potential for skeletal health; however, physical activity is quantitatively a more important factor in affecting bone than calcium intake (93). Calcium has a permissive effect on bone mineral accrual and maintenance, while physical activity has a modifying effect.

Evidence for a calcium/exercise interaction in adults is conflicting. Some studies in adults support a threshold effect of calcium intake, and others report no evidence of an interaction (94;95). In adult young women, exercise, but not calcium intake, resulted in a significant bone adaptation (96). A review of available studies from 1995 revealed that calcium and exercise might not act independently on bone; for example, a positive effect of physical activity was apparent only when calcium intake was greater than 1000 mg/day, and the benefits of high calcium intakes were only evident in the presence of physical activity (97). There appears to be a threshold of calcium intake, suggested to be over 1000mg per day, which may optimize the effects of mechanical loading on bone in adults. The bulk of existing evidence supports the theory that calcium intake interacts (at a not yet well-defined level) with physical activity to affect bone mineral accrual in children and adolescence, bone only supports maintenance in adults, and a reduction in the rate of bone loss in the elderly.

Estrogen

In vivo and in vitro studies have revealed that the bone cell response to mechanical strain requires the activity of the estrogen receptor (ER-α) (98). It has been suggested that the ER- α receptor plays a key role in the relationship between mechanical strain and bone adaptation, and that decreased ER- α activity in postmenopausal women results in a reduction in the responsiveness of bone cells to mechanical strain, which ultimately leads to bone loss (98;99). In mice lacking functional ER- α, the response to strain was reduced three-fold compared to mice with normal ER- α function, but it was not completely obliterated, suggesting that bone cells can respond to strain using pathways independent of ER- α (98;99).

Several studies have evaluated whether estrogen and exercise in combination are more beneficial to the skeleton than either alone. The results have been inconsistent: some studies demonstrate that hormone replacement therapy and exercise training have a synergistic effect on skeletal health (100;101), while others do not (102;103). A recent review suggested that the beneficial effects of estrogen supplementation and exercise in postmenopausal women may be additive (104). Since adequate calcium intake may be essential to maximize the impact of exercise on the skeleton, it may be necessary to ensure adequate calcium intake in studies investigating the effects of estrogen and exercise in combination. For example, significant increases in bone mineral density at several sites were observed in women who received supplemental calcium and participated in weight-bearing aerobic exercise combined with resistance training, compared to those who used calcium but did not exercise. When women were stratified according to HRT use, the response to exercise was significant at more sites in those who used HRT than those who did not, suggesting that the combination of HRT and exercise had an additive effect (105).

Estrogen Alternatives

The Women's Health Initiative revealed that the benefits of hormone replacement therapy may not outweigh the risks (106). Therefore, alternative therapies for reducing fracture risk, either alone or in combination with exercise are needed. Bisphosphonates, selective estrogen receptor modulators and phytoestrogens are examples of therapies that can improve bone mass. A limited number of animal and/or human trials have investigated whether these therapies in combination with exercise have additive beneficial effects on bone. Although animal studies indicate that the combination of exercise and estrogen alternatives can benefit the skeleton, human studies demonstrate mixed results (104;107;108). Future research should clarify whether exercise and pharmacological intervention can have synergistic effects on bone.

Summary

Bone is intimately related to its loading environment: strains that are too low will cause bone loss, strains that are typical will preserve or maintain bone strength, strains that are higher than those usually encountered will cause increases in bone strength, and strains that are too high will cause accumulations in microdamage and pathologic changes in bone. Not only are the higher magnitude strains important, but a high loading cycle frequency is also important to elicit an osteogenic response. The number of loading cycles required to elicit an adaptive response is surprisingly small. With the realization of the importance of muscular loading on bone there is beginning to be a better understanding of the changes in bone strength with maturation and aging. The transformation of a mechanical signal to a biochemical signal is most likely the result of multiple signal transduction pathways, activated at the level of the bone cell membrane or cytoskeleton and the activation of these signal transduction pathways ultimately leads to changes in bone formation that aim to alter bone structure to meet the mechanical demands placed on it. Immobilization leads to dramatic losses in bone mass. Higher impact loads in unusual directions are an important condition for augmenting bone at weight-bearing sites. Childhood and adolescence are a critical time for bone accrual and at this time the skeleton is especially sensitive to mechanical stimuli. Exercise has its greatest benefit is started before or during puberty. A small number of investigations have concluded that the gains in bone mass made during childhood and adolescence are likely maintained somewhat into adulthood; however, it is clear that if physical activity levels are significantly decreased, there will be a corresponding decrease in bone mass. In adults, exercise is primarily a strategy to maintain bone mass and to maintain muscle strength to both apply higher loads on bone, and perhaps more importantly, to decrease the risk of falling. Certainly adequate calcium is required in all stages of life to allow for optimal changes in bone strength. The synergy between exercise and the new generations of anti-fracture drugs needs to be better investigated.

REFERENCES

1. Wolff J. Das gesetz der transformation der knochen. Kirschwald 1892.
2. Frost HM. Bone "mass" and the "mechanostat": a proposal. Anat Rec 1987; 219(1):1-9.
3. Frost HM. Why do marathon runners have less bone than weight lifters? A vital-biomechanical view and explanation. Bone 1997; 20(3):183-189.
4. Bourrin S, Palle S, Pupier R, Vico L, Alexandre C. Effect of physical training on bone adaptation in three zones of the rat tibia. J Bone Miner Res 1995; 10(11):1745-1752.
5. Goodship AE, Lanyon LE, McFie H. Functional adaptation of bone to increased stress. An experimental study. J Bone Joint Surg Am 1979; 61(4):539-546.

6.   Meade JB, Cowin SC, Klawitter JJ, Van Buskirk WC, Skinner HB. Bone remodeling due to continuously applied loads. Calcif Tissue Int 1984; 36 Suppl 1:S25-S30.

7.   Rubin CT, Lanyon LE. Kappa Delta Award paper. Osteoregulatory nature of mechanical stimuli: function as a determinant for adaptive remodeling in bone. J Orthop Res 1987; 5(2):300-310.

8.   Burger EH, Klein-Nulend J. Mechanotransduction in bone--role of the lacuno-canalicular network. FASEB J 1999; 13 Suppl:S101-S112.

9.   Burr DB, Robling AG, Turner CH. Effects of biomechanical stress on bones in animals. Bone 2002; 30(5):781-786.

10. Duncan RL, Turner CH. Mechanotransduction and the functional response of bone to mechanical strain. Calcif Tissue Int 1995; 57(5):344-358.

11. Ehrlich PJ, Noble BS, Jessop HL, Stevens HY, Mosley JR, Lanyon LE. The effect of in vivo mechanical loading on estrogen receptor alpha expression in rat ulnar osteocytes. J Bone Miner Res 2002; 17(9):1646-1655.

12. Rubin CT, Lanyon LE. Regulation of bone mass by mechanical strain magnitude. Calcif Tissue Int 1985; 37(4):411-417.

13. LaMothe JM, Zernicke RF. Rest insertion combined with high-frequency loading enhances osteogenesis. J Appl Physiol 2004; 96(5):1788-1793.

14. Hsieh YF, Turner CH. Effects of loading frequency on mechanically induced bone formation. J Bone Miner Res 2001; 16(5):918-924.

15. Turner CH, Forwood MR, Otter MW. Mechanotransduction in bone: do bone cells act as sensors of fluid flow? FASEB J 1994; 8(11):875-878.

16. Turner CH, Owan I, Takano Y. Mechanotransduction in bone: role of strain rate. Am J Physiol 1995; 269(3 Pt 1):E438-E442.

17. Robling AG, Hinant FM, Burr DB, Turner CH. Shorter, more frequent mechanical loading sessions enhance bone mass. Med Sci Sports Exerc 2002; 34(2):196-202.

18. Turner CH, Pavalko FM. Mechanotransduction and functional response of the skeleton to physical stress: the mechanisms and mechanics of bone adaptation. J Orthop Sci 1998; 3(6):346-355.

19. Frost HM. Why do bone strength and "mass" in aging adults become unresponsive to vigorous exercise? Insights of the Utah paradigm. J Bone Miner Metab 1999; 17(2):90-97.

20. Frost HM, Ferretti JL, Jee WS. Perspectives: some roles of mechanical usage, muscle strength, and the mechanostat in skeletal physiology, disease, and research. Calcif Tissue Int 1998; 62(1):1-7.

21. Schoenau E, Frost HM. The "muscle-bone unit" in children and adolescents. Calcif Tissue Int 2002; 70(5):405-407.

22. Rauch F, Bailey DA, Baxter-Jones A, Mirwald R, Faulkner R. The 'muscle-bone unit' during the pubertal growth spurt. Bone 2004; 34(5):771-775.

23. Beck BR, Snow CM. Bone health across the lifespan--exercising our options. Exerc Sport Sci Rev 2003; 31(3):117-122.

24. Wallace BA, Cumming RG. Systematic review of randomized trials of the effect of exercise on bone mass in pre- and postmenopausal women. Calcif Tissue Int 2000; 67(1):10-18.

25. Kohrt WM. Aging and the osteogenic response to mechanical loading. Int J Sport Nutr Exerc Metab 2001; 11 Suppl:S137-42.:S137-S142.

26. Schoenau E, Neu CM, Beck B, Manz F, Rauch F. Bone mineral content per muscle cross-sectional area as an index of the functional muscle-bone unit. J Bone Miner Res 2002; 17(6):1095-1101.

27. Bianchi ML, Mazzanti A, Galbiati E, Saraifoger S, Dubini A, Cornelio F et al. Bone mineral density and bone metabolism in Duchenne muscular dystrophy. Osteoporos Int 2003; 14(9):761-767.

28. Ralis ZA, Ralis HM, Randall M, Watkins G, Blake PD. Changes in shape, ossification and quality of bones in children with spina bifida. Dev Med Child Neurol Suppl 1976;(37):29-41.

29. Daly RM, Saxon L, Turner CH, Robling AG, Bass SL. The relationship between muscle size and bone geometry during growth and in response to exercise. Bone 2004; 34(2):281-287.

30. Heinonen A, McKay HA, Whittall KP, Forster BB, Khan KM. Muscle cross-sectional area is associated with specific site of bone in prepubertal girls: a quantitative magnetic resonance imaging study. Bone 2001; 29(4):388-392.

31. Hamrick MW, McPherron AC, Lovejoy CO, Hudson J. Femoral morphology and cross-sectional geometry of adult myostatin-deficient mice. Bone 2000; 27(3):343-349.

32. Hamrick MW, McPherron AC, Lovejoy CO. Bone mineral content and density in the humerus of adult myostatin-deficient mice. Calcif Tissue Int 2002; 71(1):63-68.

33. Beck TJ, Oreskovic TL, Stone KL, Ruff CB, Ensrud K, Nevitt MC et al. Structural adaptation to changing skeletal load in the progression toward hip fragility: the study of osteoporotic fractures. J Bone Miner Res 2001; 16(6):1108-1119.

34. Dodd JS, Raleigh JA, Gross TS. Osteocyte hypoxia: a novel mechanotransduction pathway. Am J Physiol 1999; 277(3 Pt 1):C598-C602.

35. Bakker AD, Soejima K, Klein-Nulend J, Burger EH. The production of nitric oxide and prostaglandin E(2) by primary bone cells is shear stress dependent. J Biomech 2001; 34(5):671-677.

36. Kapur S, Baylink DJ, Lau KH. Fluid flow shear stress stimulates human osteoblast proliferation and differentiation through multiple interacting and competing signal transduction pathways. Bone 2003; 32(3):241-251.

37. Giangregorio L, Blimkie CJ. Skeletal adaptations to alterations in weight-bearing activity: a comparison of models of disuse osteoporosis. Sports Med 2002; 32(7):459-476.

38. Leblanc AD, Schneider VS, Evans HJ, Engelbretson DA, Krebs JM. Bone mineral loss and recovery after 17 weeks of bed rest. J Bone Miner Res 1990; 5(8):843-850.

39. Magnusson HI, Linden C, Obrant KJ, Johnell O, Karlsson MK. Bone mass changes in weight-loaded and unloaded skeletal regions following a fracture of the hip. Calcif Tissue Int 2001; 69(2):78-83.

40. Dauty M, Perrouin VB, Maugars Y, Dubois C, Mathe JF. Supralesional and sublesional bone mineral density in spinal cord- injured patients. Bone 2000; 27(2):305-309.

41. de Bruin ED, Frey-Rindova P, Herzog RE, Dietz V, Dambacher MA, Stussi E. Changes of tibia bone properties after spinal cord injury: effects of early intervention. Arch Phys Med Rehabil 1999; 80(2):214-220.

42. Garland DE, Adkins RH. Bone loss at the knee in spinal cord injury. Topics in Spinal Cord Injury Rehabilitation 6(3):37-46, 2001 Winter (27 ref) 2001;(3):37-46.

43. Collet P, Uebelhart D, Vico L, Moro L, Hartmann D, Roth M et al. Effects of 1- and 6-month spaceflight on bone mass and biochemistry in two humans. Bone 1997; 20(6):547-551.

44. Creighton DL, Morgan AL, Boardley D, Brolinson PG. Weight-bearing exercise and markers of bone turnover in female athletes. J Appl Physiol 2001; 90(2):565-570.

45. Layne JE, Nelson ME. The effects of progressive resistance training on bone density: a review. Med Sci Sports Exerc 1999; 31(1):25-30.

46. Robinson TL, Snow-Harter C, Taaffe DR, Gillis D, Shaw J, Marcus R. Gymnasts exhibit higher bone mass than runners despite similar prevalence of amenorrhea and oligomenorrhea. J Bone Miner Res 1995; 10(1):26-35.

47. Karlsson MK, Johnell O, Obrant KJ. Bone mineral density in weight lifters. Calcif Tissue Int 1993; 52(3):212-215.

48. Bass S, Pearce G, Bradney M, Hendrich E, Delmas PD, Harding A et al. Exercise before puberty may confer residual benefits in bone density in adulthood: studies in active prepubertal and retired female gymnasts. J Bone Miner Res 1998; 13(3):500-507.

49. Nordstrom P, Pettersson U, Lorentzon R. Type of physical activity, muscle strength, and pubertal stage as determinants of bone mineral density and bone area in adolescent boys. J Bone Miner Res 1998; 13(7):1141-1148.

50. Bailey DA, McKay HA, Mirwald RL, Crocker PR, Faulkner RA. A six-year longitudinal study of the relationship of physical activity to bone mineral accrual in growing children: the university of Saskatchewan bone mineral accrual study. J Bone Miner Res 1999; 14(10):1672-1679.

51. Bailey DA, Faulkner RA, McKay HA. Growth, Physical Activity and Bone Mineral Acquisition. In: Holloszy J, editor. Exercise and Sport Science Reviews. Baltimore: Wilkins and Wilkins, 1996: 233-266.

52. Blimkie CJ, Chilibeck PD, Davison KS. Bone Mineralization Patterns: Reproductive endocrine, calcium and physical activity influences during the lifespan. In: Bar-Or O, Lamb DR, Clarkson PM, editors. Perspectives in Exercise Science and Sports Medicine. Carmel, IN: Cooper Publishing Group, 1996: 73-143.

53. Beck BR, Shaw J, Snow CM. Physical Activity and Osteoporosis. In: Marcus R, Feldman D, Kelsey J, editors. Osteoporosis. San Diego: Academic Press, 2001: 701-720.

54. Kannus P, Haapasalo H, Sankelo M, Sievanen H, Pasanen M, Heinonen A et al. Effect of starting age of physical activity on bone mass in the dominant arm of tennis and squash players. Ann Intern Med 1995; 123(1):27-31.

55. Kontulainen S, Sievanen H, Kannus P, Pasanen M, Vuori I. Effect of long-term impact-loading on mass, size, and estimated strength of humerus and radius of female racquet-sports players: a peripheral quantitative computed tomography study between young and old starters and controls. J Bone Miner Res 2003; 18(2):352-359.

56. Haapasalo H, Kannus P, Sievanen H, Pasanen M, Uusi-Rasi K, Heinonen A et al. Effect of long-term unilateral activity on bone mineral density of female junior tennis players. J Bone Miner Res 1998; 13(2):310-319.

57. Nurmi-Lawton JA, Baxter-Jones AD, Mirwald RL, Bishop JA, Taylor P, Cooper C et al. Evidence of sustained skeletal benefits from impact-loading exercise in young females: A 3-year longitudinal study. J Bone Miner Res 2004; 19(2):314-322.

58. Laing EM, Massoni JA, Nickols-Richardson SM, Modlesky CM, O'Connor PJ, Lewis RD. A prospective study of bone mass and body composition in female adolescent gymnasts. J Pediatr 2002; 141(2):211-216.

59. MacKelvie KJ, Khan KM, McKay HA. Is there a critical period for bone response to weight-bearing exercise in children and adolescents? a systematic review. Br J Sports Med 2002; 36(4):250-257.

60. McKay HA, Petit MA, Schutz RW, Prior JC, Barr SI, Khan KM. Augmented trochanteric bone mineral density after modified physical education classes: a randomized school-based exercise intervention study in prepubescent and early pubescent children. J Pediatr 2000; 136(2):156-162.

61. Morris FL, Naughton GA, Gibbs JL, Carlson JS, Wark JD. Prospective ten-month exercise intervention in premenarcheal girls: positive effects on bone and lean mass. J Bone Miner Res 1997; 12(9):1453-1462.

62. MacKelvie KJ, McKay HA, Petit MA, Moran O, Khan KM. Bone mineral response to a 7-month randomized controlled, school-based jumping intervention in 121 prepubertal boys: associations with ethnicity and body mass index. J Bone Miner Res 2002; 17(5):834-844.

63. MacKelvie KJ, Khan KM, Petit MA, Janssen PA, McKay HA. A school-based exercise intervention elicits substantial bone health benefits: a 2-year randomized controlled trial in girls. Pediatrics 2003; 112(6 Pt 1):e447.

64. Iuliano-Burns S, Saxon L, Naughton G, Gibbons K, Bass SL. Regional specificity of exercise and calcium during skeletal growth in girls: a randomized controlled trial. J Bone Miner Res 2003; 18(1):156-162.

65. Heinonen A, Sievanen H, Kannus P, Oja P, Pasanen M, Vuori I. High-impact exercise and bones of growing girls: a 9-month controlled trial. Osteoporos Int 2000; 11(12):1010-1017.

66.   Khan KM, Bennell KL, Hopper JL, Flicker L, Nowson CA, Sherwin AJ et al. Self-reported ballet classes undertaken at age 10-12 years and hip bone mineral density in later life. Osteoporos Int 1998; 8(2):165-173.

67.   Kemper HC, Twisk JW, van Mechelen W, Post GB, Roos JC, Lips P. A fifteen-year longitudinal study in young adults on the relation of physical activity and fitness with the development of the bone mass: The Amsterdam Growth And Health Longitudinal Study. Bone 2000; 27(6):847-853.

68.   Fuchs RK, Snow CM. Gains in hip bone mass from high-impact training are maintained: a randomized controlled trial in children. 2002; 141(3):357-362.

69.   Kontulainen S, Kannus P, Haapasalo H, Sievanen H, Pasanen M, Heinonen A et al. Good maintenance of exercise-induced bone gain with decreased training of female tennis and squash players: a prospective 5-year follow-up study of young and old starters and controls. J Bone Miner Res 2001; 16(2):195-201.

70.   Snow CM, Williams DP, LaRiviere J, Fuchs RK, Robinson TL. Bone gains and losses follow seasonal training and detraining in gymnasts. Calcif Tissue Int 2001; 69(1):7-12.

71.   Gustavsson A, Olsson T, Nordstrom P. Rapid loss of bone mineral density of the femoral neck after cessation of ice hockey training: a 6-year longitudinal study in males. J Bone Miner Res 2003; 18(11):1964-1969.

72.   Jones HH, Priest JD, Hayes WC, Tichenor CC, Nagel DA. Humeral hypertrophy in response to exercise. J Bone Joint Surg Am 1977; 59(2):204-208.

73.   Heinonen A, Sievanen H, Kannus P, Oja P, Vuori I. Site-specific skeletal response to long-term weight training seems to be attributable to principal loading modality: a pQCT study of female weightlifters. Calcif Tissue Int 2002; 70(6):469-474.

74.   MacDougall JD, Webber CE, Martin J, Ormerod S, Chesley A, Younglai EV et al. Relationship among running mileage, bone density, and serum testosterone in male runners. J Appl Physiol 1992; 73(3):1165-1170.

75.   Slemenda CW, Johnston CC. High intensity activities in young women: site specific bone mass effects among female figure skaters. Bone Miner 1993; 20(2):125-132.

76.   Wolff I, van Croonenborg JJ, Kemper HC, Kostense PJ, Twisk JW. The effect of exercise training programs on bone mass: a meta-analysis of published controlled trials in pre- and postmenopausal women. Osteoporos Int 1999; 9(1):1-12.

77.   Kelley GA. Exercise and regional bone mineral density in postmenopausal women: a meta-analytic review of randomized trials. Am J Phys Med Rehabil 1998; 77(1):76-87.

78.   Huuskonen J, Vaisanen SB, Kroger H, Jurvelin JS, Alhava E, Rauramaa R. Regular physical exercise and bone mineral density: a four-year controlled randomized trial in middle-aged men. The DNASCO study. Osteoporos Int 2001; 12(5):349-355.

79.   Maddalozzo GF, Snow CM. High intensity resistance training: effects on bone in older men and women. Calcif Tissue Int 2000; 66(6):399-404.

80. Grove KA, Londeree BR. Bone density in postmenopausal women: high impact vs low impact exercise. Med Sci Sports Exerc 1992; 24(11):1190-1194.

81. Nelson ME, Fiatarone MA, Morganti CM, Trice I, Greenberg RA, Evans WJ. Effects of high-intensity strength training on multiple risk factors for osteoporotic fractures. A randomized controlled trial. JAMA 1994; 272(24):1909-1914.

82. Turner CH. Exercising the skeleton: Beneficial effects of mechanical loading on bone structure. The Endocrinologist 2000; 10:164-169.

83. Bass SL, Saxon L, Daly RM, Turner CH, Robling AG, Seeman E et al. The effect of mechanical loading on the size and shape of bone in pre-, peri-, and postpubertal girls: a study in tennis players. J Bone Miner Res 2002; 17(12):2274-2280.

84. Petit MA, McKay HA, MacKelvie KJ, Heinonen A, Khan KM, Beck TJ. A randomized school-based jumping intervention confers site and maturity-specific benefits on bone structural properties in girls: a hip structural analysis study. J Bone Miner Res 2002; 17(3):363-372.

85. Bradney M, Pearce G, Naughton G, Sullivan C, Bass S, Beck T et al. Moderate exercise during growth in prepubertal boys: changes in bone mass, size, volumetric density, and bone strength: a controlled prospective study. J Bone Miner Res 1998; 13(12):1814-1821.

86. Adami S, Gatti D, Braga V, Bianchini D, Rossini M. Site-specific effects of strength training on bone structure and geometry of ultradistal radius in postmenopausal women. J Bone Miner Res 1999; 14(1):120-124.

87. Jarvinen TL, Kannus P, Sievanen H, Jolma P, Heinonen A, Jarvinen M. Randomized controlled study of effects of sudden impact loading on rat femur. J Bone Miner Res 1998; 13(9):1475-1482.

88. MacIntyre NJ, Bhandari M, Blimkie CJ, Adachi JD, Webber CE. Effect of altered physical loading on bone and muscle in the forearm. Can J Physiol Pharmacol 2001; 79(12):1015-1022.

89. Heaney RP. The importance of calcium intake for lifelong skeletal health. Calcif Tissue Int 2002; 70(2):70-73.

90. Tylavsky FA, Anderson JJ, Talmage RV, Taft TN. Are calcium intakes and physical activity patterns during adolescence related to radial bone mass of white college-age females? Osteoporos Int 1992; 2(5):232-240.

91. Wosje KS, Binkley TL, Fahrenwald NL, Specker BL. High bone mass in a female Hutterite population. J Bone Miner Res 2000; 15(8):1429-1436.

92. VandenBergh MF, DeMan SA, Witteman JC, Hofman A, Trouerbach WT, Grobbee DE. Physical activity, calcium intake, and bone mineral content in children in The Netherlands. J Epidemiol Community Health 1995; 49(3):299-304.

93. Anderson JJ. Exercise, dietary calcium, and bone gain in girls and young adult women. J Bone Miner Res 2000; 15(8):1437-1439.

94. Lohman T, Going S, Pamenter R, Hall M, Boyden T, Houtkooper L et al. Effects of resistance training on regional and total bone mineral density in

premenopausal women: a randomized prospective study. J Bone Miner Res 1995; 10(7):1015-1024.

95. Uusi-Rasi K, Sievanen H, Vuori I, Pasanen M, Heinonen A, Oja P. Associations of physical activity and calcium intake with bone mass and size in healthy women at different ages. J Bone Miner Res 1998; 13(1):133-142.

96. Friedlander AL, Genant HK, Sadowsky S, Byl NN, Gluer CC. A two-year program of aerobics and weight training enhances bone mineral density of young women. J Bone Miner Res 1995; 10(4):574-585.

97. Specker BL. Evidence for an interaction between calcium intake and physical activity on changes in bone mineral density. J Bone Miner Res 1996; 11(10):1539-1544.

98. Lee K, Jessop H, Suswillo R, Zaman G, Lanyon L. Endocrinology: bone adaptation requires oestrogen receptor-alpha. Nature 2003; 424(6947):389.

99. Tobias JH. At the crossroads of skeletal responses to estrogen and exercise. Trends Endocrinol Metab 2003; 14(10):441-443.

100. Kohrt WM, Snead DB, Slatopolsky E, Birge SJ, Jr. Additive effects of weight-bearing exercise and estrogen on bone mineral density in older women. J Bone Miner Res 1995; 10(9):1303-1311.

101. Milliken LA, Going SB, Houtkooper LB, Flint-Wagner HG, Figueroa A, Metcalfe LL et al. Effects of exercise training on bone remodeling, insulin-like growth factors, and bone mineral density in postmenopausal women with and without hormone replacement therapy. Calcif Tissue Int 2003; 72(4):478-484.

102. Cheng S, Sipila S, Taaffe DR, Puolakka J, Suominen H. Change in bone mass distribution induced by hormone replacement therapy and high-impact physical exercise in post-menopausal women. Bone 2002; 31(1):126-135.

103. Heikkinen J, Kyllonen E, Kurttila-Matero E, Wilen-Rosenqvist G, Lankinen KS, Rita H et al. HRT and exercise: effects on bone density, muscle strength and lipid metabolism. A placebo controlled 2-year prospective trial on two estrogen-progestin regimens in healthy postmenopausal women. Maturitas 1997; 26(2):139-149.

104. Chilibeck PD. Exercise and estrogen or estrogen alternatives (phytoestrogens, bisphosphonates) for preservation of bone mineral in postmenopausal women. Canadian Journal of Applied Physiology 2004; 29(1):59-75.

105. Going S, Lohman T, Houtkooper L, Metcalfe L, Flint-Wagner H, Blew R et al. Effects of exercise on bone mineral density in calcium-replete postmenopausal women with and without hormone replacement therapy. Osteoporos Int 2003; 14(8):637-643.

106. Writing Group for the Women's Health Initiative Investigators. Risks and benefits of estrogen plus progestin in healthy postmenopausal women. Principal results from the Women's Health Initiative Randomized Controlled Trial. JAMA 2002; 288:321-333.

107. Braith RW, Magyari PM, Fulton MN, Aranda J, Walker T, Hill JA. Resistance exercise training and alendronate reverse glucocorticoid-induced osteoporosis in heart transplant recipients. J Heart Lung Transplant 2003; 22(10):1082-1090.

108. Uusi-Rasi K, Kannus P, Cheng S, Sievanen H, Pasanen M, Heinonen A et al. Effect of alendronate and exercise on bone and physical performance of postmenopausal women: a randomized controlled trial. Bone 2003; 33(1):132-143.

THE DIAGNOSIS OF OSTEOPOROSIS
IN POSTMENOPAUSAL WOMEN

M. Janet Barger-Lux
and
Robert R. Recker

Osteoporosis Research Center
Creighton University School of Medicine
601 North 30th Street, Suite 5766, Omaha, Nebraska, USA
E-mail addresses
jbarger@creighton.edu
rrecker@creighton.edu

Estrogen deprivation reduces bone mass, accelerates bone remodeling, and weakens bone structure. Under current guidelines, the diagnosis of osteoporosis rests heavily upon bone mass, measured as BMD. This approach can be questioned, however, by the facts that fracture resistance is more dependent on age than BMD, and treatment agents with antifracture efficacy have little effect on bone mass. We outline a comprehensive set of considerations to exclude other possibilities and support a diagnosis of osteoporosis.

1. Introduction

Osteoporosis is a condition that leads to the structural failure of the human skeleton. It can occur in men as well as women, in younger adults as well as those who are older. It can also occur as a complication of the conditions, diseases, and medications that, over time, undermine bone strength.

In its most recent consensus statement on the subject, the National Institutes of Health identified osteoporosis simply as "a skeletal disorder characterized by compromised bone strength predisposing to an increased risk of fracture."[1] Perhaps the most widely cited definition dates to an earlier consensus conference that identified osteoporosis as "a systemic skeletal disease characterized by low bone mass and microarchitectural deterioration of bone tissue, with a consequent increase in bone fragility and susceptibility to fractures."[2]

This chapter, however, is limited to the diagnosis of osteoporosis in postmenopausal women. Other chapters in this volume will describe the pathogenesis, prevention, and clinical management of osteoporosis in postmenopausal women, as well as cases that result from different causal paths.

2. Skeletal Consequences of Estrogen Deprivation

2.1 *Effects on Bone Mass*

In any discussion of low bone mass, it is important to note that this finding may reflect an earlier failure to accrue bone (i.e., low peak bone mass in early adult life) as well as bone loss later on.

Sustained estrogen deprivation at any time after the usual age of puberty means that a woman's bone mass will diminish. Without estrogen replacement, total skeletal weight gradually decreases. Most of the bone loss associated with estrogen withdrawal occurs during the first three to five years.

In recent work, Recker *et al.* gathered longitudinal data that described changes in bone mass, regionally and for the total-body, from 2 to 3 years before the last menses to 3 to 4 years after. These data showed that bone loss began before the final menses.[3] Over the entire period of observation, total bone loss that could be attributed to estrogen deprivation averaged 10.5, 7.7, and 5.3 percent, respectively, for the lumbar spine, total-body, and femoral neck.[4]

2.2 *Effects on Bone Remodeling*

In earlier work, Heaney, *et al.* followed a group of women across the menopausal transition with measurements of bone resorption and accretion at 5-year intervals using radiocalcium kinetics.[5] On their own self-selected diets, the subjects were, on average, in negative calcium balance before menopause. After menopause, calcium balance did not change among the women who were taking estrogen. However in those who were not, the rate of bone loss had increased by an average of 80 percent. These studies measured the net effect of bone remodeling throughout the skeleton, in cortical as well as cancellous bone.

In the trans-menopausal study cited earlier, Recker *et al.* also examined paired transilial bone biopsies before and about a year after the last menses.[6] The key histomorphomorphetric change was an increase in activation frequency (Ac.f) in the women who were not estrogen-replaced.

We believe that, through mechanisms now being elucidated,[7] the menopausal transition changes the response threshold of bone remodeling to PTH. Ac.f rises and the bone at each remodeling site is only partially replaced.

2.3 *Effects on Bone Structure*

Kimmel *et al.* compared histomorphometric data from postmenopausal women with untreated osteoporosis and in others who had no evidence of osteoporosis.[8] Compared to the healthy women, those with osteoporosis had: significantly fewer trabeculae (as Tb.N); slightly thinner trabeculae (as Th.Th); and trabeculae that were more widely spaced (as Tb.Sp) Together these findings indicate that, rather than general thinning of trabeculae, entire trabecular elements had probably been lost. This could occur when trabeculae are transected by osteoclasts; the "loose ends," no longer loaded, would themselves be eventually resorbed away. Differences were also found in cortical bone. In the women with osteoporosis, the inner and outer cortices (Ct.W1 and Ct.W2) were about 30 and 37 percent thinner, respectively, than the corresponding measures in the healthy women.[8]

In postmenopausal women with osteoporosis, cortical bone loss occurs at the corticoendosteal surface, where resorption cavities enlarge and coalesce. The result is a thinner cortex and a characteristic transitional zone of coarse trabeculae.[9]

3. Quantitative Criteria for Identifying Osteoporosis

3.1 The WHO Criteria

Bone mineral density (BMD) has been very widely used as a surrogate for bone fragility, both in published research and in clinical practice. In 1994, a committee of the World Health Organization (WHO) went a step further by proposing measurable criteria for defining and diagnosing osteoporosis. The reference was the distribution of BMD among healthy young women. The following criteria were set forth:[10]

Osteopenia or *low bone mass:* BMDs from –1.0 down to –2.5 standard deviations (SD) below the reference mean. These limits correspond to T-scores of –1.0 and –2.5, respectively.

Osteoporosis: BMDs that are at least 2.5 standard deviations (SD) below the mean.

Established osteoporosis: BMDs that meet the criterion for osteoporosis in persons who have already have had at least one fragility fracture.

The WHO criteria have provided common standards, but many scientists have called attention to their shortcomings.

3.2 Refinements of the WHO Criteria

In 2000, Kanis and Glüer published an examination of WHO criteria *vis á vis* scanning site, equipment issues, and fracture risk. Among their several recommendations were the following:[11]

Equipment and scanning site: Use of the WHO criteria for diagnosing osteoporosis should be limited to DXA (dual-energy X-ray absorptiometry) scans of the total hip.

Reference database: Until persuasive data indicates otherwise, NHANES III data for women aged 20 to 29 years should be used as the *international* reference group for generating the T-scores of both women *and men.*

Decision to treat: While supporting the use of a single measure for diagnosis, the decision to treat should be based upon "comprehensive assessment."

In 2001, Lu, *et al.* proposed a more complex way of using BMD to define osteoporosis.[12] They calculated absolute fracture risk by use of data from nearly 7,700 postmenopausal women who participated in the Study of Osteoporotic Fractures (SOF). Their fracture risk variable could be refined by incorporating BMD at more than one site, a reference group of older women, and the subject's age. The authors proposed that any case with a calculated fracture risk (at the hip or spine) greater than 14.6 percent be recognized as osteoporosis.

It is important to recognize that BMD is an imperfect surrogate for bone fragility. In 1988, Hui, *et al.* reported that, despite *identical* BMDs at the midradius, an 80-year-old has as much as 15 times the fracture risk as does a 45-year-old.[13] Thus age-dependent factors, taken together, are a far stronger determinant of fracture risk than is BMD. Also, for subjects in any age category, the relationship between BMD and fracture risk is continuous; there is no "fracture threshold."

4. A Comprehensive Approach to Diagnosis

Clear-cut, measurable criteria are obviously helpful for defining osteoporosis in the research setting. In the clinic, however, the diagnosis of individual patients does merit a comprehensive assessment, including more data and the professional judgment of an experienced clinician.

4.1 A Broad Index of Suspicion

We have urged orthopedists to consider osteoporosis in every patient who suffers (a) a wedge or crush vertebral fracture at any age or (b) any fracture after reaching age 45.[14] This approach casts a wide net for identifying established osteoporosis.

We believe that a wide net should also be employed in the evaluation of middle-aged women whose fracture history is still negative.

4.2 A Diagnosis of Exclusion

Osteoporosis in women of postmenopausal age is a diagnosis of exclusion. The clinician must arrive at reasonable certainty that no other problem is largely or entirely responsible for a particular patient's findings. The possibilities include other bone diseases and osteoporosis that is clearly and predominantly secondary to another health problem or its treatment. Another chapter in this volume will discuss secondary osteoporosis in detail.

4.3 Authoritative Resources

The section that follows supplements – but does not supplant – authoritative resources such as the most recent consensus conference report cited earlier[1] and the Physician's Guide available through the National Osteoporosis Foundation.[15] Also, scientific symposia, such as that recently held by the US Department of Health and Human Services,[16] provide useful and detailed updates.   Below we offer a practical interpretation of these and other sources, enriched by ample experience in the clinic and in clinical research and open to new insights as they develop.

5. Clinical Diagnosis

Diagnosis may begin at any of several points, e.g., at a follow-up clinic visit after screening in the community, when a relatively minor mishap results in fracture, or when a clinic visit follows a woman's rising concerns about changes in her height and posture.

5.1 The Patient Interview

Table 1, on the next page, gathers a number of items that should be included in the patient interview. As Table 1 indicates, positive findings suggest established osteoporosis and/or exposure to several of the putative causes of osteoporosis. The latter have been identified in studies by epidemiologists (as summarized elsewhere, e.g.,[17-18]), and examined further in clinical work. All are physiologically plausible contributors to bone fragility in postmenopausal women, and some are themselves responsible for secondary osteoporosis.

Table 1. The patient interview should include the items listed below. As the checkmarks indicate, each item suggests either established osteoporosis or significant exposure to several groups of putative causes. Occurrences need not be recent to be significant, and the list is not exhaustive.

	Established Osteoporosis	Genetic vulnerability	Poor nutrition	Hypovitaminosis D	Poor skeletal loading	Harmful bone effects	Hypogonadism
Any fracture after age 45	√						
Height loss of an inch or more as an adult	√						
Postural changes, difficulty in the fit of clothing	√						
Osteoporosis, height loss, or fractures in relatives		√					
Malabsorption or another long-term GI problem			√				
Habitual avoidance of calcium-rich foods			√				
Little or no direct exposure of skin to sunlight				√			
Persistent underweight (~BMI <19) as an adult					√		
Extended periods of bed rest as an adult					√		
Little or no standing, walking, or physical work					√		
Exposure to drugs associated with bone loss						√	
Cigarette smoking and/or alcohol abuse						√	
Taking thyroxine, irregular or no monitoring						√	
Hyperparathyroidism, bone mass not monitored						√	
Extended oligomenorrhea or amenorrhea							√
Menopause without estrogen replacement							√

Adapted from Recker RR, Barger-Lux MJ. In: *Orthopædics*. St. Louis, Mosby, 2002, pp. 203-204

A consistent finding in studies of postmenopausal women is that fractures predict fractures. A recent paper by Delmas, *et al.* showed further that the *severity* of prevalent vertebral fractures predict fracture risk over the next 3 years.[19] Subjects of the analysis were postmenopausal participants who had been allocated to the placebo group in the Multiple Outcomes of Raloxifene Evaluation (MORE) trial. Table 2 summarizes the results.

Most of the patients who visit our osteoporosis clinic have complex situations. Unfortunately, osteoporosis treatment trials typically exclude most of them, leaving the subjects who participate in these trials quite unlike the patients with osteoporosis who visit our bone clinic.[20]

A specialty clinic in an academic medical center may attract a higher proportion of complex cases. However, owing to widespread hypovitaminosis D[21], poor calcium intake[22], other nutritional problems[23], sedentary living[24], thyroid problems[25], and so on, it seems likely that very few cases of osteoporosis in postmenopausal women can be attributed to estrogen deficiency alone.

Table 2. Percent of subjects with incident fractures over an observation period of 3 years. The subjects were postmenopausal women with prevalent vertebral fractures, classified by severity.

		Incident fractures	
		Vertebral	Non-vertebral
Severity of prevalent vertebral fractures	Mild	10.50%	7.20%
	Moderate	23.60%	7.70%
	Severe	38.10%	13.80%

Adapted from Delmas PD, Genant HK, Crans GG, *et al. Bone* 2003 33:522-32.

5.2 Physical Examination

The physical examination should include careful measurement of height without shoes and weight in light clothing. Ideally, replicate measurements should be made by use of a balance-beam scale and a calibrated stadiometer.

During the patient encounter, the clinician should be alert to:

Evidence of other bone diseases. Examples are osteomalacia, Paget's disease of bone, primary hyperparathyroidism, multiple myeloma, or, occasionally, a previously unrecognized case of osteogenesis imperfecta.

Evidence of any of the diseases and conditions that can promote or complicate osteoporosis. Other health problems can promote or complicate osteoporosis by: directly damaging the skeleton; requiring medications that can damage the skeleton; creating nutritional problems; making an adequate level of physical activity impossible, difficult or dangerous; causing hormone problems; and so on. In some cases the result would be considered a secondary osteoporosis.

Characteristic postural changes. The presence of kyphosis and/or a definite short-waisted appearance, usually with a prominent tummy, suggest wedged or crushed vertebrae.

Changes in stature. Height carefully measured (in duplicate) in the clinic should be compared with the patient's recalled peak adult height.[26] A height loss greater than about 2 cm should not be ignored. In the absence of anatomical change (e.g., worsened scoliosis or crushed vertebrae), there is only a trivial loss of height in the decade after menopause.[27]

5.3 Assessment of Bone Mass

Bone Densitometry: Measurement of bone mass is an important part of the evaluative process, even when there is other evidence of skeletal fragility. However BMD measurements by dual-energy X-ray absorptiometry (DXA), are neither foolproof nor perfectly reproducible. In older patients, degenerative changes (i.e., osteophytes and endplate sclerosis) can confound measurements of BMD at the lumbar spine; when such changes are present, greater weight should be given to peripheral measurements of BMD.[28]

Lodder, *et al.* recently reported figures for the smallest detectable difference (SDD) in duplicate measurements of BMD by DXA; each set of measurements was made on the same day.[29] The SDDs for BMD of the lumbar spine (L1-L4) and BMD of the total hip were ±0.05 g/cm^2 and ±0.04 g/cm^2, respectively. The authors conclude that inter-individual changes of at least these magnitudes should be considered significant. The clinician, however, would presumably want to follow a individual patients over time. Day-to-day variation in BMD, not included in this research protocol, would surely raise the SDDs, perhaps to obscure actual changes occurring in those individuals.

5.4 Assessment of Bone Morphology

A set of two images of the lateral spine by, covering the thoracic and lumbar spine and obtained by use of conventional x-ray, are typically used to assess the spine for wedge fractures, crush fractures, and degenerative changes (i.e., osteophytosis and endplate sclerosis). DXA instruments can also produce detailed images of the lateral spine; the patient is positioned on her side, supported by bolsters. When DXA is used for this purpose, the additional radiation exposure is trivial, and additional equipment is not required.

Severe crush fractures are obvious in any lateral image of sufficient resolution and good quality. However, despite the efforts of several researchers,[30] a consensus on just what should "count" as a wedge or a less-severe crush fracture has failed to emerge.

The presence of wedged or crushed vertebrae can indicate that these bones were excessively fragile when the deformities occurred. However auto accidents, falls from horses or ladders, athletic mishaps, and overuse injuries earlier in life may also be responsible for such deformities. In general, however, as the number of vertebral deformities increases, the likelihood of underlying osteoporosis also increases.

5.5 Laboratory Tests

A number of blood and urine tests can be useful in the diagnostic and evaluative process.

Screening laboratory work. A complete blood count and a serum chemistry panel (preferably on a fasting blood specimen), may suggest other conditions that can mimic or complicate osteoporosis (e.g., primary hypoparathyroidism, multiple myeloma, or poor nutritional status). Estrogen deprivation does not affect any of these analyses.

Thyroid function. Measurements of T4 and TSH are useful for evaluating thyroid status and monitoring thyroid medications.

Parathyroid hormone. Elevated levels of PTH suggest a restricted calcium intake, vitamin D deficiency, or primary hyperparathyroidism.

Vitamin D status. Vitamin D status can be evaluated by measuring serum 25-hydroxyvitamin D. For many adults, the combined effects of occasional direct exposure to sunlight and limited dietary sources of vitamin D yields a serum 25-hydroxyvitamin far below the desirable level of about 75 nmol/L.[31] In our experience, a daily multivitamin supplies too little vitamin D_3 to produce a measurable improvement in 25-hydroxyvitamin D.

Ovarian function and menopausal status. If ovarian function or menopausal status is in doubt, E_2 and FSH can also be measured in blood specimens.

Urine calcium. The calcium-to-creatinine ratio in first-morning urine after a 10-hour fast reflects calcium intake, calcium absorption efficiency, and bone resorption. However in most cases current sodium intake is the strongest determinant of the result; as sodium intake increases, urinary output of calcium and sodium increase.

Researchers have identified many analytes ("bone markers") that reflect total-body osteoclast or osteoblast activity. Clinical trials of drugs used to treat osteoporosis now usually include bone markers. Among those found most useful are the bone resorption markers phenazo-pyridine crosslinks and related telopeptides (all measured in urine) and the bone formation markers osteocalcin, bone-specific alkaline phosphatase, and the N-terminal propeptide of type 1 procollagen (all measured in serum).[32] To date, bone markers are not useful for screening or diagnostic purposes. However effective treatments in adherent patients do yield discernable changes when baseline and 3 to 6 month results are compared.

5.6 Dietary Evaluation

Because another chapter in this volume covers the nutritional aspects of osteoporosis, this section is brief.

In the US, dairy products are the major source of dietary calcium. Assessments of calcium intake can be based upon a few questions in the clinic, a food-frequency questionnaire, or a careful and complete 7-day food diary, interpreted and analyzed by a trained dietitian. We have found that a poor calcium intake is a marker for a diet deficient in many nutrients.[33] It is probably the case that few postmenopausal women maintain an ample calcium intake without attention and effort. As Table 1 indicates, we believe that the woman's long-term intake of calcium-rich foods, particularly milk and other dairy products, is the principal issue. A diet without calcium-rich foods provides a daily calcium intake of only about 350 mg, less than one-fourth of the recommended intake for postmenopausal women.

6. Conclusions and Outlook

In the not-so-distant past, the diagnosis of osteoporosis – in postmenopausal women and in others – was delayed until fragility fractures occurred. In 1994, the WHO report[10] approved a language – osteoporosis vs. established osteoporosis – that recognized the obvious fact that fragility develops before fracture.

The WHO criteria have become widely accepted as a basis for defining and diagnosing osteoporosis. We argue that the diagnosis of osteoporosis in the clinical setting should be based on more information than a single threshold value for BMD.

Early in the present paper, we referred to osteoporosis as structural failure. Heaney has noted that the strength of a structure, as understood by engineers, is a function of three things: [34]
- mechanical properties of the component material;
- arrangement of the material in 3-dimensional space;
- massiveness of the structure.

To define and diagnose osteoporosis by use of BMD alone is to ignore completely the first two of these factors. (In bone research, these two involve what has been called the "elusive" concept of bone quality[35] and skeletal microstructure, respectively.) In osteoporosis, it is possible that skeletal massiveness (as assessed by densitometry) is the least important of the three.[34]

Ongoing research has shed further light on sources of bone fragility that cannot be assessed by densitometry. In 2002, researchers in this area gathered at symposium on bone quality. At meeting, Jepsen noted that, over time, changes occur in matrix composition as well as bone microstructure; the result is a reduction in *whole-bone toughness*.[36] A the same meeting, Burr explained that, also over time, lamellae accumulate in cortical bone and cement lines degrade; the result is an increase in *bone damageability*, which favors the propagation of cracks.[37] Heaney believes that high levels of bone remodeling – higher still in the early postmenopause – are a major source of the bone fragility of osteoporosis.[34]

Bone remodeling can already be assessed by use of bone markers, but the assays are not as reproducible as we would like. If problems of biological variation can be solved (e.g., by uniform preparation and timing for specimen collection) and the assays themselves improved, they may become useful in the diagnosis of individual patients. Unfortunately, however, bone markers assess only the patient's present rate of bone turnover; they offer no insight into her skeletal history.

A promising source of additional insight into osteoporosis lies in the genetics work now underway. Considering what we have already learned, a better understanding of gene-environment interactions could become useful for identifying women who are particularly vulnerable to bone fragility before they suffer fractures.

REFERENCES

1. NIH Consensus Development Panel. 2001, JAMA 285:785-95.
2. Consensus Development Conference. 1991, Am J Med 90:107-110.
3. Recker RR, Lappe JM, Davies KM, Kimmel DB. J Bone Miner Res 1992 7:857-62.
4. Recker R, Lappe J, Davies K, Heaney R. J Bone Miner Res 2000 15:1965-73.

5.　Heaney RP, Recker RR, Saville PD. J Lab Clin Med 1978 92:964-970.

6.　Recker RR, Lappe JM, Davies M, Heaney RP. J Bone Miner Res 2003 18 (Suppl 2):S298-299.

7.　Pacifici R. In Marcus R, Feldman D, Kelsey J (eds): Osteoporosis Second Edition (Vol 2). San Diego, Academic Press, 2001, pp. 85-101.

8.　Kimmel DB, Recker RR, Gallagher JC, Vaswani AS, Aloia JF. Bone Miner 1990; 11:217-235.

9.　Keshawarz NM, Recker RR. Metab Bone Dis Relat Res 1984; 5:223-228.

10.　World Health Organization. WHO technical report series 843. Geneva: World Health Organization, 1994.

11.　Kanis JA, Gluer CC. Osteoporos Int 2000; 11:192-202.

12.　Lu Y, Genant HK, Shepherd J, et al. J Bone Miner Res 2001 15:901-10.

13.　Hui SL, Slemenda CW, Johnston CC. J Clin Invest 1988 81:1804-9.

14.　Recker RR, Barger-Lux MJ. In Fitzgerald RH, Kauter H, Malkani AL (eds): Orthopædics. St. Louis, Mosby, 2002, pp. 201-207.

15.　National Osteoporosis Foundation. Physician's Guide to Prevention and Treatment of Osteoporosis. 2003. On-line at *www.nof.org*.

16.　Office on Women's Health, US Dept of Health and Human Services. Clinician 2004 22(3):1-17.

17.　Cooper C. Osteoporos Int 1999 2:S2-S8.

18.　Cummings SR, Melton LJ. Lancet 2002 359:1761-7.

19.　Delmas PD, Genant HK, Crans GG, et al. Bone 2003 33:522-32.

20.　Dowd R, Recker RR, Heaney RP. Osteoporos Int 2000 11:533-06.

21.　Malabanan AO, Holick MF. J Womens Health 2003 12:151-6.

22.　Heaney RP. J Am Coll Nutr 2000 19(2 Suppl):83S-99S.

23.　Miller KK. J Womens Health 2003 12:145-50.

24.　Pultila E, Kroger H, Lakka T, et al. Bone 2001 29:442-6.

25.　Schindler AE. Gynecol Endocrinol 2003 17:79-85.

26.　Heaney RP, Ryan R. N Engl J Med 1988 319:795-6.

27.　Davies KM, Recker RR, Stegman MR, Heaney RP. J Bone Miner Res 1991 6:1115-20.

28.　Lodder MC, Lems WF, Ader HJ, et al. Ann Rheum Dis 2004 63:285-9.

29.　Davies KM, Recker RR, Heaney RP. Osteoporos Int 1993 3:265-70.

30.　Holick MF. Curr Opin Endocrinol Diabetes 2002 9:87-98.

31.　Souberbielle JC, Cormier C, Kindermans C. Curr Opin Rheumatol 1999 11:312-9.

32.　Barger-Lux MJ, Heaney RP, Packard PT, Lappe JM, Recker RR. Clin Appl Nutr 1992 2(4):39-44.

33.　Heaney RP. Bone 2003 33:457-65.

34.　Watts NB. J Bone Miner Res 2002 7:1148-50.

35.　Jepsen KJ. Osteoporos Int 2003 14(Suppl 5):S57-S66.

36.　Burr D. Osteoporos Int 2003 14(Suppl 5):S67-S72.

CHAPTER 7

BIOCHEMICAL MARKERS OF BONE TURNOVER: ASSAY METHODS AND CLINICAL APPLICATION

Chun-Yuan Guo

Department of Worldwide Clinical Development
Hearth Care Research Center, Box 36
8700 Mason-Montgomery Road
Mason, Ohio 45040, USA
Email: guo.cy@pg.com
Telephone: 1-513-622-1597

1. Introduction

Bone, as a metabolically active tissue, undergoes continuous turnover (also known as remodeling) through life. Bone turnover is a function of the complex interactions between skeletal cells. Bone turnover consists of a coupled sequence of events, namely bone resorption followed by bone formation. Osteoblasts are the cells responsible for bone formation whereas osteoclasts are the cells responsible for bone resorption. Bone mass depends on the balance between resorption and formation within a remodeling unit in bone tissue and on the number of remodeling units which are activated within a given period of time in a defined area of bone. Systemic and local regulators such as hormones, growth factors and interleukins regulate the process of bone turnover. Bone turnover can be measured by invasive techniques such as bone biopsy which assesses bone turnover at local level of bone tissue. Unlike biopsy sampling, the measurement of circulating biochemical markers of bone turnover can be used to assess bone turnover at whole body skeletal level. Circulating biochemical markers of bone turnover can be widely applied in most targeted populations and the measurements can be repeated several times in a single patient. The rate of formation or degradation of the bone matrix can be assessed either by measuring a prominent enzymatic activity of the bone forming or resorption cells, or by measuring bone matrix components released into the circulation during formation or resorption. Alteration in whole body bone turnover may be evaluated by an increase or decrease in the concentration of circulating biochemical markers of bone formation or bone resorption. Recently, the clinical use of bone turnover markers has been assessed extensively in population based clinical trials. The biggest concern for clinical application of biochemical markers is their huge biological and pathological variability. Nevertheless, physicians and clinical researchers believe that biochemical markers of bone turnover may play a crucial role in some clinical aspects such as monitoring response to drug therapy and predicting risks for future bone loss and fracture.

This chapter will introduce basic and clinical knowledge and most recent progress in biochemical markers of bone turnover.

2. Biochemical markers of bone formation

Currently available bone formation markers include total alkaline phosphatase (total ALP), bone specific alkaline phosphatase (bone ALP), osteocalcin (OC), procollagen type I caboxyterminal propeptide (PICP), and procollagen type I aminoterminal propeptide (PINP). Biochemical markers of bone formation are listed in table 1.

Table 1. Biochemical markers of bone formation

Formation Markers	Samples	Origin	Specificity
Total ALP	blood	Bone, liver, intestine, kidney, placenta	+
Bone ALP	blood	Bone	+++
OC	blood	Bone	+++
PICP	blood	Bone, soft tissue, skin	++
PINP	blood	Bone, soft tissue, skin	++

2.1. Enzymes

Total alkaline phosphatase

Alkaline phosphatases are plasma membrane enzymes which include several isoenzymes: placental, intestinal, germ cell, kidney, liver, and bone etc. Over 90% of the total ALP measured in serum is derived from liver and bone. Methods for the measurement of serum total ALP are based on heat inactivation, chemical inhibition or electrophoresis [1]. Since these methods are commonly available in most laboratories, the measurement of serum total ALP has some place in the management of osteoporosis and metabolic bone diseases. However, due to the fact that total ALP is not bone specific and that liver function impairs serum total ALP significantly, bone ALP provides better index of bone formation. Detection of the bone ALP is increasingly preferred.

Bone specific alkaline phosphatase

Approximately half of the total ALP activity in serum is derived from bone ALP [2]. Bone ALP is localized primarily in the membranes of osteoblasts and its biological half-life is from 1 to 2 days. Bone ALP is released from osteoblasts during bone formation but the mechanisms of bone ALP release into the extracellular fluid remain unclear. Bone ALP plays a role in osteoid formation and mineralization. It is reported that bone ALP measurements correlate with the rates of bone mineralization significantly [3]. Many techniques have been developed to quantitate bone ALP from total ALP such as heat inhibition, electrophoresis, precipitation, selective inhibition etc. Precipitation of bone ALP with wheat germ lectin is a simple technique to quantitate bone ALP and this method used to be used widely, but the method has poor reproducibility. Measurement of bone ALP using antibodies specific for this isoform has been developed recently. In these methods, the mass of the bone ALP is measured by an immunoradiometric assay or the activity is measured after capturing the bone ALP using specific antibodies immobilized onto a plate. These methods can be easily automated, have acceptable precision and the specificity is reasonable, although have 10-20% cross-reactivity with the liver isoform [1].

2.2. Bone matrix protein

Osteocalcin

Osteocalcin, also known as bone Gla-protein, is a 5.8kDa hydroxyapatite-binding protein which contains 49 amino acids in human. OC is a unique product of osteoblasts and odontoblasts [3,4] and is the most abundant non-collagenous protein in bone. Considering the predominance of osteoblasts, OC is highly specific for bone. OC contains 3 vitamin K-dependent γ-carboxyglutamic acid residues (Gla) which are responsible for the calcium-binding properties of the molecule. Although the function of OC in bone formation has yet to be fully cleared, OC is thought to be involved in the regulation of bone mineralization [5]. Approximately 30% of the newly synthesized OC is released into the circulation and the other 70% is incorporated into the bone matrix [7]. Circulating OC can be either released from osteoblasts directly during bone formation or released from bone matrix during bone resorption. The half-life of OC in serum is extremely short, only 4 minutes in rats, the circulating OC being cleared rapidly by glomerular filtration. It is proposed that retention of OC fragments occurs if the glomerular filtration rate is below 30 ml/min [7]. Evidence indicates that this circulating OC is a specific and sensitive index of bone formation and that serum OC correlates very well with the rate of bone formation as assessed by histomorphometry [7, 28]. The intact molecule represents about a third of the immunoreactivity of the potential circulating immunoreactive forms of OC in the adult serum/plasma. Another third is represented by several small fragments, and the final third by a large N-terminal midmolecule fragment 1-43 [6] (Figure 1).

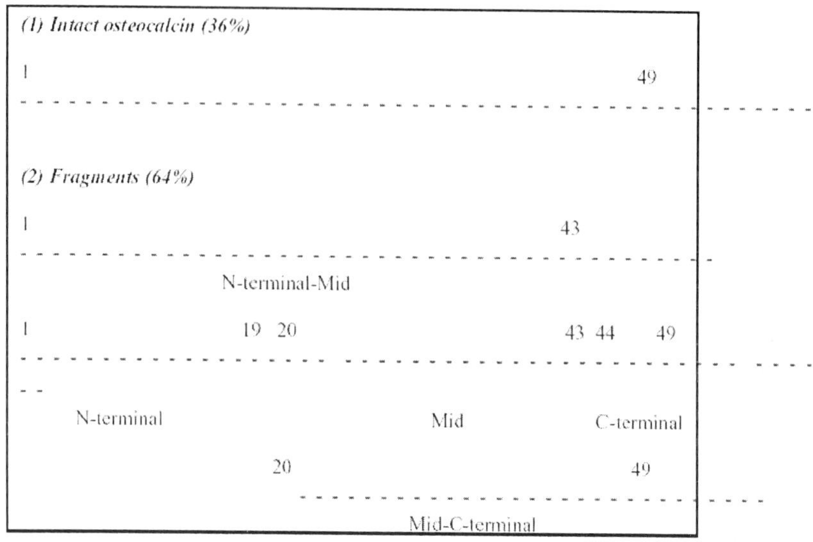

Figure 1. Fragments of circulating osteocalcin

It is not clear if the fragmentation of the intact molecule occurs in the blood, or in bone matrix during bone resorption, or both. To avoid problems associated with OC fragments in serum, newer assays are immunometricassays designed to measure either the intact molecule or a large N-terminal midregion fragment 1-43. The intact molecule is highly recommended for all studies dealing with human subjects. Storage of samples can lead to degradation of the peptides. Blood samples for OC assay is recommended to be collected on ice, and serum should be kept at - 20 °C for short-term storage and at - 70°C for long term storage [6]. Samples should be thawed only once to prevent degradation of fragments. As a large portion of OC is cleared by the kidneys, the serum concentration can be increased in renal failure. However, it must be borne in mind that there is increased bone turnover in chronic renal failure patients [4].

Procollagen type I caboxy- and amino-terminal propeptides

In bone, type I collagen makes up 90% of the organic matrix. Type I collagen is synthesized by osteoblasts and secreted as a procollagen precursor molecule. The procollagen molecule contains both C- and N-terminal extension peptides, which are cleaved by specific endoproteases before the formation of the collagen fibril and then released into the circulation (figure 2).

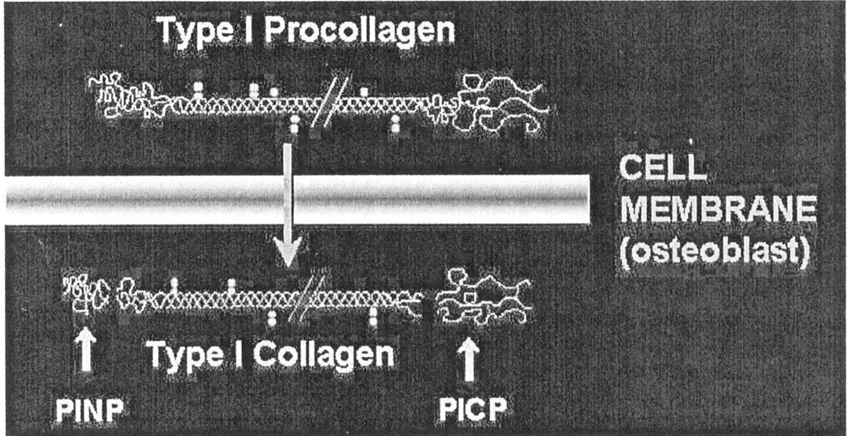

Figure 2. PINP and PICP are cleaved from type I procollagen

Both cleaved C- and N-terminal peptides (PICP and PINP) can be measured in circulation as markers of bone formation. PICP and PINP are not specific to bone because type I collagen is also existed in other issues such as in fibrocartilage and skin. Since the rate of bone turnover is way faster than collagen turnover in any other tissues, serum pool of PICP and PINP is assumed to reflect primarily type I collagen turnover in bone.

PICP has a serum half-life of 6-8 minutes. Both PICP and PINP are thought to be cleared from circulation through a specific receptors in the hepatic endothelial cells. Since serum PICP and PINP are not filtered at the glomerulus, their concentrations in serum are not affected by renal function. PICP and PINP are stable in serum and can be reliably measured by immunoassay in specimens which has been frozen and thawed a number of times. Clinically, however, it seems neither of them is as useful as bone ALP or OC because PICP and PINP are not sensitive to detect small changes in bone turnover such as those seen during menopause [8]. This may partly due to the inability of current assay to distinguish bone source PICP and PINP from other source PICP and PINP. Although both PICP and PINP can be found in the circulation, where their concentration in principle reflects the synthesis rate of type I collagen, the biochemical structure and metabolism may be different. PICP is cleaved shortly after synthesis, whereas part of the PINP can still be found on the surface of collagen fibres. It is possible that the removal of PINP regulates the further growth of the fibres. Compared to serum PICP, serum PINP appears to be more sensitive therefore serum PICP has been gradually replaced by serum PINP for the evaluation of type I collagen synthesis.

3. Biochemical markers of bone resorption

Bone resorption markers can be divided into 2 categories, enzyme products released from osteoclasts and type I collagen degradation products. Currently available markers of bone resorption are listed in table 2.

Table 2. Biochemical markers of bone resorption

Resorption Markers	Samples	Origin	Specificity
TRAP	blood	Bone	++
Oyp	urine	Bone, cartilage, dentin, blood vessel	+/-
Gal-Hyl	urine	bone, skin	++
Pyr	urine	bone, cartilage, dentin	+
D-Pyr	blood/urine	bone, cartilage, dentin	+++
NTx	blood/urine	bone, cartilage, dentin	+++
CTx	blood/urine	Bone, cartilage, dentin	+++
ICTP	blood	Bone , other tissues	+
Bone Sialoprotein	blood	bone, dentin	+

Tartrate-resistant acid phosphatase (TRAP) is an enzyme released from osteoclasts. Type I collagen degradation products include hydroxyproline (Hyp), galactosyl hydroxylysine (Gal-Hyl), pyridinoline (Pyr), deoxypyridinoline (D-Pyr), amino-terminal telopeptide of type I collagens (NTx) and carboxy-terminal telopeptide of type I collagen (CTx), and cross-linked C-telopeptide of type I collagen (ICTP). Bone sialoprotein (BSP) is a non collagen bone matrix degradation product which is reported to be potentially useful but not widely available.

3.1. Ezymes

Tartrate-resistant acid phosphatase

Acid phosphatases are lysosomal enzymes that are composed of several isoforms present primarily in bone, prostate, platelets, erythrocytes, and spleen etc. The bone acid phosphatase is resistant to L(+)-tartrate, whereas the prostatic isoenzyme is inhibited by this organic acid, TRAP is type 5 isoenzyme of acid phosphatase. TRAP may be resolved further into type 5a and type 5b, the latter appears to be specific to osteoclasts. Osteoclasts secrete TRAP during bone resorption therefore TRAP may be a useful marker of bone resorption. However, circulating TRAP can also be released from other cells such as macrophages. Serum TRAP can be measured by either kinetic methods based on resistance to tartrate or enzymatic assays based on antibodies raised against TRAP. Current assays cannot separate bone subform of TRAP from other subform of TRAP. Although TRAP has been reported preliminarily that it can be useful to assess bone resorption, TRAP has not been extensively studied as a marker of bone resorption in osteoporosis due to the lack of specificity of serum TRAP activity for bone, its instability in frozen samples, and the presence of enzyme inhibitors in serum.

3.2. Collagen degradation products

In bone matrix, 90% of collagen protein is type I collagen. Type I Collagen degradation products are commonly used biochemical markers of bone resorption. During bone resorption, these products of type I collagen degradation are released into the circulation and can be measured in blood or urine samples.

Hydroxyproline

Hyp is the predominant amino acid of type I collagen. About 85-90% of Hyp is liberated during the degradation of bone collagen which presents approximately half of the total body collagen. Hyp cannot be reutilized, therefore, circulating Hyp is derived from collagen breakdown. In the urine, 90% of Hyp appears in peptide-bound form [8]. Circulating Hyp can be measured as a marker of collagen breakdown by using colorimetric or high-performance liquid chromatography (HPLC) methods. However, Hyp is not specific to bone. Circulating Hyp can be from other sources as well, such as from skin and diet. Since diet Hyp contributes a large potion of circulating Hyp, measurement of the urinary Hyp has to be performed after 1-3 days of collagen-free diet. Because of its non-specificity in bone, Hyp has been largely replaced by more specific bone resorption markers.

Galactosyl Hydroxylysine

Hydroxylysine is produced by a post-translational modification of lysine during collagen synthesis. Hydroxylysine can undergo further modification by glycosylation giving rise to Gal-Hyl and glucosyl galactosyl hydroxylysine (Glu-Gal-Hyl). Gal-Hyl is released into circulation during type I collagen degradation but is not reutilized in type I pro-collagen synthesis. Gal-Hyl is 5-7 fold more concentrated in collagen of bone than in collagen of skin and measurements of Gal-Hyl are thought to reflect mainly resorption of bone collagen. Gal-Hyl predominates in bone where the ratio of Gal-Hyl/Glc-Gal-Hyl is 7:1, whereas in the skin the ratio of Gal-Hyl/Glc-Gal-Hyl is approximately 1:2. Since bone has much higher concentration of Gal-Hyl than skin does and diet does not influence on circulating Gal-Hyl, circulating Gal-Hyl can be used as a specific marker of bone resorption. Circulating Gal-Hay measured by HPLC has been reported to be a sensitive marker of bone resorption in studies in postmenopausal women and in patients with primary hyperparathyroidism [9].

Pyridinium crosslinks of collagen

Pyr and D-Pyr are the most important means of stabilizing collagenmoleculesby intramolecular cross-links. Pyr and D-Pyr are formed during the extracellular maturation of fibrillar collagen and are derived from non-reducible pyridinium cross-links found between neighboring mature collagen molecules (Figure 3).

Similar to Hyp and Gal-Hyl, Pyr and D-Pyr are liberated during the degradation of mature collagen. Pyr is found not only in type I collagen but also in type II collagen. Apart from bone, Pyr is found in cartilage, ligaments and vessels, the highest concentration being in cartilage [2]. Compared to Pyr, D-Pyr is less abundantly present in bone collagen, only 21% of the total cross-links is D-Pyr in bone collagen [3], but is highly specific to bone tissues. D-Pyr is present almost exclusively in bone even though a very small portion may from dentin. Pyr and D-Pyr are only found in mature collagen, the excretion of these molecules in the urine reflects degradation of mature collagen and are not reused following collagen degradation [2]. As cross-links released from collagen breakdown further metabolized in liver and kidney, 60% of cross-links are peptide-bound forms and 40% is in free forms in the urine. Pyr and D-Pyr can be measured by HPLC, enzyme immunoassay and automated imm unoassay. When using HPLC assay, total (free + peptide-bound) cross-links are measured following acid hydrolysis of urine sample. The free forms of D-Pyr can be detected by immunoassays. It is reported that D-Pyr, as a marker of bone resorption, is correlated very well with bone biopsy and calcium kinetics.

Cross-linked telopeptides of type I collagen

Specific crosslink-containing regions of type I collagen have also been isolated and can be measured in serum and urine as sensitive markers of bone resorption. These specific cross-link containing regions of type I collagen are called cross-linked telopeptides. Type I collagen has two cross-link forming sites, one in the amino-terminal and the other in the carboxy-terminal region of the molecule (see Figure 3). Immunoassays have been developed to measure NTx and CTx, (also known as Cross-laps) in serum and urine. Since NTx and CTx measured in serum are easy to handle for sample collection and do not require creatinine correction, it is believed serum assays have less variability as compared to urine assays. In addition to NTx and CTx, another specific crosslink-containing region of type I collagen is called cross-linked C-telopeptide of type I collagen (ICTP). ICTP can be measured by immunoassay in serum but this assay is poorly correlated with other bone turnover markers in osteoporosis and the component of ICTP is not fully characterized. Cross-links and specific cross-link containing regions of type I collagen including NTx, CTx and D-Pyr are currently considered the best markers for the assessment of bone resorption [10].

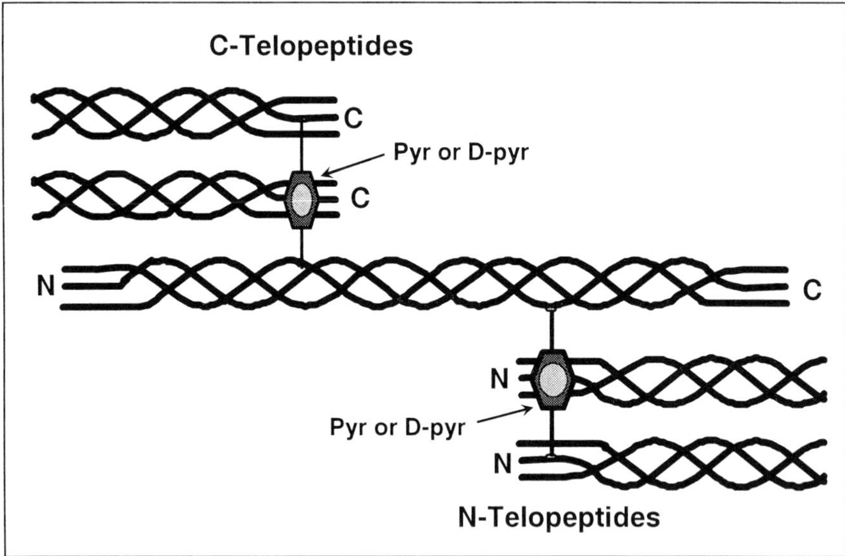

Figure 3. Type I collagen breakdown products as markers of bone resorption. Type I collagen molecules in the bone matrix are linked by pyridinoline crosslinks (Pyr or D-Pyr) in the region of N- and C-telopeptides.

3.3. Non collagen bone matrix degradation product

Bone sialoprotein

Bone sialoprotein (BSP) is a phosphorylated glycoprotein that accounts for 5-10% of the noncollagenous matrix of bone. Recent studies suggest serum BSP predominantly reflect processes related to bone resorption [11] but data are lacking to assess the utility of this new bone resorption marker.

4. Variability – a consideration when using biochemical markers

It is critical that variability should be taken into account when biochemical makers of bone turnover are used in osteoporosis clinically. Clinical interpretation of biochemical markers can be interfered by biological variability such as age and circadian rhythm, pathological variability such as drugs and diseases, and technical variability such as analytical precision and sample handling etc. (see table 3).

In an individual patient, ideally the changes generated from noise (variability) in biochemical markers over a period of follow-up should not be greater than the real biological changes, otherwise the statistical conclusion will be confounded by the noise. Hannon and Eastell have reviewed the variability of biochemical markers extensively to elucidate

Table 3. Variability in biochemical markers of bone turnover

Biological Variability	Pathological Variability	Technical Variability
Circadian	Fractures	Analytical precision
Day to day	Diseases	Sample handling
Food intake	Drugs	
Gender	Immobility	
Menstrual		
pregnancy		
lactation		
Seasonal		
Growth		
Aging		
Ethnicity		
Physical activity		

its importance in clinical interpretation of the results of biochemical markers [12]. In general, bone resorption markers are more variable than bone formation markers. Serum assays are usually less variable than urine assays. Analytical assay variability is small in comparison with biological and pathological variability.

Many biochemical markers of bone turnover, such as serum OC and PICP and urinary Pyr, D-Pyr, NTx and CTx [13-18], show a peak level in the early morning hours and a nadir in the afternoon and evening (figure 4).

This circadian paten can be established very early in life. Circadian rhythm in plasma OC is observed in 8 day old infant piglets [33] that parallel 2 months old human infants in terms of growth in body weight and length. Some biochemical markers of bone turnover such as serum bone ALP do not show a diurnal paten, possibly due to longer half-lives. Since the apparent circadian rhythms exist in most biochemical markers, the consistence of timing on sampling during a study is of important. Serum samples are recommended to be taken in the morning on a fasting status whereas a urinary sample collected in 24 hours is recommended for the measurement of urinary markers. If a 24 hour urine sample is not possible, the alternative is to collect a second void morning urine sample in which urinary creatinine (Cr) excretion should be measured to adjust for the levels of urinary biochemical marker excretion. Biochemical markers of bone resorption measured in urine, no matter collected from 24 hour urine or from morning second void urine, are predominantly expressed as a ratio to urinary Cr. Therefore, the variability in urinary Cr is largely contributed to the variability in biochemical markers measured in urine. Because urinary Cr excretion is primarily a function of muscle mass which may change remarkably within individuals over short or long term periods, therefore, it should be kept in mind that the percent change in urinary biochemical markers of bone resorption over the period of follow-up can be affected by Cr excretion. Apart from muscle mass, kidney function may also contribute to the changes in urinary Cr excretion. Recent developed biochemical markers of bone resorption measured in serum, NTx and CTx, may lead to lower variability because Cr correction is eliminated in these serum assays.

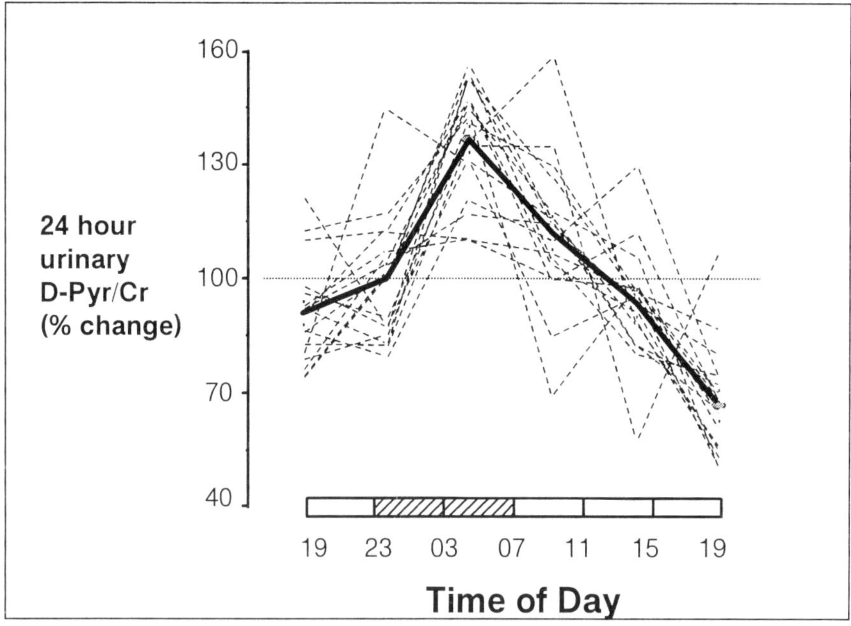

Figure 4. Twenty-four hour circadian rhythm in urinary D-Pyr/Cr, the thick solid line represents mean the doted lines individual data. The shaded are in x-axis represents night time.

Other commonly seen factors that contribute to the biological variability in biochemical markers of bone turnover are gender, age, menopause status, and ethnicity. These factors contribute to biological variability seen between individuals. When establish a normative reference data range for a biochemical marker, these factors have to be considered. Pathological variability in biochemical markers of bone turnover can be from various sources. Certain diseases, drug therapies and fractures are all contribute to the variability remarkably.

5. Clinical application of biochemical markers in osteoporosis

5.1. Monitoring response to antiresorptive drugs

Monitoring response to antiresorptive therapy is the best established clinical use for biochemical markers of bone turnover. Measurement of bone mineral density (BMD) is a traditional standard approach used to monitor bone response to treatment. However, bone mass changes slowly over time, it may take 12-24 months to detect a statistically significant change in BMD. Biochemical markers change more rapidly to therapeutic interventions than BMD does. In antiresorptive therapies, a significant reduction in biochemical markers of bone resorption usually can be observed in one month, whereas this reduction in biochemical markers of bone formation is usually observed a little late, in 2 to 3 months [19]. Studies show that the long term increase in bone mass is correlated with the short term decrease in biochemical markers of bone turnover measured during antisorptive therapy. It is reported that the

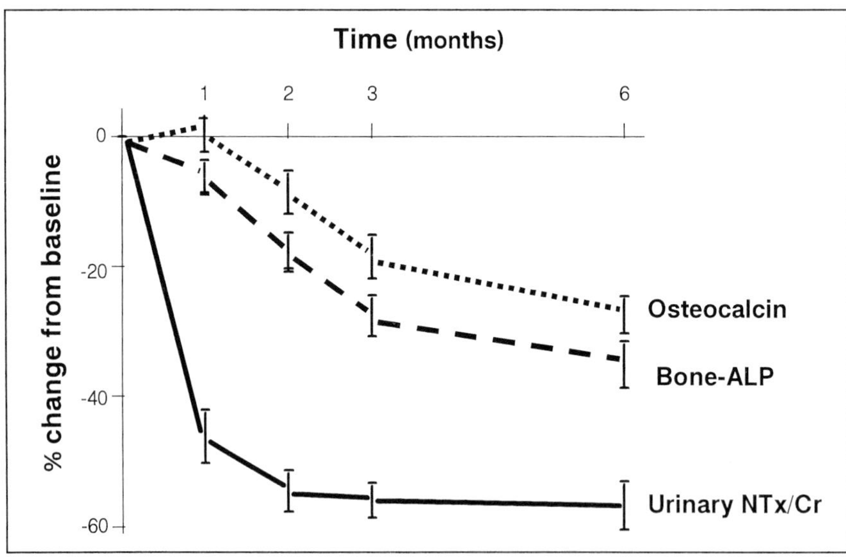

Figure 5, Changes in serum bone ALP and Osteocalcin and urinary NTx/Cr in patients with postmenopausal osteoporosis treated with risedronate. Values are means ± SEM.

decrease in biochemical markers of bone turnover in 3 to 6 months after the initiation of hormone replacement or bisphosphonates therapies correlate with increase in BMD at 2 years [20-23]. Further more, by using Receiver Operating Characteristic (ROC) analysis [22,23], biochemical markers of bone turnover can be used to monitor the BMD response at individual level in patients treated on HRT. In a 2-year risedronate treatment study [34], urinary NTx/Cr ratio decreased within one month and serum bone ALP decreased within 3 months after the initiation of risedronate treatment, and the reduction of biochemical markers remained constant during the full treatment course. Figure 5 shows a typical deduction in biochemical markers of bone turnover in postmenopausal women treated with oral risedronate.

It should be noted that this reduction in biochemical markers of bone turnover may not happen in a small proportion of patients who receive antiresorptive therapies. This may be an indication of noncompliance with therapy, or may indicate a need to change dose or therapy.

5.2. Other potential clinical applications

Unlike monitoring response to treatment, the potential uses of biochemical markers of bone in other clinical aspects are not well established.

Select therapy

For the treatment of osteoporosis, theoretically, patients with high bone turnover should be treated with antiresoptive agents whereas patients with low bone turnover status should be treated with anabolic agents. Currently, antiresorptive agents are most commonly used for the treatment of osteoporosis. Patients with high bone turnover are likely to respond to antiresorptive treatment better than patients with low bone turnover because inhibiting bone resorption will result in a larger transient increase in bone mass (filling of the remodeling space) in high-turnover patients than that in low-turnover patients [24]. In a recent study in women with postmenopausal osteoporosis (PMO) treated with risedronate [25], the magnitude of change in lumbar spine BMD was significantly greater in patients with baseline urinary deoxyperidinoline levels above the normative median. However it is not clear what practical implication the assessment of baseline bone turnover could have on treatment decision, since patients with low bone turnover also respond to antiresorptive agents and there is no study indicating that low-turnover patients should be treated with higher doses of antiresorptive drugs [24].

Prediction of bone mass and bone loss

Negative correlation between bone mass and bone turnover exists in PMO population [26], however, the attempt to use biochemical markers in predicting bone mass in individual women is not successful so far. A woman in her early postmenopausal stage may have both high bone turnover and high bone mass because her bone mass is cumulated in her life time whereas her bone turnover status is just altered by her recent menopause. It's not recommended to use biochemical markers of bone turnover for the purpose of predicting bone mass or diagnosing osteoporosis.

In women with PMO, it is generally agreed that accelerated bone loss after menopause is resulted from elevated bone turnover. Thus, an increase in bone turnover should be valuable for the prediction of future bone loss. Although it is debatable as to if biochemical markers of bone turnover can be used to predict the rate of bone loss, studies do show that biochemical markers of bone turnover measured at baseline are correlated with the loss of bone mass measured at different skeletal sites after up to 12 years [27-29]. By using traditional markers of bone turnover, serum total ALP and urinary hydroxyproline as a ratio to creatinine, Hansen and colleagues [29] reported the bone loss as predicted by baseline biochemical markers was very similar to the actual bone loss measured 12 years later. To help understand if biochemical markers are useful in predicting rate of bone loss, further longitudinal studies with newer biochemical markers of bone turnover are needed.

Prediction of fracture risk and fracture

More and more evidence has demonstrated that higher level of biochemical markers of bone turnover, particularly markers of bone resorption, measured at baseline is associated with a higher risk of osteoporotic fracture which may be independent of BMD and age [30,31]. In the EPIDOS and OFELY studies conducted in late postmenopausal women in Europe [30], patients with higher bone turnover status were found to have a higher risk of osteoporotic fracture. When the results of the EPIDOS and the OFELY studies are analyzed, sensitivity and specificity are of the same order of magnitude for biochemical markers as for BMD [32]. Recently, a study investigating the influence of baseline bone turnover on the incidence of vertebral fracture (rather than risk of fracture) was reported in women with PMO treated with placebo and risedronate [25]. In both placebo and the risedronate-treated groups, the proportion of patients with new vertebral fractures was higher in women with pretreatment bone resorption rate above than those below the normative median.

6. Conclusion

Bone turnover at whole body skeletal level cab be assessed non-invasively by using circulating biochemical markers of bone turnover. Biological, pathological and analytical variability of biochemical markers needs to be taken into account when bone turnover is evaluated by using biochemical markers. The best established use of biochemical markers of bone turnover is in the monitoring of treatment response. Recent data suggest that biochemical markers may be used to select patients for therapy and to predict bone loss/fracture risk.

REFERENCE

1. Price CP. Ann Clin Biochem 30:355-72 (1993)
2. Green S, Anstiss CL, Fishman WH. Enzymologia, 41:9-26 (1971)
3. Calvo MS, Eyre DR, Gundberg CM. Endocrinol Rev 17:333-68 (1996)
4. Price CP, Thompson PW. Ann Clin Biochem 32:1-17 (1995)

5.   Hauschka PV, Lian JB, Cole DE, Gundberg CM. Physiological Reviews, 69: 990-1047 (1989)

6.   Lee AJ, Hodges S, Eastell R. Ann Clin Biochem 37:432-46 (2000)

7.   Delmas PD. In: Riggs BL, Melton III LJ (eds). Osteoporosis, aetiology, diagnosis, and management (2nd ed). Lippincott-Raven, Philadelphia, pp319-334 (1995)

8.   Hassager C, Fabbri-Mabelli G, Christiansen C. Osteoporosis Int 3:50-2 (1993)

9.   Guo CY, Thomas WE, al-Dehaimi AW, Assiri AM, Eastell R. J Clin Endocrinol Metab, 81:3487-3491 (1996)

10. Delmas PD Eastell R, Garnero P, Seibel MJ, Stepan J. Osteoporosis Int 6:s2-17 (2000 suppl)

11. Seibel MJ, Woitge HW, Pecherstorfer M, Karmatschek M, Horn E, Ludwig H, Armbruster FP, Ziegler R. J Clin Endocrinol Metab, 81:3289-3294 (1996) Hanon R and Eastell R. Osteoporosis Int 6:s30-44 (2000)

12. Eastell R, Simmons PS, Colwell A, Clin Sci 83:375-82 (1992)

13. Delmas PD. Bone 13:S17-21 (1992)

14. Wichers M, Schmidt E, Bidlingmaier F, KlingmiHler D. Clin Chem 45:1858-60 (1999)

15. Hart SM, Eastell R. Curr Opin Nephrol Hypertens 8:421-7 (1999)

16. Hassager C, Risteli J, Risteli L, Jensen SB, Christiansen C. J Bone Minl Res, 7:1307-1311 (1992)

17. Blumsohn A, Herrington K, Hannon RA, Shao P, Eyre DR, Eastell R. J Clin Endocrinol Metab, 79: 730-735 (1994)

18. Garnero P, Shih WJ, Gineyts E, Karpf DB, Delmas PD. J Clin Endocrinol Met, 79:1693-1700 (1994)

19. Tromp AM, Ooms ME, Popp-Snijders C, Roos JC, Lipo P. Osteoporosis Int 11:134-40 (2000)

20. Greenspan SL, Rosan HN, Parker RA. J Clin Endocrinol Metab 85:3537-40 (2000)

21. Bjamason NH, Christiansan C. Bone 26:561-9 (2000)

22. Delmas PD, Hardy P, Garnero P, Dain M-P. Bone, 26:553-560 (2000)

23. Delmas PD. Osteoporosis Int 6:s66-7 (2000 suppl)

24. Seibel MJ, Naganathan V, Barton I, Grauer A. J Bone Min Res, 19:323-9 (2004)

25. Melton LJ 3rd, Khosla S, Atkinson EJ, O'Fallon WM, Riggs BL. J Bone Min Res, 12:1083-1091 (1997)

26. Marcus R, Holloway L, Wells B, Greendale G, James MK, Wasilauskas C, Kelaghan J. J Bone Min Res, 14:1583-1595 (1999)

27. Eastell R, Delmas PD, Hodgson SF, Eriksen EF, Mann KG, Riggs BL. J Clin Endocrinol Met, 67:741-748 (1988)

28. Hansen MA, Overgaard K, Riis BJ, Christiansen C. BMJ (Clinical Research Ed.), 303:961-964 (1991)

29. Garnero, P; Hausherr, E; Chapuy, M C; Marcelli, C; Grandjean, H; Muller, C; Cormier, C; Bréart, G; Meunier, P J; Delmas PD. J Bone Minl Res, 11:1531-1538 (1996)

30.   van Daele PL, Seibel MJ, Burger H, Hofman A, Grobbee DE, van Leeuwen JP, Birkenhäger JC, Pols HA. BMJ (Clinical Research Ed.), 312: 482-483 (1996)
31.   Garnero P. Osteoporosis Int 6:s55-65 (2000 suppl)
32.   Guo CY; Ward W, Cairns P, Atkinson S. Pediatric Res, 48;238-243 (2000)
33.   Fogelman I, Ribot C, Smith R; Ethgen D, Sod E, Reginster JY. J Clin Endocrinol Metab, 85:1895-1900 (2000)

CHAPTER 8

BONE MARROW ADIPOGENESIS IN OSTEOPOROSIS

Chao Wan and Gang Li

Department of Trauma and Orthopaedic Surgery,
School of Medicine, Queen's University Belfast,
Musgrave Park Hospital, Belfast, BT9 7JB, UK

Bone marrow adipogenesis is a postnatal event during bone and marrow development. In the adult bone, marrow adipocytes occupy the largest space of the marrow cavity, and serve as a source of energy, autocrine and paracrine factors. Marrow adipocyte share a common multipotential mesenchymal stem cell with other marrow stomal lineages, and functional overlap exists among them. In the marrow stroma microenvironment, adipogenesis is closely associated with osteogenesis, hematopoiesis and osteoclastogenesis. With ageing, increased marrow adipocytes accompany with decreased trabecular bone volume. Marrow adipogenesis may be an important complication of osteoporosis. Many regulators including hormones, growth factors, proinflammatory cytokines and their receptors such as nuclear hormone receptors, trans-memberane kinase receptors and G-protein coupled receptors are involved in the signaling pathway of adipogenesis, and may present potential molecular targets for the manipulation of adipocyte differentiation. Marrow adipocyte may be considered as an important target cell for the therapeutic intervention in osteoporosis. The inhibition of marrow adipogenesis and concomitant enhancement in osteogenesis may provide a potential approach to increase bone formation and therefore provide more efficacious prevention or treatment of osteoporosis.

1. Introduction

Bone marrow stromal system is composed of different stromal cell lineages, the uncommitted mesenchymal stem cells (MSCs), committed precursors and differentiated osteoblasts, adipocytes, and hematopoietic support stromal cells, among which the adipocytes occupy the largest space in the marrow cavity. Accumulated clinical and experimental research have shown that an increase in marrow adipocytes is associated with conditions that lead to bone loss or osteoporosis, such as aging [1, 2], disuse [3, 4], long-term glucocorticoid use [5], and ovariectomy [6, 7]. Adipogenesis may be an important complication of osteopenia or osteoporosis. The elucidation of the mechanisms of marrow adipogenesis and its regulation has great importance not only for the understanding of bone cell biology, but also for possible therapeutic intervention in osteoporosis and other metabolic bone diseases.

2. Adipogenesis during bone marrow development

In the bone marrow (BM), there are two related systems: the hematopoietic system, which is the major source of adult hematopoietic stem cells (HSCs) that renew the circulating blood elements, and the stromal system, which contains mesenchymal stem cells (MSCs or bone marrow stromal stem cells, BMSSCs) and contributes to the regeneration or renewal of mesenchymal tissues such as bone, cartilage, fat, tendon, muscle, and marrow stroma [8]. The changes of different phenotypes in marrow stromal system during development, growth, and aging appear in a temporal and spatial sequence along the direction of bone growth. It is well established that chondrogenesis, osteogenesis, pre-hematopoietic stroma, myelogenesis, and adipogenesis are subsequent phases in the history of bone and marrow development, among which only adipogenesis is a post-natal event [9]. According to Neumann's law, at birth, all bone marrow cavities are occupied by red haematopoietic marrow; at skeletal maturity, the whole of long bone diaphyseal marrow cavities is normally filled with yellow adipocytic marrow and red haematopoietic marrow is restricted to the cancellous bone of metaphyses and epiphyses. With aging, the number and size of marrow adipocytes increases in a linear manner [10]. It is estimated that approximately 30% of the proportion of marrow volume in the iliac crest is occupied by adipocytes in early adulthood, 60% or more at the age of 60 [11]. And up to 90% of the marrow cavity in long bones is occupied by adipocytes. Thus, bone marrow adipogenesis or adipocytic differentiation may be considered as the end point of bone development and aging. This also implies that there is a clinical correlation between the reduced bone forming capacity and the increased bone marrow adipogenesis.

3. Function of marrow adipocytes

In the adult bone marrow, the adipocytes occupy the largest space of marrow cavity, playing an important role in maintaining the marrow stroma or marrow microenvironment. A variety of potential functions of marrow adipocytes have been proposed, as listed in several elegant reviews [12, 13, 14], even though most of their functions need to be further investigated. It is hypothesized that adipocytes act as the "space fillers" for the marrow cavity, where is not required by active hematopoiesis. The changes in number and size of adipocytes occur as a function of changes in total hematopoietic component. As a component of hematopoietic supporting stroma, they exhibit an important role in the processes of lymphohematopoiesis [15-17]. Indeed, many adipocytic products including type 1 interferons (IFNs), prostaglandins (PGs), leptin, adiponectin, and sex steroids are known modulators of lymphohematopoiesis [18-25]. In addition to support lympho-hemaetopoiesis, preadipocytes or adipocytes support osteoclastogenesis [26-30], as several stromal adipocytic cell lines were shown to induce osteoclastogenesis. Adipocytes also play an active role in energy balance, they are not only lipid storing and mobilizing cells but produce or release a vast number of so called adipokines or adipocytokines, including metabolically active molecules belonging to different functional categories like endocrine function (leptin, sex steroids, various growth factors), metabolic function (fatty acids, adiponectin, resistin), and immunity (complement factors). Therefore, adipocytes in the marrow together with the extramedullary fat cells may serve as a source of energy, paracrine, or autocrine factors [31]. One of the examples, leptin, the adipocyte-derived hormone, has been identified as a powerful inhibitor of bone formation, and its effect is mediated via a brain relay, which suggests that a regulation network exists between the adipocytes and the brain [32, 33]. The marrow adipocytes also provide a localized energy reservoir for emergency situations such as blood loss which need to be recovered by hematopoiesis, or fractures which needs to be reunited by endochondral or intramemberanous ossification processes. Adipocytes may act as support cells for the differentiation of hematopoietic cells and as a source of osteoblasts during bone regeneration. With age, marrow adipogenesis increases when osteogenesis decreases, as osteoblast and adipocyte share a common multipotential precursor, and functional overlap exists between adipocytes and other stromal cell lineages in the bone marrow.

4. Transcriptional regulation of adipocyte differentiation

It is well established that several transcription factors control the signaling pathway of adipocyte differentiation, among which peroxisome proliferator-activated receptor $\gamma2$ (PPARγ2) and CCAATT enhancer-binding protein (C/EBP) were best characterized. PPARγ2 has been shown to express early in adipogenesis and act synergistically with CCAATT enhancer-binding protein (C/EBP) to regulate the adipocyte differentiation cascades [34, 35, 36]. PPARγ2 plays important roles in the regulation of adipocyte differentiation, its overexpression in fibroblast cell lines initiates adipogenesis [37] and ES cells and embryonic fibroblastic cells from mice lacking PPARγ2 were unable to differentiate into adipocytes [38-40]. Expression of C/EBP and/or PPARγ2 in fibroblasts converts the cells into adipocytes [37, 41, 42]. A combined expression of PPARγ2 and C/EBPα in G8 myoblastic cells suppresses muscle phenotype and induces adipocyte differentiation [43]. Homozygous PPARγ-deficient ES cells failed to differentiate into adipocytes, but spontaneously differentiated into osteoblasts, and the adipogenic potentials were restored by reintroduction of the PPARγ gene into the ES cells [44]. Another family of proteins are forkhead related activators (freac), among which the hepatic nuclear factor 3 (HNF3) controls the expression of lipoprotein lipase (LPL), an early adipocyte marker gene [45]. Adipocyte determination and differentiation-dependent factor 1 (ADD1) in the rat and sterol regulatory element binding protein 1 (SREBP-I) in the human [46], are shown to regulate transcription of the low density lipoprotein receptor gene. Recently, the transcription genes such as Zinc finger E-box binding protein (ZEB) and Zinc finger protein 145 (ZNF145) have been shown to regulate adipogenic differentiation of bone marrow derived MSCs [47]. A novel gene E2F5 transcriptional factor is also identified in differentiated adipocyte [48]. Adipocyte differentiation can not be identified solely by cellular morphological changes, but requires evidence of expression of phenotype specific genes. Several downstream adipocyte specific gene products are known to be involved in triglyceride synthesis, which include the early marker of adipocyte differentiation, LPL and the late markers such as glycerol-3-phosphate dehydrogenase (G-3-PD) [49] and the fatty acid binding protein aP2 [50, 51]. Using microarray technology, numbers of related genes are identified during adipogenesis [47, 48, 52-58].

5. Relationship between adipogenesis and osteogenesis

The relationship between adipogenesis and osteogenesis has confused the investigators for many years. Accumulated evidences have shown that an inverse relationship exists between adipocytes and osteoblasts. In 1970s, clinical studies on osteoporotic patients suggested that increased bone marrow adipocytes correlates with decreased trabecular bone volume [59]. Then it was found that ectopic bone formed by the "red" and "yellow" rabbit marrow are equally well, which suggested that both the "red" and "yellow" marrow might contain osteogenic cells [60]. Further investigation demonstrated that both rabbit adipocyte or fibroblast stromal colonies displayed an osteogenic capacity when implanted in diffusion chambers in vivo. The cells that have differentiated in an adipocytic direction are able to revert to a more proliferative stage and subsequently to differentiate along the osteogenic pathway [61]. In vitro, a large number of cell lines have been used to study adipogenesis, among them, the following are used extensively: BMS2 [62], UAMS33 [63],

2T3 [64], and the cell line derived from p53 null mice [65]. In these cell models, an inverse relationship exists between the differentiation of adipocytic and osteogenic cells, enhanced expression of adipocytic phenotype is paralleled with decreased expression of osteoblastic phenotype [66]. Human cell lines that have been used include MG63, exhibiting a proven adipogenic phenotype in vitro [67, 68]; and those transformed from osteoblasts or MSCs [69-72], as well as the primary MSCs, which can be expanded rapidly in culture. The human bone-derived cells when cultured in the presence of dexamethasone (Dex) and 3-isobutyl-1-methylxanthine (IBMX) will undergo adipogenic differentiation [73]. Recent studies demonstrated that trabecular bone-derived cells display stem cell-like capabilities, characterized by a stable undifferentiated phenotype as well as the ability to proliferate extensively while retaining the potential to differentiate along the osteoblastic, adipocytic, and chondrocytic lineages, even when maintained in long-term in vitro culture [74].

On the other hand, cloned adipocytes were found to be capable of dedifferentiation into fibroblast-like cells, and subsequently differentiate into two morphologically distinct cell types, osteoblasts and adipocytes [75]. Fat-derived stem cells were also successfully isolated from Lewis rats, and induced to differentiate along adipogenic and osteogenic lineages in vitro and in vivo [76]. These findings provide evidences of *trans*-differentiation between marrow adipocytes and osteoblasts. The terminally differentiated skeletal cells may be able to de-differentiate first, returning to the status of uncommitted stromal stem cells, then the cells differentiate along any other pathway. The plasticity and inter-relationship among the precursors or fully differentiated cells of the marrow stromal lineages may be of great important in understanding the progression of osteoporosis and other skeletal diseases.

6. Relationship between adipogenesis and hematopoiesis

As one of the major components of bone marrow stroma, adipocytes originate from the same MSCs that give rise to the hematopoiesis supporting stromal cells and have been suspected to influence hematopoiesis. The stromal cells secrete many extracellular matrix proteins including proteoglycans, fibronectin, tenascin, laminin, and express cell surface transmembrane proteins including CD36, CD44, integrins and vascular cell adhesion molecule (V-CAM), mediating adhesion between the stroma and the various blood cell lineages [77, 78]. The preadipocytes display some common marks with the stromal cells, and several preadipocyte stromal cell lines support both lymphopoiesis and myelopoiesis in vitro. In fact, many factors produced by adipocyte, such as type 1 IFNs, PGs, leptin, adiponectin, and sex steroids are known modulators of lymphohematopoiesis [18-25]. Recently, it is reported that adiponectin is produced by adipocytes within human bone marrow and has an inhibitory effect on adipocyte differentiation through a paracrine mechanism [79]. The protein suppresses myelomonocytic progenitor growth and macrophage functions in culture [80] and negatively and selectively influence lymphopoiesis through induction of PG synthesis [24]. These findings suggest new mechanisms for functional interactions between adipogenesis and hematopoiesis within bone marrow. However, patterns of cytokines made by mature adipocytes and preadipocyte stromal cells differ substantially [81]. The functions of these cytokines are partially affected by adipocyte differentiation, adipogenesis alters the expression of the extracellular matrix, membrane proteins, and cytokines in stromal cells. Adipocytes within bone marrow cavities interact with surrounding cells and support the microenvironment that regulate the differentiation of hematopoietic cells.

7. Relationship between adipogenesis and osteoclastogenesis

In addition to supporting hemaetopoiesis, marrow adipocytes support osteoclastogenesis. Osteoclasts are generally believed to derive from hemopoietic precursors in the bone marrow, but their differentiation pathway is complex. Several stromal adipocytic cell lines were employed to investigate the relationship between adipocytogenesis and osteoclastogenesis. When cocultured with preadipocyte or adipocyte-enriched BMS2 stromal layers, primary bone marrow cells undergo osteoclast differentiation and maturation [82]. TMS-14 is a line of preadipocytes that supports osteoclast-like cell formation without any other bone resorbing factors. When treated with thiazolidinedione, a ligand and activator of PPARγ, the ability of TMS-14 cells to support osteoclastogenesis was prevented, together with inhibiting gene expression of osteoclast differentiation factor (ODF, also called OPGL, RANKL, and TRANCE) [83]. Using the myeloblast (M1) cells and the 14F1.1 endothelial-adipocyte stromal cell line coculture system, it was demonstrated that marrow endothelial-adipocytes may play a role in regulating the differentiation of myeloblasts into osteoclasts [84]. MC3T3-G2/PA6 cells are preadipocytes similar to bone marrow derived stromal cells, and their adipose conversion is induced by glucocorticoids. The research on coculture of PTH-prestimulated long bone cells and MC3T3-G2/PA6 cells suggested that stromal preadipocytes may create a microenvironment conductive to osteoclastogenesis through direct cell-to-cell contact and communication [85]. The soluble factors released by stromal cell lines such as M-CSF and complement component C3 are also involved in osteoclastogenesis. The presence of 1,25 dihydroxyvitamin or adipogenic agonists (hydrocortisone, indomethacin, methylisobutylxanthine) induces stromal cell production of complement C3 [86-88]. The adipocytes may also serve an active role in the energy metabolism of the resorbing osteoclasts where fatty acid oxidation appears to be the major source of acetyl-CoA to support a predominantly oxidative metabolism [89].

Recently, α-Melanocyte-stimulating hormone (α-MSH), a 13-amino acid peptide produced in the brain and pituitary gland, stimulated osteoclastogenesis, whereas its production is regulated by leptin, a factor that is secreted by adipocytes [90]. The P6 strain of senescence-accelerated mice (SAM) exhibit an early decrease in bone mass with a reduction in bone remodeling. In the bone marrow, suppressed osteoblastogenesis and osteoclastogenesis with enhanced adipogenesis are observed in SAM mice[91]. Interleukin-11 (IL-11) has been shown to potentialy inhibit adipogenesis and to stimulate osteoclastogenesis. Menatetrenone (MK4), a vitamin K(2) with four isoprene units specifically inhibit adipogenesis and osteoclastogenesis of bone marrow cells[92]. Thus, a complex regulation network exists between marrow adipocyte and osteoclastogenesis.

8. Regulators and receptors for regulating adipogenesis and their therapeutic potentials for osteoporosis

Based on the fact that aging is associated with a reciprocal decrease of osteogenesis and an increase of adipogenesis in bone marrow and that adipocytes and osteoblasts share a common multipotential mesenchymal stem cell, with a conversion relationship existing between them, marrow adipocyte may be considered as a target cell for the prevention and treatment of osteoporosis. However, the regulation of adipogenesis is very complex, and many factors are involved in the regulation pathway of adipocyte differentiation. A series of studies have shown that several hormones, cytokines or growth factors are important regulators for adipocyte differentiation, such as steroid hormones, estrogen, androgen, growth hormone (GH), leptin , 1,25 dihydroxyvitamin D, transforming growth factor-β (TGF-β) related cytokines, and some proinflammatory cytokines. These regulators may mediate cytokine communication networks between adipocytes and osteoblasts. Some receptors involved in the regulation pathway, such as nuclear hormone receptors, trans-memberane kinase receptors, and G-protein coupled receptors are also found expressed on marrow stromal cells and adipocytes, these may present potential molecular targets for the manipulation of adipogenesis. In particular, in vitro and in vivo studies have demonstrated that ligands binding to the PPARs, glutococorticoid, estrogen, androgen, and vitamin D_3 receptors regulate bone marrow stromal cell adipogenesis and osteogenesis [17, 62, 93-95].

8.1 Glucocorticoids and glucocorticoid receptor

It is well konwn that high dose glucocorticoid treatment results in osteopenia or osteonecrosis in vivo. Dexamethasone and other glucocorticoids stimulate adipocyte differentiation in vitro [96, 97]. For example, human trabeculae derived osteoblasts and marrow derived MSCs are induced to express adipocyte phenotype by Dex and IBMX treatment [73, 98]. However, dexamethasone also induce expression of osteoblast-specific mRNAs including alkaline phosphatase, osteopontin, osteocalcin, decorin, biglycan [99, 100]. The complex effects of glucocorticoid on osteogenesis and adipogenesis suggest that physiological or pharmacological glucocorticoid activities may play important roles in maintaining bone health.

Glucocorticoid receptor may also mediate the process of adipocyte differentiation. It is demonstrated that glucocorticoids potentiate the early steps of preadipocyte differentiation and promote obesity in Cushing's syndrome and during prolonged steroid therapy. In vitro, glucocorticoids stimulate extrameullary 3T3 L1 preadipocyte differentiation through a non-transcriptional mechanism, mediated through the ligand-binding domain of the glucocorticoid receptor. This enhanced the onset of CCAAT/enhancer binding protein (C/EBPα) expression by potentiating its initial transcriptional activation by C/EBPβ [101]. It is postulated that the same response exist for the preadipocytes in the marrow. The modulation of glucocorticoid receptor signaling may contribute to the therapeutic intervention in osteoporosis.

8.2 1, 25 dihydroxyvitamin D and vitamin D receptor (VDR)

Though 1,25 dihydroxyvitamin D was identified as a osteoblast-inducing factor, the effects of 1,25 dihydroxyvitamin D on adipogenesis remain controversial. In primary rat calvarial cultures, 1,25 dihydroxyvitamin D, alone or in combination with dexamethasone stimulates adipogenesis [102]. In contrast, the addition of 1,25 dihydroxyvitamin D with glucocorticoids inhibits adipogenesis in MC3T3-G2/PA6 (PA6) cells, a preadipocytic stromal cell line from newborn mouse [103]. Using the multipotent murine bone marrow stromal cell line, BMS2, and its subclones, as well as primary-derived murine bone marrow stromal cell cultures, it shows that 1,25(OH)2D3 blocked adipogenesis induced by hydrocortisone, IBMX, and indomethacin. At nanomolar concentrations, 1,25(OH)2D3, completely inhibits murine bone marrow stromal cell differentiation into adipocytes in response to glucocorticoid-based adipogenic agonists [62]. Like PA6 and 3T3-L1 cells, adipogenesis in stromal ST2 cells was inhibited by 1,25-dihydroxyvitamin D3, as well as retinoic acid, tumour necrosis factor-α (TNF-α), and TGF-β [104]. However, studies on the effects of nuclear vitamin D(3) receptor (VDR) on adipogenesis are lacking. Some reported that VDR represses the transcriptional activity of PPARα but not PPARγ in a 1,25(OH)2D3-dependent manner, VDR signaling might be considered as a factor regulating lipid metabolism via PPARα pathway [105]. This suggests that VDR signaling may be involved in the regulation of adipogenesis, and it needs further investigation.

8.3 Estrogen, its analogs, and estrogen receptor

Estrogen exhibits osteogenic agonist and adipogenic antagonist properties. In ovariectomized rat and canine models, decreased estrogen levels result in reduced bone volume, increased bone erosion surfaces, and increased marrow fat volume [106, 107]. Few studies have addressed the effects of exogenous estrogen on bone marrow adipocytes. However, treatment with exogenous estrogen reduces the size and metabolic activity of rat extramedullary adipocytes [108]. It is postulated that arrow adipocytes may exhibit a similar response. Using a mouse clonal cell line KS483, it showed that 17 β-estradiol (E2) stimulates the differentiation of progenitor cells into osteoblasts and concurrently inhibits adipocyte formation in an estrogen receptor (ER)-dependent way [109]. Treatment with bone morphogenetic protein-2 (BMP-2) stimulated both osteoblastic and adipocytic differentiation in a mouse bone marrow stromal cell line, ST-2, overexpressing either human ER α (ST2ERα) or ER β (ST2ER β). When treated with E2, alkaline phosphatase activity was enhanced and lipid accumulation suppressed in these cells, and these effects were completely reversed by an ER antagonist, ICI182780 [110].

Recently, phytoestrogens have been considered as a canditate for the purposes of intervention in osteoporosis. Phytoestrogen genistein was shown to enhance the differentiation of bone marrow stromal cells to the osteoblast lineage while reducing adipogenic differentiation and maturation via an ER-dependent mechanism, involving autocrine or paracrine TGF-β1 signaling [111]. However, the biological actions of genistein are complex. At low concentrations, genistein acts as estrogen, stimulating osteogenesis and inhibiting adipogenesis. At high concentrations, it acts as a ligand of PPARγ, leading to up-regulation of adipogenesis and down-regulation of osteogenesis [112]. Daidzein, one of the main soy phytoestrogens, was also shown to activate different amounts of ERs and PPARs, and the balance of the divergent actions of ERs and PPARs determines daidzein-induced osteogenesis and adipogenesis [113]. These findings may explain distinct effects of phytoestrogen in different tissues.

8.4 Growth hormone (GH) and growth hormone receptor (GHR)

Growth hormone (GH) has diverse effects on adipose tissue. GH inhibits adipocyte differentiation, reduces triglyceride accumulation and increases lipolyses, which in turn reduce adipose tissue mass [114]. Also, GH stimulates bone growth and mineralization by direct effects on chondrocytes and osteoblasts. In GH-deficient dwarf (dw/dw) rats, marrow adipocyte numbers were increased 5-fold and adipocyte cell size was also increased by 20%, these values returned toward normal in dw/dw rats when given GH treatment but not with insulinlike growth factor-1 (IGF-1) treatment [115]. These results suggest that GH has a specific action on marrow adipocytes that is not simply due to altered bone or fat metabolism. The adipocyte population in bone marrow is an important primary target for GH. Administration of GH to a patient with severe osteopenia resulted in an increase in biochemical markers of bone formation, osteoid and osteoblast surface and also clearly decreased adipocyte number and size [116]. Both preadipocytes and mature adipocytes possess specific GH receptors; GH may mediate its actions via these receptors, but some effects are indirectly mediated through the secretion of IGF-1 [115]. In long-term marrow stromal cells culture system, it shows that GH-receptor is present in proliferating progenitor cells, myofibroblast-like cells, large reticular fibroblast cells, adipocytes and endothelial cells [117]. This implies that GH may regulate marrow stromal cell lineages directly via its receptor pathway.

8.5 *PTH, PTHrP, and PTH/PTHrP receptor or G-protein coupling receptor*

PTH and PTHrP have been shown to have potent anabolic effects on bone. Clinically relevant doses of PTH have been documented to increase the rate of bone turnover in vivo by stimulating new bone formation in rats, monkeys, and humans, with little or no stimulation of bone resorption activity [118-123]. Young heterozygous mice carrying a targeted PTHrP-null allele display a premature form of osteoporosis characterized by decreased trabecular bone volume and increased bone marrow adiposity [124]. Both PTHrP and PTH/PTHrP receptor are expressed in cells of the adipocytic lineage [125]. In a nonhuman primate ovariectomy (OVX) model, teriparatide PTH(1-34) increased bone mass, enhanced bone structural architecture, and strengthened the hip, despite increasing cortical porosity; at the cellular level, adipocyte number reduced and osteoblast number increased [126]. In vitro, PTHrP could direct osteoblastic commitment of pluripotent mesenchymal cell line C3H10T(1/2) by increasing the expression of markers of the osteoblastic phenotype. Also, PTHrP can increase MAPK activity in 3T3-L1 cells via the PKA pathway, thereby enhancing PPARγ phosphorylation and inhibiting the expression of adipocyte-specific genes [127, 128]. Signal transduction through the parathyroid hormone receptor requires G-protein coupling. In early studies, modulation of Gs alpha activity has been shown to effect differentiation of fibroblasts to adipocytes [129]. Some rare metabolic disorders, such as progressive osseous heteroplasia (POH), exhibiting heterotopic bone formation in subcutaneous adipose tissue [130], and McCune-Albright syndrome, displaying impaired stroma development including adipogenesis [131, 132], are caused by the mutations in G-protein. Taken together, a novel mechanism for the anabolic action of PTH, PTHrP, and their analogs may be the inhibition of adipogenesis within the bone marrow. G-proteins, may therefore, be a potential target for therapeutic intervention in osteoporosis.

8.6 *Leptin and leptin receptor*

Bone marrow adipocytes may also provide a source of paracrine factors, regulating osteoblastogenesis and adipogenesis [133, 134]. The obvious example is leptin, which is known to be secreted by both extramedullary adipocytes and marrow adipocytes, a cytokine that activates a stromal cell transmembrane tyrosine kinase receptor [135, 136]. Leptin exerted a negative correlation with bone mass, dependent on serum insulin levels, whereas adiponectin did not exert any effect on bone mineral density (BMD); adipocyte derived circulating leptin is considered as a determinant of bone mass [137, 138]. Increasing serum leptin level dramatically reduces bone mass, while reducing serum leptin level by overexpressing a soluble receptor for leptin increases bone mass [136]. In vivo studies using leptin (ob/ob) and leptin receptor (db/db) -deficient mice show that functional blockade of the leptin-signaling pathway in db/db mice is associated with increased bone mass. Intracerebroventricular infusion of leptin to the leptin-deficient (ob/ob) mice causes bone loss, suggesting that leptin regulates bone formation through a central nervous system pathway [32, 33]. Moreover, marrow tissue from the femora of ob/ob mice also shows a marked increase in adipocyte number compared to that of normal mice, and few adipocytes are observed in bone marrow from lumbar vertebrae, suggesting that the ob/ob mouse may be a useful animal model for studying the relationship between bone marrow adipogenesis and osteopenia or osteoporosis [139]. In vitro studies demonstrated that leptin promotes differentiation of human mesenchymal stem cells into osteoblasts rather than adipocytes [136, 140]. This may suggest that the effect of leptin on bone is mediated through both the central nervous system and peripheral receptors at the stromal cell level.

8.7 *TGF-βs, BMPs and their receptors*

Transforming growth factor-Beta (TGF-β) family members, including TGF-βs and bone morphogenetic proteins (BMPs), play important roles in directing committment and differentiation of mesenchymal stem cells.

TGF-β family members signal via specific serine/threonine kinase receptors and their nuclear effectors, named Smad proteins. While TGF-β is a potent adipogenic antagonist at all concentration [141], BMPs exhibit a dose dependent action in vitro [142, 143]. It is demonstrated that both bone marrow stromal preadipocytes and adipocytes express receptors for the BMPs and other related TGF-β family members [144, 145]. Recent evidence shows that TGF-β provide competence for early stages of chondroblastic and osteoblastic differentiation, with inhibiting myogenesis, adipogenesis, and late-stage osteoblast differentiation, and BMPs also inhibit adipogenesis and myogenesis [146]. Another TGF-β family member, Myostatin, was demonstrated to prevent BMP7 but not BMP2 mediated adipocytic differentiation by binding to its receptors. BMP7-induced heteromeric receptor complex formation was blocked by myostatin through competition for the common type II receptor, ActRIIB, suggesting that myostatin may be an important regulator of adipogenesis [147]. BMP Type IB and IA receptors play essential roles for commitment and differentiation of osteoblasts and adipocytes. Introduction of a constitutively active BMP type IB receptor forces stromal cells to differentiate into osteoblasts. In contrast, introduction of the constitutively active BMP type IA receptor forces the same cells to undergo adipocyte differentiation. Moreover, expression of truncated BMPR-IA suppresses PPARγ mRNA expression, and expression of truncated BMPR-IB enhances PPARγ mRNA expression [148]. These findings suggest that PPARγ may be one of the important downstream target genes for BMPR-IA signaling during adipocyte differentiation.

8.8 Proinflammatory factors and gp130 containing receptors

In the bone marrow microenvironment, many proinflammatory cytokines are involved in regulating adipogenesis, bone resorption and remodeling [149]. Among them, TNFα and IL-1 are mainly from macrophage-lineage cells, and both of them are potent adipogenic antagonists. Recent evidence shows that expression of IL-1 and TNF-α in bone marrow may alter the fate of pluripotent mesenchymal stem cells, directing cellular differentiation towards osteoblasts rather than adipocytes by suppressing PPARγ function through NF-kappaB activated by the TAK1/TAB1/NIK cascade [150]. Cytokines that share the gp130 protein in their receptor complex, including IL-6, IL-11, leukemia inhibitory factor (LIF), oncostatin M and ciliary neurotrophic factor, are mainly secreted by stromal-derived cells. These cytokines exhibit a potential autocrine effect, inhibiting stromal cell adipogenesis in a dose dependent manner in vitro [151]. It is demonstrated that IL-11 stimulated transcription of the target gene for BMP via STAT3, leading to osteoblastic differentiation in the presence of BMP-2, but inhibited adipogenesis in bone marrow stromal cells [152]. Preadipocyte, bone marrow and calvarial-derived stromal cells express receptor complexes containing the gpl30 protein [153], suggesting that some of the proinflammatory cytokines may serve as stimulatory factors for bone formation and inhibitors for adipogenesis, possibly via gp130 containing receptors signaling pathway.

9. Summary

Based on the evidence presented, osteoporosis may be attributable to increased adipogenesis at the expense of osteogenesis. Marrow adipogenesis exhibits a complex relationship with osteogenesis, hematopoiesis, and osteoclastogenesis. Marrow adipocyte may be considered as a crucial target cell for the therapeutic intervention in osteoporosis, and the signaling pathways implicated in the process of adipogenesis may become potential molecular targets for drug design. The key point, however, is to identify specific molecular targets that inhibit marrow adipogenesis and concomitantly increase osteoblastogenesis with no adverse effects on extramedullary tissues. The inhibition of marrow adipogenesis and concomitant enhancement in osteogenesis may provide a potential approach to enhance overall osteogenesis and bone mass, and therefore, as a stand-alone therapy or in combination with an antiresorptive medication, may provide more efficacious prevention or treatment of osteoporosis.

REFERENCES

1. Burkhardt, R, Kettner, G, Bohm, W, Schmidmeier, M, Schlag, R, Frisch, B, Mallmann, B, Eisenmenger, W, and Gilg, T, Bone, 8 (1987).
2. Justesen, J, Stenderup, K, Ebbesen, EN, Mosekilde, L, Steiniche, T, Kassem, M, Biogerontology, 2 (2001).
3. Minaire, P, Meunier, PJ, Edouard, C, Bernard, J, Courpron, J, and Bourret, J, Calcif Tiss Res, 17 (1974).
4. Jee, WSS, Wronski, TJ, Morey, ER, and Kimmel, DB, Am J Physiol, 244 (1983).
5. Kawai, K, Tamaki, A and Hirohata, K, J Bone Joint Surg Am, 67 (1985).
6. Martin, RB, Chow, BD, and Lucas, PA, Calcif Tiss Int, 46 (1990).
7. Martin, RB and Zissimos, SL, Bone, 12 (1991).
8. Pittenger, MF, Mackay, AM, Beck, SC, Jaiswal, RK, Douglas, R, Mosca, JD, Moorman, MA, Simonetti, DW, Craig, S, Marshak, DR, Science, 284 (1999).
9. Bianco, P and Riminucci, M, In Marrow stromal cell culture, Ed. Beresford, JN and Owen, ME (Cambridge University Press, Cambridge, United Kingdom, 1998), p19-23.
10. Neumann, E, Centr Med Wiss, 20 (1882).
11. Custer, RP and Ahlfeldt, FE, J Lab Clin Med, 17 (1932).
12. Gimle, JM, New Biol, 2 (1990).
13. Gimble, JM, Robinson, CE, Wu, X and Kelly, KA, Bone, 19 (1996).
14. Nuttall, ME and Gimble, JM, Bone, 27 (2000).
15. Tavassoli, M, Exp Hematol, 12 (1984).
16. Pietrangeli, CE, Hayashi, S and Kincade, PW, Eur J Immunol, 18 (1988).
17. Gimble, JM, Youkhana, K, Hua, X., Bass, H, Medina, K, Sullivan, M, Greenberger, J and Wang, CS, J Cell Biochem, 50 (1992).
18. Wang, J, Lin, Q, Langston, H and Cooper MD, Immunity, 3 (1995).
19. Shimozato, T and Kincade PW, J Immunol, 158 (1997).
20. Shimozato, T and Kincade, PW, Cell Immunol, 198(1999).
21. Umemoto, Y, Tsuji, K, Yang, FC, Ebihara, Y, Kaneko, A, Furukawa, S and Nakahata, T, Blood, 90 (1997).
22. Mazur, EM, Richtsmeier, WJ and South, K, J Interferon Res, 6 (1986).
23. Ouchi, N, Kihara, S, Arita, Y, Okamoto, Y, Maeda, K, Kuriyama, H, Hotta, K, Nishida, M, Takahashi, M and Muraguchi, M, et al, Circulation, 102 (2000).
24. Yokota, T, Meka, CS, Kouro, T, Medina, KL, Igarashi, H, Takahashi, M, Oritani, K, Funahashi, T, Tomiyama, Y, Matsuzawa, Y and Kincade, PW, J Immunol, 171 (2003).

25. Kincade, PW, Medina, KL and Smithson, G, Immunol Rev, 137 (1994).

26. Dodds, RA, Gowen, M, and Bradbeer, JN, J Histochem Cytochem, 42 (1994).

27. Hussain, MM, Mahley, RW, Boyles, JK, Lindquist, PA, Brecht, WJ and Innerarity, TL, J Biol Chem, 264 (1989).

28. Sakaguchi, K, Morita, I and Murota, S, Prostaglandins Leukot Essent Fatty Acids, 62 (2000).

29. Benayahu, D, Peled, A and Zipori, D, J Cell Biochem, 56 (1994).

30. Kelly, KA, Tanaka, S, Baron, R, and Gimble, JM, Endocrinology, 139(1998).

31. Klaus, S, Curr Drug Targets, 5 (2004).

32. Ducy, P, Amling, M, Takeda, S, Priemel, M, Schilling, AF, Beil, FT, Shen, J, Vinson, C, Rueger, JM, and Karsenty, G, Cell, 100 (2000).

33. Elefteriou, F and Karsenty G, Pathol Biol (Paris), 52 (2004).

34. Tontonoz, P, Hu, E, Graves, RA, Budavari, AI and Spiegelman, BM, Genes Dev, 8(1994).

35. Chawla, A, Schwartz, EJ, Dimaculangan, DD and Lazar, MA, Endocrinology, 135 (1994).

36. Birkenmeier, EH, Gwynn, B, Howard, S, Jerry, J, Gordon, JI, Lanschulz, WH, and McKnight, SL, Genes Dev, 3 (1989).

37. Tontonoz, P, Ha, E and Spiegelman, BM, Cell, 79 (1994).

38. Barak, Y, Nelson, MC, Ong, ES, Jones, YZ, Ruiz-Lozano, P, Chien, KR, Koder, A, Evans, RM, Mol Cell, 4 (1999).

39. Kubota, N, Terauchi, Y, Miki, H, Tamemoto, H, Yamauchi, T, Komeda, K, Satoh, S, Nakano, R, Ishii, C, Sugiyama, T, Eto, K, Tsubamoto, Y, Okuno, A, Murakami, K, Sekihara, H, Hasegawa, G, Naito, M, Toyoshima, Y, Tanaka, S, Shiota, K, Kitamura, T, Fujita, T, Ezaki, O, Aizawa, S and Kadowaki, T, et al, Mol Cell, 4 (1999).

40. Rosen, ED, Sarraf, P, Troy, AE, Bradwin, G, Moore, K, Milstone, DS, Spiegelman, BM and Mortensen, RM, Mol Cell, 4 (1999).

41. Freytag, SO, Paielli, DL and Gilbert, JD, Genes Dev, 8 (1994).

42. Lin, FT and Lane, MD, Proc Natl Acad Sci USA, 91 (1994).

43. Hu, E, Tontonoz, P and Spiegelman, BM, Proc Natl Acad Sci USA, 92 (1995).

44. Akune, T, Ohba, S, Kamekura, S, Yamaguchi, M, Chung, UI, Kubota, N, Terauchi, Y, Harada, Y, Azuma, Y, Nakamura, K, Kadowaki, T and Kawaguchi, H, J Clin Invest, 113 (2004).

45. Tontonoz, P, Kim, JB, Graves, RA, and Spiegelman, BM, Mol Cell Biol, 13 (1993).

46. Yokoyama, C, Wang, X, Briggs, MR, Admon, A, Wu, J, Hua, X, Goldstein, JL and Brown, MS, Cell, 75 (1993).

47. Sekiya, I, Larson, BL, Vuoristo, JT, Cui, JG, Prockop, DJ, J Bone Miner Res, 19 (2004).

48. Burton, GR and McGehee, RE, J Nutrition, 20 (2004).

49. Wise, LS and Green, H, J Biol Chem, 254 (1979).

50. Ailhaud, G, Grimaldi, P and Negrel, R, Annu Rev Nutr, 12 (1992).

51. Spiegelman, BM, Trends Genetics, 4 (1988).
52. Urs, S, Smith, C, Campbell, B, Saxton, AM, Taylor, J, Zhang, B, Snoddy, J, Jones Voy, B and Moustaid-Moussa, N, J Nutr, 134 (2004).
53. Burton, GR, Nagarajan, R, Peterson, CA, McGehee, RE Jr, Gene, 329 (2004).
54. Seshi, B, Kumar, S and King, D, Blood Cells Mol Dis, 31 (2003).
55. Ross, SE, Erickson, RL, Gerin, I, DeRose, PM, Bajnok, L, Longo, KA, Misek, DE, Kuick, R, Hanash, SM, Atkins, KB, Andresen, SM, Nebb, HI, Madsen, L, Kristiansen, K and MacDougald, OA, Mol Cell Biol, 22 (2002).
56. Burton, GR, Guan, Y, Nagarajan, R and McGehee, RE Jr, Gene, 293 (2002).
57. Boeuf S, Klingenspor, M, Van Hal, NL, Schneider, T, Keijer, J and Klaus, S, Physiol Genomics, 7 (2001)
58. Guo, X and Liao, K, Gene, 251 (2000)
59. Meunier, P, Aaron, J, Edward, C, and Vignon, G, Clin Orthop, 80 (1971).
60. Tavassoli, M and Crosby, WH, Science, 169 (1970).
61. Bennett, JH, Joyner, CJ, Triffit, JT, and Owen, ME, J Cell Sci, 99 (1991).
62. Kelly, KA and Gimble JM, Endocrinology, 139 (1998).
63. Lecka-Czernik, B, Gubrij, I, Moerman, EJ, Kajkenova, O, Lipschitz, DA, Manolagas, SC and Jilka, RL, J Cell Biochem, 74 (1999).
64. Ghosh-Choudhury, N, Windle, JJ, Koop, BA, Harris, MA, Guerrero, DL, Wozney, JM, Mundy, GR and Harris, SE, Endocrinology, 137 (1996).
65. Thompson, DL, Lum, KD, Nygaard, SC, Kuestner, RE, Kelly, KA, Gimble, JM and Moore EE, J Bone Miner Res, 13 (1998).
66. Beresford, JN, Bennet, JH, Devlin, C, Leboy, PS, and Owen, ME, J Cell Sci, 102 (1992).
67. Nuttall, ME, Olivera, DL and Gowen, M, J Bone Miner Res, 9 (Suppl l)A (1994).
68. Patton, AJ, Olivera, DL, Nuttall, ME, and Gown, M, J Bone Miner Res, 10 (Suppl l) (1995).
69. Bodine, PV, Trailsmith, M and Komm, BS, J Bone Miner Res, 11 (1996).
70. Colter, DC, Sekiya, I and Prockop, DJ, Proc Natl Acad Sci USA, 98 (2001).
71. Gronthos, S, Zannettino, AC, Hay, SJ, Shi, S, Graves, SE, Kortesidis, A and Simmons, PJ, J Cell Sci, 116 (2003).
72. Prabhakar, U, James, IE, Dodds, RA, Lee-Rykaczewski, E, Rieman, DJ, Lipshutz, D, Trulli, S, Jonak, Z, Tan, KB, Drake, FH and Gowen, M, Calcif Tissue Int, 63 (1998).
73. Nuttall, ME, Patton, AJ, Olivera, DL, Nadeau, DP and Gowen, M, J Bone Miner Res, 13 (1998).
74. Tuli, R, Tuli, S, Nandi, S, Wang, ML, Alexander, PG, Haleem-Smith, H, Hozack, WJ, Manner, PA, Danielson, KG and Tuan, RS, Stem Cells, 21 (2003).
75. Park, SR, Oreffo, ROC and Triffitt, JT, Bone, 24 (1999).
76. Lee, JA, Parrett, BM, Conejero, JA, Laser, J, Chen, J, Kogon, AJ, Nanda, D, Grant, RT and Breitbart, AS, Ann Plast Surg, 50 (2003).

77. Ashina, I, Sampath, TK and Huascbka, PV, Exp Cell Res, 222 (1996).

78. Klein, G, Beck, S and Muller, CA, J Cell Biol, 123 (1993).

79. Yokota, T, Meka, CS, Medina, KL, Igarashi, H, Comp PC, Takahashi, M, Nishida, M, Oritani, K, Miyagawa, J and Funahashi, T, et al, J Clin Invest,109 (2002).

80. Yokota, T, Oritani, K, Takahashi, I, Ishikawa, J, Matzuyama, A, Ouchi, N, Kihara, S, Funahashi, T, Tenner, AJ, Tomiyama, Y and Matsuzawa, Y, Blood, 96 (2000).

81. Nishikawa, M, Ozawa, K, Tojo, A, Yoshikubo, T, Okano, A, Tani, K, Ikebuchi, K, Nakauchi, H and Asano, S, Blood, 81 (1993).

82. Kelly, KA, Tanaka, S, Baron, R and Gimble, JM, Endocrinology, 139 (1998).

83. Sakaguchi, K, Morita, I and Murota, S, Prostaglandins Leukot Essent Fatty Acids, 62 (2000).

84. Benayahu, D, Peled, A and Zipori, D, J Cell Biochem, 56 (1994).

85. Katoh, M, Kitamura, K and Kitagawa, H, Bone, 16 (1995).

86. Jin, CH, Shinki, T, Hong, MH, Sato, T, Yamaguchi, A, Ikeda, T, Yoshiki, S, Abe, E and Suda, T, Endocrinology, 131 (1992).

87. Hong, ME, Jin, CH, Sate, T, Ishimi, Y, Abe, E and Soda, T, Endocrinology, 129 (1991).

88. Sato, T, Abe, E, He Jin, C, Hong, MH, Katagiri, T, Kinoshita, T, Amizuka, N, Ozawa, H, and Suds, T, Endocrinology, 133 (1993).

89. Dodds, RA, Gowen, M and Bradbeer, JN, J Histochem Cytochem, 42 (1994).

90. Cornish, J, Callon, KE, Mountjoy, KG, Bava, U, Lin, JM, Myers, DE, Naot, D and Reid, IR, Am J Physiol Endocrinol Metab, 284 (2003).

91. Kodama, Y, Takeuchi, Y, Suzawa, M, Fukumoto, S, Murayama, H, Yamato, H, Fujita, T, Kurokawa, T and Matsumoto, T, J Bone Miner Res, 13 (1998).

92. Takeuchi, Y, Suzawa, M, Fukumoto, S and Fujita, T, Bone, 27 (2000)

93. Gimble, JM, Robinson, CE, Wu, X, Kelly, KA, Rodriguez, BR, Kliewer, SA, Lehmann, JM and Morris, DC, Mol Pharmacol, 50 (1996).

94. Cui, Q, Wang, GJ, Su, CC and Balian, G, Clin Orthop, 344 (1997).

95. Couse, JF and Korach, KS, Ann Endocrinol (Paris), 60 (1999).

96. Leboy, PS, Beresford, JN, Devlin, C and Owen, ME, J Cell Physiol, 146 (1991).

97. Locklin, RM, Williamson, MC, Beresford, JN, Triffitt, JT and Owen, ME, Clin Orthop, 313 (1995).

98. Beresford, JN, Joyner, CJ, Devlin, C and Triffitt, JT, Arch Oral Biol, 39 (1994).

99. Kimoto, S, Cheng, SL, Zhang, SF and Avioli, LV, Endocrinology, 135 (1994).

100. Rickard, DJ, Kassem, M, Hefferan, TE, Sarkar, G, Spelsberg, TC and Riggs, BL, J Bone Miner Res, 11 (1996).

101. Wiper-Bergeron, N, Wu, D, Pope, L, Schild-Poulter, C and Hache, RJ, EMBO J, 22 (2003).

102. Bellows, CG, Wang, YH, Heersche, JNM, and Aubin, JE, Endocrinology, 134 (1994).

103. Shionome, M, Shinki, T, Takahashi, N, Hasegawa, K and Suda, T, J Cell Biochem, 48 (1992).
104. Ding, J, Nagai, K and Woo, JT, Biosci Biotechnol Biochem, 67, (2003)
105. Sakuma, T, Miyamoto, T, Jiang, W, Kakizawa, T, Nishio, SI, Suzuki, S, Takeda, T, Oiwa, A and Hashizume, K, Biochem Biophys Res Commun, 312 (2003)
106. Martin, RB, Chow, BD and Lucas, PA, Calcif Tissue Int, 46 (1990).
107. Martin, RB and Zissimos, SL, Bone, 12 (1991).
108. Pedersen, SB, Borglum, JD, Moller-Pedersen, T and Richelsen, B, Mol Cell Endocrinol, 85 (1992).
109. Dang, ZC, van Bezooijen, RL, Karperien, M, Papapoulos, SE and Lowik, CW, J Bone Miner Res, 17 (2002).
110. Okazaki, R, Inoue, D, Shibata, M, Saika, M, Kido, S, Ooka, H, Tomiyama, H, Sakamoto, Y and Matsumoto, T, Endocrinology, 143 (2002).
111. Heim, M, Frank, O, Kampmann, G, Sochocky, N, Pennimpede, T, Fuchs, P, Hunziker, W, Weber, P, Martin, I and Bendik, I, Endocrinology, 145 (2004)
112. Dang, ZC, Audinot, V, Papapoulos, SE, Boutin, JA and Lowik, CW, J Biol Chem, 278 (2003).
113. Dang, Z and Lowik, CW, J Bone Miner Res, 19 (2004).
114. Richelsen, B, Horm Res, 48 Suppl 5 (1997).
115. Gevers, EF, Loveridge, N and Robinson, IC, Endocrinology, 143 (2002).
116. Kroger, H, Soppi, E and Loveridge, N, Calcif Tissue Int, 61 (1997).
117. Lincoln, DT, Sinowatz, F, Gabius, S, Gabius, HJ, Temmim, L, Baker, H, Mathew, TC and Waters, MJ, Anat Histol Embryol, 26 (1997)
118. Cosman, F and Lindsay, R, Calcif Tissue Int, 62 (1998).
119. Sato, M, Grese, TA, Dodge, JA, Bryant, HU and Turner, CH, J Med Chem, 42 (1999).
120. Marcus, R, Clin Lab Med, 20 (2000).
121. Jerome, CP, Burr, DB, Van Bibber, T, Hock, JM and Brommage, R, Bone, 28 (2001)
122. Hock, JM, J Musculoskel Neuron Interact, 2 (2001).
123. Dempster, DW, Cosman, F, Parisien, M, Shen, V and Lindsay, R, Endocr Rev, 14 (1993).
124. Amizuka, N, Karaplis, AC, Henderson, JE, Warshawsky, H, Lipman, ML, Matsuki, Y, Ejiri, S, Tanaka, M, Izumi, N, Ozawa, H and Goltzman, D, Dev Biol, 175 (1996).
125. Reeve, J, J Bone Miner Res, 11 (1996).
126. Sato, M, Westmore, M, Ma, YL, Schmidt, A, Zeng, QQ, Glass, EV, Vahle, J, Brommage, R, Jerome, CP and Turner, CH, J Bone Miner Res, 19 (2004).
127. Chan, GK, Miao, D, Deckelbaum, R, Bolivar, I, Karaplis, A and Goltzman, D, Endocrinology, 144 (2003).
128. Chan, GK, Deckelbaum, RA, Bolivar, I, Goltzman, D, Karaplis, AC, Endocrinology, 142 (2001)

129. Wang, HY, Watkins, DC and Malbon, CC, Nature, 358 (1992).

130. Shore, EM, Li, M, Hebela, N, Jan de Beur, SM, Eddy, MC, Whyte, MP, Levine, MA and Kaplan, FS, J Bone Miner Res, 14 (Suppl 1) (1999).

131. Riminucci, M, Fisher, LW, Majolagbe, A, Lala, R, Robey, P G and Bianco, P, J Bone Miner Res, 14 (Suppl 1) (1999).

132. Bianco, P, Riminucci, M, Majolagbe, A, Kuznetsov, SA, Collins, MT, Mankani, MH, Corsi, A, Bone, HG, Weintroub, S, Spiegel, AM, Fisher, LW and Gehron Robey, P, J Bone Miner Res, 15 (2000).

133. Trayhurn, P and Beattie, JH, Proc Nutr Soc, 60 (2001).

134. Manolagas, SC and Jilka, RL, N Engl J Med, 332(1995).

135. Laharrague, P, Larrouy, D, Fontanilles, AM, Truel, N, Campfield, A, Tenenbaum, R, Galitzky, J, Corberand, JX, Penicaud, L and Casteilla, L, FASEB J, 12 (1998).

136. Thomas, T, Gori, F, Khosla, S, Jensen, MD, Burguera, B and Riggs, BL, Endocrinologyl, 140 (1999).

137. Kontogianni, MD, Dafni, UG, Routsias, JG and Skopouli, FN, J Bone Miner Res, 19 (2004).
Elefteriou, F, Takeda, S, Ebihara, K, Magre, J, Patano, N, Kim, CA, Ogawa, Y, Liu, X, Ware, SM, Craigen, WJ, Robert, JJ, Vinson, C, Nakao, K, Capeau, J and Karsenty, G, Proc Natl Acad Sci U S A, 101 (2004).

138. Hamrick, MW, Pennington, C, Newton, D, Xie, D and Isales, C, Bone, 34 (2004).
Kliewer, SA, Forman, BM, Blumberg, B, Ong, ES, Borgmeyer, U, Mangelsdorf, DJ, Umesono, K and Evans, RM, Proc Natl Acad Sci USA, 91 (1994).

139. Gimble, JM, Dorheim, MA, Cheng, Q, Pekala, P, Enerback, S, Ellingsworth, L, Kincade, PW and Wang, CS, Mol Cell Biol, 9 (1989).

140. Ashina, I, Sampath, TK and Huascbka, PV, Exp Cell Res, 222 (1996).

141. Gimble, JM, Morgan, C, Kelly, K, Wu, X, Dandapam, V, Wang, CS and Rosen, V, J Cell Biochem, 58 (1995).

142. Wu, X, Robinson, CE, Fong, HW, Crabtree, JS, Rodriguez, BR, Roe, BA and Gimble, JM, Biochem Biophys Res Commun, 216 (1995).

143. Wu, X, Robinson, CE, Fong, HW and Gimble, JM, J Cell Physiol, 168 (1996).

144. Roelen, BA and Dijke, P, J Orthop Sci, 8 (2003).

145. Rebbapragada, A, Benchabane, H, Wrana, JL, Celeste, AJ and Attisano, L, Mol Cell Biol, 23 (2003).

146. Chen, D, Ji, X, Harris, MA, Feng, JQ, Karsenty, G, Celeste, AJ, Rosen, V, Mundy, GR and Harris SE, J Cell Biol, 142 (1998).

147. Manolagas, SC and Jilka, RL, New Engl J Med, 332 (1995).

148. Suzawa, M, Takada, I, Yanagisawa, J, Ohtake, F, Ogawa, S, Yamauchi, T, Kadowaki, T, Takeuchi, Y, Shibuya, H, Gotoh, Y, Matsumoto, K and Kato, S, Nat CellBiol,5(2003).

149. Gimble, JM, Wanker, F, Wang, CS, Bass, H, Wu, X, Kelly, K, Yancopoulos, GD and Hill, MR, J Cell Biochem, 54 (1994).
150. Takeuchi, Y, Watanabe, S, Ishii, G, Takeda, S, Nakayama, K, Fukumoto, S, Kaneta, Y, Inoue, D, Matsumoto, T, Harigaya, K and Fujita T, J Biol Chem, 277 (2002).
151. Bellido T, Stahl N, Farruggella TJ, Borba V, Yancopoulos GD, Manolagas SC, J Clin Invest, 97 (1996).

CHAPTER 9

STATISTICAL METHODS IN OSTEOPOROSIS RESEARCH

Ying Lu[1,2]

Hua Jin[1,3]

Department of Radiology;

Department of Epidemiology and Biostatistics,

University of California, San Francisco,

San Francisco, CA 94143-0946, USA

Department of Mathematics, South China Normal University,

Guangzhou 510631, China

The chapter briefly introduces some statistical methods used to develop osteoporosis diagnosis techniques, to assess fracture risk, to evaluate and compare diagnostic markers, quality control, clinical trials, and cost-effectiveness analysis. It focuses on statistical concepts and gives references for their applications in osteoporosis without mathematical details.

1. Introduction

"Statistics is a body of methods for learning from experience -usually in the form of numbers from many separate measurements showing individual variations."[1] Different from Newton's Laws of Motion that allow exact relationship of variables, statistics studies the relationships that may hold true on average, but vary for different sampling subjects or conditions.

"Osteoporosis is a disease characterized by low bone mass and micro-architectural degradation of bone tissue, leading to enhanced bone fragility and a consequent increase in fracture risk."[2] As a silent, chronic, and epidemic disease, statistics has been used from the very beginning of disease definitions[3], diagnosis[4], and development of treatment strategies. In this chapter, we introduce statistical tools that have been used in osteoporosis research literature, including relevant concepts and methods, and practical considerations for their uses. We do not, however, give all the technical details of these methods. With the extensive list of references given in this chapter, readers should be able to find all these technical details whenever there is a need.

The chapter briefly introduces some statistical methods used to develop osteoporosis diagnosis techniques, to assess fracture risk, to evaluate and compare diagnostic markers, quality control, clinical trials, and cost-effectiveness analysis. It focuses on statistical concepts and gives references for their applications in osteoporosis without mathematical details.

2. Basic Concepts of Statistics

Statistics methods can be characterized into descriptive and inference. Descriptive statistics has a long history to summarize population characteristics to give people an overview of the population distribution based on few key parameters. Statistical inference is a relative new scientific technique developed in the last century. It uses random data to support a scientific hypothesis. In this subsection, we provide a summary of basic concepts of both statistical techniques.

2.1. Descriptive Statistics

Descriptive statistics are usually used to numerically examine the characteristics of a collected data set from a particular study population. An example of a study *population* could be elderly postmenopausal Chinese women. While it is difficult, if not impossible, to measure bone mineral density (BMD) of all Chinese postmenopausal women, we often select some *samples* (women in our example) from the *sample population* to estimate the distribution of BMD. Usually a sample population is smaller than the study population. For example, the Study of Osteoporosis Fracture (SOF) wanted to investigate risk factors for hip fracture of postmenopausal white women in US. Instead of selecting samples from all post-menopausal white women from US, SOF selected study participants from four US metropolitan areas. We use these samples to study distribution parameters of the study population, such as location, scale, and shape, to characterize the population distribution.

To make a valid statistics estimation, the samples must be representative of the study population. If you only select women within age range of 50-60 or only those working in hospitals, your estimated distribution will be different from your study population. Such difference is called *sampling bias*. The only guaranteed way to avoid such sampling bias is to select *random samples* from the population. Unfortunately, random samples are not often used because of the costs or the logistic difficulties. Many alternative sampling methods have been developed to reduce the potential sampling bias.

Suppose we have n randomly selected subjects from a study population, denote as $X_1, X_2, \cdots, X_n$, we want to use these sample data to understand the overall distribution properties of BMD in the population. The following descriptive statistics are introduced to estimate the location, scale, and shape of the population:

Measures of Central Tendency (or *Location*)

Measures of central tendency provide an indication of the location of a population. They are useful in determining the expected value of a sample, or where (on average) an observation tends to lie. The sample mean is the most common measure of location, which is simply the arithmetic average of the observations:.

$$\overline{X} = \frac{1}{n} \sum_{i=1}^{n} X_i$$

It's attractive as a conceptually straightforward estimate. However, it's very sensitive to outlying observations. So we often use it in conjunction with robust measures of location such as median, which is defined to be the middle value of the sorted observations in ascending order if the number of subjects n is odd, or the average of the two middle values of the sorted observations if n is even. Other robust measures of location include trimmed mean, mode, and more general M-estimators[5].

Measures of Dispersion (or Scale)

Measures of dispersion provide an indication of the variability, or scatteredness, of the collected data points. Many of them are based on averaging the distance of each observation from the center of the data. The most used one is the *standard deviation*, the square root of the *variance* that is the average value of the squared deviation from the sample mean. The formula is given by $s = \sqrt{\dfrac{1}{n-1}\sum_{i=1}^{n}(X_i - \bar{X})^2}$. Like the sample mean, it's very sensitive to outliers. As a result, it's often used in conjunction with robust measures of scale such as median absolute deviation, defined as the median distance from the observations to the center. Other measures of scale include range, inter-quartile range, and two robust measures of scale based on M-estimators of location: bisquare A-estimates and Huber τ estimators [5,6].

Measures of Shape

Measures of shape describe the overall pattern in the distribution of data values. The most popular measures of shape, skewness and kurtosis, compare a particular data set to a normal distribution, and indicate how similar or different the data is to a Gaussian density function. Skewness is a signed measure that describes the degree of symmetry in a distribution. For a sample with second and third central moments, m_2 and m_3, the coefficient of skewness is defined to be $b_1 = \dfrac{m_3}{m_2^{3/2}}$ with the rth central moment $m_r = \dfrac{1}{n}\sum_{i=1}^{n}(X_i - \bar{X})^r$. Positive values of b_1 indicate skewness (or long-tailedness) to the right, negative values of b_1 indicate skewness to the left, and values close to zero indicate a nearly-symmetric distribution. Kurtosis describes the degree of peakedness in a distribution. For a sample with second and fourth central moments, m_2 and m_4, the coefficient of kurtosis is defined to be $b_2 = \dfrac{m_4}{m_2^2}$. Large values of b_2 usually imply a high peak at the center of the data while small values imply a broad peak at the center.

Example of Descriptive Statistics in Osteoporosis Research

In the National Health and Nutritional Study (NHANS) III, 14646 adults were randomly selected from the US population[7]. Among them, there were 2930 non-Hispanic white men and 3251 white women. We use the values of femoral neck BMD (g/cm^2) for men and women aged 20-29 years to illustrate the ideas. The means of peak BMD for these young non-Hispanic white men and women in US were 0.934 g/cm^2 and 0.858 g/cm^2 respectively. The corresponding standard deviations were 0.137 g/cm^2 and 0.120 g/cm^2 respectively. This suggested that, on average, the peak BMD of non-Hispanic white men are higher than that of women. There are more differences among men than women. Other descriptive statistics for peak BMD for these two groups are the 25th, 50th (median), and 75th percentiles, which were 0.836 g/cm^2, 0.929 g/cm^2, and 1.029 g/cm^2 for men, and 0.774 g/cm^2, 0.845 g/cm^2 and 0.944 g/cm^2 for women. The interval between the 25th and 75th percentiles is the inter-quartile range, another commonly used statistics to describe dispersions.

Box Plot

Boxplots have proven to be quite a good exploratory tool to summarize descriptive statistics of continuous variables, especially when several boxplots are placed side by side for comparison[8]. The most striking visual feature is the box of the inter-quartiles that shows the limits of the half of the data as well as the median (the line inside the box). Extreme points are also highlighted. Boxplots show not only the location and spread of data but indicate skewness, as well. Figure 2.1 is the boxplots for femoral neck BMD of Non-Hispanic white men and women aged 20-29 years old in NHANSE study. Another example of a boxplot in osteoporosis research can be found in Jowitt, et al.[9]. Other plots very similar to the boxplots are the diamond plots used in JMP software.

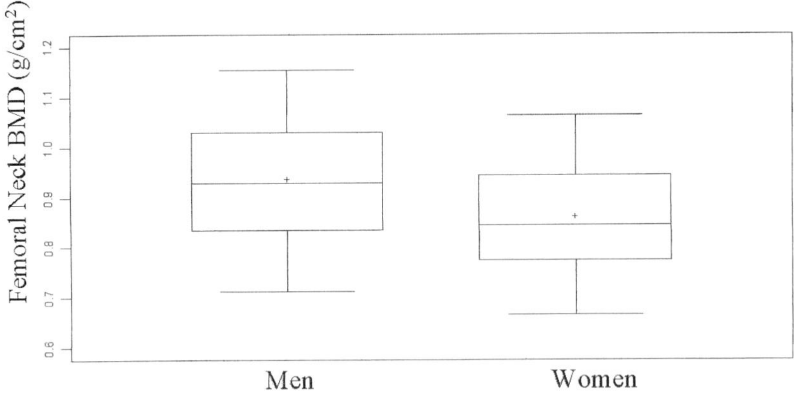

Men   Women

Fig. 2.1 Box plot for femoral neck BMD of Non-Hispanic white men and women aged 20-29 years in NHANSE Study. The five horizontal lines from top to bottom correspond to the 95th ,75th, 50th (i.e. median), 25th, and 5th percentiles of the Femoral Neck BMD of Non-Hispanic White Men and Women Aged 20-29 Years in NHANSE Study respectively. The height of the box is equal to the inter-quartile distance (IQD). "+" correspond to the mean values of the Femoral Neck BMD.

Descriptive Statistics for Categorical Data

Instead of summarized by central location, scale, and shape for continuous variables, frequency distributions are used to characterize categorical data. Sometimes, values of categorical variables aren't comparable, i.e., there is no order of their values. In other applications, categorical values can be ordered, such as the severity of spinal fractures[10]. In a study on risk factors of vertebral fractures in Chinese women, 400 postmenopausal women age 50 years or older were randomly selected from the four central districts of Beijing[10]. They were divided into four groups based on the years of education they had taken: (1) No education; (2) 1 to 6 years of education; (3) 7 to 12 years; (4) more than 12 years. So a categorical variable Education could be used to describe their education status, which took four values: 0,1,2,3 for the specified groups above respectively. And the frequency distributions of this categorical variable were 44.7%, 34.5%, 14.8%, and 6.0%.

A special case of categorical data is the binary data. We summarize the binary data in the probability of the event of interest. The probability can be estimated by the proportion of subjects with that event in the samples, denoted as p. For example, a binary outcome is osteoporosis disease status of a woman. Prevalence of osteoporosis is defined as the proportion of women in the population who have osteoporosis. According to WHO criteria, women with BMD below 2.5SD from the peak bone mass of young normals have osteoporosis. Use the NHANSE[11] as our example, 20% US non-Hispanic white women age over 50 years were estimated to have femoral neck BMD below 2.5 SD from the mean of the peak BMD. The standard error of this estimate was

$$\sqrt{p(1-p)/n} = \sqrt{0.20(1-0.20)/1880} = 1\%.$$

Graphical description of categorical data is the bar chart that showed percentages of each category in the population. Also we use the pie chart to describe the proportion of multiple level categories. An example of such application is in Lu et al.[12] that examined the percentage of elderly non-Hispanic white women in SOF who had osteoporosis at AP spine, total hip, femoral neck, Ward's triangle, trochanteric, distal and proximal forearm, and calcaneal BMD according to the WHO criterion (See Figure 2.2).

2.2. Statistical Inferences

Formal methods of *statistical inference* provide probability-based statements about population parameters such as the mean, variance, and correlation coefficient for the data. To address limitations of a point estimate that neither conveys any uncertainty about the value of the estimate, nor indicates whether a hypothesis about the population parameter should be rejected, we usually use *confidence intervals* or *hypothesis tests* or both methods for statistical inference.

2.2.1. Confidence Intervals

A $1-\alpha$ confidence interval for the unknown parameter θ is any interval of the form (L, U), such that (L, U) has the probability of $1-\alpha$ to contain θ. Here $1-\alpha$ is called the *confidence level* of the confidence interval. Common values of α are 0.01 or 0.05, that correspond to the 99% or 95% confidence intervals.

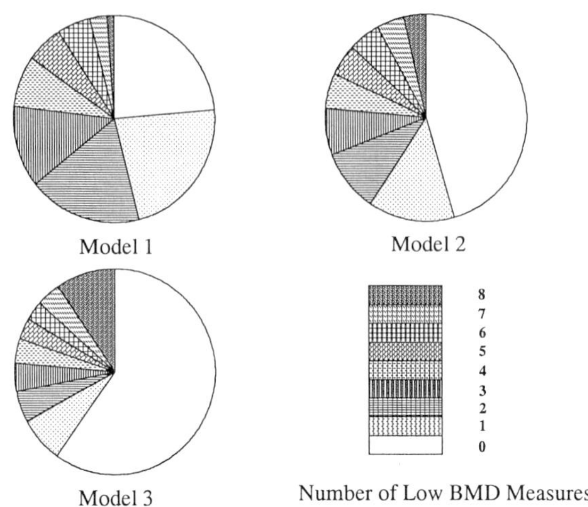

Fig. 2.2 Pie chart for the distribution of the number of low BMD sites. The pie chart consists of SOF participants in nine categories according to their number of osteoporotic sites. The area of each category represents the percentage of participants in it. Participants who are classified consistently by eight BMD measurement sites had either no low BMD sites or eight low BMD sites. Model 1 used WHO criterion, Model 2 used there reference of SOF participants aged 65 years. Model 3 used risk based classifications. Details can be found in Lu et. al.[12]

<u>Example 2.2.1</u>. Suppose a random sample of size n, $X_1, X_2, \cdots, X_n$, is drawn from a normal distribution $N(\mu, \sigma^2)$ with σ unknown. A $1 - \alpha$ confidence interval for the parameter μ is $[\overline{X} - t_{n-1}^{(1-\frac{\alpha}{2})} \cdot \frac{s}{\sqrt{n}}, \overline{X} + t_{n-1}^{(1-\frac{\alpha}{2})} \cdot \frac{s}{\sqrt{n}}]$, where $\overline{X}$ and s are respectively the sample mean and standard deviation, and $t_{n-1}^{(1-\frac{\alpha}{2})}$ is the $(1 - \alpha/2)th$ percentile of the t distribution with $n - 1$ degrees of freedom.

One example of 95% confidence interval is *"the least significant change" (LSC)* for bone densitometry. For clinical decision making it is important to know the minimum magnitude of measured change that is not caused by measurement errors. Let X_1 and X_2 be two successive measurements of a subject. If there is no change in the two measurements, the difference between them is the result of longitudinal measurement errors, which is also called *precision*. If we assume the longitudinal measurement error follows a normal distribution with a variation σ, the standard error of the difference is $\sqrt{2}\sigma$. Based on the normal distribution of the difference, $\Pr\left(\left|X_1 - X_2\right| > z_{1-\alpha/2}\sqrt{2}\sigma\right) = \alpha$.

If we take $\alpha = 5\%$, $z_{1-0.05/2} = z_{0.975} = 1.96$. The interval ($-1.96 \times 1.44\,\sigma$, $1.96 \times 1.44\,\sigma$) = ($-2.88\,\sigma$, $2.88\,\sigma$) has a 95% chance to contain the mean change when there is not difference between two measurements. Thus, when we observe a difference between two visits more than $2.8\,\sigma$, we have a reason to suspect that the change in BMD is beyond chance of the measurement error. The least significant change is also called the "biologically significant change" in laboratory medicine[13]. Some more detailed discussions about LSE can be found in Lu and Zhao[14].

2.2.2. Hypothesis Testing

A hypothesis test is a probability-based method for making a decision concerning the value of a population parameter θ (for example, the population mean μ in a one-sample problem), or the relative values of two population parameters θ_1 and θ_2 (for example, the difference between the population means $\mu_1 - \mu_2$ in a two-sample problem). We begin by forming a *null hypothesis* and an *alternative hypothesis*, then choose a "good" test statistic T, and calculate the *p-value,* which is the probability that the statistic T "exceeds" the observed value t_{obs} when the null hypothesis is true. Our decision to accept or reject the null hypothesis in favor of the alternative is based on the *p*-value. We reject the null hypothesis if the *p*-value is less than a pre-specified *level of significance*, the probability of rejecting the null hypothesis when it is in fact true. Otherwise, we accept the null hypothesis. The most commonly used significant level is 5%, although there is no specific biological reason to use this specific level.

The statistical hypothesis testing theory is most easily described using the American legal system. In such a system, a defendant (here a research question) is assumed not guilty (null hypothesis) until the evidence (the test statistics) shows inconsistency to the innocent assumption (*p*-values). We then reject the assumption of innocence (reject null hypothesis) and accept the alternative hypothesis of guilty of the defendant. The error of claiming defendant guilty when the defendant actually is innocent (rejecting null hypothesis when it is true) is called type I error. The chance of making type I error is called significant level or *p*-value, usually denoted by α. The error of claiming defendant innocent when the defendant actually is guilty (accepting null hypothesis when it is false) is called type II error. Its chance is usually denoted by β. $1-\beta$ is the power, the probability of rejecting the null hypothesis when the alternative is true. Like our legal system, we place higher standard for type I error than the type II error. We usually place the alternative hypothesis as the clinical hypothesis that we believe to be true and want to prove.

Example 2.2.1 (continued). Suppose we want to test the null hypothesis $\mu = \mu_0$ against the alternative one $\mu \neq \mu_0$. A suitable test statistic is

$$T = \left| \frac{\sqrt{n-1}(\bar{X} - \mu_0)}{s} \right| , \qquad \text{and} \qquad \text{the} \qquad p\text{-value} \qquad \text{is}$$

$P\{T > t_{obs} \mid \mu = \mu_0\} = 2\left(1 - t_{n-1}(t_{obs})\right)$, where t_{obs} is the observed value of T and t_{n-1} is the cumulative *t*-distribution function with *n-1* degrees of freedom. If this *p*-value is 2%, for example, we will reject $\mu = \mu_0$ at a significance level of 5%, but will accept it at a significance level of 1%.

Classical methods of statistical inference, such as *Student's t* methods in Example 2.2.1, rely on the assumptions of normally distributed and serially uncorrelated data. If our data contain outliers or are strongly non-normal (such as bi-mode or heavily skewed), we should use robust and/or non-parametric methods to derive reliable statistical inference[15,16]. Special methods are needed for dealing with data that are not independently collected, such as multiple vertebrae from the same subjects, or repeated observations from the same subjects, etc.[17].

Example 2.2.2. In a study to compare the non-invasive bone mineral measurements in assessing age-related bone loss, Grampp et al.[18] compared BMD values between healthy pre-and post-menopausal women using several commonly available techniques. The mean (*m*) and standard deviation (*s*) of QCT trabecular BMD were 178 mg/cm^3 and 33 mg/cm^3 for 47 (n_1) healthy pre-menopausal women, and 106 mg/cm^3 and 30 mg/cm^3 for 41 (n_1) healthy post-menopausal women. The null hypothesis was that there was no difference in QCT trabecular BMD between pre and post-menopausal women. The pre-specified significant level was 5%. Using the t-test statistics for two independent samples,

$$t = (m_1 - m_2)\bigg/ \sqrt{\left[(n_1 - 1)s_1^2 + (n_2 - 1)s_2^2\right]/(n_1 + n_2 - 2)}$$

$$= (178 - 106)\bigg/ \sqrt{(46 \times 33^2 + 40 \times 30^2)/86} = 2.2756.$$ The chance to observe such a t-statistics value (p-value) was 2.5% when there was truly no difference between pre- and post-menopausal healthy women. This was less than 5%. Thus, we were willing to take this small chance to make type I error and rejected the null hypothesis. We concluded that there were significant differences in trabecular BMD between pre- and post-menopausal women.

3. Statistics for Osteoporosis Diagnosis

Osteoporosis is a silent disease. Most patients with low bone mineral density have no acute clinical symptoms. When patients develop spinal or hip fracture, they have already had osteoporosis for a long time. For that reason, diagnose of osteoporosis has been relying on bone densitometry, such as dual X-ray absorptiometry, CT, or quantitative ultrasound, etc. Hui et al first proved that baseline BMD can prospectively predict hip fracture risks[4]. Therefore, WHO has defined women with BMD 2.5 SD below population mean peak BMD as osteoporotic patients[2].

3.1. Diagnosis of Osteoporosis

As described previously, summary descriptive statistics, such as mean and standard deviation, are usually reported in osteoporosis literature. Such information is always important and should be presented in an organized format[19]. Usually summary statistics depend on the unit of the measurement. Therefore, any efforts of comparisons of summary statistics should be based on comparable measurement unit and physical meaningfulness.

The most commonly used descriptive statistics in osteoporosis diagnosis are the Z-Score and the T-Score. The Z-score for a patient by a particular technique is defined as the deviation of the observed value from the mean of the age matched controls expressed in a standard deviation unit by the same age matched controls:

$$\text{Z-score} = \frac{\text{observed value - mean of age matched normals}}{\text{standard deviation of age matched normals}}.$$

T-score is defined similarly but using the young controls (having peak bone mass) as the reference group:

$$\text{T-score} = \frac{\text{observed value - mean of young normals}}{\text{standard deviation of young normals}}.$$

The advantage of Z-score and T-score are that they are independent of measurement units and can be used across different instruments if their reference parameters are derived from the same group of controls. Usually, a Z-score or T-score should be based on either normative data collected by the manufacturers or from some large scale and properly sampled epidemiological data[7,11,20].

The T-score is different from the t-statistics normally referred in statistical literature. Initially, T-score has been used to define osteoporosis. Women with a T-score of any BMD below -2.5 have osteoporosis[2,21]. Based on this cut-off value, approximately 30% white women in US are having osteoporosis in their lifetime.

Sometimes, Z-score or T-score is used in cross-sectional studies. These scores when averaged over a group of patients represent the mean Z-score and mean T-score for that group with respect to the distribution in their respective reference groups. The magnitude of these means could provide indication of which technique more efficiently discriminates the high-risk group from the controls (bigger absolute mean Z-score is an indication of better discrimination). However it is not advisable to draw conclusions based on these scores[22]. It is because the probability of misclassifying between the high-risk group and the controls depends on the characteristics of the measurements other than T-scores or Z-scores[23].

When population distributions of the interesting parameters follow normal distribution[24], comparisons between means and standard deviations of two groups of subjects can use t-test, paired t-test, and analysis of variance (ANOVA) depending on the study design[19]. For example, when we compare the mean difference of SOS between normal and osteoporotic patients, we can use t-test. In the use of a t-test, it is important to examine whether the variances of two groups are equal. A t-test statistics will be calculated differently based on equal or unequal variances in the two groups. When we compare mean differences of SOS before and after a treatment for the same individual, we can use paired t-test. When compare the means of more than two groups, we can use ANOVA. Sometimes, transformation of a variable may be helpful to improve the normality of the data[25,26]. It may be important for studies with few patients. It is less important, however, when the sample size of a study is over 30 due to the large sample theory. Alternative approach would be to use non-parametric statistical methods, such as Wilcoxon rank test, paired Wilcoxon signed rank test, and Kruskal-Wallis test, etc.

3.2. Sensitivity and Specificity and ROC Curves

The traditional measures to quantify the diagnostic accuracy of a diagnostic test are sensitivity and specificity[27,28]. The sensitivity or true positive rate (TPR) describes the rate of diseased patients that actually has a positive test result. The specificity or true negative rate (TNR) describes the fraction of a negative test result in non-diseased individuals. Because the lower SOS and/or BUA indicate the low bone mass, one way to use QUS parameters for the diagnosis of osteoporosis is to classify an individual positive if his/her SOS or BUA is less than a pre-specified cut-off value. The sensitivity and specificity of QUS and SOS depend on the liberal or conservative choices of cut-off values. A method with good diagnostic ability should be high in both sensitivity and specificity. However, it is difficult to achieve both because of a reciprocal relationship between them, that is to say, an increase in sensitivity is associated with a decrease in specificity.

As Swet[29] pointed out, the sensitivity and specificity values associated with a diagnostic test are subject to two types of variations: (1) the test's capacity to discriminate a given disease from non-disease, and (2) the decision criterion that is adopted for declaring a test result to be positive (high risk of fracture). Use of sensitivity and specificity does not allow us to compare two diagnostic tests because the differences may depend on the choices of cut-off values. To obtain the global assessment of diagnostic ability, receiver operating characteristic (ROC) curves have been adapted in radiology literature[30,31].

ROC analysis is a procedure derived from statistical decision theory. It plots the true positive rate (sensitivity) as a function of the false positive rate (one minus specificity). Thus, it shows the trade off between the sensitivity and specificity of a test. Because an ROC curve removes the effect of different choices of decision criteria and represents them as different points on the same curve, ROC analysis allows direct comparisons between two diagnostic techniques[32-35].

There are several procedures available to fit data into an ROC curve. SAS, a widely used statistical package, provides a list of estimated true and false positive rates in its logistic regression analysis procedure[36]. These data can be plotted to form an ROC curve. Alternatively, a maximum of binormal likelihood approach is available from Metz[37]. The curves from SAS and Metz's algorithm are not identical, but very close. Several summary statistics have been used in ROC analysis[38-40]. The most common one, however, is the area under an ROC curve (AUC), with a larger AUC indicating a better test for discriminating between two populations. Estimation of area under the curve and comparison of it from two ROC curves can be based on non-parametric approach[32], or parametric approach[37]. The advantages of area under curve are that it reflects the diagnostic accuracy over the whole range of possible operating points and has convenient and well-studied statistical properties[41].

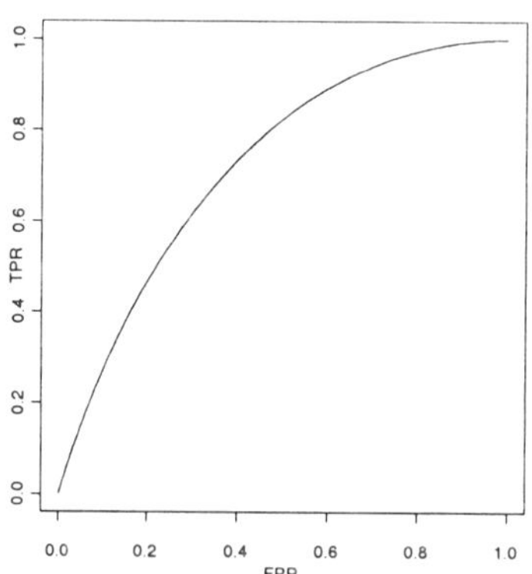

Figure 3.1 Typical ROC Curve in Osteoporosis Research

A disadvantage, however, is that such area covers useless ranges of both sensitivity and specificity. Area under the curve becomes unreasonable when two ROC curves cross to each other and the gain in the area of one ROC curve is due to the differences in very low specificities or sensitivities. An alternative index would be focusing the comparison of the true positive rates (sensitivity) in a reasonable range of false positive rates[39]. Detailed issues in study design for ROC analysis, such as the sample size determinations, patient selections, number of readers, etc., can be found in an extensive review by Hanley[30]. More recent developments in this area include an introduction of generalized linear regression models to ROC analysis[35,42,43] and methods to deal with imperfect data[44-46]. A recent published text book by Zhou, McClish, and Obuchowski[47] gave great detailed information for the design and use of ROC in diagnostic studies.

3.3. Combination of Multiple Diagnostic Predictors

Multiple alternative diagnostic tests for one disease are commonly available to clinicians. While several tests exist, none of them may be sufficiently sensitive and specific on its own for diagnosis of disease. Combination use of multiple tests is likely to substantially improve the statistical utility. So it's important to use all the available diagnostic predictors simultaneously to establish a new predictor with higher statistical utility.

The linear functions of multiple predictors are often of particular interest to people for its mathematical simplicity. One of the most classic methods to find the best linear combination is linear discriminant analysis (LDA) based on multivariate normal distribution theory[48]. It is a technique designed to create a classification rule that minimizes the probability of misclassification between two or more groups. Explanatory variables (also called risk factors), such as age, BMD, or QUS parameters, are combined in an optimum linear fashion, which is called the linear discriminant function, such that the difference between the two groups with respect to this linear combination is maximized. When the risk factors follow multivariate normal distributions, it has been proven that the linear discriminant function is also the best linear combination of risk factors among all possible linear choices that maximizes the area under the ROC curve[49].

Binary regression methods are routinely used in practice to develop optimal linear diagnostic score. McIntosh and Pepe[50] provided a justification for their use. Specially, under the generalized linear model for binary outcomes, the linear combination of multiple predictors is proved optimal in the sense that its area under the receiver operating characteristic (ROC) curve is the largest among all possible linear combination. Other methods for finding linear combinations of markers may refer to Pepe and Thompson[51].

Both logistic regression and discriminant analysis provide effective methods for combination use of multiple tests. In many applications, these two approaches give similar results. For example, if we consider the relationship between age, the femoral neck BMD and loss of height with the hip fracture within 5 years (from baseline) based on the data from the Study of Osteoporotic Fractures (SOF)[52], the standard software S-plus or SAS can easily result in the following logistic regression model:

$$P\left(Z = 1 \mid (X_1, X_2, X_3)\right) = 1 - \frac{1}{1 + \exp(-3.89 + 0.075 X_1 - 8.90 X_2 + 0.100 X_3)}$$

where $Z = 1$ stands for hip fracture, X_1, X_2 and X_3 denote age, femoral neck BMD and loss of height respectively. Thus $0.075 X_1 - 8.90 X_2 + 0.100 X_3$ is the optimal linear combination under the ROC criterion with coefficients proportional to (1, -119, 1.33). Meanwhile, the linear discriminant analysis results in the best coefficients proportional to (1, -103, 1.05). So it's not surprising that the two corresponding area under ROC (AUC) are both empirically estimated as 0.805.

When the risk factors are normally distributed in both the groups with equal variances and equal between variable correlation (this also implies that none of the covariates are discrete), a discriminant analysis is more efficient and has a greater statistical power than a logistic regression. In the presence of discrete covariates and departures from normality assumptions, logistic regression is more efficient. The comparison between logistic regression and discriminant analysis has been studied in great detail by various authors including Efron[53] and Baron[54].

In some cases, we may be interested in nonlinear combinations of multiple predictors, which can be explored by non-parametric statistical procedures such as the recursive partitioning methods, including the classification and regression tree analysis (CART)[55] and tree structured survival analysis (TSSA)[56,57]. A recursive partitioning method involves splitting and pruning steps. A split is to partition the subjects into two groups by a risk factor, such as age, SOS, etc., according to their values below or above a particular cutoff point. In every group of the tree that is to be subdivided, all the risk factors are examined at all possible cut-off points, and the optimal split is finally selected such that the two resulting subgroups have the largest difference in the summary statistics. Typically, this splitting procedure generates a large sized tree with many subgroups. A subsequent pruning algorithm is used to reduce the tree size to avoid over fitting of the learning data. The pruning can use either another testing samples or by cross-validation techniques. Finally, based on the cutoff points and each subject's risk factor values, the subject is classified into a subgroup with each subgroup having different risk for osteoporosis or osteoporotic fracture, depending on the goal of original study.

There are both advantages and disadvantages of recursive partitioning methods over more traditional regression based methods in construction of combinations of multiple tests. Both CART and TSSA requires no specific model assumptions while the regression-based methods depend on the validity of their assumptions. Because of different use of risk factors, the tree-based methods sometimes can identify some structures of risk factors that were not obvious from linear models[58]. Because the recursive partitioning methodology is computationally intensive, software to perform such analysis is not widely available. Given the relative advantages and disadvantages of the regression based models and recursive partitioning methods, they should be used as complimentary tools in the analysis. Detailed discussions and two applications of CART and TSSA to predict risk of hip fractures can be found from Jin, et al.[59] and Lu, et al.[60].

Backing to the problem of looking for the best way to combine multiple tests, the likelihood ratio score leads to the best theoretical combination of multiple testing results that achieves the largest area under the ROC curve[61]. Baker directly approximated the likelihood ratio function from nonparametric estimation of the false positive rate (FPR) and the true positive rate (TPR)[62]. McIntosh and Pepe[50] proposed an alternative approach using standard binary regression methodology. Further research would be of interest. The remaining question is, however, how to get good estimation of the likelihood ratio score for higher number of diagnostic tests and without prior knowledge of their joint distributions. Furthermore, we are also interested in when a simpler version of combination, such as linear combination, can replace the optimum but complicated likelihood ratio score without loss much efficiency.

3.4. Assessment of Agreements

In osteoporosis research, we often want to assess the agreement of measurements. For example, during a longitudinal osteoporosis trial, a study site might upgrade its DXA machine. Because the change of BMD from baseline is the key measurement, we must be certain that the BMD values measured by the old and new machines are equivalent or in agreement. Also in clinical trials that require a radiologist's assessment of outcomes, we must be certain that readings from different radiologists are the same, and that readings at the beginning and the end of the study are similar. All these require assessment of agreement.

The concept of agreement is related to but different than association. Agreement means interchangeability of two measurements. In other words, a patient's BMD should be the same whether measured on an old DXA scanner or a new one; and the spine fracture grade of a vertebra should be the same regardless by whom or when it is read. An association, on the other hand, suggests that two machines or two readers tend to agree in the same directions. In other words, for two patients with different BMD values, both DXA machines will find the same lower and higher BMD subjects but their BMD measurements can be different.

The best example of the difference between agreement and association is the correlation coefficient of two continuous variables[63,64]. A correlation coefficient can apply to any two continuous variables regardless of their scales, such as height and weight. Even if there is a high association between height and weight, they are not interchangeable because they measure completely different things. Even when X and Y are two continuous variables that measure the same physical properties in the same units, an association still cannot indicate agreement. In fact, $Cor(X,Y) = Cor(a+bX,Y)$. Thus, the correlation is invariant for a shift of mean or a change of scale. Further, the estimation of the correlation depends on the range of the true quantity in the sample: the wider the range, the higher the correlation coefficient. Also, the null hypothesis in testing for a correlation coefficient is for independence of two variables, which is not relevant to the agreement. Therefore, the use of correlation to assess agreement is inappropriate. On the other hand, a high correlation of two continuous variables in the same scale suggests that it is possible to calibrate variables so that they agree with each other.

The most commonly used statistical tools to assess the associations are the Pearson's correlation coefficients and regression analysis[65]. However, study of agreement can only be meaningful for the same physical measurements. It needs special statistical methods different from the traditional approaches, such as coefficients and regressions.

Cohen[66] proposed the use of Kappa statistic to evaluate agreement between two categorical variables and obtained its maximum likelihood estimate. Kraemer[67] and Fleiss and Davies[68] derived alternative estimation of the Kappa statistic based on jackknife technique. Although all these formulas are asymptotically equivalent, there are still differences when using them for small samples. A simulation study[69] compared the different estimates and gave guidance in methods to estimate and construct confidence intervals for Cohen's Kappa statistic for small samples. Agreement of categorical variables is most commonly applied to qualitative evaluations of health or disease status by two readers or by the same reader at two different sessions, which are referred as inter-reader and intra-reader agreement respectively. We want to ensure that the inter-reader agreement and/or the longitudinal intra-reader Kappa statistics are above an acceptable pre-specified level before we start the study. However, the subject of Kappa applications is very broad, including agreement for ordinal or multinomial data[70-73]; for case-control studies[74]; for multiple readers or correlated samples[75-77]; and for using logistic regression models to adjust for the effects of covariates on Kappa statistics[78]. Interested readers should investigate the literature.

As for comparing the agreement of two continuous measurements, Bland and Altman[63] proposed a procedure base on regression of pair differences of two measures to their mean. A zero intercept and a zero slope for such a regression line imply the agreement of distribution characteristics, i.e., the agreement in their means and variances. A simultaneous statistical test for both parameters to be zero was given by Bradley and Blackwood[79]. On the other hand, if the regression line has a non-zero intercept or slope, the two measurements have different distribution parameters, and therefore, not equivalent. Application of Bland and Altman methods in bone densitometry can be found in papers of Lu, et al.[80] and Abrahamsen, et al.[81].

A bivariate normal distribution has 5 parameters: two means, two standard deviations, and a correlation coefficient. The Bland-Altman regression compares four of the five parameters. We can have two normal random variables with the same mean and standard deviation but a negative correlation coefficient, such as Y and $-Y$, when mean Y is 0. Thus, the Bland-Altman regression alone is inadequate for evaluating agreement. We still need to examine the correlation coefficient between the two measurements, in addition to the Bland-Altman regression. Only a high correlation and a zero for both intercept and slope in the Bland-Altman regression can suggest that the two measurements are equivalent.

An alternative measurement for agreement of continuous variables is the intraclass correlation coefficient (ICC)[82], which is simply the percentage of between readers/techniques variance in the total variance of the sum of between and within reader/technique variations. A high ICC means less difference between two readers as well as less measurement error. Lee et al. suggested a cut-off value of 0.75 beyond which the readers or measurement devices are considered to be in agreement[82]. Fleiss and Shrout[83] derived an approximate formula for the confidence interval of ICC. The advantage of ICC over the Bland-Altman regression is that it is easier to evaluate agreement among three or more readers or devices using ICC, although there exist some deficiencies of ICC for evaluation of agreement[84], including its dependence on sample variations. Bartko[85] developed an altered version of ICC, which is simplified and has an exact formula for confidence intervals.

3.5. *Comparisons Between Diagnostic Methods*

Besides assessing agreement of two measurements on the same subjects, we also want to compare their diagnostic accuracies. For example, suppose we have BMD as well as SOS measurement on the same subjects. In such paired-sample study design, we may want to know (1) if there is significant difference between these two measurements; (2) if SOS is non-inferior or equivalent to BMD. The first is a common/traditional hypothesis test with the null hypothesis of no difference against the alternative of a difference while the second test considers non-equivalence or inferior as the null hypothesis with equivalence or non-inferior as the alternative. The test (1) for no difference does not mean equivalence in the test (2). Because the statistical inference paradigm protects the null hypothesis, test (1) is usually used to determine significant difference between the two measurements. When no significant difference is found, we may need use test (2) to examine their equivalence.

The test statistics depend on the accuracy index employed to describe the compared techniques. First we discuss the comparison of sensitivity and/or specificity. If only sensitivity or specificity is to be compared, a McNemar test can be used to test for significant difference[86](p389-392). However, when exact equality in sensitivity and specificity are both considered, a different test such as 2 degrees-of-freedom Chi-square test may be preferred[87].

As for testing the non-inferiority or equivalence of sensitivity and/or specificity, several methods have been proposed recently[88-90]. Nam[91] and Tango[92], nearly simultaneously, derived improved statistical tests for non-inferiority of two treatments based on the score or the restricted maximum likelihood methods. All of these studies considered the non-inferiority or equivalence of sensitivity or specificity separately. Because sensitivity and specificity are two equally important parameters used to characterize a diagnostic test, we must consider both parameters simultaneously when assessing the non-inferiority of a diagnostic test to another one. Lu, et al[93] proposed a statistical testing procedure based on an intersection union test (IUT)[94] for such a comparison for both case-control and prospective cohort study design. Monte Carlo simulation studies suggest that the proposed IUT test can correctly control the type I errors and the proposed sample size calculation can assure the desired power.

Let's see a real example from the Study of Osteoporotic Fractures (SOF)[59]. We want to use forty-three previously documented predictive variables to predict osteoporotic hip fracture within 5 years. The SOF data were randomly separated into two data sets: sixty percent were used for splitting and forty percent were used for pruning. First, using an algorithm similar to CART, we generated a robust optimum classification rule for subjects with elevated risk of 5-year hip fracture without consideration of the cost of the predictive variables. The variables included bone mineral density (BMD) of the hip by dual x-ray absorptiometry (DXA), age, functional status assessment, and walking speed, which had 61.4% sensitivity and 77.2% specificity for the testing samples. We then generated an alternative cost saving rule with equivalent diagnostic utility, but using only hip BMD by DXA scan, age, height loss, and body mass index (BMI). The corresponding sensitivity and specificity were 64.8% and 76.6%, respectively. A 6-fold cross-validation design was used to compare the two algorithms and proved that the cost-saving alternative classification is statistically non-inferior to the optimal CART tree based on the method proposed by Lu, et al[93]. The result suggests that a DXA hip scan and information available from clinical examinations can identify subjects with elevated risk of osteoporotic hip fracture within 5 years without loss of efficiency to more costly and complicated algorithms.

As we described earlier, AUC of ROC is a better index than single values of sensitivity and specificity for diagnostic efficiency. We often want to directly compare two ROC curves. This can be done by either parametric or non-parametric methods. We may fit a parametric model to the data, such as the binormal model[95], and then test the equality of the parameters[96]. If the parametric model does not fit the data well, we may follow Venkatraman and Begg's non-parametric method to directly test the equality of two correlated ROC curves based on a permutation test[97].

Alternate method is to test the equality of a summary measure from the ROC curves, such as the area under the curve, obtained either from a parametric model or non-parametrically. The non-parametric version of the area test was developed by Hanley and McNeil[98] for paired data. The test was then refined by Delong, Delong, and Clarke-Pearson[32] with their derivation of a jackknife estimate of the variance for the area under the ROC curve of one or more diagnostic predictors from the same subjects. Their test was based on the well-known non-parametric Wilcoxon/Mann-Whitney test statistic, and is now used extensively with a public domain program available for calculation[37]. One should note, however, that this method is less powerful than Venkatraman and Begg's method. It takes fairly large differences in area before these become significant.

In the end of this subsection, we'd like to refer interested readers to a new book written by Zhou, McClish, and Obuchowski[47]. This book provides a comprehensive account of statistical methods for design and analysis of diagnostic studies, including sample size calculations, estimation of the accuracy of a diagnostic test, comparison of accuracies of competing diagnostic tests, and regression analysis of diagnostic accuracy data. It also discusses recently developed methods for correction of verification bias and imperfect reference bias, methods for analysis of clustered diagnostic accuracy data, and meta-analysis methods.

3.6 Universal Standardization of BMD

Bone mineral density (BMD) is commonly used for the diagnosis of osteoporosis[2] and in other epidemiological and clinical studies. Its uses range from evaluation of risk of fracture to assessment of intervention efficacy. Dual X-ray absorptiometry (DXA) is the most commonly used technology to measure BMD. Because of differences in the analysis algorithms, region of interest definitions and calibration standards, DXA scanners from different manufacturers present systematically different disease status from the same patient. Such differences may classify a subject into different diagnostic status and will introduce variations in epidemiological studies as well as clinical trials. To resolve such difficulties, the International Committee for Standards in Bone Measurement (ICSBM) was established to develop calibration formulas to convert BMD from one manufacturer to another and to set up a standard BMD (sBMD). To distinguish from BMD obtained from usual DXA, the sBMD uses the unit of mg/cm^2.

To establish the sBMD and cross-calibration formula, we first need to collect data of BMD of the same subjects measured by DXA scanners from all manufacturers. The design of such study has to cover age and BMD ranges for which the formulas will be used. Furthermore, we have to exclude subjects with know bone diseases that may affect the measurement accuracy. We should not, however, to exclude subjects with low BMD because we want to make correct calibration not only for healthy but also osteoporotic subjects. For example, a cross-calibration study of three DXA densitometers was conducted at the University of California at San Francisco under the auspices of the ICSBM in 1994. The study consisted of 100 healthy, non-pregnant, white women with age evenly distributed over 20-80 years. Data from this cohort has been used to derive the standardization formula for AP spine and femoral neck BMD[99,100]. A more recent study recruited another 100 women, aged 20 to 80 with about 16 women in each age decade[101]. One hundred and one subjects were actually recruited with 13 to 19 subjects in each decade. This population was chosen to provide a broad range of clinically observed forearm BMD values. The self-declared racial breakdown was

74% Caucasian/Hispanic, 18% Asian, 4% African-American, 4% Pacific Islander/Indian. The following exclusion criteria were used: women known to be pregnant, women with a history of fracture at the distal radius of either arm, the known presence of generalized bone diseases of bone other than osteoporosis including hyperparathyroidism, hypoparathyroidism, Paget's disease, renal osteodystrophy, Cushing's disease, and steroid-induced osteoporosis, or other metabolic diseases, a history of malignant diseases localized to bone or treatment by local resection, the presence of rheumatoid arthritis or other arthritic processes that severely limit patient mobility, and the presence of senile dementia severe enough to hinder adequate compliance and understanding of the study. This later data set was used to establish calibration formulas for forearm BMD[101].

The statistical procedure to derive the standardized BMD and convert measurement from one scanner to another is called *cross-calibration*. The proper calibration formulas should be simple, optimum, and internal consistent. The original calibration formula for spine BMD was developed using pair-wise linear regression[99,100]. This method was internally inconsistent and not optimum. For example, if one calibrates BMD from Hologic scanner to Luner scanner and then calibrate backwards, the value of double calibrated BMD is different from the original values. To overcome their limitations, Lu, et al.[80] and Hui, et al.[102] developed two statistical models that derived simple, consistent, and optimum formulas.

The model of Lu, et al.[80] was based on assumption of normal distributions of population BMD and measurement errors. It assumes for each subject, there is only one true standardized BMD. The observed BMD is a linear function of that standardized unobserved BMD plus measurement errors. Using the maximum likelihood method, this algorithm simultaneously estimates the regression parameters as well as model parameters. This method derived an improved formula for calculating standardized spine BMD as well as new formulas for hip BMD[103,104].

The alternative model by Hui, et al.[102] did not require normal distributions. It assumes that standardized BMD is a linear function of observed BMD measured by different DXA scanners. It then minimizes the sum of pair-wise differences of standardized BMD between different scanners. Lu, et al.[80] proved that when the measurement errors of different scanners are approximately equal, two methods derived identical formulas to obtain sBMD and calibrations between manufacturers. Hui's method has been used also in the standardization of forearm BMD[101].

While there is no difference in derived formulas in most cases, the two models are different. Hui's method is relatively simple because it doesn't impose distribution assumptions. When the BMD did not follow normal distributions, Hui's method is a better choice. On the other hand, Lu's method provides additional information, such as 95% confidence intervals of calibration formulas and is more accurate when the measurement errors are not equal among different manufacturers. Details of these methods can be found in their original papers as well as in Lu, et al.[14].

The following Table 3.1 lists the formulas to calculate sBMD for Hologic, Lunar, and Norland DXA scanner from BMD at AP spine, total hip, femoral neck (FN), trochanteric (TR), and Ward's triangle (WT). In this table, sBMD = (a+b*BMD)*100 for each manufacturer device. The cross-calibration formulas between manufacturers can be obtained by converting one manufacturer BMD to sBMD and then converting sBMD backwards to BMD by other manufacturer devices. For example, to convert a femoral neck BMD value (x) measured by a Hologic scanner to its corresponding value by a Lunar scanner, we first convert it to sBMD by $(0.019+1.087x)*100$. We then convert this value to a Lunar scanner, i.e., $(0.019+1.087x)/0.939+0.023=0.043+1.158x$.

Table 3.1 Universal Standardization Formulas for AP Spine and Femoral BMD

Manufacturer	Parameter	AP Spine	Total Hip	FN	TR	WT
Hologic	a	0.015	0.006	0.019	-0.017	0.101
	b	0.917	1.008	1.087	1.105	0.940
Lunar	a	0.055	-0.031	-0.023	-0.042	-0.106
	b	1.000	0.979	0.939	0.949	0.980
Norland	a	-0.070	0.026	0.006	0.057	0.001
	b	0.995	1.012	0.985	0.961	1.091

Standardization calibration formulas are not designed for individual BMD conversion rather to summarize population characteristics in clinical studies so that studies using scanners from different manufacturers can be compared and pooled. Example in Lu, et al.[104]

demonstrated the standardization formula helped to reduce variations in hip BMD in clinical trials. Another application is to develop common cut-off values for hip BMD based on the NHANSE study. Because this is the only population-based sample of BMD in US, the WHO cut-off values of osteoporosis was determined based on the peak mean and standard deviation of NHASE population. On the other hand, only Hologic scanners were used to measure BMD in NHASE study. For subjects measured by Lunar or Norland scanners, the cut-off values have to be converted using the standardization formulas above. The following Table 3.2 gave the WHO cut-off values of osteoporosis and osteopenia at total hip and femoral neck BMD for non-Hispanic white women in US.

Table 3.2 WHO Cut-off Values of Total Hip and Femoral Neck BMD
for Non-Hispanic White Women

Manufacturer	Cut-off Points for Total Hip BMD		Cut-off Points for Femoral Neck BMD	
	T-score <-1	T-score <-2.5	T-score <-1	T-score <-2.5
Hologic	0.820 g/cm^2	0.637 g/cm^2	0.738 g/cm^2	0.558 g/cm^2
Lunar	0.882 g/cm^2	0.693 g/cm^2	0.898 g/cm^2	0.690 g/cm^2
Norland	0.797 g/cm^2	0.615 g/cm^2	0.827 g/cm^2	0.629 g/cm^2

4. Statistics for Osteoporosis Clinical Trials

4.1. General Issues in Osteoporosis Clinical Trials

The ultimate purpose of osteoporosis research is to prevent and treat osteoporosis. Drug development for osteoporosis treatment is no different from all other drug development[105]. From its initial discovery to final marketing, a new drug in the United States has to go through various stages of development. Typically, preclinical animal studies are the first step to determine the toxicity and carcinogenicity potential of a new compound. If these studies offer no suggestion of toxicity and evidence of carcinogenicity, small phase I studies on human volunteers are conducted to determine the metabolism and pharmacologic actions of the drug in humans, dose dependent side effects, and if possible evidence of effectiveness. The information collected will permit the design of well-controlled, scientifically valid studies in Phase 2. The clinical studies in Phase 2 are conducted to evaluate the effectiveness of the drug for a particular indication or indications in patients with the disease or condition under study and to determine the common short-term side effects and risks associated with the drug. In addition, for serious diseases such as cancer, a drug may be approved conditionally based on acceptable surrogate efficacy endpoints in phase 2. The information gathered in these early phases is used to guide the drug sponsor in the planning of phase 3 clinical trials. Phase 3 studies are expanded controlled and uncontrolled studies carried out to obtain additional effectiveness and safety information that is needed to evaluate the benefit-risk relationship of the drug and to provide adequate basis for physician labeling[106].

One of the critical requirements for pre-marketing approval of a new drug in the United States is the demonstration of the effectiveness of the drug through phase 3 clinical trials. The United States Code of Federal Regulations[106] requires that to establish the efficacy of a new drug, the sponsor must produce reports of adequate and well-controlled clinical trials that demonstrate its effectiveness. Generally, the evidence of effectiveness is based on at least two adequate and well-controlled studies. Some of the characteristics of an adequate and well-controlled study are described in the regulation[106]. Another critical requirement for pre-marketing approval of a new drug is safety. The safety of the drug is evaluated on the basis of the entire database obtained from all three phases of drug development prior to approval, and continues to be evaluated through phase 4 clinical trials, if required as a condition for approval. To be approved, the drug sponsor must demonstrate that there is sufficient information to show that the drug is safe for use under the conditions prescribed, recommended, or suggested in its proposed labeling. Once approved, the safety of the new drug continues to be monitored through post-marketing adverse reaction reports.

Minimization of the potential for bias and control of the probability of the overall type I error (that is to make a false positive conclusion) are two fundamental statistical principles that are central to the quality of a trial. They are intimately related to the design, conduct and analysis of the trial, as well as the final interpretation of the trial results. Potential biases include confounding, operational bias during trial execution, evaluation bias in outcome measurement, structural bias in the trial design, and statistical bias in the method of analysis. In any given situation, bias could come from one or more or event a combination of these sources. Interesting readers can find a detailed overview in Chi, et al.[105].

While the general principles and methods are the similar for all therapeutic areas, some specific design issues are raised in osteoporosis trials. They are addressed in the FDA guidelines[107]. Substantial discussions have been given in previous chapters on pre-clinical animal studies and our focus of this chapter will be on the clinical evaluations.

FDA guideline divided osteoporosis into two separate syndromes (Type I and Type II) for selecting a treatment regimen. Type I osteoporosis affects women after menopause and results from an accelerated rate of bone loss (mainly trabecular) due to factors related to menopause. Type II (age-related) osteoporosis involves both men and women over age 70 and is characterized by gradual (over several decades) loss of both trabecular and cortical bone mass due to aging. The guideline also classified an intervention according to the indication of prevention or treatment. It provided an outline for clinical evaluations of a drug that affects the rate of fracture occurrence (treatment) or the underlying rate of bone loss (prevention), but not for a drug to affect symptoms directly.

Phase I studies focus on pharmacokinetic and pharmacodynamic studies based on healthy volunteers. This is not different from other general drug development phase I studies. Phase II studies should include twelve month, double blind, placebo-controlled, parallel group studies. The primary endpoints are the minimal effective dose and dose-response curve. The measurements of such studies include AP spine BMD, biochemical markers, as well as pharmacodynamic of a drug. Trials to investigate the biologic actions of a drug and the mechanism involved in actions are usually performed in representative a subset of trial participants who are carefully studied under a separate protocol.

All phase III study of prevention or treatment of osteoporosis trial should be double-blind and randomized, with either placebo or active drug in control group. A relatively unique feature of osteoporosis trial is the selection of the primary efficacy endpoints. For prevention trials or treatment trials using estrogens, bone mineral density at spine and femoral is the only the efficacy endpoint necessary to be demonstrated. For treatment trials for non-estrogens, the primary efficacy endpoint should be the reduction of spinal fractures at 3 years after the intervention. Ordinarily, BMD alone as an endpoint will be sufficient for approval of the prevention indication only if efficacy has already been demonstrated in a treatment study with a fracture endpoint.

Both primary endpoints in BMD and fracture require blindly serial assessments by radiologists and/or experience technicians. By the nature of interventions, the slow change in BMD, and the low incident fracture rates, most phase III osteoporosis trials are long term studies (at least 3 years for treatment trials) involving multiple clinical sites[22,108-111]. The quality of BMD readings as well as evaluation of fracture will affect the efficiency of these trials[112-114].

Statisticians play important roles in all phase clinical trials. They are responsible of or provide supports for the design of the study, selection of the primary and secondary endpoints, determination of the sample size, development of sampling/dose escalating schemes, development of data analysis plan, clinical database design and case report forms, protocol development, quality control and quality assurance, interim and final data analysis, final reports, etc. They are also in the protocol review and data safety monitoring committees, etc. The data analysis plan has to be prospectively developed before final lock the clinical data and revealing the blindness of the treatment assignment to avoid subjective bias.

In the next section we will discuss some statistical techniques for quality control and quality assurance for these radiological based primary endpoints.

4.2. Quality Control and Quality Assurance in Osteoporosis Clinical Trials

Quality control and quality assurance for BMD measurements and fracture assessments are critical components for a successful osteoporosis trial. Quality has many connotations. Quality control is a very limited function that "controls" the product, primarily by testing, while quality assurance regulates the systems and methods for "assuring" the quality of the product [115].

The primary tool to measure BMD is the DXA scanner. Quantitative ultrasound (QUS) also provide alternatives to DXA to measure not only the bone quantity but also quality. As with all machinery, products of different manufacturers vary in quality. Over time, machine may draft and age can affect performance. Furthermore, precision errors are always to be expected in any radiological equipments or technique; even when the same patient is scanned under identical conditions the results will be different. Last but not least, many radiological assessments are based on the experience of reader and are relatively subjective. It is common to have different readers to give different interpretations of the same image. Therefore, many factors will affect the results of radiological assessments. The statistical principles discussed here can resolve the conflicts among results from different devices and improve interpretation of the results.

Good Clinical Practice (GCP) is an international quality standard for the design, conduct, recording, and reporting of clinical trials with human subjects. GCP guidelines not only provide a framework for protecting the rights of participating patients or volunteers, they also set standards to safeguard the integrity of data that are used to evaluate treatment efficacy and submitted to regulatory agencies[116]. In radiology, GCP includes training documents and standard operating procedures, imaging device quality control, image acquisition protocols, software validation, record keeping, and reporting, etc.[117]. Obviously, this is not only a statistical process. Successful quality control and quality assurance require good leadership from department chairs or principal investigators and, importantly, a team of multi-disciplinary experts. The expert team should always include a statistician. Statisticians are important in planning quality control, including determining appropriate sampling to avoid bias in selecting test samples, calculating the sample sizes, analyzing results to identify deficiencies, planning the processing control charts for monitoring machine performance, reassessing the results of quality improvement, and in reporting data and study results.

There are many aspects of quality control and quality assurance that are not directly related to statistics[114,118,119]. Here, we only present some statistical tools for longitudinal quality control for DXA scanner and the assessment of agreement for radiologist assessment of fracture status.

The key component of quality control is to control measurement errors. Measurement errors describe the limits of a quantitative or qualitative assessment of a disease using a particular technique or procedure. Measurement errors have many sources, but mainly accuracy and precision errors. *Precision errors* reflect the reproducibility of the technique. The most commonly used measure of relative precision error is the coefficient of variation (CV), defined as the ratio of the standard deviation to the mean measurement. It is usually given on a percentage basis. CV is unit free and therefore can be used with different techniques and instruments.

Long-term precision errors are used to evaluate instrument stability, including additional sources of random variation attributable to small drifts in instrumental calibration, variations in patient characteristics, change of technicians and other technical changes related to time. The quality control and assurance for BMD measurement in osteoporosis trial focus on this long-term precisions over time. Because of randomization and blindness of both phase II and III osteoporosis trials, it is not expect the precision error to cause biased estimates of relative differences between treated and controlled arms. However, it may introduce noises that reduces statistical power and creates difficulty to interpret the trial results.

In an osteoporosis trial, it is commonly recommend establish a centralized quality control and quality assurance center to monitor the quality of BMD results across all clinical sites. Precision errors are always assessed before the beginning of clinical trials[113,114]. Although the manufacturer's service personnel can set up the device so that precision errors are within appropriate limits at baseline, it is very important to monitor the equipment to assure that imprecision remains within acceptable limits. Despite the remarkable accuracy and reproducibility of radiological equipment, measurements can still vary because of changes in equipment, software upgrades, machine recalibration, X-ray source decay, hardware aging and/or failure, or operator errors.

In an ideal setting, a well maintained equipment produce values that are randomly spread around a reference value. A change point is defined as the point in time at which the measured values start to deviate from the reference value. To evaluate measurement stability and identify change points, radiologists develop phantoms that simulate human measurements but, unlike humans, do not change over time[114,120]. Variations in phantom measurements should reflect variations in human measurements. Phantoms are measured regularly to detect one or more of the following events: (1) The mean values before and after the change point are statistically significantly different; (2) The standard deviations of measurements before and after the change point are statistically significantly different; (3) The measurements after the change point show a gradual but significant departure from the reference value.

Statistical process control (SPC) is a powerful collection of problem solving tools for achieving process stability and improving capacity through reduction of variability[121]. Here we give an overview of these methods.

Visual Inspection Method: Potential change points in the data can be determined after careful visual inspection. This can be done by plotting longitudinal phantom data over time and using visual judgment to identify the potential change points created by drifts or sudden jumps. Statistical tests, such as the t-test, can be used to confirm the significance of the changes. It is important to note that there can be multiple potential change points observed for a given period of time. Careful control for type one errors for repeated tests is recommended for the t-tests.

Only experienced medical physicists or radiologists should perform periodic visual inspections. The role of primary evaluator should always be taken by the same individual to avoid subjective variations. The selection of the change points is based on reading of the scatter plot in the most recent data. Once a change point has been identified, its cause should be investigated to determine if the change is machine related.

Visual inspection is not recommended because its efficiency depends on the experience of the reviewer and may not be reproducible.

Shewhart Control Chart: A Shewhart chart is a graphic display of a quality that has been measured over time. The chart contains a central horizontal line that represents the mean reference value. Three horizontal lines above and three below the central line indicate 1, 2, and 3 standard deviations from the reference value. By plotting the observed quality control measurements on the chart, we can determine if the machine is operating within acceptable limits.

The reference values can be derived from theoretical values for the phantom, or from the first 25 observations measured at baseline. The reference value changes whenever the Shewhart chart indicates an out of control signal and the machine is recalibrated. The new reference value will then be the mean of the first 25 observations after scanner recalibration by the manufacturer service personnel. The number of observations needed to calculate the reference value may vary; the number 25 was chosen based on practical experience to balance the stability of the reference value with the length of time needed to establish it.

The standard deviation varies among individual devices, and manufacturers should be selected accordingly. For example, in one osteoporosis study, we sometimes use the BMD of a Hologic phantom to monitor DXA scanner performance. We usually assume the coefficient of variation for Hologic machines to be 0.5% and Lunar to be 0.6%, based on reported data on long-term phantom precision[122]. Therefore, the standard deviation for the scanner was calculated as 0.005 and 0.006 times the reference value for Hologic and Lunar machines respectively.

The original Shewhart chart will signal that there is a problem if the observed measurement is more than 3 standard deviations from the reference value. Although intuitive and easy to apply, the chart is not very sensitive to small but significant changes[123]. Therefore, a set of sensitizing tests for assignable causes has been developed to improve the sensitivity of Shewhart charts. Eight of the tests are available in the statistical software package SAS[36]. The tests are listed in Table 4.1.

The sensitizing rules can be used in total or in part depending on the underlying processes of interest. For example, for quality control of DXA machines, we used four tests—1, 2, 5 and 6[121]. Once a change point has been identified by any one of the tests, the manufacturer's repair service should be called to examine the causes and to recalibrate the machine. We then use the next 25 observations to generate new reference values and apply the tests to the subsequent data according to the new reference value.

Table 4.1. Definition of Tests for Assignable Causes for Shewhart Charts

Tests	Pattern Description
1	One point is more than 3 standard deviation from the central line
2	Nine points in a row on one side of the central line
3	Six points in a row steadily increasing or steadily decreasing
4	Fourteen points in a row alternating up and down
5	Two out of 3 points in a row more than 2 standard deviation from the central line
6	Four out of 5 points in a row more than 1 standard deviation from the central line
7	Fifteen points in a row all within 1 standard deviation from the central line on either or both sides of the line
8	Eight points in a row all beyond 1 standard deviation from the central line on either or both sides of the line

Figure 4.1 shows the application of a Shewhart chart. In this chart, the dots are the observed BMD. The six lines are the control limits 1, 2 and 3 standard deviations away from the central reference line. There is a problem with Test 2 from April 10, 1989.

The sensitizing rules increase the sensitivity of the Shewhart Chart, but also increase the number of clinically insignificant alarms, which is not desirable. To overcome this problem, a threshold based on the magnitude of the mean shift can also be implemented. For example, we can select ten consecutive scans from after the possible change point identified on the Shewhart chart, and then calculate their mean values. If the mean differs by more than one standard deviation (which equals 0.5% times the reference value, in our example) from the reference value, the change point is confirmed as a true change point. Otherwise, the signal from the Shewhart chart is ignored and the reference value is unchanged. This approach filters out small and clinically insignificant changes. However, the true difference must be more than one standard deviation for this approach to be effective, and this approach can delay the recognition of true change points.

More advanced methods, such as moving average chart, cumulative sum (CUSUM) chart and exponentially weighted moving-average (EWMA) control chart, etc. can also be applied for quality assurance of DXA scanners in osteoporosis trials. Because we don't want to present detailed mathematics in this book, we recommend interesting readers to read detailed descriptions in Lu and Zhao[14].

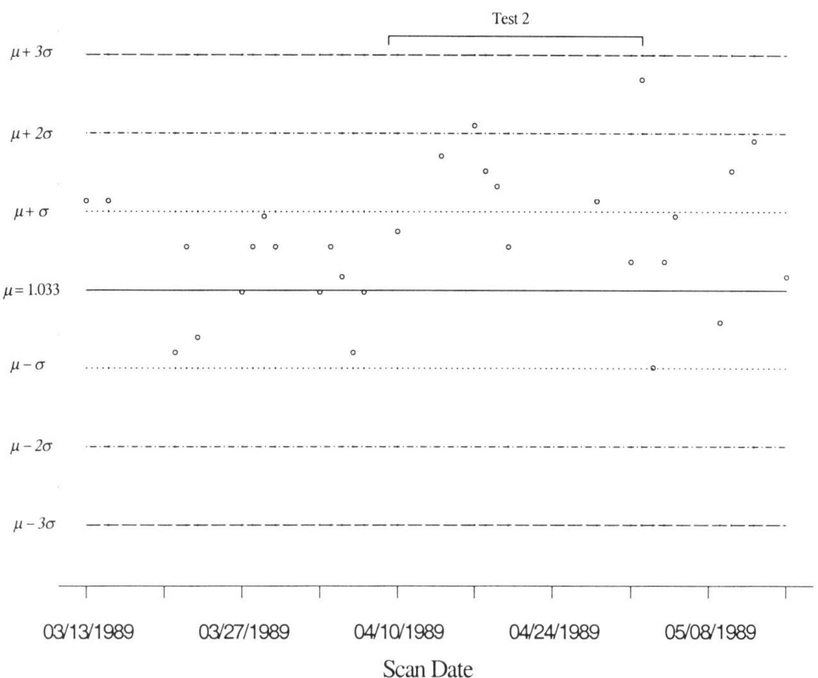

Fig. 4.1. Shewhart Chart for QC Data.

Lu, et al.[121] compared several statistical process control procedures and their applications to monitoring DXA scanners based on daily scans of a Hologic spine phantom. The comparisons were based on their results on longitudinal quality control data from 5 clinical trial sites as well as simulation studies. They concluded that visual inspection is relatively subjective and depends on the operator's experience and alertness. The regular Shewhart chart with sensitizing rules has a high false alarm rate. The Shewhart chart with sensitizing rules and an additional filter of clinically insignificant mean changes has the lowest false alarm rate but relatively low sensitivity. This method does not require a lot of statistics and can be easily applied to clinical study sites. The CUSUM approach has the best combination of sensitivity, specificity, and identification of the time and magnitude of change. It is recommended for use in quality control centers in clinical trials, especially if patient data must be recalculated to adjust for change points[112]. Combining a moving average chart and a moving standard deviation chart comes closest to the performance of the CUSUM method as a quality control procedure for monitoring DXA scanner performance.

Different from BMD quality control that focuses on precision errors, the quality control for fracture assessment focus on the agreement between two radiologists in calling incident fractures. The Kappa statistics discussed in subsection 3.4 is the most commonly used statistics. Periodic review of inter- and intra-reader agreement is a part of quality control of clinical trials. Readers should always be blinded of clinical information as well as time order of the films if possible. The sequence of subjects to be reviewed should be randomly mixed. The testing films should have a complete spectrum of potential cases, including easy ones and the most difficulty ones. Sufficient time between two QC readings of the same set of testing films should be allowed to avoid recall effect. If the readers disagree with each other, re-training is necessary. The minimum level of inter-reader agreement should be specified prospectively before the study starts. Details of these methods and their applications in quality control studies can be found in Lu and Zhao[14].

5. Cost-Effective Analysis (CEA) for Osteoporosis Treatment

As discussed in earlier chapters, osteoporosis is a prevalent disease. Osteoporosis and, in particular, the consequent fracture cost substantial health care resources. While there are increasing options for treatment options to reduce the incidence of fracture, these new pharmaceutical interventions are expensive and require relatively long-term uses. Because the healthcare resources are always limited (both for developed and more for developing countries), healthcare policies need to be developed and evaluated to balance the benefits and constrains. Cost-effectiveness analysis (CEA) is a research method designed to help determine which health interventions provide the most effective and affordable medical care. It identifies the tradeoff between the resources expended on osteoporosis intervention and health benefits that result. Thus, CEA provides scientific bases for rational healthcare policy development[124,125].

There have been many CEA studies to evaluate and compare therapeutic options, treatment thresholds, and screening strategies. In this section, we want to provide an overview of the CEA methodology, in particular, the Markov Models that have been used for CEA in many studies. We describe the parameters needed for such a study and review literature that established these parameters for CEA for osteoporosis.

5.1 An Overview of Cost-Effective Analysis (CEA)

Different from the efficacy that measures the ability of a treatment to reduce the fracture or the ability to detect low bone mass in a clinical setting, the effectiveness measures the overall risks and benefits of a health intervention in the real world. Studies for the effectiveness need to specify three components: the health intervention, health status, and health costs. In our case, we need to specify whether we want to compare interventions, such as vitamin D, hormone replacement therapy (HRT), bisphosphonate, and raloxifene, etc. We need to specify the cohorts of interests, such as bone mineral density (BMD) values, age groups, and menopausal status for women, etc. The health states for subjects in the cohort will transit after intervention and during the follow-up, including fracture, recovery from the fracture, other chronicle diseases, and death. The health costs normally include diagnostic costs, intervention costs, costs to monitor the treatment, costs to treat adverse effects of interventions, averted costs because of the reducing fractures, quality of life gains, etc. Benefit of intervention is normally expressed in a cost effective ratio (CER)[125]. The numerator of the CER is the cost of the intervention minus the costs averted by an intervention. The denominator of the CER is usually the QALY gain, number of fractures averted, etc.

There are three primary types of economic studies for medical interventions: the cost-effective analysis (CEA), cost-benefit analysis (CBA), and the cost-utility analysis (CUA)[126]. All CEA, CUA, and CBA

                                        Y. Lu & H. Jin

use the tool of incremental ratio (IR): that is the ratio of cost differences over the health outcome differences. Table 5.1 is adopted from Tella, Feinglass, and Chang[126] to illustrate three different analyses in their incremental ratios.

Table 5.1. Calculating the Incremental Ratio in CEA, CUA, and CBA (Tella, et al.)[126]

	Cost	Health outcome (effectiveness, utility, or benefit)
Health service A	Ca	Ea or Ua or Ba
Health service B	Cb	Eb or Ub or Bb
Cost-effectiveness ratio (CER)	(Cb-Ca) (Eb-Ea)	
Cost-utility ratio (CUR)	(Cb-Ca) (Ub-Ua)	
Cost-benefit ratio (CBR)	(Cb-Ca) (Bb-Ba)	

Cost benefit analysis involves calculating the total costs associated with a specific choice, estimating the benefits of the choice in monetary values and comparing the total costs with the total benefits. Cost benefit analysis is used to compare actual or ascribed costs of one activity with another. Because the elusive nature of perceived benefits can make them difficult to quantify, this method hasn't been used in osteoporosis research.

"Cost effectiveness analysis (CEA) is used to determine the costs and patient benefits of medical treatments in order to identify the treatments that produce the greatest benefits for the least amount of money."[124] It attempts to determine the relative benefit of no medical intervention versus intervention or the relative benefit of one treatment over another. The benefits here are often directly quantifiable, objectively observed, such as the average number of life-year gained or fracture events averted. It is the most common cost analysis used in health care.

Cost utility analysis (CUA) compares costs of health costs with the benefits not only in the length of life but also the quality of life. The quality of life is usually determined by the health related quality of life (HRQL) score that will be briefly explained later. Because CUA and CEA use the identical analytical methods, they have been used interchangeably[125]. Almost all CEA in osteoporosis research are the CUA.

5.2 Markov Models

CEA studies often use the Markov models to describe health status and their relationships. In such a model, we usually start an artificial cohort of interest. The cohort can be healthy women at age 50-60, or post-menopausal women aged 65 or more, or healthy male aged 75 or more, etc. The model will list all related health states in chronicle orders and put links among them[127,128]. Figure 5.1 shows a possible model for osteoporosis CEA.

The health states included in the model will have great impact on the final CEA analysis. Because of osteoporotic fractures mostly occur among old people who may have other chronic diseases, we may want to consider them as separate health states if they will affect the chances of fracture or if the intervention will affect not only osteoporosis but also other diseases, such as cardiovascular disease (CAD) or Breast Cancer, etc. Also, various types of osteoporotic fractures have different impact on quality of life and mortalities and may need to be separately listed in a Markov Model.

Moving between health states will depend on probabilities obtained from epidemiological studies, clinical trials, and prognostic studies. An accurate probability distribution of risk factors, such as age distribution of BMD and risk of fracture, will allow calculations for when and what type of fractures occur among what proportion of subjects in the cohort. Treatment efficacy will alter the chance of fracture and hopefully extend time to stay on the fracture-free states when an intervention is applied. Regardless the use of intervention or not, fracture will occur among some subjects. After a fracture occurs, information from prognostic studies will help to determine the chance of death or other recovery states. A Markov property means that each transition from one state to another one only depends on the current health state but not the history prior to the current state[127].

 Y. Lu & H. Jin

Table 5.2. Summary of Health States in Review Papers

Study Year	Cohort	Interventions	Fracture/ Disease States	Recovery States
1[129] 1999	Age groups 50-80 post-menopausal women by 10 year increments	(1) 5-year universal use of HRT (2) 5-year universal use of Bisphosphonates (3) no treatment	Hip Fracture CAD Breast Cancer	Not Specified (no 2nd fracture)
2[130] 2001	50 years old healthy post-menopausal women	(1) Life time universal use of HRT (2) lifetime universal use of Raloxifene (3) no treatment	CAD, Hip Fx, Spine Fx, Breast and Endometrial Cancer, Thromboemb olism	Not Specified
3[131] 2002	50 years old post-menopausal Japanese	(1) No treatment (2) universal HRT (no screening) (3) HRT for osteopenia women (4) HRT for osteoporotic women.	Hip Fracture	Good Poor (no 2nd fracture)
4[132] 2002	75-year-old women who with a mild prevalent VT Fx and low BMD 3 years after treatment of Risendronate	(1) continue Risendronate (2) stop Risendronate	hip,vertebral, wrist or other Fx	Healthy post Fx
5[133] 2002	Age groups 50-70 post-menopausal women by 10 year increments	(1) Calcium and vitamin D3	Hip Fracture	History of Hip Fracture
6[134] 2002	Age groups 50-70 post-menopausal women by 5 year increments	Generic treatments with efficacy 50%, 35%, 20%, and 10% and treat for subjects with different relative risk of hip fracture.	Hip Fracture	Not specified
7[135] 2002	PM Canadian Women age 65+ with low BMD and prev. VT Fx	5-year nasal calcitonin, Alendronate, Etidronate	Hip, Wrist, Spine Fx	1-year post hip Fx
8[136] 2003	PM Swedish Women age 71 with low BMD and prev. VT Fx	5-year Alendronate versus no trtment	Hip, Wrist, and Spine Fx	Post-hip Fx State

Table 5.2 reviewed six recent publications in CEA and their corresponding list of states[129-134]. Because these studies used different epidemiological data, their transitional rates and prognostic rates varied and could not be summarized in tables.

5.3 Interventions

Interventions should be specified in a CEA analysis. CEA of an intervention can be derived by incremental CER in comparison to no-intervention. Two interventions can be compared based on the incremental CER from one intervention to another. Cost-effectiveness of an intervention can also determine based on a prespecified threshold of CER, i.e., the dollars per quality-adjusted life-year (QALY) gained. If an

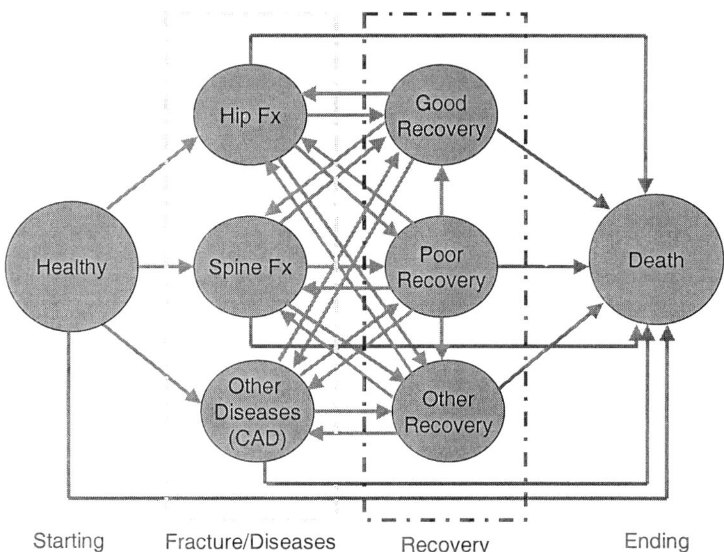

Fig. 5.1. An illustration of health states of a Markov model. The figure shows possible states of a Markov model in Osteoporosis CEA. The immediate state after healthy state include all fracture status, including non-trauma or low-trauma fractures in hip, spine, wrist, etc. and other competing diseases, such as cardiovascular disease or breast cancer, etc. Subject can also go to the death state without fracture or disease listed in the model. Once a subject experienced a fracture or disease, he/she can recover in either good or poor or any intermediate recovery state or die without the second fracture. The transition between models will follow a Markov property with transition rates from epidemiological studies, clinical trials, and prognostic studies.

intervention reduces costs with a positive gain in quality of life against another one, it is considered "dominant" choice[125]. More often, we have the expensive intervention with a positive gain in QALY (discussed later). We can compare two intervention based on the CER.

An intervention may be selectively applied to a subset of the cohort. The distribution of risk factors and chance of receiving intervention will chance the transition rates. For example, Nagata-Kobayashi, Shimbo, and Fujui[131] assumed HRT reduced hip incident fracture rate 25%. Thus, the transition rate of a HRT treated subject from healthy to hip fracture was only 75% of untreated subjects with the same BMD and age.

While most osteoporosis interventions are relatively long-term, it is possible that the fracture risk will be reversed after the stop of the interventions. The offset may take for several years and linear models have been used to describe such offset effects[129].

5.4 Costs

Costs in CEA analyses associate with the health states in a model. Allocating costs in CER requires economic studies of the direct costs, indirect costs, and intangible costs[125]. For CEA for osteoporosis, costs need to be determined including diagnostic test to select who to treat, the costs of intervention and monitoring, the costs resulted from fractures. Most time, we calculate the direct costs, rather than indirect costs and intangible costs. The most common used method is to use matched case-control study based either on retrospective review or prospective follow-up designs.

Gabriel, et al.[137] used a population-based cohort of men and women 50 years of age or older with incident fracture during 1989-1991 due to minimal or moderate trauma. For each case, a control of same age (± 1 year) and sex who attended in the local medical system in the same year was identified as control. The incremental costs in the year after fracture was estimated based on the differences between cases and controls. Because this cohort has their medical treatment information almost exclusively captured in the Mayo Cost Data Warehouse, it is possible to provide a standardized, inflation-adjusted estimate to reflect the national average cost of providing the service. It showed that the median incremental cost was $11,241 for hip fracture, $1,955 for clinical spine fracture, and $1,628 for wrist fracture. Regression analysis revealed that age, prior year costs, and type of fracture were significant predictors of incremental costs.

De Laet, et al.[138] used a matched case-control design within a longitudinal follow-up study. Both incident hip and morphological spine fractured patients were matched with randomly selected controls in age, gender, self-perceived health, ability to perform activities of daily live, living situation and general practitioner. Medical expenditure included healthcare usages (hospital, surgery, nursing home, physician visits) and pharmaceutical consumptions. The mean incremental cost in the first year after hip fracture was $9,540 for all subjects and $10,157 for surviving subjects. The second year mean incremental cost was $1,017 for all subjects and $1,943 for surviving subjects. Incremental yearly costs for morphological fractures were divided based on years before first radiograph ($508), years between radiographs ($431 in between mean 2.2 years), and years after fracture ($1,057).

In another Belgium study, Autier and colleagues[139] used a case-control prospective study design of 1-year duration. In this study, 4 hospitals provided hip fracture women (cases). Controls were searched using the "nearest neighborhood" method matched for age ($\pm$5 years). The 1-year follow-up started just after hospital discharge. Costs was calculated based on daily provided by patients, including hospital costs for hip fracture, transportations, orthopedic wards, surgery, rehabilitation, convalescent homes, geriatric care, nursing homes, physiotherapy, and assistance at home. The mean incremental cost per hip fracture in this study was €6,636. The costs depend on age group (<=80, >80) and nursing home usage.

Table 5.3 summarizes these studies. It at least illustrates the differences in costs between countries, including items to be counted and values. Depending on the purpose, the costs instead of charges should be used. For a long-term study, inflation adjustment will help standardizing the costs for comparisons. A Chinese specific study is necessary.

5.5 Quality of Life Evaluations

Pharmaceutical interventions not only reduce deaths because of hip fracture but most importantly improve morbidity and the quality of life

Table 5.3. Summary of Studies for Costs

Study Year	Design	Fractures	Type of Costs	Total Incremental Costs
1[138] 1999	1. Matched case-control study within a longitudinal prospective cohort study. 2. Medical costs data retrieved from medical records of GP. Pharmaceutical consumption retrieved from central pharmacy.	Hip fracture and morphological spine fracture for women	1. Pharmacy 2. Orthopedic surgery 3. Other hospital admissions 4. Nursing home 5. Physician visits	Mean cost: 1st year after hip fx: $9,540 2nd year after hip fx: $1,017 Mean cost for morphological spine fx: Years before 1st X-ray film: $508(NS) Years between films: $431(NS) Years after 2nd X-ray: $1,057 (NS)
2[139] 2000	1. Matched case-control prospective study design of 1-year duration based on patients in 4 regional hospitals 2. Costs determined by dairy	Hip fracture for women	1. Acute hospital stay 2. Rehabilitation 3. Nursing home 4. Fee for physician 5. Physiotherapy 6. Home assistance by nurse 7. Extra hospital stay 8. One-day clinic 9. No inflation adjustment	Mean cost 1-year after fx: €6,636 Age 50-80: €6,254 Age >80: €6,771 In a nursing home before fx: Yes: €3,479 No: €9,914
3[137] 2002	1. Population-based matched case-control retrospective review of a cohort of men and women 50 years of age in a county in US 2. Costs determined by Mayo Cost Data Warehouse.	No-trauma or low-trauma fractures in hip, clinical spine, wrist, like a hip, like a spine, and like a wrist, like a finger/toe for men and women	Standardized, inflation-adjusted (1995$) unit cost (not the charge) for all medical care services, except outpatient prescription drug, durable medical equipment, dental care, ambulance service, and nursing home care	Median after one year fx: Hip: $11,241 Spine: $1,955 Wrist: $1,628 Like a hip: $4,159 Like a spine: $581 Like a wrist: $1,996 Like a finger/toe: $542

by avoiding hip, spine, and other fractures. Thus, CEA for osteoporosis are almost always measured by gain in quality adjusted life year (QALY).

Essentially, the QALY values are composed of health state preference values covering six domains and subsequent 24 facets[140]. The best way to determine the values attached to specific health status is based on direct measurements from patients. Two most commonly used methods are time trade-off (TTO) method and standard gambling (SG) method.

The TTO method asks a patient to estimate how many years of "perfect health" they would be willing to trade to be cured of a specific condition[141]. The SG method asks a patient to choose between living with a specified condition and "gambling" on a treatment that, if successful, would restore full health; but if unsuccessful, would result in death. "The odds are then varied to determine at what point the respondent decides the gamble is not worth taking."[142] Dolan compared TTO and SG methods and concluded that TTO is a better method[143].

The quality adjusted life year is calculated by multiplying these preference values for a particular condition by the amount of time the patient is likely to spend in that condition. Thus, using a scale in which one represents full health and zero represents death, results in a lower value being placed on time spent with impaired function than in full health[142].

Most CEA studies for osteoporosis research used the HRQL scores provided by National Osteoporosis Foundation based on a panel of experts[144]. Other studies reported utility for different countries, such as Dolan, Torgerson, and Kakarlapudi from UK[145], Salkeld, et al. from Australia[146], Cranney, et al. from Canada[147], Martin, et al.[148] from France, etc.

The source of preference scores has an impact on the cost-effectiveness of osteoporosis interventions. In a study by Gabriel, et al.[149], three groups of subjects aged $\geq$ 50 years women with (183 women) and without (199 women) osteoporotic fractures were studied. TTO method was used to assess two preference-classification systems: Health Utilities Index preference-classification system and direct utility assessment in patients. The preference scores for hypothetical osteoporosis health states of the non-fracture subjects were approximately 50% lower than those of the women who had actually experienced the health state. The Health Utilities Index preference-classification system may provide an efficient and inexpensive alternative to direct utility assessment in this patient group. Cost-utility analyses based solely on fracture patients' preferences for osteoporotic health states may undervalue prevention.

5.6 Sensitivity Analysis

We have demonstrated that a CEA involves several steps and uses data from population BMD distribution and other risk factors, the mortality of the population, the intervention costs and costs for fractures, the efficacy of treatments and their impact on other competing diseases, the health related quality of life scores, etc. Changing values of one parameter may affect the study conclusions. Therefore, it is critical to perform sensitivity analysis in CEA to investigate whether the study conclusion is reliable[125]. Usually, the population parameters are derived from large epidemiological study and should not be altered. Depending on the source of HRQL score, it may or may not be subject to variations. The treatment costs and efficacy usually vary in sensitivity analysis. To determine intervention thresholds, alternating of eligibility for treatments can also provide useful information. Other factors to be considered include varying discount rates, inflation rates, and percentage compliance of patients to the treatment, etc.

5.7 Use of CEA

The primary use of CEA is to determine whether a treatment should be implemented. In our review of six papers, five compared specific intervention strategies[129-133] and one evaluated unspecified blanket intervention strategies[134]. Using $30,000/QAYL as the cost-effective threshold, Jonsson et al.[129] concluded that 5-year HRT was cost-effective from age 60 or above who has double risk of hip fracture ($20,000/QALY) and was more cost-effective than bisphosphonates. Based on Armstrong et al.[130] study and recent knowledge about HRT on CAD and breast cancer, raloxifene is more cost-effective

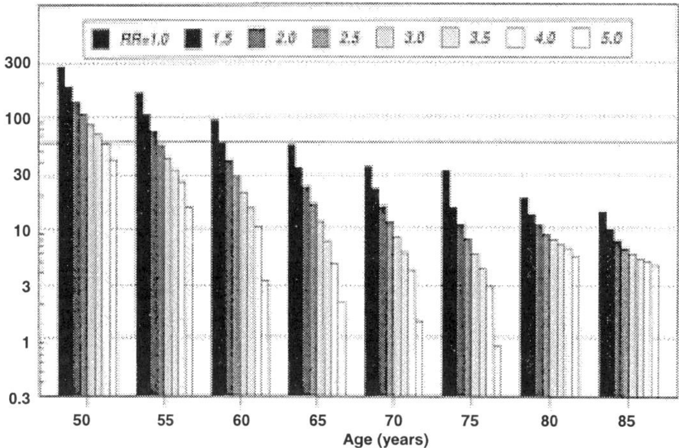

Fig. 5.2. Cost-effectiveness of an intervention costing $500 per annum with an efficacy of 35% according to age and relative risk. The threshold for cost effectiveness is set at $60,000 per QALY gained (solid horizontal line) [From Figure 1 of Kanis, et al. (Bone, 2002)].

(<$43,056/QALY) for all postmenopausal women. Nagata-Kobayashi, et al.[131] reported CER of HRT reference to no-treatment from 5,400,000 yen/QALY for screening and treating osteoporosis subjects only to 41,700,000 yen/QALY for universal treatments without screening. Iglesias, et al.[132] showed continuing risendronate 3 additional years for a particular cohort who have prevalent fracture and had been treated by risendronate for three years was cost-effective (£1,187.5/QALY) and was dominant to continue risendronate for them over a lifetime. Willis[133] concluded that treatment using Calcium and Vitamin D3 was cost saving of 70-year-old women and was cost-effective for 50- (ranged from 89,400-147,220SEK/QALY) and 60-year old (ranged from C/S to 11,000SEK/QALY) cohorts against alternative of no treatment. Kanis, et al.[134] used the Markov model to investigate the blanket treatment options under various intervention strategies. In their analysis, no specific intervention was investigated. Instead, several cost options and efficacies of any interventions and different cut-off values for receiving treatments were investigated. A threshold of $60,000/QALY is considered cost effective. Their analysis showed when an intervention is cost-effective versus the no-treatment in Figure 5.2. They concluded that the cost-effective intervention thresholds vary with age and relative risk of hip fracture and the available treatments can be cost-effectively targeted to individuals at moderately increased risk. Table 5.4 summarizes conclusions of these studies.

5.8 Conflicts of Interests

Most CEA studies are scientifically and scholarly. However, readers should still pay attention to disclosure statements of such studies. Because the model assumptions and parameter selections can potentially alter the conclusions, conscious or unconscious biases of investigators can still greatly affect the objectivity of the study. Several studies have been sponsored by pharmaceutical companies. CEA studies use parameters derived from population records or epidemiological studies should give more weight than small clinical trial cohorts sponsored by pharmaceutical companies in development of healthcare polices for osteoporosis.

5.9 CEA for Screening Strategies

Many studies have also investigated cost-effective or cost-saving strategies to screen osteoporosis. None of them have linked to cost-effective therapeutic decisions and none of them related to health-related quality-of-life (HRQL). NOF has recommended hip dual X-ray absorptiometry (DXA) scan for postmenopausal US women aged 65 and older or younger women with a least one risk factor of osteoporosis[150]. Recent studies have explored alternatives to identify osteoporosis using other low cost instruments. For example, Langton, et al.[151] proposed the use of quantitative ultrasound (QUS) to screen patients before their DXA scans. The study mostly related to China is an osteoporosis self-

Table 5.4. Summary of CER in Review Papers

Study Year	CER (Costs/QALY)	Conclusions
[1]129 1999	Bisphosphonates ($625/year) 50- with hip fx RR$\geq$2: $370,000 60- with hip fx RR$\geq$2: $110,000 70- with hip fx RR$\geq$2: $ 26,000 HRT ($250/year) 50- with hip fx RR$\geq$2: $118,000 60- with hip fx RR$\geq$2: $ 20,000	1. Intervention in elderly is preferred at the time of the menopause. 2. Treatment efficacy offset time is a critical component of cost-effectiveness, particularly in younger women.
[2]130 2001	Raloxifene vs HRT overall Long-term therapy: HRT dominant 5-y therapy: $37,029 10-y therapy: $32,992 Raloxifene vs HRT on Breast Cancer Breast Cancer Risk 15%: $43,056 Breast Cancer Risk 30%: $ 3,830	1. Both HRT and Raloxifene are cost-effective relative to no therapy. 2. If HRT prevents CAD (not true), HRT is a better choice. 3. Raloxifene is cost-effective for women average risk of CAD and major risk of breast cancer.
[3]131 2002	HRT versus no therapy for post-menopausal women from age 50: BMD T-score $\leq$ -2.5: 5,360,000 yen BMD T-score $\leq$ -1.0: 14,700,000 yen All: 39,400,000 yen	1. Screening postmenopausal Japanese women and treating osteoporosis may be acceptable. 2. Cost-effectiveness ratio only fair.
[4]132 2002	Continue Risedronate versus no therapy: 25-year treatment: dominant 3-year treatment: £1,187.5	1. The use of risedronate therapy improves quality of life with cost savings.

[5]133 2002	Calcium and Vitamin D3 versus no therapy for postmenopausal Sweden Women:
	Age 50-: Efficacy 15%: SEK 359,733
	          20%: 204,075
	          27%: 89,400
	Age 60-: 15%: 193,667
	          20%: 67,200
	          27%: C/S
	Age 70-: 15%: 74,600
	        $\geq$20%: C/S
		Treatment may be cost saving or at least cost-effective for many cohorts of high-risk 50 and particularly 60-year-old women, in particularly those with osteoporosis or a maternal family history of hip fracture.

[6]134 2002	Figure 5.2	1. Inclusion of all osteoporotic fractures has a marked effect on CEA. 2. Available treatments can be cost-effectively targeted to individuals at moderately increased risk.
[7]135 2002	5-year therapy (Against no treatment): Nasal Calcitonin: $Can46,500 Alendronate: $Can52,742 Etidronate: $Can269,000	1. Nasal calcitonin is cost-effective 2. Nasal calcitonin is more cost-effective than etidronate. 3. Nasal calcitonin versus alendronate is inconclusive.
[8]136 2003	71-year-old OP women with prior spine fracture: SEK 76,384 Starting age 65: SEK172,520 Starting age 77: SEK 52,348	1. Alendronate is more cost-effective to treat older than younger osteoporotic women. 2. Alendronate is more cost-effective to treat osteoporotic women with than without prior spine fracture.

assessment tool (OSAT)[152] derived from 8 participated Asian countries to identify women who has osteoporosis in femoral neck based on the WHO criterion. This tool is still relatively complicated for individual women to use and has a low specificity (45%) for the given sensitivity of 91%. In another study in Belgium, Ben Sedrine and colleagues[153] used 10 questions covering lifestyle data, reproductive history, medical history, and mediations to screen subjects who should received DXA scans. Again, their focus was identifying women and men who have osteoporosis or osteopenia defined by WHO criterion. The sensitivity of presence of at least one risk factor was 75% and specificity was 37%. Kanis, et al.[154] studied 2113 women aged 75 years or more from UK. Only 21% of them had 10-year fracture probability predicted by clinical factors in between 20% to 80%. A strategy that only uses DXA for these individuals would only misclassify 8% of all women. An extensive review on this topic can be found from the meta-analysis of Nelson, et al.[155]. A recent discussion about screening for Chinese women in Hong Kong can be found in Hui[156].

The strategy of population screening of osteoporosis should depend on the subsequent therapeutic actions and costs associated with the treatment strategies. Unfortunately, except Nagata-Kobayashi et al.[131], none of the current studies link the screening strategy with the treatment options. Information from Nelson, et al.[155] and CEA strategies summarized in previous sections can lead to models for such studies.

Another factor to be considered the value of a DXA scan is the interaction of an intervention with BMD. Reported observations suggest that BMD measured by DXA not only provides information about risk of fracture, and thus to make the treatment decision, but also predicts possible responses to an intervention. Whether the ability of clinical factors can predict treatment responses is unclear.

Table 5.5 itemizes the reviewed articles by their corresponding tasks.

5.10 Summary

As we have pointed out at the beginning, CEA studies depend on the population, culture, health care system and are not directly transferable from one country to another. Proper CEA studies should specify the intervention strategies, model assumptions, and model parameters. They are very useful to help determining which health interventions provide the most effective and affordable medical care and support the development of health care policies. Proper CEA studies are very important for managing osteoporosis. Such studies by definition should be multi-disciplinary to include government agents, health economists, health care provides, epidemiologists, and statisticians, etc.

Table 5.5. List of Review Papers by Categories

Categories	References
CEA Methodology	124,125,128,140
Therapeutic Interventions	129-136
Determining Costs	137-139
Health-Related Quality-of-Life	140-149
Screening Strategies	151-159
Chinese Studies	10,160-169

6. Conclusion

In this chapter we provide a brief overview of statistical methods that are applicable to osteoporosis research. Like many other medical fields, statistics play an important role in clinical research, drug development, and establishments of healthcare policy. Statistics is a scientific language to describe random phenomenon and a tool to separate information from random noises. Statisticians should be involved in planning stages for any of above tasks to maximize the power of these methods.

REFERENCES

1.   Moses, L. in *Medical Uses of Statistics* (ed. III JCB, M. F., eds) 5-26 (NEJM Books, Boston, 1992).
2.   WHO. (World Health Organization, Geneva, 1994).
3.   Kanis, J. A., Melton, L. J., Christiansen, C., Johnston, C. C. & Khaltaev, N. The diagnosis of osteoporosis. *Journal of Bone and Mineral Research* 9, 1137-1141 (1994).

4. Hui, S., Slemenda, C. & Johnston, C. Baseline measurement of bone mass predicts fracture in white women. *Ann Intern Med* 111, 355-361 (1989).

5. Wilcox, R. R. *Introduction to Robust Estimation and Hypothesis Testing* (Academic Press, San Diego, 1997).

6. Yohai, V. J. & Zamar, R. (Department of Statistics, University of Washington, Seattle, 1986).

7. Looker, A. *et al.* Updated data on proximal femur bone mineral levels of US adults. *Osteoporosis International* 8, 468-89 (1998).

8. Tukey, J. W. Data-based graphics: visual display in the decades to come. *Statistical Science* 5 (1990).

9. Jowitt, N., MacFarlane, T., Devlin, H., Klemetti, E. & Horner, K. The reproducibility of the mandibular cortical index. *Dentomaxillofacial Radiology* 28, 141-144 (1999).

10. Xu, L. *et al.* Vertebral fractures in Beijing, China: the Beijing Osteoporosis Project. *Journal of Bone and Mineral Research* 15, 2019-2025 (2000).

11. Looker, A. C. *et al.* Prevalence of low femoral bone density in older U.S. adults from NHANES III [see comments]. *Journal of Bone and Mineral Research* 12, 1761-8 (1997).

12. Lu, Y. *et al.* Classification of Osteoporosis Based on Bone Mineral Densities. *Journal of Bone and Mineral Research* 16, 901-910 (2001).

13. Strike, P. W. *Statistical Methods in Laboratory Medicine* (Butterworth-Heinemann Ltd., Oxford, 1991).

14. Lu, Y. & Zhao, S. in *Advanced Medical Statistics* (eds. Lu, Y. & Fang, J.-Q.) 101-156 (World Sceintific Publication Co. Pte. Ltd., Singapore, 2003).

15. Conover, W. J. *Practical Nonparametric Statistics* (John Wiley & Sons, Inc., New York, 1980).

16. Snedecor, G. W. & Cochran, W. G. *Statistical Methods* (Iowa State university Press, Ames, IA, 1980).

17. Heidelberger, P. & Welch, P. D. A spectral method for confidence interval generation and run-length control in simulations. *Communications of the ACM* 24, 233-245 (1981).

18. Grampp, S. *et al.* Comparisons of non-invasive bone mineral measurements in assessing age-related loss, fracture discrimination, and diagnostic classification. *Journal of Bone and Mineral Research* 12, 697-711 (1997).

19. Altman, D. & Bland, J. Presentation of numerical data. *British Medical Journal* 312, 572 (1996).

20. Looker, A. C. *et al.* Prevalence of low femoral bone density in older U.S. women from NHANES III. *Journal of Bone and Mineral Research* 10, 796-802 (1995).

21. Kanis, J. & Gluer, C. An update on the diagnosis and assessment of osteoporosis with densitometry (for the Committee of Scientific Advisors, International Osteoporosis Foundation). *Osteoporosis International* 11, 192-202 (2000).

22. Black, D., Palermo, L., Genant, H. & Cummings, S. Four reasons to avoid the use of BMD T-scores in treatment decisions for osteoporosis. *Journal of Bone and Mineral Research* 11, S118 (1996).

23. Lu, Y., Mathur, A. & Genant, H. Pitfalls of using Z-score, T-score for discriminant purpose. *Journal of Bone and Mineral Research* 11, S264 (1995).

24.   Altman, D. G. The normal distribution. *BMJ* 310, 298 (1995).

25.   Bland, J. M. & Altman, D. G. Transforming data. *BMJ* 312, 770 (1996).

26.   Bland, J. M. The use of transformation when comparing two means. *BMJ* 312, 1153 (1996).

27.   Sox, H. Probability theory in the use of diagnostic tests. *Ann Intern Med* 104, 60-66 (1986).

28.   Sox, H. C., Blatt, M. A., Higgins, M. C. & Marton, K. I. *Medical Decision Making* (Butterworths, Boston, 1988).

29.   Swets, J. A. Sensitivities and specificities of diagnostic tests. *JAMA* 248, 548-549 (1982).

30.   Hanley, J. Receiver operating characteristic (ROC) methodology: the state of the art. *CRC Crit Rev Diagn Imag* 29, 307-335 (1989).

31.   Gatsonis, C., Begg, C. & Wieand, S. Introduction. *Academic Radiology* 2, S1-S3 (1995).

32.   DeLong, E. R., DeLong, D. M. & Clark-Pearson, D. L. Comparing the areas under two or more correlated receiver operating characteristic curves: a nonparametric approach. *Biometrics* 44, 837-845 (1988).

33.   Metz, C. E. ROC methodology in radiology imaging. *Invest Radiol* 21, 720-733 (1986).

34.   Tosteson, A. & Begg, C. A general regression methodology for ROC curve estimation. *Medical Decision Making* 8, 204-215 (1988).

35.   Pepe, M. S. A regression modelling framework for receiver operating characteristic curves in medical diagnostic testing. *Biometrika* 85, 595-608 (1997).

36.   *SAS/QC User's Guide (for SAS V8)* (SAS Research Institute, Cary, NC, 2000).

37.   Metz, C. (Department of Radiology, University of Chicago, 1988).

38.   Hanley, J. & McNeil, B. The meaning and use of the area under the receiver operating characteristic (ROC) curve. *Radiology* 143, 29-36 (1982).

39.   Wieand, H., Gail, M., Barray, R. & James, K. A family of nonparametric statistics for comparing diagnostic markers with paired or unpaired data. *Biometrika* 76, 585-92 (1989).

40.   Lee, W. C. & Hsiao, C. K. Alternative summary indices for the receiver operating characteristic curve. *Epidemiology* 7, 605-611 (1996).

41.   Swets, J. A. & Pickett, R. M. Assessing diagnostic technologies: reply to Habicht. *Science* 207, 1415 (1980).

42.   Pepe, M. S. Three approaches to regression analysis of receiver operating characteristic curves for continuous test results. *Biometrics* 54, 124-135 (1998).

43.   Roe, C. A. & Metz, C. E. Variance-component modeling in the analysis of receiver operating characteristic index estimates. *Academic Radiology* 4, 587-600 (1997).

44.   Zhou, X. H. & Gastonis, C. A. A simple method for comparing correlated ROC curves using incomplete data. *Statistics in Medicine* 15, 1687-1693 (1996).

45.   Zhou, X. Empirical Bayes combination of estimated areas under ROC curves using estimating equations. *Medical Decision Making* 16 (1996).

46.   Metz, C. E., Herman, B. A. & Roe, C. A. Statistical comparison of two ROC-curve estimates obtained from partially-paired datasets. *Medical Decision Making* 18, 110-121 (1998).

47. Zhou, X.-H., Donna K. McClish & Obuchowski, N. A. *Statistical Methods in Diagnostic Medicine* (, 2002).

48. Lachenbruch, P. A. *Discriminant Analysis* (Hafner Press, Nerw York, USA, 1975).

49. Su, J. & Liu, J. Linear combinations of multiple diagnostic markers. *Journal of American Statistical Association* 88, 1350-1355 (1993).

50. McIntosh, M. & Pepe, M. Combining several screening tests: optimality of the risk score. *Biometrics* 58, 657-664 (2002).

51. Pepe, M. S. & Thompson, M. L. Combing diagnostic test results to increase accuracy. *Biostatistics* 1, 123-140 (2000).

52. Cummings, S. *et al.* Bone density at various sites for prediction of hip fractures: the study of osteoporotic fractures. *Lancet* 341, 72-75 (1993).

53. Efron, B. The efficiency of logistic regression compared to normal discriminant analysis. *Jounral of the American Statistical Association* 70, 892-898. (1995).

54. Baron, A. E. Misclassification among methods used for multiple group discrimination - the effects of distribution properties. *Statistics in Medicine* 10, 757-766. (1991).

55. Breiman, L., Friedman, J., Olshen, R. & Stone, C. *Classification And Regression Trees.* (Wadsworth & Brooks Cole, Monterey, CA, 1984).

56. Segal, M. Regression trees for censored data. *Biometrics* 44, 35-47 (1988).

57. Segal, M. & Bloch, D. A comparison of estimated proportional hazards models and regression trees. *Statistics in Medicine* 8, 539-550 (1989).

58. Sevin, B.-U. *et al.* Surgically defined prognostic parameters in early cervical carcinoma: a tree structured survival analysis. *Cancer* 78, 1438-1446 (1996).

59. Jin, H. *et al.* Classification algorithms for hip fracture prediction based on recursive partitioning methods. *Medical Decision Making*, in press (2004).

60. Lu, Y., Black, D., Mathur, A. & Genant, H. Study of hip fracture risk using tree structured survival analysis. *J. Miner. Stoffwechs* 10, 11-16 (2003).

61. Baker, S. Evaluating multiple disgnostic tests with partial verification. *Biometrics* 51, 330-337 (1995).

62. Baker, S. G. Identifying combinations of cancer markers for further study as triggers of early intervention. *Biometrics* 56, 1082-1087 (2000).

63. Bland, J. M. & Altman, D. G. Statistical methods for assessing agreement between two methods of clinical measurement. *The Lancet* i, 307-310 (1986).

64. Bland, J. M. & Altman, D. G. Comparing two methods of clinical measurement: a personal history. *International Journal of Epidemiology* 24, S7-S14 (1995).

65. Kleinbaum, D. G., Kupper, L. L. & Muller, K. E. *Applied Regression Analysis and Other Multivariable Methods.* (PWS-KENT Publishing Company, Boston, 1988).

66. Cohen, J. A. A coefficient of agreement for nominal scales. *Educ. Psychol Meas* 20, 37-46 (1960).

67. Kraemer, H. C. Extension of the kappa coefficient. *Biometrics* 36, 207-216 (1980).

68. Fleiss, J. L. & Davies, M. Jacknifing functions of multinomial frequencies, with an application to a measure of concordance. *American Journal of Epidemiology* 115, 841-845 (1982).

69. Blackman, N. J.-M. & Koval, J. J. Interval estimation for Cohen's kappa as a measure of agreement. *Statistics in Medicine* 19, 723-741 (2000).

70. Cohen, J. Weighted Kappa: nomial scale agreement with provision for scaled disagreement or partial credit. *Psycological Bulletin* 70, 213-219 (1968).

71. Fleiss, J. L. *Statistical Methods for Rates and Proportions* (Wiley, New York, 1981).

72. Barlow, W., Lai, M.-y. & Azen, S. P. A comparison of methods for calculating a stratified Kappa. *Statistics in Medicine* 10, 1465-1472 (1991).

73. Donner, A. & Eliasziw, M. A hierachical approach to inferences concerning interobserver agreement for multinomial data. *Statistics in Medicine* 16, 1097-1106 (1997).

74. Kraemer, H. C. & Bloch, D. A. A note on case-control sampling to estimate Kappa coefficients. *Biometrics* 46, 49-59 (1990).

75. Posner, K. L., Sampson, P. D., Caplan, R. A., Ward, R. J. & Cheney, F. W. Measuring interrater reliability among multiple raters: an example of methods for nominal data. *Statistics in Medicine* 9, 1103-1115 (1990).

76. Oden, N. L. Estimating Kappa from binocular data. *Statistics in Medicine* 10, 1303-1311 (1991).

77. Shoukri, M. M. & Martin, S. W. Maximum likelihood estimation of the Kappa coefficient from models of matched binary responses. *Statistics in Medicine* 14, 83-99 (1995).

78. Shoukri, M. M. & Mian, I. U. H. Maximum likelihood estimation of the Kappa coefficient from bivariate logistic regression. *15* Statistics in Medicine, 1409-1419 (1996).

79. Bradley, E. L. & Blackwood, L. G. Comparing paired data: A simultaneous test of means and variances. *The American Statistician* 43, 234-235 (1989).

80. Lu, Y. *et al.* Comparative calibration without a gold standard. *Statistics in Medicine* 16, 1889-1905 (1997).

81. Abrahamsen, B., Hansen, T. B., Jensen, L. B., Hermann, A. P. & Eiken, P. Site of Osteodensitometry in perimenopausal women: correlation and limits of agreement between anatomic regions. *Journal of Bone and Mineral Research* 12, 1471-1479. (1997).

82. Lee, J., Koh, D. & Ong, C. N. Statistical evaluation of agreement between two methods for measuring a quantitative variable. *Comput. Biol. Med.* 19 (1989).

83. Fleiss, J. L. & Shrout, P. E. Approximate interval estimation for a certain intraclass correlation coefficient. *Psychometrika* 43, 259-262 (1978).

84. Bland, J. M. & Altman, D. G. A note on the use of the intraclass correlation coefficient in the evaluation of agreement between two methods of measurements. *Comput. Biol. Med.* 20, 337-340 (1990).

85. Bartko, J. J. General methodology II measures of agreement: a single procedure. *Statistics in Medicine* 13, 737-745 (1994).

86. Kleinbaum, D., Kupper, L. & Morgenstern, H. *Epidemiologic Research, Principles and Quantitative Methods.* (Van Nostrand Reinhold, New York, 1982).

87. Lachenbruch, P. & Lynch, C. Assessing screening tests: extensions of McNemar's test. *Statistics in Medicine* 17, 2207-17 (1998).

88. Lu, Y. & Bean, J. A. On the sample size for studies of bioequivalence based upon McNemar's test. *Statistics in Medicine* 14, 1831-1839 (1995).

89.   Morikawa, T. & Yishida, M. A useful testing strategy in phase II trials: combined test of superiority and test of equivalence. *Journal of Biopharmaceutical Statistics* 5, 297-306 (1995).

90.   Liu, J.-p., Hsueh, H.-m., Hsieh, E. & Chen, J. J. Tests for equivalence or non-inferiority for paired binary data. *Statistics in Medicine* 21, 231-245 (2002).

91.   Nam, J. M. Establishing equivalence of two treatments and sample size requirements in matched-pairs design. *Biometrics* 53, 1422-30 (1997).

92.   Tango, T. Equivalence test and confidence interval for the difference in proportions for the paired-sample design. *Statistics in Medicine* 17, 891-908 (1998).

93.   Lu, Y., Jin, H. & Genant, H. K. On the non-inferiority of a diagnostic test based on paired observations. *Statistics in Medicine* 22, 3029-3044 (2003).

94.   Berger, R. L. & Hsu, J. C. Bioequivalence trials, intersection-union tests and equivalence confidence sets. *Statistical Science* 11, 283-319 (1996).

95.   Dorfman, D. D. & Alf, E. Maximum likelihood estimation of parameters of signal detection theory and determination of confidence intervals; rating method data. *Journal of Mathematical Psychology* 6, 487-496 (1969).

96.   Metz, D. E., Wang, P. L. & Kronman, H. B. in *Information Processing in Medical Imaging* (ed. Deconick, F.) 432-445 (Nijhoff, The Hague, 1984).

97.   Venkatraman, E. S. & Begg, C. B. A distribution-free procedure for comparing receiver operating characteristic curves from a paired experiment. *Biometrika* 83, 835-848 (1996).

98.   Hanley, J. & McNeil, B. A method of comparing the area under two ROC curves derived from the same cases. *Radiology* 148, 839-843 (1983).

99.   Genant, H. K., Grampp, S., Gluer, C. C. & et.al. Universal standardization for dual x-ray absorptiometry: patient and phantom cross-calibration results. *Journal of Bone and Mineral Research* 9, 1503-1514 (1994).

100.   Genant, H. K. Universal standardization for dual x-ray absorptiometry: patient and phantom cross-calibration results [letter]. *Journal of Bone and Mineral Research* 10, 997-998 (1995).

101.   Shepherd, J. *et al.* Universal Standardization of Forearm Bone Densitometry. *Journal of Bone and Mineral Research* 17, 734-45 (2002).

102.   Hui, S. L. *et al.* Universal standardization of bone density measurements: a method with optimal properties for calibration among several instruments. *Journal of Bone and Mineral Research* 12, 1463-1470 (1997).

103.   Hanson, J. Standardization of femur BMD [letter]. *Journal of Bone and Mineral Research* 12, 1316-7 (1997).

104.   Lu, Y., Fuerst, T., Hui, S. & Genant, H. K. Standardization of bone mineral density at femoral neck, trochanter and Ward's triangle. *Osteoporosis International* 12, 438-444 (2001).

105.   Chi, G., Jin, K., Chen, G. & Cui, L. in *Advanced Medical Statistics* (eds. Lu, Y. & Fang, J.-Q.) (World Sceintific Publications Co. Pte. Ltd., Singapore, 2003).

106.   Fisher, L. & Moye, L. Carvedilol and the Food and Drug Administration approval process: an introduction. *Controlled Clinical Trials* 20, 1-15 (1999).

107.   FDA. 1-23 (Division of Metabolic and Endocrine Drug Products, Food and Drug Administration, Rockville, Maryland, 1994).

108.   Cummings, S. R. *et al.* Effect of Alendronate on risk of fracture in women with low bone density but without vertebral fractures. *JAMA* 280, 2077-2082 (1998).

109.   Harris, S. *et al.* Effects of risedronate treatment on vertebral and nonvertebral fractures in women with postmenopausal osteoporosis: a randomized controlled trial. Vertebral Efficacy With Risedronate Therapy (VERT) Study Group. *JAMA* 282, 1344-52 (1999).

110.   Ettinger, B. *et al.* Reduction of vertebral fracture risk in postmenopausal women with osteoporosis treated with raloxifene: Results from a 3-year randomized clinical trial. *JAMA* 282, 637-645 (1999).

111.   McClung, M. *et al.* Effect of risedronate on the risk of hip fracture in elderly women. Hip Intervention Program Study Group. *New England Journal of Medicine* 344, 333-40 (2001).

112.   Lu, Y. *et al.* in *International Conference on Statistical Methods and Statistical Computation for Quality and Productivity Improvement* 474-480 (Seoul, Korea, 1995).

113.   Faulkner, K. M., MR. Quality control of DXA instruments in multicenter trials. *Osteoporosis International* 5, 218-27 (1995).

114.   Fuerst, T., Lu, Y., Hans, D. & Genant, H. K. in *Bone Densitometry and Osteoporosis* (eds. Genant, H. K., Guglielmi, G. & Jergas, M.) 461-476 (Springer-Verlag, Berlin Heidelberg New York, 1998).

115.   Huxsoll, J. F. in *Quality Assurance for Biopharmaceuticals* (ed. Huxsoll, J. F.) 2-13 (John Wiley and Sons, Inc., New York, 1994).

116.   Switula, D. Principles of good clinical practice (GCP) in clinical research. *Sci Eng Ethics* 6, 71-7 (2000).

117.   van Kuijk, C. Good clinical practice in clinical trials: what does it mean for a radiology department? *Radiology* 209, 625-627 (1998).

118.   Fraass, B. D., K; Hunt, M; Kutcher, G; Starkschall, G; Stern, R; Van Dyke, J. American Association of Physicists in Medicine Radiation Therapy Committee Task Group 53: quality assurance for clinical radiotherapy treatment planning. *Medical Physics* 25, 1773-829 (1998).

119.   Laurila, J. S.-N., CG; Suramo, I; Tolppanen, EM; Tervonen, O; Korhola, O; Brommels, M. The efficacy of a continuous quality improvement (CQI) method in a radiological department. Comparison with non-CQI control material. *Acta Radiologica* 42, 96-100 (2001).

120.   Kalender, W. *et al.* The European spine phantom - a tool for standardization and quality control in spine bone mineral measurements by DXA and QCT. *Eur J Radiol* 20, 83-92 (1995).

121.   Lu, Y. *et al.* Dual X-ray absorptieometry quality control: comparison of visual examination and process-control charts. *Journal of Bone and Mineral Research* 11, 626-637 (1996).

122.   Jergas, M. & Genant, H. K. Current methods and recent advances in the diagnosis of osteoporosis. *Arthrit Rheum* 36, 1649-1662 (1993).

123.   Montgomery, D. C. *Introduction to Statistical Quality Control* (Wiley, New York, 1992).

124.   Russell, L. B., Gold, M. R., Siegel, J. E., Daniels, N. & Weinstein, M. C. The role of cost-effectiveness analysis in health and medicine. *JAMA, The Journal of the American Medical Association* 276, 1172-7 (1996).

125.   Muennig, P. *Designing and Conducting Cost-Effectiveness Analyses in Medicine and Health Care* (Jossey-Bass, San Francisco, 2002).

126. Tella, M., Feinglass, J. & Chang, R. Cost-effectivenss, cost-utility, and cost-benefit studies in rheumatology: a review of the literature, 2001-2002. *Current Opinion in Rheumatology* 15, 127-131 (2003).

127. Chiang, C. L. *An Introduction to Stochastic Processes and Their Applications* (Robert E. Krieger Publishing Company, Huntington, New York, 1980).

128. Li, C. & Fang, J.-Q. in *Advanced Medical Statistics* (eds. Fang, J.-Q. & Lu, Y.) (People's Health Publishing Company, Beijing, 2001).

129. Jonsson, B., Kanis, J., Dawson, A., Oden, A. & Johnell, O. Effect and offset of effect of treatments for hip fracture on health outcomes. *Osteoporosis International* 10, 193-199 (1999).

130. Armstrong, K., Chen, T.-M., Altert, D., Randall, T. & Schwartz, J. Cost-effectivenss of Raloxifene and hormone replacement therapy in postmenopausal women: inpact of breast cancer risk. *Obstetrics and Gynecology* 98, 996-1003 (2001).

131. Nagata-Kobayashi, S., Shimbo, T. & Fukui, T. Cost-effectiveness analysis of screening for osteoporosis in postmenopausal Japanese women. *Journal of Bone and Mineral Metabolism* 20, 350-357 (2002).

132. Iglesias, C., Torgerson, D., Bearne, A. & Bose, U. The cost utility of bisphosphonate treatment in established osteoporosis. *Q J Med* 95, 305-311 (2002).

133. Willis, M. S. The health economics of calcium and vitamin D3 for the prevention of osteoporotic hip fractures in Sweden. *International Journal of Technology Assessment in Health Care* 18, 791-807 (2002).

134. Kanis, J. A. *et al.* Intervention thresholds for osteoporosis. *Bone* 31, 26-31 (2002).

135. Coyle, D., Cranney, A., Lee, K., Welch, V. & Tugwell, P. Cost effectiveness of nasal calcitonin in postmenopausla women: use of Cochrane Collaboration methods for meta-analysis within economic evaluation. *Pharmacoeconomics* 19, 565-575 (2002).

136. Johnell, O., Jonsson, B., Jonsson, L. & Black, D. Cost effectiveness of Alendronate (Fosamax) for the treatment of osteoporosis and prevention of fractures. *Pharmacoeconomics* 21, 305-314 (2003).

137. Gabriel, S. E. *et al.* Direct medical costs attributable to osteoporotic fractures. *Osteoporosis International* 13, 323-330 (2002).

138. De Laet, C. E. D. H. *et al.* Incremental cost of medical care after hip fracture and first vetebral fracture: the Rotterdam study. *Osteoporosis Internationl* 10, 66-72 (1999).

139. Autier, P. *et al.* Cost induced by hip fracture: a prospective controlled study in Belgium. *Osteoporosis International* 11, 373-380 (2000).

140. Hao, Y. & Fang, J.-Q. in *Advanced Medical Statistics* (eds. Fang, J.-Q. & Lu, Y.) 118-149 (People's Health Publication, Beijing, 2001).

141. Dolan, P., Gudex, C., Kind, P. & Williams, A. The time trade-off method: results from a general population study. *Health Econ* 5, 141-54 (1996).

142. Greenhalgh, T. How to read a paper. Papers that tell you what things cost (economic analyses). *British Medical Journal* 315, 596-9 (1997).

143. Dolan, P., Gudex, C., Kind, P. & Williams, A. Valuing health states: a comparison of methods. *Journal of Health Economics* 15, 209-31 (1996).

144. National Osteoporosis Foundation. Review of the evidence for prevention, diagnosis and treatment and cost-effectiveness analysis. *Osteoporosis International* 8, 1-88 (1998).

145. Dolan, P., Torgerson, D. & Kakarlapudi, T. Health-related quality of life of Colles' fracture patients. *Osteoporosis International* 9, 196-199 (1999).

146. Salkeld, G. *et al.* Quality of life related to fear of falling and hip fracture in older women: a time trade off study. *BMJ - British Medical Journal* 320, 341-346 (2000).

147. Cranney, A. *et al.* The psychometric properties of patient preferences in osteoporosis. *The Journal of Rheumatology* 28, 132-7 (2001).

148. Martin, A. *et al.* The impact of osteoporosis on quality-of-life: the OFELY cohort. *Bone* 31, 32-36 (2002).

149. Gabriel, S. *et al.* Health-related quality of life in economic evaluations for osteoprosis: whose values should we use? *Medical Decision Making* 19, 141-8 (1999).

150. NOF. Osteoporosis: review of the evidence for prevention, diagnosis, and treatment and cost-effectiveness analysis. Status report. *Osteoporosis International* 8, S3-S80 (1998).

151. Langton, C. M., Ballard, P. A., Langton, D. K. & Purdie, D. W. Maximising the cost effectiveness of BMD referral for DXA using ultrasound as a selective population pre-screen. *Technology and Health Care* 5, 235-41 (1997).

152. Koh, L. *et al.* A Simple Tool to Identify Asian Women at Increased Risk of Osteoporosis. *Osteoporosis International* 12, 699-705 (2001).

153. Ben Sedrine, W. *et al.* Interest of a prescreening questionaire to reduce the cost of bone densitometry. *Osteoporosis International* 13, 434-442 (2002).

154. Kanis, J. *et al.* in *ASBMR 25th Annual Meeting* Abstract 1222 (Minneapolis, MN, 2003).

155. Nelson, H., Helfand, M., Woolf, S. & Allan, J. Screening for postmenopausal osteoporosis: a review of the evidence for the U.S. Preventive Services Task Force. *Annuals of Internal Medicine* 137, 529-41 (2002).

156. Hui, Y. Osteoporosis: should there be a screening programme in Hong Kong? *Hong Kong Meidcal Journal* 8, 270-277 (2002).

157. Falasca, G., Dunston, C. & Banglawala, Y. Further validation of a questionnaire to identify women likely to have low bone density. *Journal of Clinical Densitometry* 6, 231-6 (2003).

158. Diez-Perez, A. *et al.* Evaluation of calcaneal quantitative ultrasound in a primary care setting as a screening tool for osteoporosis in postmenopausal women. *Journal of Clinical Densitometry* 6, 237-46 (2003).

159. Berg, A. Screening for osteoporosis in postmenopausal women: recommendations and rationale. *American Journal of Nursing* 103, 73-80 (2003).

160. Kung, A., Yeung, S. & Chu, L. The efficacy and tolerability of alendronate in postmenopausal osteoporotic Chinese women: a randomized placebo-controlled study. *Calcified Tissue International* 67, 286-90 (2000).

161. Lau, E., Woo, J., Chan, Y. & Griffith, J. Alendronate prevents bone loss in Chinese women with osteoporosis. *Bone* 27, 677-80 (2000).

162. Xu, S. *et al.* Reference data and predictive diagnostic models for calcaneus bone mineral density measured with single-energy X-ray absorptiometry in 7428 Chinese. *Osteoporos Int.* 12, 755-62 (2001).

163. Woo, J., Li, M. & Lau, E. Population bone mineral density measurements for Chinese women and men in Hong Kong. *Osteoporos International* 12, 289-95 (2001).

164. Liu, Z. *et al.* The diagnostic criteria for primary osteoporosis and the incidence of osteoporosis in China. *Journal of Bone Mineral and Metabolism* 20, 181-9 (2002).

165. Li, N., Ou, P., Zhu, H., Yang, D. & Zheng, P. Prevalence rate of osteoporosis in the mid - aged and elderly in selected parts of China. *Chinese Medical Journal (Engl)* 115, 773-5 (2002).

166. Liao, E. *et al.* Age-related bone mineral density, accumulated bone loss rate and prevalence of osteoporosis at multiple skeletal sites in Chinese women. *Osteoporos Int.* 13, 669-76 (2002).

167. Haines, C. *et al.* A prospective, randomized, placebo-controlled study of the dose effect of oral oestradiol on menopausal symptoms, psychological well being, and quality of life in postmenopausal Chinese women. *Maturitas* 44, 207-14 (2003).

168. Liao, E. *et al.* Establishment and evaluation of bone mineral density reference databases appropriate for diagnosis and evaluation of osteoporosis in Chinese women. *J Bone Miner Metab* 21, 184-92 (2003).

169. Kung, A., Ho, A., Sedrine, W., Reginster, J. & Ross, P. Comparison of a simple clinical risk index and quantitative bone ultrasound for identifying women at increased risk of osteoporosis. *Osteoporosis International* 14, 716-721 (2003).

CHAPTER 10

PREVENTION AND TREATMENT OF POSTMENOPAUSAL OSTEOPOROSIS

Lu Amy Sun and Arkadi Chines

Procter & Gamble Pharmaceuticals, Inc.
8700 Mason Montgomery Road
Mason, Ohio 45040 USA
E-mail: sun.la@pg.com, chines.aa@pg.com

Osteoporosis is a growing health problem affecting many postmenopausal women. The overall goal of postmenopausal osteoporosis (PMO) management is the prevention of fracture. The prevention strategy includes increased calcium and vitamin D intake, exercise, and fall prevention. For patients with a high-risk of osteoporosis, the Food and Drug Administration (FDA) approved pharmacological agents including estrogen may be considered. Drugs approved by the FDA for the treatment of PMO include calcitonin, raloxifene, alendronate, risedronate, and teriparatide. This chapter reviews current understanding of PMO prevention and treatment.

1. Postmenopausal Osteoporosis Prevention

1.1. *Risk Factors Modification*

A comprehensive risk factor assessment is necessary to initiate behavior and/or lifestyle changes to reduce the risk of fracture, and to prevent the development of postmenopausal osteoporosis (PMO). Table 1 summarizes the osteoporosis-related risk factors identified by The National Osteoporosis Foundation.[1] Patients should be thoroughly evaluated and educated to reduce the likelihood of any modifiable risk

261

factors associated with bone loss and fracture. For patients with significant risk factors of fracture, bone mineral density (BMD) measurement may be considered (Table 2).

Table 1. Risk Factors for Osteoporosis

Non-modifiable Risk Factors	Modifiable Risk Factors
Family history of osteoporosis	Current cigarette smoking
Personal history of osteoporotic fracture	Low calcium and vitamin D intake
Caucasian or Asian race	Alcoholism
Advanced age	Impaired vision
Female	Poor health/frailty/inadequate physical activity
Low body weight (< 127 lbs)	Estrogen deficiency (early menopause or bilateral ovariectomy)

Table 2. Recommendations for Measuring BMD in Women for Assessing Risk of Fracture

National Osteoporosis Foundation[1]

- Postmenopausal women 65 years or older, regardless of additional risk factors; includes women 65 years or older who have been taking osteoporosis therapy and have not had a BMD test.
- Postmenopausal women younger than 65 years and with one or more additional risk factors for osteoporosis.
- Postmenopausal women who have had a fracture of any type as an adult after age 45 years.

U.S. Preventive Services Task Force[2]

- All women 65 years of age and older should be screened routinely for osteoporosis.
- Routine screening beginning at 60 years of age for women at increased risk for osteoporotic fractures.

1.2. *Adequate Dietary Calcium and Vitamin D*

The recommended calcium intake for women and men over 51 years old is 1200 mg/day (Table 3).[3] However, optimal daily calcium intake is higher for postmenopausal women who require an average of

1500 mg/day of calcium.[4] The preferred source of calcium is from dairy products (milk, yogurt, and cheese) and fortified foods such as certain cereals, waffles, snacks, juices, and crackers. If tolerated, calcium supplementation may be helpful for women with suboptimal dietary intake. Calcium supplement should be taken in doses of < 600 mg at a time to ensure a good absorption as the calcium absorption fraction decreases at higher doses. Most available calcium salts exhibit similar bioavailability.[5] Calcium carbonate is the salt most widely used in the United States (U.S.), and is best taken with food since it requires acid for solubility. Calcium citrate supplements can be taken at any time. Calcium supplements are generally well tolerated. Patients with a history of kidney stones should have a 24-hour urine calcium determination prior to calcium supplementation to avoid hypercalciuria, although there is no evidence calcium supplementation increases the risk of kidney stone formation.

Table 3. Adequate Calcium Intake

Life-Stage Group	Estimated Adequate Daily Calcium Intake
Infants	210-270 mg/day
Young children (1-3 years)	500 mg/day
Older children (4-8 years)	800 mg/day
Adolescents and young adults (9-18 years)	1300 mg/day
Men and women (19-50 years)	1000 mg/day
Men and women (51 and older)	1200 mg/day

Vitamin D supplementation in a combination with calcium has been shown to reduce the risk of fractures in the elderly population.[6] Vitamin D is synthesized in skin under the influence of heat and ultraviolet. In elderly postmenopausal population, with the decrease of cutaneous production from solar exposure, oral vitamin D supplementation may be required to ensure adequate daily intake. The Institute of Medicine recommends daily intakes of 200 IU for adults less than 50 years, 400 IU for those from 50-70 years, and above 600 IU for those more than 70 years.[3] For patients who are malnourished, or who have intestinal malabsorption, or who are receiving long-term anticonvulsant (e.g., phenytoin, phenobarbital) or glucocorticoid therapy, 800 IU/day of vitamin D is required. It is important to remember though, in postmenopausal women and men, calcium and vitamin D supplementation alone may not be sufficient to provide maximal prevention of fracture.

1.3. *Regular Weight-Bearing Exercise*

Exercise in young individuals helps maintain the maximal genetically determined peak bone mass. In postmenopausal women, weight-bearing exercise may slow bone loss attributable to disuse. Exercise also has beneficial effect on neuromuscular function, mobility, coordination, and balance, all of which may help reduce the risk of falls. The type of exercise has to be based on the patients' physical ability. Walking is a practical way to start. Other exercises include dancing, racquet sports, and swimming. Exercise should be consistent, at least a few times a week. It is important to note in patients with established osteoporosis, heavy weight-bearing exercise or vigorous activity may trigger a fracture, therefore, lower-impact exercises such as walking or water aerobics is recommended for these patients. The focus should be primarily on mild weight-bearing exercise.

1.4. *Fall Prevention*

Fall prevention is important at all ages. Over 90% of hip and wrist fractures result from a fall.[7] Varieties of reasons attributed to falls in the elderly include visual and cognitive impairment, impaired gait and muscular weakness, sedative medications, and environmental hazards. Elimination of environmental hazards is one of the easily modifiable risk factors, and is applicable to any patient with osteoporosis risk factors or osteoporosis per se.

1.5. *Pharmacological Prevention*

Pharmacological agents may be considered for PMO prevention in postmenopausal women who are at high risk of developing osteoporosis and for whom the desired clinical outcome is to maintain bone mass and to reduce the risk of future fracture. Drugs approved by the Food and Drug Administration (FDA) for PMO prevention indication are listed in Table 4. Among the listed pharmacologic agents, only estrogen prevention is discussed in this chapter.

Table 4. Drugs Approved by the FDA for PMO Prevention Indication

Drug Name	Dose (mg) and Regimen
Estrogen*	0.3-0.625 mg/day conjugated equine estrogens (CEE) 0.3-0.625 mg/day CEE and 1.5-5.0 mg/day medroxyprogesterone acetate (MPA)
Raloxifene	60 mg/day
Alendronate	10 mg/day or 70 mg/weekly
Risedronate	5 mg/day or 35 mg/weekly

* Other FDA approved estrogen and progestin products for PMO prevention indication are listed in Table 5.

1.5.1. Estrogen

For many years, estrogen has been the sole FDA-approved pharmacologic therapy for the prevention and management of osteoporosis. Results from the Women's Health Initiative (WHI) showed hormone replacement therapy (HRT) prevents fractures but has an overall unfavorable risk-benefit profile.

1.5.1.1. Mechanism of Action

It has been known for many years that estrogen prevents or slows the bone loss in postmenopausal women. The mechanism of its action on bone is still not fully understood. Estrogen binds to its nuclei estrogen receptor and activates gene expression of cytokine and growth factor in both osteoclasts and osteoblasts, resulting in suppression of osteoclastic bone resorption.[8] Estrogen may also affect calcium homeostasis through actions on bone, kidney, and gastrointestinal tract; and may alter the response of bone to calcitropic hormones.[9] The minimum dose of estrogen for bone effect has not been established. Premarin[®] at dose of 0.625 mg or higher was previously considered as an optimal dose, but a recent study of esterified estrogens showed a typical dose response with 0.3 mg daily being effective for prevention bone loss.[10]

1.5.1.2. Pharmacokinetic Profile

There are many types of estrogen and progestin products available. In this section discussion is limited to oral and transdermal products only. The FDA approved estrogens and progestins for PMO prevention indication are summarized in Table 5. The list is not inclusive; however, the strengths and regimens listed in the table are only for PMO prevention.

Estrogens from oral or transdermal formulations are rapidly absorbed from gastrointestinal tract or skin, reach maximum plasma concentration within 6-9 hours (Premarin) and 4 hours (Vivelle®). The half-life of Premarin is about 12-26 hours and the half-life of Vivelle is about 4 hours. Oral estrogen is normally administered daily, transdermal estrogen like Vivelle delivers consistent amount of estrogen over 3-4 days of wear period.[11,12]

The distribution of exogenous estrogens is similar to that of endogenous estrogens. Estrogens are widely distributed in the body and are generally found in higher concentration in the sex hormone target organs. Estrogens circulate in the blood largely bound to sex hormone binding globulin (SHBG) and albumin, with only the unbound fraction being biologically active. Because estrogen itself raises levels of SHBG, measurements of total estrogens or estradiol are of limited clinical importance.

Exogenous estrogens are metabolized in the same manner as endogenous estrogens. Circulating estrogens exist in a dynamic equilibrium of metabolic interconversions. These transformations take place mainly in the liver. Estradiol is converted reversibly to estrone, and both can be converted to estriol, which is the major urinary metabolite. *In vitro* and *in vivo* studies have shown estrogens are metabolized partially by cytochrome P450 3A4 (CYP3A4), therefore, inducers or inhibitors of CYP3A4 may affect estrogen drug metabolism.

1.5.1.3. Effects on BMD and Fracture Risk

Clinical trials evaluating the efficacy of estrogen therapy on bone date back to the 1970s, when the first controlled clinical trial demonstrated long-term estrogen therapy was associated with preservation of bone mass and beneficial effect on vertebral fractures.[13] Most of the studies showing estrogens reduce the risk of fractures were observational studies and only a few were interventional. The WHI report was the first clinical trial to convincingly demonstrate that HRT significantly reduces the risk of both hip and spine fractures.[14] The WHI enrolled over 16,000 postmenopausal women aged 50-79 with an intact uterus at baseline at 40 U.S. clinical centers in 1993-1998. The study's primary objective was to assess the major health benefits and risks of the most commonly used combined hormone preparation in the U.S. Estrogen and progestin treatment increased total hip BMD by 3.7% compared to 0.14% with placebo (p < 0.001).[15] Treatment with estrogen and progestin also significantly reduced the risk of any clinical fracture by 24% and hip fracture by 33%. The WHI data are consistent with the other observational data and limited data from clinical trials[16] and are also consistent with known ability of estrogen (with or without progestin) to maintain BMD.[17]

1.5.1.4. Indications and Regimen

While HRT has a clear fracture reduction benefit in women with PMO, this benefit must be weighted against data on the risks associated with HRT (see details below). Most organizations with guidelines on postmenopausal HRT have recently revised their recommendations in light of the findings of recently reported WHI clinical trials. The American College of Obstetricians and Gynecologists[18] and the North American Menopause Society (Report from the NAMS) recommend caution in using HRT solely to prevent osteoporosis and suggest alternative therapies should also be considered. When HRT is indicated, patients should be treated with the lowest effective dose of HRT.

Table 5. The FDA Approved Estrogens and Progestins for the Prevention of PMO

Product	Active Ingredients	Doses (mg/day)
Premarin	CEE	0.3
		0.45
		0.625
Prempro™	CEE/MPA	0.3/1.5
		0.45/1.5
		0.625/2.5
		0.625/5.0
Activella®	Estradiol/norethindrone	1.0/0.5
Femhrt®	Ethinyl estradiol/norethindrone	0.5/1.0
Ortho-Prefest®	Estradiol/norethindrone	1.0/0.09
Estrace®	Estradiol	0.5/1.0/2.0
Ogen®	Estropipate	0.75
Ortho-Est	Estropipate	0.75
Vivelle (patch)	Estradiol	0.025-0.1 (weekly)
Climara® (patch)	Estradiol	0.025-0.1 (twice weekly)

CEEs are most commonly used for unopposed estrogen therapy. Estrone sulfate found in both human and horses are the major component of CEEs.   Premarin, one the most popularly prescribed estrogen products, has been typically started at 0.625 mg/day in the past. This dose should be periodically reassessed by the healthcare provider depending on individual clinical and bone mineral density responses. Premarin therapy may be given continuously with no interruption in therapy, or in cyclical regimens (regimens such as 25 days on drug followed by 5 days off drug) as medically appropriate on an individualized basis. Other commonly prescribed oral or transdermal estrogen preparations are listed in Table 5.

A progestin is usually added for women with an intact uterus, but progestin by itself is of no known bone effect. In the U.S., MPA is the most commonly used oral progestin due to the nature that MPA is less androgenic than other progestin such as norethindrone and norethindrone acetate. MPA can be given cyclically or continuously. The most common dosage of cyclic MPA is 2.5-10 mg/day for 10-13 days. A dose of 2.5 mg/day is commonly used for continuous therapy.

Combination estrogen/progestin products offer convenience for the patients. Prempro, consisting of 0.625 mg of estrogen and 2.5 or 5 mg of medroxyprogesterone, is taken daily for continuous therapy. Premphase® on the other hand, is a cyclic form of combined estrogen/progestin therapy. Premphase tablets taken for the first 14 days contain only 0.625 mg of Premarin, and tablets taken on days 15-28 contain 0.625 mg Premarin and 5 mg of MPA.

When prescribing estrogens and progestins solely for the prevention of PMO, therapy should only be considered for women at significant risk of osteoporosis and non-estrogen medications should be carefully considered. Patients should be treated with the lowest effective dose. Generally women should be started at 0.3 mg/1.5 mg Prempro daily. Dosage may be adjusted depending on individual clinical and bone mineral density responses. This dose should be periodically reassessed by the healthcare provider.

1.5.1.5. Side Effects

The prescribed estrogen products are normally well-tolerated; the commonly reported side effects of estrogens include vaginal bleeding, nausea, and breast tenderness. The effect of estrogen on cardiovascular disease, strokes, and risk for breast and ovary cancer is evaluated in the WHI studies.

Over the past 20 years, numerous observational studies have consistently suggested estrogen replacement therapy in postmenopausal woman may reduce the risk of coronary heart disease (CHD) and strokes. Contrary to previous beliefs, the WHI results demonstrated that, even though overall CHD rates were low, the rate of women experiencing CHD events was increased by 29% for women taking estrogen plus progestin relative to placebo. Most CHD events were nonfatal myocardial infarction (MI) within the first year of treatment. No significant differences were observed in CHD deaths or revascularization procedures.[14] In the majority of subgroups evaluated (i.e., smokers, hypertensives, preexisting CHD), there was no significant difference in the risk of CHD with estrogen and progestin treatment.[19] The analysis clearly demonstrated treatment with estrogen and progestin should not be used for primary prevention of CHD.

Stroke rates were also higher in women receiving estrogen plus progestin, a 41% increasing in the risk of stroke over 5.2 years of follow-up, with most of the elevation occurring in nonfatal events. An additional 4 months of stroke-related outcomes from women included in the WHI study demonstrated treatment with estrogen/progestin significantly increased the risk of total stroke by 31% and ischemic stroke by 44%. This increased risk was evident across all patient types, even after adjusting for related factors such as hypertension and baseline stroke risk, and age.[20]

The effects of treatment of estrogen and progestin on breast and gynecologic cancer were also evaluated in women included in the WHI study. Women in the estrogen/progestin group experienced a 24% increase in the risk of both total breast cancer and invasive breast cancer cases compared with placebo (p < 0.001 and p = 0.003, respectively). Cancers diagnosed in the treatment group were also significantly larger (1.7 vs. 1.5 cm, p = 0.04) and more advanced (25% vs. 15%, p = 0.04) than those diagnosed in the placebo group. Additionally, more women receiving estrogen and progestin had at least one abnormal mammogram compared to those in the placebo group (31.5% vs. 21.2%, p < 0.001). Collectively, the data suggested short-term treatment with estrogen and progestin increases the risk of breast cancer and number of abnormal mammograms.[21] Although not significant, the risk of ovarian cancer was elevated in the estrogen and progestin group. There was no significant difference in the risk of endometrial cancers between the estrogen/progestin group and the placebo group. Additionally, the distributions of tumor histology, stage, or grade for either cancer site were not appreciably different for either cancer site. Endometrial biopsies were performed in women taking estrogen plus progestin (33%) compared to placebo (6%, p < 0.001); however, the proportion of normal findings was similar between groups.[22] These data provided additional support that estrogen and progestin should not be used to prevent chronic diseases.

The effects of estrogen plus progestin on dementia and global cognitive function were also evaluated. Treatment with estrogen and progestin increased the risk of probable dementia by greater than 2-fold.[23] Additionally, women receiving treatment with estrogen and progestin were more likely to experience substantial declines (≥ 2 standard deviation [SD]) in modified Mini Mental State Exam scores compared to placebo.[24]

In summary, the WHI study reported increased risks of MI, stroke, invasive breast cancer, pulmonary emboli, and deep vein thrombosis in postmenopausal women during 5 years of treatment with CEEs (0.625 mg) combined with MPA (2.5 mg) relative to placebo. Other doses of conjugated estrogens and MPAs and other combinations of estrogens and progestins were not studied in the WHI and, in the absence of comparable data, these risks should be assumed to be similar. Because of these risks, estrogens with or without progestins should be prescribed at the lowest effective doses and for the shortest duration consistent with treatment goals and risks for the individual woman.

2. PMO Treatment

Drugs approved by the FDA for the treatment of PMO are summarized in Table 6.

Table 6. The FDA Approved Drugs for PMO Treatment

Drug Name	Indication	Regimen
Calcitonin	PMO (> 5 years postmenopausal)	200 IU/day intranasal or 100 IU SC or IM
Raloxifene	PMO	60 mg/day
Alendronate	PMO	10 mg/day or 70 mg/week
Risedronate	PMO	5 mg/day or 35 mg/week
Teriparatide	PMO with high risk of fracture	20 μg/day SC

2.1. Calcitonin

Calcitonin is a polypeptide hormone secreted by the parafollicular cells of the thyroid gland in mammals. Miacalcin® (calcitonin-salmon) was approved by FDA for the treatment of PMO in women who are at least

5 years postmenopausal. Miacalcin is not approved for osteoporosis prevention.

2.1.1. Mechanism of Action

The actions of calcitonin on bone and its role in normal human bone physiology are still not completely elucidated, although calcitonin receptors have been discovered in osteoclasts and osteoblasts.

Calcitonin secretion is stimulated by high plasma calcium levels. Calcitonin's ability to lower serum calcium concentration is associated with an inhibition of osteoclastic activity. Single injection of calcitonin causes a marked transient inhibition of the ongoing bone resorptive process. With prolonged use, there is a persistent, smaller decrease in the rate of bone resorption. Histologically, the decrease in bone resorption is associated with decreased number of osteoclasts and an apparent decrease in their resorptive activity. It has been observed that after exposure to calcitonin *in vitro*, osteoclasts undergo flattening of their ruffled border and withdraw from sites of bone resorption.[25] Calcitonin has analgesic benefit in patients with acute painful vertebral fractures. The mechanism of bone pain relief by calcitonin is not completely understood but it is believed through its central effect. The possible analgesic mechanism of calcitonin includes increases in circulating beta endorphins, inhibition of prostaglandin synthesis, and a direct effect on CNS receptors.[26] Miacalcin has been proven to be analgesic for acute or chronic pain of vertebral fractures.[27]

2.1.2. Pharmacokinetic Profile

Two formulations of calcitonin were approved by the FDA; injectable and nasal formulation. The discussion of pharmacokinetic profile below is limited to nasal spray formulation Miacalcin.

Miacalcin nasal spray is absorbed rapidly by the nasal mucosa. Peak plasma concentrations of drug appear 31-39 minutes after nasal administration. The bioavailability of nasal calcitonin is about 25% of that administered by intramuscular or subcutaneous injection.[28] The half-life of elimination of Miacalcin is about 43 minutes. There is no accumulation of the drug on repeated nasal administration at 10-hour intervals for up to 15 days.

No drug interaction studies have been performed with Miacalcin nasal spray ingredients.

2.1.3. Effects on BMD and Fracture Risk

Two randomized, placebo controlled trials were conducted with 325 postmenopausal females with spinal, forearm, or femoral BMD at least 1 SD below normal for healthy pre-menopausal females. Subjects who received 200 international units (IU) daily of Miacalcin nasal spray for 2 years had increases in lumbar vertebral BMD relative to baseline and relative to placebo. Miacalcin nasal spray produced statistically significant increases in lumbar vertebral BMD in osteoporotic females who were more than 5 years postmenopausal compared to placebo as early as 6 months after initiation of therapy with persistence of this level for up to 2 years of observation.[29]

The effect of Miacalcin nasal spray on fracture was evaluated in the Prevent Recurrence of Osteoporotic Fracture (PROOF) study,[30] a large 5-year, multicenter, double blind, randomized study of the efficacy of nasal calcitonin on patients with 1-5 previous vertebral fractures and low vertebral BMD. Patients were randomized to daily Miacalcin at doses of 100, 200, or 400 IU, or placebo. All patients received daily supplement of calcium and vitamin D. The data have shown a significant 36% vertebral fracture reduction in the 200 IU group and a 45% reduction in the number of patients with multiple new vertebral fractures. The reduction in vertebral fracture incidence was seen after year 3 and was sustained through year 5 with 200 IU. There was no significant effect on fracture risk with other doses in the study. There was a non-significant 46% reduction in hip/femur fractures in the 200 IU group compared with placebo. There was also no effect on nonvertebral fracture incidence.

2.1.4.   Indications and Regimen

Miacalcin nasal spray is indicated for the treatment of PMO in women who are more than 5 years postmenopausal and for women who refuse or cannot tolerate bisphosphonates or raloxifene.

The recommended dose of Miacalcin nasal spray in postmenopausal osteoporotic women is 200 IU daily administered intra-nasally in alternating nostrils. Nasal calcitonin may be taken at any time of day. Miacalcin nasal spray should be taken in conjunction with an adequate calcium (at least 1000 mg elemental calcium per day) and vitamin D (400 IU per day) intake to retard the progressive loss of bone mass.

2.1.5.   Side Effects

Miacalcin nasal spray is well tolerated. In all postmenopausal patients treated with Miacalcin nasal spray, the most commonly reported nasal adverse events included rhinitis (12%), epistaxis (3.5%), and sinusitis (2.3%). Flushing, nausea, local irritation, and possible allergic reactions have also been reported.

2.2. *Raloxifene*

Raloxifene (Evista®) is a selective estrogen receptor modulator (SERM) approved by the FDA for PMO prevention and treatment.

2.2.1.   Mechanism of Action

Decreases in estrogen levels after oophorectomy or menopause lead to increases in bone resorption and accelerated bone loss. Raloxifene has selective estrogen agonist effect on estrogen responsive tissues (reduces bone loss and lowers total and LDL cholesterol), but has antagonistic effect on breast tissue and uterine mucosa. After binding to its receptors, raloxifene produces different expression of estrogen-regulated genes in different tissues, activating certain estrogenic pathways and blockading others.[31,32] In clinical trials, raloxifene prevents bone loss, and lowers serum cholesterol levels without increasing the risk of endometrial cancer or breast tenderness.

2.2.2. Pharmacokinetic Profile

Raloxifene is absorbed rapidly after oral administration. Approximately 60% of an oral absorbed dose undergoes extensive first-pass metabolism in the liver, resulting in about 2% bioavailability.[33] Raloxifene can be administered without regard to meals.

Protein binding is high; about 95% of raloxifene binds to both albumin and (alpha) 1-acid glycoprotein, but not to sex-steroid binding globulin. Raloxifene is primarily excreted in feces and less than 0.2% is excreted unchanged in urine.[34] Other than interference of cholestyramine absorption, no significant drug-drug interactions have been identified.

2.2.3. Effects on BMD and Fracture Risk

The effects of raloxifene on BMD in postmenopausal women were examined in 3 randomized, placebo-controlled, double blind osteoporosis prevention trials involving 1764 patients. Women enrolled in these studies had a median age of 54 years and a median time since menopause of 5 years. The majority of the women were Caucasian (93.5%). The principal outcome measures of these clinical trials were BMD of the spine, hip, and total body. Compared with placebo, raloxifene 60 mg administered once daily produced statistically significant increases in BMD for each of the 3 studies at 12 months and the effect was maintained at 24 months. The placebo groups lost approximately 1% of BMD over 24 months.[35]

The effects of raloxifene on fracture incidence in postmenopausal women with osteoporosis were examined in a large randomized, placebo-controlled, double blind, multinational osteoporosis treatment trial. All vertebral fractures were confirmed radiographically; some of these fractures also were associated with symptoms (i.e., clinical fractures). The study population consisted of 7705 postmenopausal women with osteoporosis as defined by low BMD (vertebral or hip BMD at least 2.5 SD below the mean value for healthy young women) or one or more baseline vertebral fractures. All women in the study received calcium (500 mg/day) and vitamin D (400 to 600 IU/day). Women enrolled in this study had a median age of 67 years (range: 31 to 80 years) and a median time since menopause of 19 years. Subjects who received either 60 mg or 120 mg of raloxifene experienced significantly less new fractures than the placebo group.[36] Raloxifene decreased the incidence of the first vertebral fracture from 4.3% for placebo to 1.9% for raloxifene (relative risk reduction = 55%) and subsequent vertebral fractures from 20.2% for placebo to 14.1% for raloxifene (relative risk reduction = 30%). There was no significant effect on hip fractures or other nonvertebral fractures.

2.2.4. Effects of Raloxifene on Cardiovascular Disease and Breast Cancer

Raloxifene has beneficial effects on lipid metabolism. Raloxifene decreases total and LDL cholesterol levels but does not increase triglyceride levels. It does not change total HDL cholesterol levels. These results suggest raloxifene not only prevents bone loss in postmenopausal women, but also might have a cardio-protective effect.[37]

In the Multiple Outcomes of Raloxifene Evaluation (MORE) trial, 13 cases of breast cancer were diagnosed in the treatment group, compared with 27 cases in the placebo group, a 76% risk reduction principally due to a reduction in estrogen receptor positive breast cancer.[38] Although this study cannot be directly compared with the larger Breast Cancer Prevention Trial, the data suggest raloxifene may be an alternative to estrogen for the prevention of osteoporosis in women at high-risk or with familial history of breast cancer.

2.2.5. Indications and Regimen

Raloxifene is indicated for the treatment and prevention of osteoporosis in postmenopausal women. For either osteoporosis treatment or prevention, supplemental calcium and/or vitamin D should be added to the diet if daily intake is inadequate. The recommended dosage is one 60 mg raloxifene tablet daily, which may be administered any time of day without regard to meals.

2.2.6. Side Effects and Contraindication

Raloxifene was well tolerated in clinical trials. The side effects associated with raloxifene administration are generally mild and did not result in discontinuation. Leg cramps occurred approximately 2-3 times more often with raloxifene than with placebo. Raloxifene is associated with a low but statistically significant increased risk of thrombophlebitis and pulmonary emboli similar to that observed with estrogen treatment. Raloxifene is contraindicated in women with active or past history of venous thromboembolic events, including deep vein thrombosis, pulmonary embolism, and retinal vein thrombosis.

2.3. *Bisphosphonates*

Bisphosphonates are structural analogs of pyrophosphates that have high affinity for hydroxyapatite, a major inorganic component of bone. The general chemical structure shows that two phosphonic acids joined to a carbon. The R1 side chain determines the affinity of bisphosphonates for bone and the R2 chain contributes to its antiresorptive potency. Modification of these two side chain results in a variety of agents.[39]

2.3.1. Mechanism of Action

Bisphosphonates have an affinity for hydroxyapatite crystals in bone and acts as an antiresorptive agent. At the cellular level, bisphosphonates preferentially localizes to sites of bone resorption and inhibits osteoclasts.[40] Osteoclasts adhere normally to the bone surface, but show evidence of reduced active resorption (e.g., lack of ruffled border). Induction of osteoclast apotosis has been shown in vitro and in vivo studies in mice.[41] Bisphosphonates interfere with protein prenylation by inhibiting farnesyl pyrophosphatase, an enzyme in the HMG-CoA reductase pathway,[42] leading to prevention of post-translational prenylation of guanosine triphosphate (GTP)-binding proteins, which in turn cause reduced resorptive activity of osteoclasts and accelerated apoptosis (programmed cell death).

2.3.2.   Pharmacokinetic Properties

The discussion below is limited to the two most commonly prescribed orally administered bisphosphonates.   Alendronate (Fosamax[®]), a nitrogen-containing bisphosphonate, and risedronate (Actonel[®]), a pyridinyl bisphosphonate.

Bisphosphonates have a rapid absorption phase. After an oral dose, the time to maximum plasma concentration is relatively rapid with t_{max} about 1 hour and occurring throughout the upper gastrointestinal tract. The bioavailability of bisphosphonates is generally very low. The mean oral bioavailability of alendronate in women was 0.64% for doses ranging from 5 to 70 mg when administered after an overnight fast and 2 hours before a standardized breakfast.[43] The mean oral bioavailability of risedronate was 0.63% ranging from 2.5-30 mg.[44] The extent of absorption of both alendronate and risedronate was decreased by approximately 40-50% when administered 0.5-1 hour before breakfast.

Following a single IV dose of [^{14}C] alendronate, approximately 50% of the radioactivity was excreted in the urine within 72 hours and little or no radioactivity was recovered in the feces. Approximately half of the absorbed risedronate dose is excreted in urine within 24 hours. The estimated terminal half-life of alendronate and risedronate in humans is different; more than 10 years for alendronate and about 20 days for risedronate. There is no evidence of systemic metabolism of alendronate or risedronate.

2.3.3.   The Effect of Bisphosphonates on BMD and Fractures

2.3.3.1. Alendronate

Alendronate was the first bisphosphonate approved by the FDA for PMO indication. In a pivotal Phase III study involving over 900 patients, postmenopausal women receiving 10 mg/day alendronate had significant, progressive increases in BMD at all skeletal sites, whereas those receiving placebo had decreases in BMD. At 3 years, the mean ($\pm$ SE) differences in bone mineral density between the women receiving 10 mg of alendronate daily and those receiving placebo were 8.8 $\pm$ 0.4% in the spine, $5.9 \pm 0.5\%$ in the femoral neck, $7.8 \pm 0.6\%$ in the trochanter, and $2.5 \pm 0.3\%$ in the total body ($p < 0.001$ for all comparisons).[45] Hosking and colleagues compared the treatment effects of alendronate with HRT on BMD of the lumbar spine, hip, and forearm. The study recruited 1174 postmenopausal women under the age of 60 years with pre-existing osteoporosis. Patients were randomized to alendronate or HRT groups. The placebo group had a loss of BMD at all sites, while the alendronate group had a mean increase in BMD ranging from 3.5% at the lumber spine to 1.9% at the hip, compatible to the HRT group, demonstrating alendronate is efficacious in preventing bone loss[46].

Fracture Intervention Trial (FIT),[47] the first study to show the beneficial effect of alendronate on bone fracture endpoints, was a large-scale (over 2000 patients), double-blind clinical trial designed to assess the effect of alendronate on the frequencies of vertebral and nonvertebral fractures in postmenopausal women with low bone mass. 2027 women were randomly assigned placebo (1005) or alendronate (1022) and followed for 36 months. The dose of alendronate (initially 5 mg daily) was increased (to 10 mg daily) at 24 months, with maintenance of the double-blind. Lateral spine radiography was done at baseline and at 24 and 36 months. New vertebral fractures, the primary endpoint, were defined by morphometry as a decrease of 20% (and at least 4 mm) in at least one vertebral height between the baseline and latest follow-up radiograph. 78 (8.0%) women in the alendronate group had one or more new morphometric vertebral fractures compared with 145 (15.0%) women in the placebo group. For clinically apparent vertebral fractures, the corresponding numbers were 23 (2.3%) women in the alendronate group and 50 (5.0%) women in the placebo group. The risk of hip fracture and wrist fracture was also lower in the alendronate group than in the placebo group. This study indicated alendronate is well tolerated and substantially reduces the frequency of morphometric and clinical vertebral fractures, as well as other clinical fractures. Other studies have also confirmed the antifracture benefit of alendronate.[48,49]

2.3.3.2. Risedronate

Risedronate was shown to be effective for prevention of bone loss and increasing BMD in postmenopausal women in the two studies where change in mean lumbar spine BMD was the primary endpoint.[50,51] In one study, women with a mean lumbar spine T-score of -2 or less (n = 543) received 24 months of placebo or risedronate (2.5 or 5 mg/day). All received calcium (1 g/day). The principal outcome measures were BMD at the lumbar spine, femoral neck, and femoral trochanter. At 24 months, lumbar spine BMD increased from baseline by 4% with 5 mg risedronate and 1.4% in the 2.5 mg group, compared with no change in the placebo group. At 24 months, 5 mg risedronate had also increased BMD at the femoral neck and trochanter, whereas BMD decreased in the placebo group. BMD increases were seen at all three sites with 5 mg risedronate after only 6 months of therapy.

Effects of risedronate treatment on vertebral and nonvertebral fractures in women with PMO was evaluated in 2 large clinical trials involving a total of 3684 patients.[52,53] Women with at least 1 vertebral fracture at baseline were enrolled. Subjects were randomly assigned to receive oral treatment for 3 years with risedronate (2.5 or 5 mg/day) or placebo. All subjects received calcium, 1000 mg/day. Vitamin D (cholecalciferol, up to 500 IU/day) was provided if baseline levels of 25-hydroxyvitamin D were low. Incidence of new vertebral fractures as detected by quantitative and semiquantitative assessments of radiographs; incidence of radiographically confirmed nonvertebral fractures and change from baseline in BMD as determined by dual x-ray absorptiometry (DXA). The 2.5 mg group was discontinued after 1-2 years. Risedronate caused statistically significant reduction in vertebral fractures in these 2 clinical trials. Compared with placebo, there was a 41% and 49% reduction in risk of new vertebral fractures, and a 39% and a 33% reduction in the incidence of nonvertebral fractures in patients receiving 5 mg/day of risedronate. Additionally, a 65% and 61% reduction in vertebral fracture risk was seen within the first year of treatment.

The efficacy of risedronate treatment in preventing hip fracture was evaluated in the largest prospective randomized trial of osteoporosis therapy, enrolling almost 9500 women.[54] This is also the only prospective trial where reduction of hip fracture was the primary endpoint. Patients were stratified into 2 groups. Group 1 included patients 70-79 years with osteoporosis based on low BMD and Group 2 included patients 80 years or older with at least one clinical risk factor for hip fracture or low BMD at the femoral neck. Overall, the incidence of hip fracture among all the women assigned to risedronate was 2.8%, as compared with 3.9% among those assigned to placebo (relative risk, 0.7; 95% confidence interval, 0.6 to 0.9; p = 0.02). In Group 1 (women with osteoporosis between 70 to 79 years old), the incidence of hip fracture among those assigned to risedronate was 1.9%, as compared with 3.2% among those assigned to placebo. In Group 2 (women selected primarily on the basis of risk factors and were at least 80 years of age), the incidence of hip fracture was 4.2% among those assigned to risedronate and 5.1% among those assigned to placebo (p = 0.35). Across both groups, risedronate produced a significant overall hip fracture risk reduction over the 3 years of the study.

2.3.4.   Indications and Regimens

Alendronate is approved for prevention and treatment of PMO, treatment of corticosteroid-induced osteoporosis in men and women, and treatment of osteoporosis in men. The recommended dose for prevention and treatment of PMO is 10 mg daily or 70 mg once weekly.

Risedronate is approved for prevention and treatment of PMO and the treatment of corticosteroid-induced osteoporosis in men and women. The FDA approved dose for prevention and treatment of PMO is 5 mg daily or 35 mg once weekly.

2.3.5.   Adverse Effects and Cautions

Bisphosphonates are relatively well tolerated with gastrointestinal complaints being the most commonly reported adverse events. Bisphosphonates should not be given to patients who have esophageal emptying disease, including esophageal strictures, achalasia, or severe dysmotility. Bisphosphonates should be taken at least 30 minutes before the first food or drink of the day other than water. To facilitate delivery to the stomach, bisphosphonates should be swallowed while the patient is in an upright position and with a full glass of plain water (6 to 8 oz). Other beverages (including mineral water), food, and some medications are likely to reduce the absorption of bisphosphonates. Patients should not lie down for 30 minutes after taking the medication.

Patients should receive supplemental calcium and vitamin D if dietary intake is inadequate. Calcium supplements and calcium-, aluminum-, and magnesium-containing medications may interfere with the absorption of bisphosphonates and should be taken at a different time of the day. Bisphosphonates are not recommended for use in patients with severe renal impairment (creatinine clearance < 30 mL/min). No dosage adjustment is necessary in patients with mild-to-moderate renal insufficiency (creatinine clearance 35-60 mL/min).

Table 7. Other Bisphosphonates

Name of Bisphosphonate	Regulatory Approved Indications
Clodronate	Not available in the United States. In Europe and Canada, clodronate is approved for treatment of hypercalcemia of malignancy
Etidronate	Approved in Canada and many European countries for treatment of osteoporosis. In the United States, etidronate is sometimes used "off label" for patients who cannot tolerate other oral bisphosphonates. Etidronate is approved by the FDA for the treatment of symptomatic Paget's disease of bone and in the prevention of heterotopic ossification following total hip replacement or due to spinal cord injury.
Ibandronate	Ibandronate is the newest bisphosphonates for osteoporosis indication. 2.5 mg/day orally is approved by the FDA for osteoporosis indication.
Pamidronate	In the United States, pamidronate is approved by the FDA for the treatment of hypercalcemia of malignancy, osteolytic lesions in multiple myeloma or metastatic cancer to bone, and Paget's disease of bone. Pamidronate is not approved in the United States for osteoporosis. It is sometimes used "off label" for patients who can not tolerate other oral bisphosponates
Tiludronate	Approved in the United States for treatment of Paget's disease of bone.
Zoledronate	Approved by the FDA for treatment of hypercalcemia of malignancy and osteolytic lesions in multiple myeloma or metastatic cancer to bone.

2.3.6. Other Bisphosphonates

Other bisphosphonates approved by either the FDA, or Europe or Canada regulatory authorities, are summarized in Table 7.

2.4. *Teriparatide [rhPTH (1-34)]*

Teriparatide [rhPTH (1-34)] (FORTEO™) contains recombinant human parathyroid hormone (1-34), which has an identical sequence to the 34 N-terminal amino acids (the biologically active region) of the 84-amino acid human parathyroid hormone (PTH). Teriparatide has been recently approved by the FDA with indication of osteoporosis.

2.4.1. Mechanism of Action

Endogenous 84-amino-acid parathyroid hormone is the primary regulator of calcium and phosphate metabolism in bone and kidney. Physiological actions of PTH include regulation of bone metabolism, renal tubular re-absorption of calciumand phosphate, and intestinal calcium absorption. The biological actions of PTH and teriparatide are mediated through binding to specific high-affinity cell-surface receptors. Teriparatide and the 34 N-terminal amino acids of PTH bind to these receptors with the same affinity and have the same physiological actions on bone and kidney. Teriparatide is not expected to accumulate in bone or other tissues.

The skeletal effects of teriparatide depend upon the pattern of systemic exposure. Once-daily administration of teriparatide stimulates new bone formation on trabecular and cortical bone surfaces by preferential stimulation of osteoblastic activity over osteoclastic activity.[55,56] By contrast, continuous excess of endogenous PTH, as occurs in hyperparathyroidism, may be detrimental to the skeleton because bone resorption may be stimulated more than bone formation.[57]

2.4.2. Pharmacokinetic Profile

Teriparatide is extensively absorbed after subcutaneous injection; the absolute bioavailability is approximately 95%. The rates of absorption and elimination are rapid. The peptide reaches peak serum concentrations about 30 minutes after subcutaneous injection of a 20 μg dose and declines to non-quantifiable concentrations within 3 hours. The half-life of teriparatide in serum is 5 minutes when administered by intravenous injection and approximately 1 hour when administered by subcutaneous injection. The longer half-life following subcutaneous administration reflects the time required for absorption from the injection site. No metabolism or excretion studies have been performed with teriparatide. Peripheral metabolism of PTH is believed to occur by non-specific enzymatic mechanisms in the liver followed by excretion via the kidneys.[58]

2.4.3. Effects on BMD and Fracture Risk

The effect of teriparatide on BMD and fractures was evaluated in 1637 postmenopausal women with osteoporosis who were treated for a median of 19 months. Patients were randomized to receive daily subcutaneous injection of 20 or 40 μg of parathyroid hormone (1-34) or placebo, along with calcium and vitamin D supplementation. Daily treatment at doses of 20 and 40 μg increased the BMD by 9 and 13 percentage points in the spine and by 3 and 6 percentage points in the femoral neck than did placebo. The treatment reduced the risk of new vertebral fractures by 65% and 69%, respectively, as compared with placebo. Daily injection with parathyroid hormone reduced the risk of nonvertebral fractures by 35% at the 20 μg dose and by 40% at the 40 μg dose, and reduced the risk of nonvertebral fragility fractures by 53% and 54%, respectively. In summary, treatment of PMO with parathyroid hormone (1-34) decreases the risk of vertebral and nonvertebral fractures; increases vertebral, femoral, and total-body BMD. The 40 μg dose increased BMD more than the 20 μg dose but has similar effects on the risk of fractures and was more likely to have side effects.[59]

2.4.4. Indications and Regimen

Teriparatide is indicated for the treatment of osteoporotic patients who are at high risk for fracture including women with a history of osteoporotic fracture, or who have multiple risk factors for fracture, or who have failed or are intolerant of previous osteoporosis therapy.

Teriparatide should be administered as a subcutaneous injection into the thigh or abdominal wall. The recommended dosage is 20 μg once a day.

2.4.5. Side Effects and Cautions

Teriparatide was very well tolerated. Most side effects reported were mild and included nausea, dizziness, and leg cramps. Transient episodes of symptomatic orthostatic hypotension were observed infrequently, and was relieved by placing the person in a reclining position.

In clinical trials, the frequency of urolithiasis was similar in patients treated with teriparatide and placebo. However, teriparatide has not been studied in patients with active urolithiasis. If active urolithiasis or pre-existing hypercalciuria is suspected, measurement of urinary calcium excretion should be considered. Teriparatide should be used with caution in patients with active or recent urolithiasis because of the potential to exacerbate this condition.

Teriparatide transiently increases serum calcium and should be used with caution in patients taking digitalis because sporadic case reports have suggested hypercalcemia may predispose patients to digitalis toxicity.

In animal studies, teriparatide showed an increase in the development of osteosarcoma. In human clinical trial, there were no cases of osteosarcoma reported.[59]

3. Summary

Osteoporosis is recognized as a major growing health problem affecting more than 8 million postmenopausal women in the U.S. Osteoporosis A to H is one way of remembering the clinical management pertaining to osteoporosis[60] as shown in Table 8 below.

Table 8. Osteoporosis A to H

A	Assess risk factors
B	Bone densitometry, as clinically indicated, using NOF and regulatory guidelines, as applicable
C	Calcium intake
D	Vitamin D supplement
E	Exercise
F	Fall prevention
G	Glandular and other secondary disorders to be considered, as clinically indicated
H	Hormone therapy, bisphosphonates, calcitonin, raloxifene and teriparatide

The most comprehensive set of guidelines for the management of osteoporosis comes from the National Osteoporosis Foundation. Other resources found on the internet for osteoporosis and bone metabolism are listed in Table 9.

Table 9. Internet Resources for Osteoporosis and Bone Metabolism

Organization	Web Address
International Osteoporosis Foundation	www.osteofound.org
American Diabetes Association Nutrition Resources	www.eatright.org
American Society of Bone and Mineral Research	www.asbmr.org
BoneKey-Osteovision Site of the International Bone and Mineral Society (IBMS)	www.bonekey-ibms.org

Acknowledgments

The authors appreciably thank Ms. Barbara McCarty-Garcia for her assistance in preparing this manuscript.

REFERENCES

1. NOF: Physician's Guide to Prevention and Treatment of Osteoporosis, (Excerpta Medica, Inc., Belle Meade, New Jersey, 1998).
2. U.S. Preventive Services Task Force, Ann. Intern. Med., 526 (2002).
3. Food and Nutritional Board, Standing Committee of the Scientific Evaluation of Dietary Reference Intakes, (Institute of Medicine, Washington, DC, 1997).
4. Council on Scientific Affairs, American Medical Association, Arch. Fam. Med., 495 (1997).
5. R. P. Heaney, M. S. Dowell, J. Bierman, C. A. Hale, A. Bendich, J. Am. Coll. Nutr., 239 (2001).
6. R. J. Heikinheimo, J. A. Inkovaara, E. J. Harju, M. V. Haavisto, R. H. Kaarela, J. M. Kataja, A. M. Kokko, L. A. Kolho, S. A. Rajala, Calcif. Tissue Int., 105 (1992).
7. J. A. Grisso, J. L. Kelsey, B. L. Strom, G. Y. Chiu, G. Maislin, L. A. O'Brien, S. Hoffman, F. Kaplan, N. Engl. J. Med., 1326 (1991).
8. R. T. Turner, B. L. Riggs, T. C. Spelsberg, Endocr. Rev., 275 (1994).
9. R. L. Prince, J. Clin. Endocrinol. Metab., 301 (1994).
10. H. K. Genant, J. Lucas, S. Weiss, M. Akin, R. Emkey, H. McNaney-Flint, R. Downs, J. Mortola, N. Watts, H. M. Yang, N. Banav, J. J. Brennan, J. C. Nolan, Arch. Intern. Med., 2609 (1997).
11. B. R. Bhavnani, Proc. Soc. Exp. Biol. Med., 6 (1998).
12. Physician's Desk Reference, 2095 (1999).
13. R. Lindsay, D. M. Hart, C. Forrest, C. Baird, Lancet, 1151 (1980).
14. J. E. Rossouw, G. L. Anderson, R. L. Prentice, A. Z. LaCroix, C. Kooperberg, M. L. Stefanick, R. D. Jackson, S. A. Beresford, B. V. Howard, K. C. Johnson, J. M. Kotchen, J. Ockene; Writing Group for the Women's Health Initiative Investigators, JAMA., 321 (2002).
15. J. A. Cauley, J. Robbins, Z. Chen, S. R. Cummings, R. D. Jackson, A. Z. LaCroix, M. LeBoff, C. E. Lewis, J. McGowan, J. Neuner, M. Pettinger, M. L. Stefanick, J. Wactawski-Wende, N. B. Watts; Women's Health Initiative Investigators, JAMA., 1729 (2003).
16. D. J. Torgerson, S. E. Bell-Seyer, JAMA., 2891 (2001).
17. The Writing Group for the PEPI, JAMA., 1389 (1996).
18. Guidelines for Women's Health Care, 2nd ed., American College of Obstetricians and Gynecologists, (American Coll. of Obstetricians and Gynecologists, Washington, DC, 2002) pp. 130, 171, 314.
19. J. E. Manson, J. Hsia, K. C. Johnson, J. E. Rossouw, A. R. Assaf, N. L. Lasser, M. Trevisan, H. R. Black, S. R. Heckbert, R. Detrano, O. L. Strickland, N. D.

Wong, J. R. Crouse, E. Stein, M. Cushman; Women's Health Initiative Investigators, N. Engl. J. Med., 523 (2003).

20.   S. Wassertheil-Smoller, S. L. Hendrix, M. Limacher, G. Heiss, C. Kooperberg, A. Baird, T. Kotchen, J. D. Curb, H. Black, J. E. Rossouw, A. Aragaki, M. Safford, E. Stein, S. Laowattana, W. J. Mysiw; WHI Investigators, JAMA., 2673 (2003).

21.   R. T. Chlebowski, S. L. Hendrix, R. D. Langer, M. L. Stefanick, M. Gass, D. Lane, R. J. Rodabough, M. A. Gilligan, M. G. Cyr, C. A. Thomson, J. Khandekar, H. Petrovitch, A. McTiernan; WHI Investigators, JAMA., 3242 (2003).

22.   G. L. Anderson, H. L. Judd, A. M. Kaunitz, D. H. Barad, S. A. Beresford, M. Pettinger, J. Liu, S. G. McNeeley, A. M. Lopez; Women's Health Initiative Investigators, JAMA., 1739 (2003).

23.   S. A. Shumaker, C. Legault, S. R. Rapp, L. Thal, R. B. Wallace, J. K. Ockene, S. L. Hendrix, B. N. Jones 3rd, A. R. Assaf, R. D. Jackson, J. M. Kotchen, S. Wassertheil-Smoller, J. Wactawski-Wende; WHIMS Investigators, JAMA., 2651 (2003).

24.   S. R. Rapp, M. A. Espeland, S. A. Shumaker, V. W. Henderson, R. L. Brunner, J. E. Manson, M. L. Gass, M. L. Stefanick, D. S. Lane, J. Hays, K. C. Johnson, L. H. Coker, M. Dailey, D. Bowen; WHIMS Investigators, JAMA., 2663 (2003).

25.   T. J. Chambers, A. Moore, J. Clin. Endocrinol. Metab., 819 (1983).

26.   S.L. Silverman, M. Azria, Osteoporos. Int., 858 (2002).

27.   G. P. Lyritis, I. Paspati, T. Karachalios, D. Ioakimidis, G. Skarantavos, P.G. Lyritis, Acta. Orthop. Scand., 112 (1997).

28.   K. Overgaard, D. Agnusdei, M. A. Hansen, E. Maioli, C. Christiansen, C. Gennari, J. Clin. Endocrinol. Metab., 344 (1991).

29.   S. L. Silverman, in Osteoporosis: an evidence based guide to prevention and management, Ed. S. R. Cummings, F. Cosman, S. A. Jamal, (American College of Physicians, Philadelphia, PA, 2002), p. 197.

30.   C. H. Chesnut 3rd, S. Silverman, K. Andriano, H. Genant, A. Gimona, S. Harris, D. Kiel, M. LeBoff, M. Maricic, P. Miller, C. Moniz, M. Peacock, P. Richardson, N. Watts, D. Baylink, Am. J. Med., 267 (2000).

31.   A. M. Brzozowski, A. C. W. Pike, Z. Dauter, R. E. Hubbard, T. Bonn, O. Engström, L.Öhman, G. L. Greene, J. A. Gustafsson, M. Carlquist, Nature, 753 (1997).

32.   K. Paech, P. Webb, G. G. J. M. Kuiper, S. Nilsson, J. Å. Gustafsson, P. J. Kushner, T. S. Scanlan, Science, 1508 (1997).

33.   T. A. Grese, L. D. Pennington, J. P. Sluka, M. D. Adrian, H. W. Cole, T. R. Fuson, D. E. Magee, D. L. Phillips, E. R. Rowley, P. K. Shetler, L. L. Short, M. Venugopalan, N. N. Yang, M. Sato, A. L. Glasebrook, H. U. Bryant, J. Med. Chem., 1272 (1998).

34.   J. A. Balfour, K. L. Goa, Drugs Aging, 335 (1998).

35.   P. D. Delmas, N. H. Bjarnason, B. H. Mitlak, A. C. Ravoux, A. S. Shah, W. J. Huster, M. Draper, C. Christiansen, N. Engl. J. Med., 1641 (1997).

36. B. Ettinger, D. M. Black, B. H. Mitlak, R. K. Knickerbocker, T. Nickelsen, H. K. Genant, C. Christiansen, P. D. Delmas, J. R. Zanchetta, J. Stakkestad, C. C. Gluer, K. Krueger, F. J. Cohen, S. Eckert, K. E. Ensrud, L. V. Avioli, P. Lips, S. R. Cummings, JAMA., 637 (1999).

37. B. W. Walsh, L. H. Kuller, R. A. Wild, S. Paul, M. Farmer, J. B. Lawrence, A. S. Shah, P. W. Anderson, JAMA., 1445 (1998).

38. S. R. Cummings, S. Eckert, K. A. Krueger, D. Grady, T. J. Powles, J. A. Cauley, L. Norton, T. Nickelsen, N. H. Bjarnason, M. Morrow, M. E. Lippman, D. Black, J. E. Glusman, A. Costa, V. C. Jordan, JAMA., 2189 (1999).

39. N. B. Watts, Clin. Geriatr. Med., 395 (2003).

40. H. Fleisch, Endocr. Rev., 80 (1998).

41. D. E. Hughes, K. R. Wright, H. L. Uy, A. Sasaki, T. Yoneda, G. D. Roodman, G. R. Mundy, B. F. Boyce, J. Bone. Miner. Res., 1478 (1995).

42. M. J. Rogers, J. C. Firth, S. P. Luckman, F. P. Coxon, H. L. Benford, J. Monkkonen, S. Auriola, K. M. Chilton, R. G. Russell, Bone, 73S (1999).

43. G. Porras, S. D. Holland, B. J. Gertz, Clin. Pharmacokinet., 315 (1999).

44. D. Y. Mitchell, R. A. Eusebio, D. W. Axelrod, K. R. Hicks, D. A. Russell, L. C. Kamra, J. H. Powell, Bone, 100S (1997).

45. U. A. Liberman, S. R. Weiss, J. Broll, H. W. Minne, H. Quan, N. H. Bell, J. Rodriguez-Portales, R. W. Downs Jr, J. Dequeker, M. Favus, N. Engl. J. Med., 1437 (1995).

46. D. Hosking, C. E. Chilvers, C. Christiansen, P. Ravn, R. Wasnich, P. Ross, M. McClung, A. Balske, D. Thompson, M. Daley, A. J. Yates, N. Engl. J. Med., 485 (1998).

47. D. M. Black, S. R. Cummings, D. B. Karpf, J. A. Cauley, D. E. Thompson, M. C. Nevitt, D. C. Bauer, H. K. Genant, W. L. Haskell, R. Marcus, S. M. Ott, J. C. Torner, S. A. Quandt, T. F. Reiss, K. E. Ensrud, Lancet, 1535 (1996).

48. S. R. Cummings, D. M. Black, D. E. Thompson, W. B. Applegate, E. Barrett-Connor, T. A. Musliner, L. Palermo, R. Prineas, S. M. Rubin, J. C. Scott, T. Vogt, R. Wallace, A. J. Yates, A. Z. LaCroix, JAMA., 2077 (1998).

49. H. A. P. Pols, D. Felsenberg, D. A. Hanley, J. Stepán, M. Muñoz-Torres, T. J. Wilkin, G. Qin-sheng, A. M. Galich, K. Vandormael, A. J. Yates, B. Stych, Osteoporos. Int., 461 (1999).

50. Fogelman, C. Ribot, R. Smith, D. Ethgen, E. Sod, J. Y. Reginster, Clin. Endocrinol. Metab., 1895 (2000).

51. M. McClung, W. Bensen, M. Bolognese, S. Bonnick, M. Ettinger, S. Harris, H. Heath, R. Lang, P. Miller, E. Pavlov, S. Silverman, G. Woodson, K. Faulkner, P. Bekker, D. W. Axelrod, J. Bone Miner. Res., S169 (1997).

52. S. T. Harris, N. B. Watts, H. K. Genant, C. D. McKeever, T. Hangartner, M. Keller, C. H. Chesnut 3rd, J. Brown, E. F. Eriksen, M. S. Hoseyni, D. W. Axelrod, P. D. Miller, JAMA., 1344 (1999).

53. J. Y. Reginster, H. W. Minne, O. H. Sorensen, M. Hooper, C. Roux, M. L. Brandi, B. Lund, D. Ethgen, S. Pack, I. Roumagnac, R. Eastell, Osteoporos. Int., 83 (2000).

54. M. R. McClung, P. Geusens, P. D. Miller, H. Zippel, W. G. Bensen, C. Roux, S. Adami, I. Fogelman, T. Diamond, R. Eastell, P. J. Meunier, J. Y. Reginster; Hip Intervention Program Study Group, N. Engl. J. Med., 344 (2001).

55. R. Podbesek, C. Edouard, P. J. Meunier, J. A. Parsons, J. Reeve, R. W. Stevenson, J. M. Zanelli, Endocrinology, 100 (1983).

56. J. M. Hock, I. Gera, J. Bone Miner. Res., 65 (1992).

57. C. S. Tam, J. N. Heersche, T. M. Murray, J. A. Parsons, Endocrinology, 506(1982).

58. Physician's Desk Reference® Electronic Library.

59. R. M. Neer, C. D. Arnaud, J. R. Zanchetta, R. Prince, G. A. Gaich, J. Y. Reginster, A. B. Hodsman, E. F. Eriksen, S. Ish-Shalom, H. K. Genant, O. Wang, B. H. Mitlak, N. Eng. J. Med., 1434 (2001).

60. S. Petak, personal communication, (1999).

CHAPTER 11

NOVEL POTENTIAL DRUG TARGETS FOR THE ANTI-RESORPTIVE TREATMENT OF OSTEOPOROSIS

Jiake Xu, Shek Man Chim and Ming Hao Zheng

Molecular Orthopaedic Laboratory,
School of Surgery and Pathology,
The University of Western Australia,
QE II Medical Centre, M Block,
Nedlands, Western Australia, 6009 Australia
Tel:618 9346 4051
Fax:618 9346 3210
Email:jiakexu@cyllene.uwa.edu.au

Osteoclasts are bone resorbing cells. The increased formation and activation of osteoclasts underlies many common bone lytic disorders such as osteoporosis, Paget's disease, bone metastatic diseases, arthritis, and aseptic bone loosening. Currently, drugs used in management of osteoporosis are limited to bisphosphonates, calcium and vitamin D. Although there is evidence that hormone replacement therapy prevents bone loss in postmenopausal women, its beneficial effect on bone is overshadowed by its association with increased risks in breast cancer and cardiovascular disease. Unravelling the genetic regulation of osteoclastogenesis and osteoclast activation and discovering therapeutic agents to control these processes are critical for the development of effective treatment for osteoporosis. This chapter reviews novel potential targets for anti-resorptive drugs and determines the viability of these targets, giving special consideration to specificity to bone and any side effects. Several groups of targets have been identified as being promising: including the RANKL/RANK/OPG axis; intracellular signalling molecules, such as c-Src; integrins, especially the $\alpha_v\beta_3$ integrin, and enzymes, such as cathepsins and vacuolar H+ATPase. A significant amount of in vitro data concerning many of these targets have been generated, yet there is still little research investigating the capacity for drugs to manipulate these targets and to provide beneficial and non-toxic therapy in a clinical setting. It is clear that some targets are more promising than others, namely RANKL/RANK/OPG axis, cathepsin K and c-Src tyrosine kinase. However, additional research is required before any one target or therapy can be pursued clinically.

Introduction

An imbalance between bone resorption and formation, in favour of bone resorption, is the mechanism underlying many bone diseases, such as osteoporosis, malignancy-related osteolysis and various inflammatory conditions of bone. These conditions are significant problems because they cause much morbidity and mortality. Of concern is that osteoporotic fractures in the elderly have been correlated with increased mortality rates (1). Additionally, diseases of excess bone resorption place a significant financial burden on the health care system.

Currently, most research into bone diseases is centred on the development of agents that counter bone resorption. So far the clinically viable anti-resorptive pharmaceuticals in current use are limited to bisphosphonates, calcium and vitamin D. Although these agents have had reasonable success, there are still issues of toxicity and dosing that are yet to be rectified. For instance, the required dosing regimes and gastrointestinal side effects of bisphosphonates have often raised issues of compliance (2). Furthermore, the problems of excess bone resorption are worsening, indicating that current anti-resorptive agents are not ultimately successful in preventing the clinical outcomes of bone disease. In fact, the number of osteoporosis related fractures is expected to increase in greater proportion than the population increase during the next century given the current treatments available (3).

Fortunately, recent discoveries in the field of osteoclast biology and physiology are uncovering new targets for potential anti-resorptive agents that may not have the same problems of efficacy and toxicity. This chapter reviews these new targets and the viability of agents that could manipulate these targets. Osteoclast lifespan can be divided into three phases: osteoclast differentiation, osteoclast resorption of bone and cessation of osteoclast function and apoptosis. Each phase is highly regulated by osteoclastogenic factors, intracellular signalling molecules, integrins and enzymes and in these regulators lie the basis of the potential targets for anti-resorptive therapy. Some targets may have to be excluded from potential therapeutics because of lack of specificity to bone, but others are very promising.

The Origin and Characteristics of Osteoclasts

Osteoclasts are responsible for the resorption of bone. In coupling with osteoblasts, osteoclasts form the foundation on which bone turnover and skeletal integrity are based. Osteoclasts were initially thought to develop from specific osteoprogenitors, however, through experiments during the 1970s involving parabiosis, tissue grafting and bone marrow transplantation, have now been shown to be of haemopoeitic lineage. This was demonstrated in humans after cure of an osteopetrotic female was achieved through transplantation of bone marrow derived from her brother (4). In vitro experiemtns have shown that peripheral blood monocytes and macrophages when cultured under the appropriate conditions, formed cells that expressed the phenotypic characteristics of osteoclasts (5,6). Studies have also been conducted to determine when during the macrophage maturation process the osteoclastogenetic pathway is undertaken, which is accompanied by the upregulation of a number of genes differentially expressed by osteoclasts. A mature osteoclast expresses very high levels of tartrate-resistant acid phosphatase (TRAP), vitronectin, pp60c-src, carbonic anhydrase and calcitonin receptors, but lacks many of the antigens that are characteristic of macrophages and inflammatory polykaryons, with Fc and C3 receptors antigens notably absent (7,8). These differences determine the ultimate distinguishing features between macrophages and osteoclasts – only osteoclasts excavate bone.

Osteoclastogenic Factors

Osteoclast differentiation and function are regulated by osteoclastogenic factors, intracellular signalling molecules, integrins and enzymes. There have been many exciting breakthroughs in recent times with respect to the way that osteoclastogenic factors control bone, with the finding that many of the previously known cytokines, such as interleukins and tumour necrosis factor, may be influential. However, the major breakthrough in knowledge of bone metabolism is the establishment of the RANKL/RANK/OPG axis as the main determinant of bone mass. The receptor activator of NF-κB (RANKL, also known as TRANCE, ODF and OPGL) is a type 1 transmembrane protein and a member of the tumour necrosis factor (TNF) superfamily. RANKL is a ligand present on the surface of osteoblasts and stromal cells that bind to its receptor (RANK) on osteoclast precursor cells and mature osteoclasts. The binding of RANKL to RANK results in the final transition of the precursor cell into a fully-fledged osteoclast, a process that can be blocked by osteoprotegerin (OPG) , a soluble decoy receptor for RANKL. Essentially, it is the balance between RANKL and OPG that determines how much bone is resorbed.

RANKL/RANK/OPG

RANKL stimulates the pool of M-CSF-expanded precursors to commit to the osteoclast phenotype (9,10). Further studies also associate RANKL with activation of mature osteoclasts *in vivo* and regulation of calcium honeostasis (11,12). RANKL shows widespread expression outside bone, with mRNA and protein found to be present in megakaryocytes, brain, heart, kidney, skeletal muscle and skin as well as also being expressed in abundance by activated T lymphocytes. Most, if not all, osteotropic factors (eg. PTH, vitamin D_3, PGE_2, IL-1α and TNF-α) that induce osteoclast formation act indirectly by binding to marrow stromal cells which in turn induce upregulation of RANKL expression leading to the juxtaposition of RANKL with its receptor RANK on osteoclasts and their precursors, inducing further osteoclast formation (13). The expression of RANK is, like RANKL, widespread having been identified in mammary epithelium (14), heart, lung, brain, skeletal muscle, kidney, liver and skin (15). Mice with deficient RANKL showed severe osteopetrosis and a defect in tooth eruption with a complete loss of osteoclasts (16). Similarly, deletion of the gene coding for RANK leads to osteopetrosis and failure of lymph node development (17-19), indicating that

RANKL/RANK are essnetial molecules for osteoclast differentiation and function.

OPG is a soluble 'decoy' receptor that compete with RANK for RANKL. It acts by exerting a restraining action on bone resorption both *in vivo* and *in vitro* (20,21). Overexpression of OPG in transgenic mice results in a profound but nonlethal osteopetrosis (20), whereas deletion of OPG results in osteoporosis (22). In addition, human mutation of OPG causes an idiopathic hyperphosphatasia phenotype (23). OPG strongly inhibits osteoclast formation induced by vitamin D_3, PTH or PGE_2, in a dose-dependent manner, and suppresses PTH-mediated activation of osteoclast in osteoblast-osteoclast co-cultures (24). In addition to its action on osteoclasts, OPG shows widespread expression in skin, bones, large arteries and gastrointestinal tract suggest that it plays a role in tissues other than bone.

The importance of RANKL in osteoclasts is manyfold. It has a role in osteoclast differentiation and survival, as well as activation of the mature osteoclast (9-11). Undoubtedly, RANKL is an essential component of every step in the physiological functioning of the osteoclast. RANK is expressed on the surface of osteoclast precursors and interacts with RANKL on osteoblasts and stromal cells (13,19,25). This differentiation process includes the induction of genes that are characteristic of osteoclasts, such as c-Src, tartrate resistant acid phosphatase, beta3 integrin, calcitonin receptor and cathepsin K (9,11). Subsequently, although M-CSF is necessary (in conjunction with RANKL) to expand the population of differentiated cells (26), RANKL alone is required for the survival of osteoclasts and the ultimate production of multinucleated cells with the ability to resorb bone (11,16). Both membrane bound and soluble forms have been identified and are capable of stimulating osteoclastogenesis in vitro (27,28). The vast majority of RANKL is more than likely confined to the cell membrane, as several experiments have shown a requirement for cell-to-cell contact between osteoblasts and osteoclast precursors for stimulation of osteoclast differentiation (13). However, soluble RANKL appears to be a significant predictor of nontraumatic fracture (29).

To fully understand the interaction between RANKL and OPG, it is best to analyse the relative ratio of RANKL to OPG because this is what ultimately determines osteoclast activity and, hence, bone resorption (7,30,31). For instance, giant cell tumour of bone involves overexpression of RANK and RANKL (32), while multiple myeloma induces RANKL and inhibits OPG via release of IL-6 and PTHrP (33). Recent studies also showed that serum OPG levels decline consistently following initiation of immunosuppressive therapy in patients of posttransplantation and this leads to bone loss at the lumbar spine and femoral neck (34).

OPG is an exciting prospect in the development of new anti-resorptive drugs because it is a natural anti-resorptive molecule. By opposing RANKL-mediated osteoclastogenesis, OPG can be thought of as a triple threat to osteoclasts; it inhibits osteoclast formation, activity and survival (31). Several studies have dealt with the experimental use of recombinant OPG or other compounds with OPG activity. OPG has been shown to be very effective in a variety of situations in vitro and as part of animal studies. OPG administration can reduces trabecular bone loss in ovariectomized mice via impairment of the structure and bone resorbing activity of osteoclasts (31,35,36). In animal models of malignancy administration of OPG can rectify abnormalities in the RANKL:OPG ratio, resulting in a reversal in bone complications of malignancies (33). It also diminishes chronic ethanol-induced bone loss in mice (37). In a rat adjuvant arthritis model, OPG was effective in preventing bone loss but could not reduce inflammation (30). Other studies showed that OPG may be useful against hyperparathyroidism and inflammatory bone diseases (24) and is effective in preventing and reducing hypercalcemia and bone metastases present in many neoplastic diseases (14,24,33). However, further study is still needed to determine the effect of OPG on clinical outcomes like bone mineral density (BMD) and fracture incidence in humans, and to evaluate any side effect on the immunological system.

Clinical trials on OPG in a human population have been conducted. One report elucidated the results of a randomised, double-blinded, placebo-controlled study in which a group of 52 postmenopausal women, between 40 and 70 years old, were given a single subcutaneous dose of OPG (38). The OPG used was a genetically engineered fusion molecule that had similar binding affinity for RANKL as native OPG. This study used urinary N-telopeptide (NTX) and deoxypyridinoline as markers of bone resorption to determine the impact of OPG, and it was found that OPG produced a dose-dependent reduction in bone resorption as indicated by these bone resorption markers. Subjects were followed up for 84 days. OPG was found to cause a decrease in bone resorption compared to placebo within 12 hours of subcutaneous administration. The maximum reduction in bone resorption was measured at 5 days post-administration. At six weeks, there was still an average reduction of 14% in NTX. Thus, this study confirmed that OPG is profoundly and rapidly effective in reducing bone turnover in humans and may be effective in treating diseases characterised by increased resorption of bone. Importantly, no serious toxicity was reported. Ideally, the findings of this study should be verified in a much larger study. Furthermore, osteoporotic patients and others with diseases favouring bone resorption should be included in the trials to obtain data on the influence of OPG in pathologic states. The participants were selected using various exclusion criteria that made the study an unrealistic analysis of the female population. Future studies should follow up subjects for a longer period to gain more knowledge regarding the long term effects of OPG in the human body (39), with special attention to relevant clinical endpoints such as BMD and fracture incidence (33).

In addition to its relationship with RANKL, OPG also interacts with TRAIL, a ligand that causes cell apoptosis by binding to its receptors (13). OPG has been shown to act as a decoy receptor of TRAIL, inhibiting apoptosis in Jurkat cells (40). Conversely, TRAIL may act as an inhibitor of OPG. However, it is unlikely that the significance of the reciprocal relationship between TRAIL and OPG extends to osteoclastogenesis (14,15,31).

The other roles of RANKL and OPG in the body are important to consider because alteration of the delicate balance between these molecules may lead to unwanted side effects that rule out the use of some potential anti-resorptives. Aside from the crucial role in bone metabolism, the RANKL/RANK/OPG axis has also been implicated in development of lymph nodes (41,42), mammary gland growth during pregnancy (43) and arterial calcification (22,44). Osteoporosis and arterial calcification are present together with a high incidence in many people, especially the elderly and postmenopausal women (45). Recent studies have found that serum OPG levels are associated with the presence and severity of coronary artery disease, and increased OPG serum levels may be involved in advanced cardiovascular disease in men (46,47). In addition, exogenous OPG IV is able to prevent the development of calcification in arteries, but it cannot reverse the problem (44).

Taken together, the significance of the RANKL/RANK/OPG system is that most, if not all, known hormones and cytokines that have any effect on bone work through this system, making it an attractive target for potential anti-resorptive drugs. Ideally, drugs could be developed that would combat RANKL-induced messages to the osteoclast and thus be able to defend against the excess bone resorption of almost any bone disease. Furthermore, human neutralizing antibodies to RANKL could be developed as an anti-resorptive agent. Recent studies have found that small molecule mimic of OPG can be used to alter the biological function of RANKL/RANK receptor complex, pointing to a potential therapeutic approach (48).

Other Osteoclastogenic Factors

Although the RANKL/RANK/OPG axis has been identified as the main determinant of bone mass, there are other cytokines that potentially modulate the activity of this system. For instance, Burgess et al (11) concluded that something other than RANKL is required to regulate osteoclast resorption because they observed that osteoclasts possess a basal level of activity even in the presence of excess OPG.

In fact, several interleukins have been observed to have a potential role in bone metabolism, indicating an important role for this group of molecules.

Of particular importance is interleukin 1 (IL-1), which is found to have higher activity in estrogen deficient states (49) and some inflammatory bone diseases, such as rheumatoid arthritis (13). IL-1 appears to be a key player in estrogen deficiency-induced bone loss as mice lacking IL-1 receptor do not lose bone mass after ovariectomy (50). Several studies have also shown that IL-1 is influential in various aspects of osteoclast development *in vitro*. It has been found that IL-1 stimulates survival (51) and activation of osteoclast-like cells in culture (52). Importantly, the action of IL-1 was not suppressed by OPG, implying a pathway for osteoclast activation outside of the RANKL/RANK/OPG axis (53). While RANKL is involved in physiological bone resorption, IL-1 may play a role in pathological resorption (13,54). However, they share intracellular pathways which mean that a single agent could be developed to target a site downstream of the RANKL or IL-1 receptor and simultaneously block both pathways. For example, proteasome inhibitors and antisense oligonucleotides to NF-kB components inhibit IL-1 mediated osteoclast-like cell survival (52).

IL-1 activity is controlled to some degree by the relative level of IL-1 receptor antagonist (IL-ra), a blocker of the IL-1 receptor and inhibitor of IL-1 induced signals (13). IL-ra administration to ovariectomised animals can block bone loss associated with their condition (49). In addition, retrovirus-mediated hIL-1Ra gene transfer can protect against ultra-high-molecular-weight polyethylene particle-induced inflammatory bone resorption (55), suggesting the potential for IL-ra as a anti-resorptive agent. However, there appears to be no relationship between IL-ra gene polymorphisms and BMD in postmenopausal women (49,56).

Other interleukins have also been implicated in control of bone resorption. For example, IL-6 has been shown to play an important role in the local regulation of bone turnover and, IL-6 deficient female mice have a normal amount of trabecular bone, but higher rates of bone turnover than control littermates (57). Ovariectomy does not induce any change in either bone mass or bone remodeling rates in the IL-6 deficient mice indicating that IL-6 is essential for the bone loss caused by estrogen deficiency (57). IL-11 has been shown to promote osteoclast formation by RANKL-independent processes (58). Overexpression of human IL-11 gene in transgenic mice, however resulted in the stimulation of bone formation to increase cortical thickness and strength of long bones, and in the prevention of cortical bone loss with advancing age, suggesting that IL-11 may be a new therapeutic target for senile osteoporosis (59). IL-12 (individually or in synergy with IL-18) results in the inhibition of osteoclast formation *in vitro* (60,61). IL-17 is present in synovial fluids from patients with rheumatoid arthritis with potent effect on osteoclastogenesis, and is capable of promoting bone erosion in murine collagen-induced arthritis through loss of the RANKL/OPG balance (62,63).

TNF-α has been proposed as a mediator of osteoclastogenesis and bone resorption. Studies have demonstrated that TNF-α stimulates osteoclast differentiation in the presence of M-CSF via a mechanism independent of the RANKL/RANK system, but osteoclasts induced by TNF-α formed resorption pits on dentine slices only in the presence of IL-1α (64). However, other studies have found that TNF-α alone does not induce osteoclastogenesis, but synergizes with RANKL to promote osteoclastogenesis (65). Cenci et al (66) reported that TNF-α can enhances M-CSF and RANKL-induced osteoclastogenesis. In RANK deficient mice, Li et al (19) has shown that TNF-α can induce osteoclast-like cell formation and, like IL-1, transient hypocalcemia. Since TNF-α is pivotal to the pathogenesis of inflammatory osteolysis, it might serves as a convenient target in combating inflammatory osteolysis.

TGF-β is another player in bone resorption involved in cell proliferation, differentiation, migration and apoptosis (67). It was found that TGF-β causes upregulation of OPG, thus acting as negative feedback for the resorptive process (68). On the other hand, TGF-β acts with RANKL to direct osteoclasts towards a resorptive function (8). In epidemiological studies, polymorphisms of the TGF-β1 gene have been associated with susceptibility to osteoporosis, vertebral fracture and with outcome to vitamin D treatment for osteoporosis (69). More recent studies have found that TGF-β activates p38 MAPK in monocytes, but not in mature osteoclasts, suggesting a dual effect of TGF-beta on promoting osteoclastogenesis in monocytes through stimulation of the p38 MAPK and on abrogating osteoclastogenesis through down-regulation of RANK expression (70). These diverse effects might make TGF-β as a drug target difficult.

Prostaglandin E2 (PGE2) has been found to stimulate the formation of osteoclast-like multinucleated cells and bone resorption (71,72). PGE2 does this by down-regulating the expression of OPG mRNA, probably via an increase in cAMP (73). Cyclo-oxygenase-2 (COX-2), an inducible rate-limiting enzyme in PG biosynthesis regulates the production of PGE2, and plays an important role in the osteolysis of bone metastasis in vivo as well as in osteoclast formation in cocultures (74). Chonic administration of a selective COX-2 inhibitor blocks prostaglandin synthesis and significantly reduced tumor burden, osteoclastogenesis and bone destruction, suggesting a potential clinical utility in the management of bone cancer (75).

It is worth pointing out that osteoclasts grown *in vitro* do not behave identically to those *in vivo*. For instance, *in vitro* osteoclasts responded to IL-1 by forming actin rings, while this did not happen in ex vivo cells Feige (30). TNF-α, which has been observed to work directly to cause osteoclast formation *in vitro*, appears only to work through RANKL induction *in vivo* (8). At least two explanations exist: either the cells grown in culture do not represent the osteoclast phenotype accurately; or osteoclasts *in vivo* exist in heterogenous forms (8,76). Therefore, *in vitro* results never substitute the effects of cytokines *in vivo* and in clinical trials.

Intracellular Signalling Molecules

Upon binding of RANKL to RANK, a set of intracellular signalling pathways is triggered, resulting ultimately in maturation of the osteoclast precursor and activation of the osteoclast with resorptive capacity. The initial step following RANKL binding to RANK involves down stream interaction of the cytoplasmic portion of RANK to a family of zinc finger cytoplasmic adaptor molecules within the cell (15). Several versions of these adaptor molecules, called tumor necrosis factor receptor-associated factors (TRAFs), have been identified. RANK has potential binding sites for TRAF1, 2, 3, 5 and 6 (77,78). In any case, TRAF6 appears to have the largest role in the transduction of signals induced by RANKL binding. This is manifested in the development of osteoporosis in TRAF6 knockout mice (79). Mice completely lacking TRAF6 possessed similar phenotypes to mice lacking RANKL and RANK (79), indicating the critical role TRAF6 plays in the osteoclast. However, deletion of this TRAF6 binding region does not fully inhibit activation of another transcription factor, JNK (13,14), suggesting that other molecules may be able to partially compensate for the absence of TRAF6 during osteoclastogenesis. Following binding of RANKL to the RANK, several intracellular cascades are initiated, involving the activator protein-1 (AP-1) transcription factor complex, NF-κB, serine-threonine kinase Akt/PKB, NF-AT, and c-Src.

AP-1 Pathway

The AP-1 transcription factor complex, comprised of various combinations of Fos and Jun family members, is intimately involved in osteoclastogenesis via DNA binding and gene expression. Four separate Fos family members (c-Fos, FosB, Fra-1 and Fra-2) and two Jun members (c-Jun, JunB, JunD) have been described (52). Fos protein is a major component of the AP-1 transcription factor complex in the members of the jun family. Severe osteopetrotic phenotypes have been observed in mice lacking c-Fos (80,81). In fact, lack of c-Fos causes overproduction of macrophages and a deficiency in osteoclasts, implicating it as a factor essential in the differentiation of monocyte precursors into osteoclasts instead of macrophages. This is supported by the finding that c-Fos is absolutely required to activate the c-Jun N-terminal kinase (JNK) (54). Activation of JNK1, but not JNK2, is required for efficient osteoclastogenesis from bone marrow monocytes of mice lacking JNK1 or JNK2 (82).

NF-kB Pathway

The nuclear factor-kB (NF-kB) family is a key player in controlling osteoclast formation and activation (7). NF-kB proteins are present in the cytoplasm in association with inhibitory proteins that are known as inhibitors of NF-kB (IkBs). Upon activation, the IkB proteins become phosphorylated, ubiquitylated and, subsequently, degraded by the proteasome. NF-kB proteins are released from their binding to IkBs, translocate to the nucleus and bind their cognate DNA binding sites to regulate the transcription of a large number of down stream target genes (83,84). Over the past decade or so, intensive studies have provided many new insights into the singaling pathways linking ligand/receptor family with NF-kB activation. At the molecular level, the structure and components of NF-kB are highly complex. The core components of NF-kB have been well modelled and consist of five mammalian reticuloendotheliosis family (REL)/nuclear factor kB (NF-kB) proteins that belong to two groups (85,86). The first group consists of p65 (also known as RELA), c-REL and RELB that do not require proteolytic processing. The second group includes p105 (also known as NF-kB1) and p100 (also known as NF-kB2), which are processed to produce the mature p50 and p52 proteins, respectively. These two groups form dimers - the most commonly detected NF-kB dimer is p50-p65. p50 and p52 are essential for normal osteoclast development, as deletion of both results in osteopetrosis caused by arrested generation of osteoclasts (87,88). As its name would suggest, RANKL activates NF-kB, another transcription factor involved in the regulation of gene expression during osteoclastogenesis. In the cytoplasm, NF-kB is bound to IκBα and is comprised of dimers of subunits, most commonly the p50 and p65 subunits (26). RANK, via its interaction, with TRAF6, activates the Inhibitor of $\kappa\beta$ Kinase (IKK) complex, which is responsible for the serine phosphorylation and subsequent degradation of IκBα. This facilitates the release of NF-kB and the translocation of the NF-kB subunits into the nucleus where they act by binding to specific sites on DNA (26).

NF-kB acitivation is obligatory for osteoclast differentiation. Delinearization of the NF-kB signaling pathways will certainly facilitate the development of anti-resorptive agents. Recent studies have found that p62, a down stream target of TRAF6 is an important mediator for RANK-activated osteoclastogenesis (89). Interestingly, p62 or SQSTM1 has been associated with Peget's disease (90-92), suggesting that p62 could serve as a novel target for anti-resoptive therapy.

The author's laboratory has recently studied the effects of NF-kB inhibitors from natural compounds and found that inhibition of NF-kB reduced osteoclastogenesis and bone resorption *in vitro* and blocked lipopolysaccharide-induced osteolysis *in vivo* (93). In addition, We have found that protein kinase C (PKC) activity is also invloved in NF-kB pathway of osteoclasts (94), suggesting that selective modulation of PKC pathway may have important therapeutic implications for the treatment of bone diseases associated with enhanced bone resorption. There is the possibility that separate functions of NF-kB may be differentially blocked, raising hopes that agents could be developed to target osteoclast activating pathways while maintaining other NF-kB functions.

Protein Kinase B/Akt Pathway

RANKL binding to osteoclasts initiates another cascade involving the anti-apoptotic serine/threonine kinase PKB (also known as Akt) (95). TRAF6 enhances the kinase capacity of c-Src, which subsequently phosphorylates phosphatidylinositol-3 kinase (PI3K) , leading the recruitment of PKB/Akt (95,96). Inhibition of AKT, MEK1/2, and PI3K leads to rapid apoptosis of nearly all osteoclasts, thus the AKT pathway might represent a potential target for the apoptosis in osteoclasts (97,98).

NF-AT Pathway

Recent studies have found that the gene expression of nuclear factor of activated T cells (NF-AT) was upregulated during the early stage of osteoclastogenesis (99). Knock down expression of NF-AT inhibits osteoclastogenesis whereas overexpression of a constitutive form of NF-AT induces the formation of osteoclasts in vitro, indicating that NF-AT is an important signalling pathway of osteoclastogenesis (100). Furthermore, inhibition of calcineurin, an upstream molecule of NF-AT with either the immunosuppressant drugs cyclosporin A and FK506 potently inhibits the RANKL-induced differentiation of the RAW264.7 monocyte-macrophage cell line into mature multinucleated osteoclasts (100). Unravelling the NF-AT signalling pathway in osteoclastogenesis might help to design novel drugs for anti-resorptive treatment.

c-Src

c-Src provides another intervention point for therapeutics in bone lytic disorders. They belong to a family of non-receptor tyrosine kinases that are ubiquitously expressed throughout the body, having their highest levels of expression on platelets, neurons and osteoclasts. The recurrent theme in the activation of c-Src is G-protein coupled receptor-induced ras-dependent signalling, responsible for growth-factor and integrin-mediated signal transduction, and probably also in mitotic progression of cells (101). Studies have revealed a functional duality of c-Src in growth factor-mediated signal transformation and kinase-independent scaffolding (102).

In osteoclasts, c-Src expression is essential for the formation of ruffled borders, a requirement for bone resorption, identified through experiments with c-Src-deficient mice showing an osteopetrotic phenotype (103,104). Deficiency of this integrin-mediated signalling pathway was characterised by normal numbers of osteoclasts but with deficient bone resorption activity, correlating with failed ruffled border formation. Of further note was the ability of the osteopetrotic phenotype, resulting from c-Src deficiency mice, to be rescued through expression of a kinase-inactive mutant of c-Src, arguing that kinase-independent functions of c-Src are more important in osteoclasts (105).

In addition, c-Src is involved in the synthesis and secretion of collagenolytic cysteine proteases (106). Hence, the proposed mechanism of action of c-Src inhibitors are regulation of the last step of bone resorption by suppressing functions such as secretion of demineralising acid and secretion, but not synthesis, of collagenolytic cysteine proteases. As there is little effect on the differentiation process, other feasible mechanisms of action of these inhibitors involve regulation of ruffled border formation through polymerisation of actin, failure to form ruffled borders through pp60^{c-src} PI3-kinase signalling pathways and suppression of H$^+$ secretion into Howship's lacuna (106).

Inhibitors of c-Src, such as the antibiotic herbimycin A and CGP77675 which inhibits c-Src tyrosine kinase activity have been found to inhibit bone resorption (107,108). Other studies have found that inhibitors isoflavone, tyrphostin, and benzoquinonoid directly inhibit osteoclast membrane hydrochloric acid transport (109). Sharma et al (110) described a non-kinase inhibitor of c-Src action experimented on mouse calvariae – UCS15A. UCS15A prevents c-Src-specific tyrosine phosphorylation of numerous proteins in v-Src-transformed cells. This mechanism differs from conventional c-Src inhibitors as it does not inhibit the tyrosine kinase activity of c-Src but rather, disrupts the interaction of proteins associated with c-Src, thereby modulating downstream events in the signal transduction pathway. Results from experiments conducted by Sharma and colleagues also determined that UCS15A inhibits the bone resorption activity of osteoclast-like multinucleated cells both *in vitro* and in organ culture systems.

The major challenge confronting development of these drugs is the issue of specificity since the binding of inhibitors to kinase domains may be non-specific and potentially unacceptable in their side effect profile. More recently, selective c-Src inhibitors pyrrolopyrimidine derivatives were found to inhibit osteoclastogenesis and resorption pit formation (111). In addition, bone-targeted c-Src tyrosine kinase inhibitors have been developed for the treatment of osteoporosis and cancer-related bone diseases; AP-22408, a novel c-Src homology (SH)-2 inhibitor and AP-23236, a novel ATP-based c-Src kinase inhibitor might represent next-generation of bone-targeted inhibitors (112). One would expect that upon advancement of current preclinical c-Src inhibitors through clinical trials, more information regarding their efficacy and side effect profile will be made available allowing an informed consensus to be formed.

In summary, intractably intertwined with the action of cytokines are intracellular signalling molecules such as transcription factors, kinases and adaptor molecules. These various molecules are responsible for the ultimate manifestation of the extracellular movements and binding of cytokines throughout the body. In general, the major problem with intracellular signalling molecules as targets for therapeutics is that they are largely ubiquitous. Thus, disruption of these pathways in cells resident in bone will have effects in other tissues. The challenge is to find the intracellular signallers that are the most specific for bone and to develop agents related to these signallers that generate the least side effects. However, exciting information exists in the finding that although downstream intracellular signalling molecules such as transcription factors c-Src, c-Fos and NF-κB are present and important in many cell types, they seem to be essential in the osteoclast (8). This is very significant because targeting of these signalling molecules to inhibit bone resorption may result in drugs with minimal side effects.

Cell Fusion Molecules

One of the most striking features of osteoclastogenesis involves the cell fusion. Although membrane fusion is a ubiquitous event that occurs in a wide range of biological processes, no other cell types have dramatic cell fusion and multinucleation as osteoclasts. This observation indicates that specific molecules are expressed to regulate these events. Using monoclonal antibodies that had the ability to block the fusion of macrophages in vitro, surface proteins of 150 kDa that regulate the fusion of macrophages in vitro were identified (113). Subsequently, macrophage fusion receptor, also called P84/SHPS-1/SIRPalpha/BIT was identified that interacts with CD47 during adhesion/fusion of macrophage (114). Further characterization of specific ligand or receptors that specifically regulate osteoclast fusion might represent a potential target for drug development.

Integrins

The alpha v beta 3 ($\alpha_v\beta_3$, vitronectin receptor) is a member of the integrin superfamily of adhesion molecules. This non-covalent multi-domain protein demonstrates its highest expression in osteoclasts. Mediation of cell adhesion to the extracellular matrix is performed through recognition by $\alpha_v\beta_3$ of the arg-gly-asp (RGD) amino acid sequence on plasma and matrix proteins – a characteristic of the α_v family of integrins. Binding to the $\alpha_v\beta_3$ integrin activates multiple signal transduction pathways involving elevation of intracellular calcium, lipid turnover and tyrosine phosphorylation (115). The activation of these intracellular pathways results in de novo gene expression and cytoskeletal rearrangement implicating it in several physiological activities that include osteoclastic adhesion to bone matrix, smooth muscle cell migration and angiogenesis (116).

$\alpha_v\beta_3$ has been identified as the dominant integrin of mature osteoclasts, both quantitatively and functionally. Extensive research into integrins and their expression on osteoclasts revealed that osteoclasts express different factors during different stages of maturation (117-119). Differentiation from osteoclastic precursors involves the replacement of the immature osteoclast marker - $\alpha_v\beta_5$ - with the mature osteoclast marker - $\alpha_v\beta_3$ - providing a means by which maturity of the osteoclast can be measured. Both $\alpha_v\beta_3$ and $\alpha_v\beta_5$ are not solely influenced by differentiation, as other signalling molecules, such as cytokines, also affect their expression. For example, GM-CSF accelerates the replacement process through enhanced β_5 mRNA degradation and induction of β_3 expression by transcriptional stimulation (117,118). Similarly, IL-4, TNF-α and 1,25-dihydroxyvitamin D also variously impact expression of $\alpha_v\beta_3$ and $\alpha_v\beta_5$ (120,121).

The essentiality of the cytoplasmic domain of the β_3 chain for the capacity to generate the complete osteoclast phenotype has been demonstrated by several studies. Osteoclasts of β_3 nude mice fail to form a ruffled membrane and moreover, and results in suboptimal capacity to resorb bone (118). This was further supported by the identification of increased numbers of osteoclasts around the bone surface with a poor capacity to spread and shallow and poorly-defined resorption pits. Additionally, deletion of the β_3 chain was shown to result in abnormal cytoskeletons in which fibular actin, within the actin ring, was diffusely distributed throughout the cytoplasm preventing effective formation of a normal ruffled membrane. Consequently, β_3 null mice were significantly hypocalcaemic compared to their heterozygous littermates.

Though $\alpha_v\beta_3$ has been shown to be highly osteoclast-specific, its interaction with a wide variety of proteins proves to be a drawback for inhibition. Upon its discovery, the name vitronectin was allocated to this integrin, as it was thought to uniquely bind to vitronectin (122), however, this has proven to be a misnomer since the $\alpha_v\beta_3$ integrin binds a number of proteins in addition to vitronectin (123).

Inhibitors of the $\alpha_v\beta_3$ integrin have been primarily focussed on mimicking the RGD sequence. Since RGD-binding mediates cell-matrix adhesion, inhibition of this process prevents formation of acidic resorption lacuna. Like many other forms of osteoporosis therapy, discovery of therapeutic agents have stemmed largely from incidental findings. Early work with antibodies raised against $\alpha_v\beta_3$ and RGD-containing peptides provided a foundation for the design and synthesis of specific and non-peptide $\alpha_v\beta_3$ antagonists (123). Echistatin, a potent inhibitor of rat osteoclast-mediated bone resorption *in vitro* and PTH-dependent rise in serum calcium *in vivo* (123), represents one of this class of non-selective inhibitors. The ability to bind to several ligands and receptors respectively provided one of the most interesting challenges in the area of design of selective antagonists since both $\alpha_v\beta_3$ and $\alpha_{IIb}\beta_3$ bind to the same RGD recognition motif (124). Subsequently, modifications to incorporate the subtle differences in ligand structure were undertaken in order to generate a more selective antagonist (124).

Similar techniques were employed by Lark and his colleagues in their design and characterisation of an orally-active integrin antagonist. Their study delivered the first orally active antagonist effective at inhibition of resorption when dosed in a pharmaceutically acceptable fashion (125). SB 265123, a non-peptide RGD-mimetic $\alpha_v\beta_3$ antagonist, was developed to maintain a high affinity for $\alpha_v\beta_3$, but to bind weakly to the related RGD-binding integrin $\alpha_{IIb}\beta_3$, resulting in minimal inhibition of human platelet aggregation. Previous agents required significantly greater amounts to undergo continuous IV infusion for delivery and proved to be an unrealistic mode of treatment for postmenopausal osteoporosis.

Other techniques of reducing multiple interactions between the $\alpha_v\beta_3$ receptor and its substrates involved structural analysis and redesign of the antagonists. Benzodiazepine-based analogues were the result of structural analysis which determined that the shortened distance between the basic benzimidazole nitrogen and the carboxylic acid groups was an important determinant for the selectivity of $\alpha_v\beta_3$ over $\alpha_{IIb}\beta_3$ (123). Similarly, centrally constrained α-phenylsulphonamide antagonists were developed from modification of high affinity ligands for the $\alpha_{IIb}\beta_3$ receptor in an attempt to identify potent ligands for $\alpha_v\beta_3$ (123).

Progression of selective agents have come a long way from their infancy only a few years ago in which *in vitro* inhibitors were minimally selective for $\alpha_v\beta_3$ to their current standing as highly-potent, selective and orally-active molecules. Despite some success in the development of $\alpha_v\beta_3$ antagonists using RGD-mimetics, there are other various means by which to inhibit the function of the integrin. The strategies for therapeutic modification of integrin function involved theoretical investigation into means of inhibition, characterised into direct approach such as the use of naturally-occurring protein inhibitors and their engineered derivatives, or indirect approaches such as altered receptor synthesis via use of antisense oligonucleotides and modification of integrin receptor function via adhesion molecule (integrin)-associated proteins (126).

Many of the outlined approaches are yet to be tackled despite antagonists of integrins being the furthest developed of any of the novel anti-resorptive agents (127-130). However, application of $\alpha_v\beta_3$ inhibitors in other clinical areas may persuade swing researchers into investing more interest into their development. Upregulation of the $\alpha_v\beta_3$ in clinical areas such as angiogenesis, melanoma and coronary artery stenosis, begs the question as to whether development of a drug, highly specific for $\alpha_v\beta_3$, could possibly have use in other associated diseases. Inhibitors, in addition to bone resorption, could be used to block coronary artery restenosis, inhibit neovascularisation in eye diseases, induce tumour death by depleting blood supply or inducing apoptosis and furthermore, target melanoma tumour or inhibit metastases (116). Possibilities surrounding these questions are nothing short of exciting for therapeutic prospects, however, history has shown that ancillary pharmacology toward other disease areas could detract from their utility in the prevention and treatment of the primary target disease (126). Ultimately, it will depend on long-term human clinical trials to determine optimal dosing schedules which counter balance the desired effects and side-effects of the drug.

Enzymes

V-H⁺-ATPase

Proton extrusion plays an important role in all eukaryotic cells for membrane trafficking, protein sorting and protein degradation (131). In bone, acidification is absolutely required for the degradation of both inorganic and organic components of bone (132). This is accomplished by a high concentration of vacuolar-type proton pumps (V-H⁺-ATPase) on the apical pole of the cell (ruffled border) (133). The pump is a multi-subunit enzyme, with an osteoclast-specific subunit (OC-116 kDa) encoded by the gene Atp6i (134,135). Proton pumping couples ATP hydrolysis to proton translocation through a rotary mechanism, where a proton gradient is utilised to synthesise ATP (136,137). The electrical potential difference created across the membrane is used to drive the movement of ions and solutes into the vacuole (133). This forms the foundation for maintenance of the acidic environment of the resorption lacuna, allowing for demineralisation and subsequent degradation of the bone matrix by cathepsin K (138). Whilst V-H$^+$-ATPase lowers the pH of the lacunae to between 4 and 5, cytosolic pH levels are regulated by Na$^+$/H$^+$ and Cl$^-$/HCO$_3^-$ exchangers (139,140).

This essential role of V-H$^+$-ATPase in bone resorption provides a basis for pharmacological intervention in the treatment of osteolytic disorders. Antisense RNA and DNA molecules targeted against 2 subunits of the V-H$^+$-ATPase inhibit bone resorption by rat osteoclasts proving that this enzyme is a major potential target for reducing osteoclast activity (141). Attempts at generating an inhibitor for V-H$^+$-ATPase has proven to be a difficult task since lack of inhibitor specificity could result in considerable toxicity and limit the safety of the compounds (142). This stems from the fact that V-H$^+$-ATPase is a ubiquitous component of eukaryotic organisms and is the major electrogenic pump of endomembranes (143).

Initial steps in developing an inhibitor for V-H$^+$-ATPase involved the structural analysis of bafilomycin A1. This compound is a macrolide antibiotic which potently inhibits all V-H$^+$-ATPases *in vitro* and *in vivo*. However, bafilomycin was not selective enough for any particular type of V-H$^+$-ATPase, leading to unacceptable systemic toxicity (133). Hence, for treatment of excess bone resorption, it is necessary to modify the structure of bafilomycin to confer high selectivity for the osteoclast enzyme compared with other essential V-H$^+$-ATPases, such as those found in the kidney.

5-(5,6-Dichloro-2-indolyl)-2-methoxy-2,4-pentadienamides or SB 242784 was discovered by Gagliardi et al in 1998 (144). It is a low nanomolar inhibitor of the bafilomycin-sensitive (vacuolar) Mg-ATPase in membrane preparations of osteoclasts obtained from egg-laying hens. It has been shown to be a very potent inhibitor of bone resorption in human osteoclasts *in vitro* and also completely prevents retinoid-induced hypercalcaemia in thyroparathyroidectomised rats (133). SB 242784 was at least as effective in preventing bone loss as an optimal dose of estrogen (133). In addition, SB 242784 had a greater than 1000-fold selectivity for the osteoclast V-H$^+$-ATPase compared with the enzyme measured in the kidney, liver, spleen, stomach, brain or endothelial cells and has no effect on other cellular ATPases (133). Evaluation of SB 242784 toxicity in ovariectomised rats during a 6-month treatment program resulted in no overt toxic effects being recorded (133). At fully active therapeutic doses, SB 242784 has no effect on urinary acid excretion. Since V-H$^+$-ATPase located on the plasma membrane in kidneys participates in urinary acidification, this finding confirms the selectivity *in vivo*.

The efficacy of this compound has been shown to be exceptional via measurements of BMD, biochemical markers of bone resorption and histomorphometry (133). This can be attributed to its extreme selectivity. However, the molecular mechanism of action of SB 242784 selectivity is still poorly understood. OC-116 kDa or Atp6i null mice had severe osteopetrosis but had normal acid-base balance in blood and urine and functional intracellular acidification (134,135). This illustrated that OC-116kDa null mutations are unlikely to affect V-H$^+$-ATPase of lysosomes, endosomes and kidney tubule cells and that OC-116 kDa is structurally and functionally different from the corresponding subunits in other V-H$^+$-ATPases. This observation of the existence of a specific osteoclast 116-kDa subunit was subsequently confirmed via in situ hybridisation and sequence analysis (145). Further more, recent studies have found that mutations in the Atp6i gene, which mediates the acidification of the bone/osteoclast interface, are responsible for a subset of human malignant infantile osteopetrosis, a genetically heterogeneous autosomal recessive disorder of bone metabolism (146), indicating that subunits of V-ATPase play a specific role in osteoclast function.

It is clear that the emergence of V-H$^+$-ATPase inhibitors is exciting news for patients and prescribers alike. Although more study into its efficacy compared with other current treatments, such as bisphosphonates, is still required, it certainly seems as though this option provides another plausible avenue by which to target enhanced bone resorption. Now that the macrolide model has been revamped for SB

242784, it gives an opportunity to further research the long-term effects of highly specific, orally available $V\text{-}H^+\text{-}ATPase$ inhibitors.

The electrogenic proton pump of the osteoclast ruffled membrane is coupled to a passive chloride channel (147). More interestingly, mice deficient for the ubiquitously expressed ClC-7 Cl(-) channel has been shown to have severe osteopetrosis and retinal degeneration. Furthermore, CLCN7 mutations have been identified in a patient with human infantile malignant osteopetrosis, indicating that the chloride conductance is required for an efficient proton pumping by the $V\text{-}H^+\text{-}ATPase$ of the osteoclast ruffled membrane (148). It remains to be seen whether chloride channel serves as a potential drug target for anti-resorptive agents.

Cysteine Protease and Cathepsin K

Cathepsins are a major group of intracellular acidic cysteine protease responsible for physiological intracellular protein and bone degradation. Pioneer studies by Gelb et al (149) have found that patients with cathepsin K mutations developed pycnodysostosis, an autosomal recessive osteochondrodysplasia characterized by osteosclerosis and short stature (149). This was further confirmed by the studies showing that knockout of cathepsin K results in osteoporosis and pycnodysostosis (150). Several other human mutations have subsequently been found in families of pycnodysostosis (151-153), and this has made cathepsin K an attractive target for therapeutic intervention to combat osteoporosis.

Cathepsin K, known also as cathepsin O, X and O2, belongs to the papain superfamily of lysosomal cysteine protease which includes cathepsins B, L, H and S. Studies involving immunocytochemistry and immunoblotting have identified cathepsin K as being almost exclusively expressed by osteoclasts. Cathepsin K has a unique, high degree of proteolytic activity against several extracellular matrix substrates and unique collagenolytic activity against type I collagen – the most abundant matrix protein in bone, comprising 90% of bone matrix. Its crucial role in bone resorption is demonstrated via studies showing that antisense DNA specific for cathepsin K results in decreased resorptive activity (154,155), In addition, specific aldehyde inhibitors of cathepsin

K inhibit bone resorption *in vivo* and *in vitro* and deletion of the cathepsin K gene in mice leads to an osteosclerotic phenotype (156).

It is important to note that cathepsin K knockout mice develop osteopetrosis due to a deficit in matrix degradation but not demineralisation. This is because demineralisation of the bone proceeds normally via a functional osteoclast vacuolar V-H^+-ATPase activity. In cathepsin K null mice, failure of osteoclasts to resorb and endocytose the bone matrix, a histologic observation described previously in pycnodysostotic bone. This finding is consistent with the expected role of cathepsin K in degrading the organic phase of the matrix during the resorptive process (150). In addition to its role in osteoclasts, cathepsin K was also expressed in the intimal smooth muscle cells, especially in cells traversing the internal elastic lamina (157). This has implications for vessel wall remodelling with inhibitors of cathepsin K potentially able to stabilise atherosclerotic plaque, providing promising therapeutic benefit in the treatment or prevention of cardiovascular disease. This same study also postulated the possible involvement of cathepsin K in cartilage breakdown in diseases such as osteoarthritis and rheumatoid arthritis.

Cysteine proteases are synthesised as latent precursors and can be either secreted as proenzymes or transported to acidic lysosomal compartments via mannose-6-phosphate (M6P) receptors where activation occurs. Rieman et al (158) studied the biosynthesis and processing of cathepsin K in cultured human osteoclasts and discovered that it is synthesised as a proenzyme undergoing post-translational modification in a time-dependent manner. Pro-cathepsin K is then subsequently transported to acidic lysosomal compartments where the pro-peptide is cleaved and the enzyme is activated. Mature, catalytically active cathepsin K is either directionally secreted into the resorption lacunae or undergoes proteolytic degradation within the lysosome (158). Although *in vitro* studies described here demonstrate that through activation of cathepsin K is constitutive, processing *in vivo* has recently shown that cathepsin K appears to be a highly regulated process.

Cysteine protease inhibitors cause the absence of concomitant proteolytic breakdown of bone matrix, the limited dissolution of bone mineral. Selective inhibitors for cathepsins have been developed over a number of years but their incorporation into standard treatment for bone-lytic disorders has been limited. Three distinct possibilities for inhibition of cathepsin K action have been reported (158):

1. Wortmannin (WT), an inhibitor of PI3-kinase (involved in growth factor signal transduction and vesicular membrane trafficking), inhibited cathepsin K processing dose-dependently. Furthermore, its role in delivering the proenzyme to lysosomal vesicles for enzymatic activation was also targeted through induction of the mis-targeting of acid hydrolases to the vesicles.

2. M6P prevents the reuptake and delivery of secreted proenzyme to the lysosomes for activation via M6P receptors. This is attributed primarily to its enhancement of WT action when used as an adjunct.

3. Since activity of cathepsin K is optimal at pH 5.5, alkalinisation of the acidic intracellular compartments resulted in complete inhibition of cathepsin K processing – confirming that activation occurs within lysosomes.

More often than not, cysteine protease inhibitors contain an inherently reactive functional group that might derivatise the side chain or backbone elements of the protein leading to undesired antigenic responses. In order to minimise potential immunological complications in drugs given chronically, design of these protease inhibitors has been to avoid the presence such intrinsically reactive groups (159). The successful design of selective, reversible inhibitors for cathepsin K based on the poorly electrophilic 1,3-bid(acylamino)-2-propanone scaffold has been underway (159). The advantage to using this model as a skeleton for design of other antagonists is through the opportunity to explore potential substrate-like binding interactions on both the primed and unprimed sides of the active site (159). In addition, a potent, nonpeptide inhibitor of rat cathepsin K, SB 331750 was identified to be efficacious in preventing bone matrix resorption in the ovariectomized rat (160). More recently, a novel series of nonpeptidic biaryl compounds has been identified as potent and reversible inhibitors of cathepsin K which exhibit an improved selectivity profile against other cathepsins (161). Other potent and selective inhibitors of cathepsin K have also been shown to attenuate PTH-stimulated hypercalcemia in the rat model (162).

In summary, cathepsin K has proven to be an ideal target through its almost exclusive expression in osteoclasts and its vital role in bone degradation. In addition, it provides several points where intervention can possibly occur (ie. during enzyme activation, inhibition of secretion). Whilst much is known about the effects of cathepsin K and hence, the therapeutic benefits of its inhibition, the ultimate assessment of its feasibility in osteoporosis treatment lies in further *in vivo* trials. Gowen et al. (142) provided one of the more recently available lists of cathepsin K (and B, L and S) inhibitors described in published literature demonstrating that the majority of cathepsin inhibitors are in the preclinical development phase. Like all other potential novel inhibitors of bone resorption, the development of potent and selective cathepsin inhibitors pends on the emergence of agents with less adverse side-effects and better pharmacodynamic properties.

Matrix Metalloproteinases

Matrix metalloproteinases (MMP) are a family of proteolytic enzymes, capable of degrading most major components of the extracellular matrix. Their participation in young bone development, arthritic conditions and pathological bone conditions has fuelled interest into its role in bone resorption with particular emphasis currently being placed on the function of MMP-9/gelatinase B.

Tezuka et al (163) identified MMP-9 to be one of the major proteases constitutively produced by osteoclasts under physiological conditions. Northern blotting showed mRNA for MMP-9 to be highly and predominantly expressed in isolated osteoclasts when compared with levels in other tissues (163). Further in situ hybridisation studies also detected significant expression of MMP-9 in in vivo osteoclasts. Though MMP-9 has been shown to be the protagonist in expanding the primitive marrow cavity of long bones, shortcomings in its function in bone resorption have been repeatedly identified. That is, the degradative role of MMP-9 on various components of the extracellular matrix (eg. collagen IV, collagen V, proteoglycans, elastin, gelatin) was not extended to type I collagen (163), implying a permissive function in facilitating osteoclast invasion. Engsig (164) found MMP-9 to be specifically required for the invasion of osteoclasts into the discontinuously mineralised hypertrophic cartilage that fills the core of the diaphysis but other MMPs were required for the passage of the cells through unmineralised type I collagen of the nascent bone collar. Histological studies in null mice also support this finding through demonstration of MMP-9 as a key proteinase for the migration of immature osteoclasts to the bone surface through basement membranes (165), but do not support its role in the actual solubilisation of mineralised matrix in osteoclasts (166). Lack of MMP-9 or its activity also leads to an accumulation of TRAP positive cells around the osteoid-cartilage interface. This demonstrates the requirement of both MMPs and cysteine proteases for the complete degradation of bone matrix during resorption.

In vitro and *in vivo* studies suggest that the degradation of bone collagen by osteoclasts is mainly carried out in concert (167) by two types of proteases – MMPs and cysteine proteases (especially MMP-9 and cathepsin K) – each with their own distinct roles (168). The cooperative action of cysteine proteases and MMPs is based on the fact that bone type I collagen may be solubilized by lysosomal cysteine proteinases and subsequently degraded by MMP-9 into small peptides by its gelatinase activity (169,170). This implicates MMP-9 in two distinct roles – recruitment of osteoclasts to developing bones and synergy with cysteine proteinases in solubilizing calcified matrix within the resorption zone (164).

Interestingly, the study conducted by Everts et al. (171), on rat and rabbit osteoclasts, determined that significant differences exist between osteoclasts of calvariae and long bones with respect to their bone resorbing activities. This brought up the question of whether functionally and phenotypically different subpopulations of osteoclasts originate from different sets of progenitors. Their results found that osteoclastic resorption of calvarial bone depended on the activity of cysteine proteases and MMPs, whereas long bone resorption relied on cysteine proteases, but not on MMP activity. This corresponded with the fact that though the functional qualities of the osteoclasts are similar, the mineralised matrices that they resorb are markedly different. Consequently, it was concluded that osteoclasts use different enzyme systems depending on the site of the skeleton.

The possibility of MMP inhibitors for the treatment of bone lytic disorders has been aired and like all other possible osteoclast targets, specifications restrict their employment. Degradation of the skeletal connective tissue is regulated, at least in part, by the balance between MMPs and tissue inhibitor of metalloproteinases (TIMPs) . These natural inhibitors provide the neutralising effect for the maintenance of bone structure, organization and integrity. It has been demonstrated that more poorly organised bone formation was present in even low levels of TIMP, and in particular its absence in osteoclasts, in pathological bone samples (172). Similar findings in other studies that the control of MMP activity by TIMP in developing human bone provided sufficient evidence to warrant attempts to mimic the effects of TIMP function through synthetic inhibitors.

It is evident that the MMP-9 is vital in the migration of osteoclasts to the resorptive surface. Theoretically, the inhibition of MMP-9 could result in arrested progress of the bone resorption process, however, in light of the findings by Everts et al (171), it could be assumed that this would only be effective for certain locations of accelerated bone resorption (ie. intramembranous bone). If this discovery holds true for human osteoclasts, bifunctional inhibitors and/or combination treatments of inhibitors against MMPs and cysteine proteases might provide the preferred therapeutic strategy for the treatment of osteoporosis (168).

Conclusion

Bone lytic disorders are a modern health epidemic amongst both Western and Eastern society. They have been proven to be of economic, emotional and physical burden to back pockets, minds and hips of society. Whilst the majority of current modes of therapy aim to prevent, or at least reduce, bone resorption, toxicity profile and dosing regimen make them less than ideal. Fortunately, osteoclasts provide a multitude of potential targets for novel anti-resorptive agents intracellularly and within the microenvironment in which they operate. Current concepts for the treatment for osteoporosis suggest that the development of new agents for resorption inhibition will be the best for the short to medium term treatment, while developing anabolic drugs or cell therapeutics is needed for the long-term therapeutic gaol.

Through investigation of osteoclast biology and pathogenesis, a number of targets were identified with the potential for reducing the accelerated rate of bone resorption seen in many bone lytic disorders (Fig. 1, Table 1). These targets provide steps throughout the life cycle and activity of the osteoclast that can be manipulated for therapeutic intervention. However, whilst current technology has enabled researchers to identify these compounds, their often ubiquitous expression in a variety of physiological systems proves to be the major challenge in designing selective modulators in bone.

Several targets emerge as the most promise for design of pharmacological agents. The RANKL/RANK/OPG axis, involved in the differentiation and maturation of osteoclasts, and cathepsin K, the protagonist in bone matrix degradation, share a number of properties that make them appropriate for further scrutiny. Their specificity and high expression on osteoclasts are essential in determining their suitability since side-effect profiles depend highly on these factors. Both agents fulfil the criteria for further investigation into their possible integration into current anti-resorptive regimens, pending progression through the rigorous process of clinical trials. In addition, bone-targeted c-Src tyrosine kinase inhibitors also show promising and are in the stage of preclinical studies.

One problem when analysing the ability of compounds to inhibit bone loss *in vivo* is that many experiments are conducted in the artificial environment of a cell culture. This is often an unavoidable problem when drug molecules are in the initial stages of testing, but results are often difficult to extrapolate to the body system. Thus, the significance of results of *in vitro* experiments to animals or humans is not always clear, especially in light of evidence that shows that osteoclasts grown *in vitro* do not behave identically to those *in vivo*. Nevertheless, although *in vitro* results are helpful, they can never substitute for proper *in vivo* and clinical trials.

Whilst it is feasible for development of these agents to be the new 'breakthrough' drugs for diseases of accelerated bone resorption, combination therapy should not be discounted. Many other conditions, such as peptic ulcer disease and HIV, subscribe to poly-drug regimens in their quest to maximise their intended effects. The advantage to this mode of treatment lies in the multi-faceted approach which minimises tolerance and utilises synergistic modes of action. By employing this philosophy to osteoporosis treatment, room may be left for the use of other aforementioned targets, despite their potential downfalls in specificity.

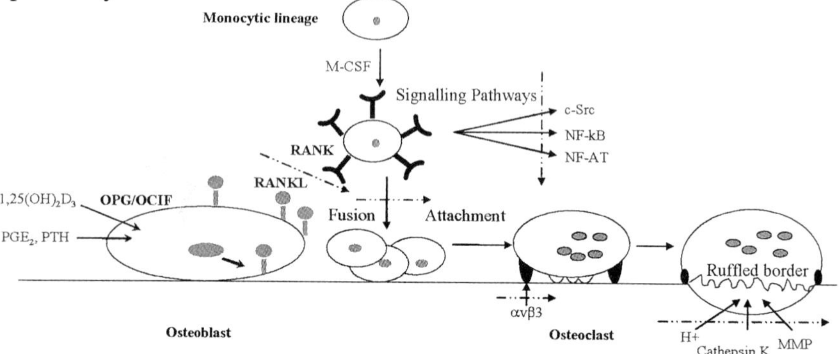

Fig. 1. An illustration of the biology of osteoclast differentiation, signalling transduction pathways, and bone resorption. Novel potential drug targets for the development of anti-resorptive agents are highlighted by arrow heads with broken lines. Among these are RANKL/RANK/OPG, c-Src, NF-kB, NF-AT, cell fusion molecules, $\alpha_v\beta_3$, V-H$^+$-ATPases, cathepsin K, and MMP.

Table 1: Novel potential targets and agents for the anti-resorptive treatment of osteoporosis

Potential Targets	Agents	Potential mechanisms of action
RANKL/RANK	Monoclonal Antibodies	Neutralizing the effect of RANKL
	OPG	Blocking the effect of RANKL
c-Scr	Herbimycin A	Inhibiting c-Src tyrosine kinase activity
	CGP77675	Inhibiting c-Src tyrosine kinase activity
	UCS15A	Disrupting the interaction of proteins associated with c-Src
	AP-22408	A novel c-Src homology (SH)-2 inhibitor
	AP-23236	A novel ATP-based c-Src kinase inhibitor
NF-kB	NF-kB inhibitors	Inhibition of NF-kB subunits and pathways
	Parthenolide	Inhibition of NF-kB activity
NF-AT	Cyclosporin A	Inhibition of calcineurin, an upsream molecule of NF-AT
	FK506	Inhibition of calcineurin, an upsream molecule of NF-AT
Cell fusion molecules	Monoclonal Antibodies	Blocking cell fusion
αvβ3	Echistatin	A potent inhibitor of bone resorption
	SB 265123	A non-peptide RGD-mimetic avb3 antagonist
V-H-ATPases	Bafilomycin	Binding and inbibitng V-ATPase
	SB 242784	Selective inhibition to osteoclast V-ATPase
Cathepsin K	Protease inhibitors	Inhibitions of proteases
	SB 331750	Preventing bone matrix resorption
	Nonpeptidic biaryl compounds	Reversible and selective inhibitors of cathepsin K
MMP	MMP inhibitors	Dimishing the effect of MMPs

REFERENCES

1. Iacovino JR 2001 Mortality outcomes after osteoporotic fractures in men and women. J Insur Med 33(4):316-20.
2. Rang HP 1999 Pharmacology / H.P. Rang, M.M. Dale, J.M. Ritter ; illustrations by Peter Lamb, 4th ed ed. Churchill Livingstone,, Edinburgh ; New York :.
3. Chipchase LS, McCaul K, Hearn TC 2000 Hip fracture rates in South Australia: into the next century. Aust N Z J Surg 70(2):117-9.
4. Coccia PF, Krivit W, Cervenka J, Clawson C, Kersey JH, Kim TH, Nesbit ME, Ramsay NK, Warkentin PI, Teitelbaum SL, Kahn AJ, Brown DM 1980 Successful bone-marrow transplantation for infantile malignant osteopetrosis. N Engl J Med 302(13):701-8.
5. Quinn JM, Neale S, Fujikawa Y, McGee JO, Athanasou NA 1998 Human osteoclast formation from blood monocytes, peritoneal macrophages, and bone marrow cells. Calcif Tissue Int 62(6):527-31.
6. Matsuzaki K, Udagawa N, Takahashi N, Yamaguchi K, Yasuda H, Shima N, Morinaga T, Toyama Y, Yabe Y, Higashio K, Suda T 1998 Osteoclast differentiation factor (ODF) induces osteoclast-like cell formation in human peripheral blood mononuclear cell cultures. Biochem Biophys Res Commun 246(1):199-204.
7. Teitelbaum SL 2000 Bone resorption by osteoclasts. Science 289(5484):1504-8.
8. Chambers TJ 2000 Regulation of the differentiation and function of osteoclasts. J Pathol 192(1):4-13.
9. Lacey DL, Timms E, Tan HL, Kelley MJ, Dunstan CR, Burgess T, Elliott R, Colombero A, Elliott G, Scully S, Hsu H, Sullivan J, Hawkins N, Davy E, Capparelli C, Eli A, Qian YX, Kaufman S, Sarosi I, Shalhoub V, Senaldi G, Guo J, Delaney J, Boyle WJ 1998 Osteoprotegerin ligand is a cytokine that regulates osteoclast differentiation and activation. Cell 93(2):165-76.
10. Yasuda H, Shima N, Nakagawa N, Yamaguchi K, Kinosaki M, Mochizuki S, Tomoyasu A, Yano K, Goto M, Murakami A, Tsuda E, Morinaga T, Higashio K, Udagawa N, Takahashi N, Suda T 1998 Osteoclast differentiation factor is a ligand for osteoprotegerin/osteoclastogenesis-inhibitory factor and is identical to TRANCE/RANKL. Proc Natl Acad Sci U S A 95(7):3597-602.
11. Burgess TL, Qian Y, Kaufman S, Ring BD, Van G, Capparelli C, Kelley M, Hsu H, Boyle WJ, Dunstan CR, Hu S, Lacey DL 1999 The ligand for osteoprotegerin (OPGL) directly activates mature osteoclasts. J Cell Biol 145(3):527-38.
12. Xu J, Tan JW, Huang L, Gao XH, Laird R, Liu D, Wysocki S, Zheng MH 2000 Cloning, sequencing, and functional characterization of the rat homologue of receptor activator of NF-kappaB ligand. J Bone Miner Res 15(11):2178-86.

13.   Suda T, Takahashi N, Udagawa N, Jimi E, Gillespie MT, Martin TJ 1999
      Modulation of osteoclast differentiation and function by the new members of
      the tumor necrosis factor receptor and ligand families. Endocr Rev 20(3):345-
      57.
14.   Theill LE, Boyle WJ, Penninger JM 2002 RANK-L and RANK: T cells, bone
      loss, and mammalian evolution. Annu Rev Immunol 20:795-823.
15.   Horowitz MC, Xi Y, Wilson K, Kacena MA 2001 Control of
      osteoclastogenesis and bone resorption by members of the TNF family of
      receptors and ligands. Cytokine Growth Factor Rev 12(1):9-18.
16.   Kong YY, Yoshida H, Sarosi I, Tan HL, Timms E, Capparelli C, Morony S,
      Oliveira-dos-Santos AJ, Van G, Itie A, Khoo W, Wakeham A, Dunstan CR,
      Lacey DL, Mak TW, Boyle WJ, Penninger JM 1999 OPGL is a key regulator
      of osteoclastogenesis, lymphocyte development and lymph-node
      organogenesis. Nature 397(6717):315-23.
17.   Hughes AE, Ralston SH, Marken J, Bell C, MacPherson H, Wallace RG, van
      Hul W, Whyte MP, Nakatsuka K, Hovy L, Anderson DM 2000 Mutations in
      TNFRSF11A, affecting the signal peptide of RANK, cause familial expansile
      osteolysis. Nat Genet 24(1):45-8.
18.   Dougall WC, Glaccum M, Charrier K, Rohrbach K, Brasel K, De Smedt T,
      Daro E, Smith J, Tometsko ME, Maliszewski CR, Armstrong A, Shen V, Bain
      S, Cosman D, Anderson D, Morrissey PJ, Peschon JJ, Schuh J 1999 RANK is
      essential for osteoclast and lymph node development. Genes Dev 13(18):2412-
      24.
19.   Li J, Sarosi I, Yan XQ, Morony S, Capparelli C, Tan HL, McCabe S, Elliott R,
      Scully S, Van G, Kaufman S, Juan SC, Sun Y, Tarpley J, Martin L, Christensen
      K, McCabe J, Kostenuik P, Hsu H, Fletcher F, Dunstan CR, Lacey DL, Boyle
      WJ 2000 RANK is the intrinsic hematopoietic cell surface receptor that
      controls osteoclastogenesis and regulation of bone mass and calcium
      metabolism. Proc Natl Acad Sci U S A 97(4):1566-71.
20.   Simonet WS, Lacey DL, Dunstan CR, Kelley M, Chang MS, Luthy R, Nguyen
      HQ, Wooden S, Bennett L, Boone T, Shimamoto G, DeRose M, Elliott R,
      Colombero A, Tan HL, Trail G, Sullivan J, Davy E, Bucay N, Renshaw-Gegg
      L, Hughes TM, Hill D, Pattison W, Campbell P, Boyle WJ, et al. 1997
      Osteoprotegerin: a novel secreted protein involved in the regulation of bone
      density. Cell 89(2):309-19.
21.   Yasuda H, Shima N, Nakagawa N, Mochizuki SI, Yano K, Fujise N, Sato Y,
      Goto M, Yamaguchi K, Kuriyama M, Kanno T, Murakami A, Tsuda E,
      Morinaga T, Higashio K 1998 Identity of osteoclastogenesis inhibitory factor
      (OCIF) and osteoprotegerin (OPG): a mechanism by which OPG/OCIF inhibits
      osteoclastogenesis in vitro. Endocrinology 139(3):1329-37.
22.   Bucay N, Sarosi I, Dunstan CR, Morony S, Tarpley J, Capparelli C, Scully S,
      Tan HL, Xu W, Lacey DL, Boyle WJ, Simonet WS 1998 osteoprotegerin-
      deficient mice develop early onset osteoporosis and arterial calcification. Genes
      Dev 12(9):1260-8.
23.   Cundy T, Hegde M, Naot D, Chong B, King A, Wallace R, Mulley J, Love DR,
      Seidel J, Fawkner M, Banovic T, Callon KE, Grey AB, Reid IR, Middleton-
      Hardie CA, Cornish J 2002 A mutation in the gene TNFRSF11B encoding

osteoprotegerin causes an idiopathic hyperphosphatasia phenotype. Hum Mol Genet **11**(18):2119-27.

24. Morony S, Capparelli C, Lee R, Shimamoto G, Boone T, Lacey DL, Dunstan CR 1999 A chimeric form of osteoprotegerin inhibits hypercalcemia and bone resorption induced by IL-1beta, TNF-alpha, PTH, PTHrP, and 1, 25(OH)2D3. J Bone Miner Res **14**(9):1478-85.

25. Hsu H, Lacey DL, Dunstan CR, Solovyev I, Colombero A, Timms E, Tan HL, Elliott G, Kelley MJ, Sarosi I, Wang L, Xia XZ, Elliott R, Chiu L, Black T, Scully S, Capparelli C, Morony S, Shimamoto G, Bass MB, Boyle WJ 1999 Tumor necrosis factor receptor family member RANK mediates osteoclast differentiation and activation induced by osteoprotegerin ligand. Proc Natl Acad Sci U S A **96**(7):3540-5.

26. Wei S, Teitelbaum SL, Wang MW, Ross FP 2001 Receptor activator of nuclear factor-kappa b ligand activates nuclear factor-kappa b in osteoclast precursors. Endocrinology **142**(3):1290-5.

27. Nagai M, Kyakumoto S, Sato N 2000 Cancer cells responsible for humoral hypercalcemia express mRNA encoding a secreted form of ODF/TRANCE that induces osteoclast formation. Biochem Biophys Res Commun **269**(2):532-6.

28. Ikeda T, Kasai M, Suzuki J, Kuroyama H, Seki S, Utsuyama M, Hirokawa K 2003 Multimerization of the RANKL isoforms and regulation of osteoclastogenesis. J Biol Chem.

29. Schett G, Kiechl S, Redlich K, Oberhollenzer F, Weger S, Egger G, Mayr A, Jocher J, Xu Q, Pietschmann P, Teitelbaum S, Smolen J, Willeit J 2004 Soluble RANKL and risk of nontraumatic fracture. Jama **291**(9):1108-13.

30. Feige U 2001 Osteoprotegerin. Ann Rheum Dis **60 Suppl 3**:iii81-4.

31. Kostenuik PJ, Shalhoub V 2001 Osteoprotegerin: a physiological and pharmacological inhibitor of bone resorption. Curr Pharm Des **7**(8):613-35.

32. Huang L, Xu J, Wood DJ, Zheng MH 2000 Gene expression of osteoprotegerin ligand, osteoprotegerin, and receptor activator of NF-kappaB in giant cell tumor of bone: possible involvement in tumor cell-induced osteoclast-like cell formation. Am J Pathol **156**(3):761-7.

33. Hofbauer LC, Neubauer A, Heufelder AE 2001 Receptor activator of nuclear factor-kappaB ligand and osteoprotegerin: potential implications for the pathogenesis and treatment of malignant bone diseases. Cancer **92**(3):460-70.

34. Fahrleitner A, Prenner G, Leb G, Tscheliessnigg KH, Piswanger-Solkner C, Obermayer-Pietsch B, Portugaller HR, Berghold A, Dobnig H 2003 Serum osteoprotegerin is a major determinant of bone density development and prevalent vertebral fracture status following cardiac transplantation. Bone **32**(1):96-106.

35. Shimizu-Ishiura M, Kawana F, Sasaki T 2002 Osteoprotegerin administration reduces femoral bone loss in ovariectomized mice via impairment of osteoclast structure and function. J Electron Microsc (Tokyo) **51**(5):315-25.

36. Kostenuik PJ, Bolon B, Morony S, Daris M, Geng Z, Carter C, Sheng J 2004 Gene therapy with human recombinant osteoprotegerin reverses established osteopenia in ovariectomized mice. Bone **34**(4):656-64.

37. Zhang J, Dai J, Lin DL, Habib P, Smith P, Murtha J, Fu Z, Yao Z, Qi Y, Keller ET 2002 Osteoprotegerin abrogates chronic alcohol ingestion-induced bone loss in mice. J Bone Miner Res **17**(7):1256-63.

38. Bekker PJ, Holloway D, Nakanishi A, Arrighi M, Leese PT, Dunstan CR 2001 The effect of a single dose of osteoprotegerin in postmenopausal women. J Bone Miner Res 16(2):348-60.

39. Rodan GA, Martin TJ 2000 Therapeutic approaches to bone diseases. Science 289(5484):1508-14.

40. Emery JG, McDonnell P, Burke MB, Deen KC, Lyn S, Silverman C, Dul E, Appelbaum ER, Eichman C, DiPrinzio R, Dodds RA, James IE, Rosenberg M, Lee JC, Young PR 1998 Osteoprotegerin is a receptor for the cytotoxic ligand TRAIL. J Biol Chem 273(23):14363-7.

41. Anderson DM, Maraskovsky E, Billingsley WL, Dougall WC, Tometsko ME, Roux ER, Teepe MC, DuBose RF, Cosman D, Galibert L 1997 A homologue of the TNF receptor and its ligand enhance T-cell growth and dendritic-cell function. Nature 390(6656):175-9.

42. Wong BR, Josien R, Choi Y 1999 TRANCE is a TNF family member that regulates dendritic cell and osteoclast function. J Leukoc Biol 65(6):715-24.

43. Fata JE, Kong YY, Li J, Sasaki T, Irie-Sasaki J, Moorehead RA, Elliott R, Scully S, Voura EB, Lacey DL, Boyle WJ, Khokha R, Penninger JM 2000 The osteoclast differentiation factor osteoprotegerin-ligand is essential for mammary gland development. Cell 103(1):41-50.

44. Min H, Morony S, Sarosi I, Dunstan CR, Capparelli C, Scully S, Van G, Kaufman S, Kostenuik PJ, Lacey DL, Boyle WJ, Simonet WS 2000 Osteoprotegerin reverses osteoporosis by inhibiting endosteal osteoclasts and prevents vascular calcification by blocking a process resembling osteoclastogenesis. J Exp Med 192(4):463-74.

45. Schoppet M, Preissner KT, Hofbauer LC 2002 RANK ligand and osteoprotegerin: paracrine regulators of bone metabolism and vascular function. Arterioscler Thromb Vasc Biol 22(4):549-53.

46. Jono S, Ikari Y, Shioi A, Mori K, Miki T, Hara K, Nishizawa Y 2002 Serum osteoprotegerin levels are associated with the presence and severity of coronary artery disease. Circulation 106(10):1192-4.

47. Schoppet M, Sattler AM, Schaefer JR, Herzum M, Maisch B, Hofbauer LC 2003 Increased osteoprotegerin serum levels in men with coronary artery disease. J Clin Endocrinol Metab 88(3):1024-8.

48. Cheng X, Kinosaki M, Takami M, Choi Y, Zhang H, Murali R 2004 Disabling of receptor activator of nuclear factor-kappaB (RANK) receptor complex by novel osteoprotegerin-like peptidomimetics restores bone loss in vivo. J Biol Chem 279(9):8269-77.

49. Keen RW, Woodford-Richens KL, Lanchbury JS, Spector TD 1998 Allelic variation at the interleukin-1 receptor antagonist gene is associated with early postmenopausal bone loss at the spine. Bone 23(4):367-71.

50. Lorenzo JA, Naprta A, Rao Y, Alander C, Glaccum M, Widmer M, Gronowicz G, Kalinowski J, Pilbeam CC 1998 Mice lacking the type I interleukin-1 receptor do not lose bone mass after ovariectomy. Endocrinology 139(6):3022-5.

51. Abu-Amer Y, Ross FP, McHugh KP, Livolsi A, Peyron JF, Teitelbaum SL 1998 Tumor necrosis factor-alpha activation of nuclear transcription factor-kappaB in marrow macrophages is mediated by c-Src tyrosine phosphorylation of Ikappa Balpha. Journal of Biological Chemistry. 273(45):29417-23.

52. Miyazaki T, Katagiri H, Kanegae Y, Takayanagi H, Sawada Y, Yamamoto A, Pando MP, Asano T, Verma IM, Oda H, Nakamura K, Tanaka S 2000 Reciprocal role of ERK and NF-kappaB pathways in survival and activation of osteoclasts. J Cell Biol **148**(2):333-42.

53. Kudo O, Fujikawa Y, Itonaga I, Sabokbar A, Torisu T, Athanasou NA 2002 Proinflammatory cytokine (TNFalpha/IL-1alpha) induction of human osteoclast formation. J Pathol **198**(2):220-7.

54. Wei S, Wang MW, Teitelbaum SL, Ross FP 2002 Interleukin-4 reversibly inhibits osteoclastogenesis via inhibition of NF-kappa B and mitogen-activated protein kinase signaling. J Biol Chem **277**(8):6622-30.

55. Yang SY, Wu B, Mayton L, Mukherjee P, Robbins PD, Evans CH, Wooley PH 2004 Protective effects of IL-1Ra or vIL-10 gene transfer on a murine model of wear debris-induced osteolysis. Gene Ther **11**(5):483-91.

56. Bajnok E, Takacs I, Vargha P, Speer G, Nagy Z, Lakatos P 2000 Lack of association between interleukin-1 receptor antagonist protein gene polymorphism and bone mineral density in Hungarian postmenopausal women. Bone **27**(4):559-62.

57. Poli V, Balena R, Fattori E, Markatos A, Yamamoto M, Tanaka H, Ciliberto G, Rodan GA, Costantini F 1994 Interleukin-6 deficient mice are protected from bone loss caused by estrogen depletion. Embo J **13**(5):1189-96.

58. Kudo O, Sabokbar A, Pocock A, Itonaga I, Fujikawa Y, Athanasou NA 2003 Interleukin-6 and interleukin-11 support human osteoclast formation by a RANKL-independent mechanism. Bone **32**(1):1-7.

59. Takeuchi Y, Watanabe S, Ishii G, Takeda S, Nakayama K, Fukumoto S, Kaneta Y, Inoue D, Matsumoto T, Harigaya K, Fujita T 2002 Interleukin-11 as a stimulatory factor for bone formation prevents bone loss with advancing age in mice. J Biol Chem **277**(50):49011-8.

60. Yamada N, Niwa S, Tsujimura T, Iwasaki T, Sugihara A, Futani H, Hayashi S, Okamura H, Akedo H, Terada N 2002 Interleukin-18 and interleukin-12 synergistically inhibit osteoclastic bone-resorbing activity. Bone **30**(6):901-8.

61. Horwood NJ, Elliott J, Martin TJ, Gillespie MT 2001 IL-12 alone and in synergy with IL-18 inhibits osteoclast formation in vitro. J Immunol **166**(8):4915-21.

62. Kotake S, Udagawa N, Takahashi N, Matsuzaki K, Itoh K, Ishiyama S, Saito S, Inoue K, Kamatani N, Gillespie MT, Martin TJ, Suda T 1999 IL-17 in synovial fluids from patients with rheumatoid arthritis is a potent stimulator of osteoclastogenesis. J Clin Invest **103**(9):1345-52.

63. Lubberts E, van den Bersselaar L, Oppers-Walgreen B, Schwarzenberger P, Coenen-de Roo CJ, Kolls JK, Joosten LA, van den Berg WB 2003 IL-17 promotes bone erosion in murine collagen-induced arthritis through loss of the receptor activator of NF-kappa B ligand/osteoprotegerin balance. J Immunol **170**(5):2655-62.

64. Kobayashi K, Takahashi N, Jimi E, Udagawa N, Takami M, Kotake S, Nakagawa N, Kinosaki M, Yamaguchi K, Shima N, Yasuda H, Morinaga T, Higashio K, Martin TJ, Suda T 2000 Tumor necrosis factor alpha stimulates osteoclast differentiation by a mechanism independent of the ODF/RANKL-RANK interaction. J Exp Med **191**(2):275-86.

65. Lam J, Takeshita S, Barker JE, Kanagawa O, Ross FP, Teitelbaum SL 2000 TNF-alpha induces osteoclastogenesis by direct stimulation of macrophages exposed to permissive levels of RANK ligand. J Clin Invest **106**(12):1481-8.

66. Cenci S, Weitzmann MN, Roggia C, Namba N, Novack D, Woodring J, Pacifici R 2000 Estrogen deficiency induces bone loss by enhancing T-cell production of TNF-alpha. J Clin Invest **106**(10):1229-37.

67. Souchelnytskyi S, Moustakas A, Heldin CH 2002 TGF-beta signaling from a three-dimensional perspective: insight into selection of partners. Trends Cell Biol **12**(7):304-7.

68. Murakami T, Yamamoto M, Ono K, Nishikawa M, Nagata N, Motoyoshi K, Akatsu T 1998 Transforming growth factor-beta1 increases mRNA levels of osteoclastogenesis inhibitory factor in osteoblastic/stromal cells and inhibits the survival of murine osteoclast-like cells. Biochem Biophys Res Commun **252**(3):747-52.

69. Yamada Y 2001 Association of polymorphisms of the transforming growth factor-beta1 gene with genetic susceptibility to osteoporosis. Pharmacogenetics **11**(9):765-71.

70. Karsdal MA, Hjorth P, Henriksen K, Kirkegaard T, Nielsen KL, Lou H, Delaisse JM, Foged NT 2003 Transforming growth factor-beta controls human osteoclastogenesis through the p38 MAPK and regulation of RANK expression. J Biol Chem **278**(45):44975-87.

71. Miyaura C, Inada M, Matsumoto C, Ohshiba T, Uozumi N, Shimizu T, Ito A 2003 An essential role of cytosolic phospholipase A2alpha in prostaglandin E2-mediated bone resorption associated with inflammation. J Exp Med **197**(10):1303-10.

72. Li X, Okada Y, Pilbeam CC, Lorenzo JA, Kennedy CR, Breyer RM, Raisz LG 2000 Knockout of the murine prostaglandin EP2 receptor impairs osteoclastogenesis in vitro. Endocrinology **141**(6):2054-61.

73. Brandstrom H, Jonsson KB, Ohlsson C, Vidal O, Ljunghall S, Ljunggren O 1998 Regulation of osteoprotegerin mRNA levels by prostaglandin E2 in human bone marrow stroma cells. Biochem Biophys Res Commun **247**(2):338-41.

74. Ono K, Akatsu T, Murakami T, Kitamura R, Yamamoto M, Shinomiya N, Rokutanda M, Sasaki T, Amizuka N, Ozawa H, Nagata N, Kugai N 2002 Involvement of cyclo-oxygenase-2 in osteoclast formation and bone destruction in bone metastasis of mammary carcinoma cell lines. J Bone Miner Res **17**(5):774-81.

75. Sabino MA, Ghilardi JR, Jongen JL, Keyser CP, Luger NM, Mach DB, Peters CM, Rogers SD, Schwei MJ, de Felipe C, Mantyh PW 2002 Simultaneous reduction in cancer pain, bone destruction, and tumor growth by selective inhibition of cyclooxygenase-2. Cancer Res **62**(24):7343-9.

76. Fox SW, Fuller K, Chambers TJ 2000 Activation of osteoclasts by interleukin-1: divergent responsiveness in osteoclasts formed in vivo and in vitro. J Cell Physiol **184**(3):334-40.

77. Kim HH, Lee DE, Shin JN, Lee YS, Jeon YM, Chung CH, Ni J, Kwon BS, Lee ZH 1999 Receptor activator of NF-kappaB recruits multiple TRAF family adaptors and activates c-Jun N-terminal kinase. FEBS Lett **443**(3):297-302.

78. Galibert L, Tometsko ME, Anderson DM, Cosman D, Dougall WC 1998 The involvement of multiple tumor necrosis factor receptor (TNFR)- associated factors in the signaling mechanisms of receptor activator of NF-kappaB, a member of the TNFR superfamily. J Biol Chem **273**(51)**:**34120-7.

79. Lomaga MA, Yeh WC, Sarosi I, Duncan GS, Furlonger C, Ho A, Morony S, Capparelli C, Van G, Kaufman S, van der Heiden A, Itie A, Wakeham A, Khoo W, Sasaki T, Cao Z, Penninger JM, Paige CJ, Lacey DL, Dunstan CR, Boyle WJ, Goeddel DV, Mak TW 1999 TRAF6 deficiency results in osteopetrosis and defective interleukin-1, CD40, and LPS signaling. Genes Dev **13**(8)**:**1015-24.

80. Wang ZQ, Ovitt C, Grigoriadis AE, Mohle-Steinlein U, Ruther U, Wagner EF 1992 Bone and haematopoietic defects in mice lacking c-fos. Nature **360**(6406)**:**741-5.

81. Johnson RS, Spiegelman BM, Papaioannou V 1992 Pleiotropic effects of a null mutation in the c-fos proto-oncogene. Cell **71**(4)**:**577-86.

82. David JP, Sabapathy K, Hoffmann O, Idarraga MH, Wagner EF 2002 JNK1 modulates osteoclastogenesis through both c-Jun phosphorylation- dependent and -independent mechanisms. J Cell Sci **115**(Pt 22)**:**4317-4325.

83. Dixit V, Mak TW 2002 NF-kappaB signaling. Many roads lead to madrid. Cell **111**(5)**:**615-9.

84. Mercurio F, Manning AM 1999 Multiple signals converging on NF-kappaB. Curr Opin Cell Biol **11**(2)**:**226-32.

85. Joyce D, Albanese C, Steer J, Fu M, Bouzahzah B, Pestell RG 2001 NF-kappaB and cell-cycle regulation: the cyclin connection. Cytokine Growth Factor Rev **12**(1)**:**73-90.

86. May MJ, Ghosh S 1997 Rel/NF-kappa B and I kappa B proteins: an overview. Semin Cancer Biol **8**(2)**:**63-73.

87. Franzoso G, Carlson L, Xing L, Poljak L, Shores EW, Brown KD, Leonardi A, Tran T, Boyce BF, Siebenlist U 1997 Requirement for NF-kappaB in osteoclast and B-cell development. Genes Dev **11**(24)**:**3482-96.

88. Iotsova V, Caamano J, Loy J, Yang Y, Lewin A, Bravo R 1997 Osteopetrosis in mice lacking NF-kappaB1 and NF-kappaB2. Nat Med **3**(11)**:**1285-9.

89. Duran A, Serrano M, Leitges M, Flores JM, Picard S, Brown JP, Moscat J, Diaz-Meco MT 2004 The atypical PKC-interacting protein p62 is an important mediator of RANK-activated osteoclastogenesis. Dev Cell **6**(2)**:**303-9.

90. Hocking LJ, Lucas GJ, Daroszewska A, Mangion J, Olavesen M, Cundy T, Nicholson GC, Ward L, Bennett ST, Wuyts W, Van Hul W, Ralston SH 2002 Domain-specific mutations in sequestosome 1 (SQSTM1) cause familial and sporadic Paget's disease. Hum Mol Genet **11**(22)**:**2735-9.

91. Ciani B, Layfield R, Cavey JR, Sheppard PW, Searle MS 2003 Structure of the ubiquitin-associated domain of p62 (SQSTM1) and implications for mutations that cause Paget's disease of bone. J Biol Chem **278**(39)**:**37409-12.

92. Johnson-Pais TL, Wisdom JH, Weldon KS, Cody JD, Hansen MF, Singer FR, Leach RJ 2003 Three novel mutations in SQSTM1 identified in familial Paget's disease of bone. J Bone Miner Res **18**(10)**:**1748-53.

93. Yip KH, Zheng MH, Feng HT, Steer JH, Joyce DA, Xu J 2003 Sesquiterpene Lactone Parthenolide Blocks Lipopolysaccharide Induced Osteolysis via the Suppression of NF-kB Activity. J Bone Miner Res (accepted).

94.   Wang C, Steer JH, Joyce DA, Yip KH, Zheng MH, Xu J 2003 12-O-tetradecanoylphorbol-13-acetate (TPA) inhibits osteoclastogenesis by suppressing RANKL-induced NF-kappaB activation. J Bone Miner Res **18**(12):2159-68.

95.   Wong BR, Besser D, Kim N, Arron JR, Vologodskaia M, Hanafusa H, Choi Y 1999 TRANCE, a TNF family member, activates Akt/PKB through a signaling complex involving TRAF6 and c-Src. Mol Cell **4**(6):1041-9.

96.   Sugatani T, Alvarez U, Hruska KA 2003 PTEN regulates RANKL- and osteopontin-stimulated signal transduction during osteoclast differentiation and cell motility. J Biol Chem **278**(7):5001-8.

97.   Gingery A, Bradley E, Shaw A, Oursler MJ 2003 Phosphatidylinositol 3-kinase coordinately activates the MEK/ERK and AKT/NFkappaB pathways to maintain osteoclast survival. J Cell Biochem **89**(1):165-79.

98.   Lee ZH, Kim HH 2003 Signal transduction by receptor activator of nuclear factor kappa B in osteoclasts. Biochem Biophys Res Commun **305**(2):211-4.

99.   Ishida N, Hayashi K, Hoshijima M, Ogawa T, Koga S, Miyatake Y, Kumegawa M, Kimura T, Takeya T 2002 Large scale gene expression analysis of osteoclastogenesis in vitro and elucidation of NFAT2 as a key regulator. J Biol Chem **277**(43):41147-56.

100. Hirotani H, Tuohy NA, Woo JT, Stern PH, Clipstone NA 2004 The calcineurin/NFAT signaling pathway regulates osteoclastogenesis in RAW264.7 cells. J Biol Chem.

101. Thomas SM, Brugge JS 1997 Cellular functions regulated by Src family kinases. Annu Rev Cell Dev Biol **13**:513-609.

102. Kay BK, Williamson MP, Sudol M 2000 The importance of being proline: the interaction of proline-rich motifs in signaling proteins with their cognate domains. Faseb J **14**(2):231-41.

103. Lowe C, Yoneda T, Boyce BF, Chen H, Mundy GR, Soriano P 1993 Osteopetrosis in Src-deficient mice is due to an autonomous defect of osteoclasts. Proc Natl Acad Sci U S A **90**(10):4485-9.

104. Boyce BF, Yoneda T, Lowe C, Soriano P, Mundy GR 1992 Requirement of pp60c-src expression for osteoclasts to form ruffled borders and resorb bone in mice. J Clin Invest **90**(4):1622-7.

105. Schwartzberg PL, Xing L, Hoffmann O, Lowell CA, Garrett L, Boyce BF, Varmus HE 1997 Rescue of osteoclast function by transgenic expression of kinase-deficient Src in src-/- mutant mice. Genes Dev **11**(21):2835-44.

106. Furuyama N, Fujisawa Y 2000 Regulation of collagenolytic protease secretion through c-Src in osteoclasts. Biochem Biophys Res Commun **272**(1):116-24.

107. Yoneda T, Lowe C, Lee CH, Gutierrez G, Niewolna M, Williams PJ, Izbicka E, Uehara Y, Mundy GR 1993 Herbimycin A, a pp60c-src tyrosine kinase inhibitor, inhibits osteoclastic bone resorption in vitro and hypercalcemia in vivo. J Clin Invest **91**(6):2791-5.

108. Missbach M, Jeschke M, Feyen J, Muller K, Glatt M, Green J, Susa M 1999 A novel inhibitor of the tyrosine kinase Src suppresses phosphorylation of its major cellular substrates and reduces bone resorption in vitro and in rodent models in vivo. Bone **24**(5):437-49.

109. Williams JP, Jordan SE, Barnes S, Blair HC 1998 Tyrosine kinase inhibitor effects on avian osteoclastic acid transport. Am J Clin Nutr **68**(6 Suppl):1369S-1374S.

110. Sharma SV, Oneyama C, Yamashita Y, Nakano H, Sugawara K, Hamada M, Kosaka N, Tamaoki T 2001 UCS15A, a non-kinase inhibitor of Src signal transduction. Oncogene **20**(17):2068-79.

111. Recchia I, Rucci N, Funari A, Migliaccio S, Taranta A, Longo M, Kneissel M, Susa M, Fabbro D, Teti A 2004 Reduction of c-Src activity by substituted 5,7-diphenyl-pyrrolo[2,3-d]-pyrimidines induces osteoclast apoptosis in vivo and in vitro. Involvement of ERK1/2 pathway. Bone **34**(1):65-79.

112. Shakespeare WC, Metcalf CA, 3rd, Wang Y, Sundaramoorthi R, Keenan T, Weigele M, Bohacek RS, Dalgarno DC, Sawyer TK 2003 Novel bone-targeted Src tyrosine kinase inhibitor drug discovery. Curr Opin Drug Discov Devel **6**(5):729-41.

113. Saginario C, Qian HY, Vignery A 1995 Identification of an inducible surface molecule specific to fusing macrophages. Proc Natl Acad Sci U S A **92**(26):12210-4.

114. Vignery A 2000 Osteoclasts and giant cells: macrophage-macrophage fusion mechanism. Int J Exp Pathol **81**(5):291-304.

115. Nakamura I, Lipfert L, Rodan GA, Le TD 2001 Convergence of alpha(v)beta(3) integrin- and macrophage colony stimulating factor-mediated signals on phospholipase Cgamma in prefusion osteoclasts. J Cell Biol **152**(2):361-73.

116. Horton MA 1997 The alpha v beta 3 integrin "vitronectin receptor". Int J Biochem Cell Biol **29**(5):721-5.

117. Inoue M, Namba N, Chappel J, Teitelbaum SL, Ross FP 1998 Granulocyte macrophage-colony stimulating factor reciprocally regulates alphav-associated integrins on murine osteoclast precursors. Mol Endocrinol **12**(12):1955-62.

118. McHugh KP, Hodivala-Dilke K, Zheng MH, Namba N, Lam J, Novack D, Feng X, Ross FP, Hynes RO, Teitelbaum SL 2000 Mice lacking beta3 integrins are osteosclerotic because of dysfunctional osteoclasts. J Clin Invest **105**(4):433-40.

119. Teitelbaum SL 2000 Osteoclasts, integrins, and osteoporosis. J Bone Miner Metab **18**(6):344-9.

120. Inoue M, Ross FP, Erdmann JM, Abu-Amer Y, Wei S, Teitelbaum SL 2000 Tumor necrosis factor alpha regulates alpha(v)beta5 integrin expression by osteoclast precursors in vitro and in vivo. Endocrinology **141**(1):284-90.

121. Mimura H, Cao X, Ross FP, Chiba M, Teitelbaum SL 1994 1,25-Dihydroxyvitamin D3 transcriptionally activates the beta 3-integrin subunit gene in avian osteoclast precursors. Endocrinology **134**(3):1061-6.

122. Pytela R, Pierschbacher MD, Ruoslahti E 1985 A 125/115-kDa cell surface receptor specific for vitronectin interacts with the arginine-glycine-aspartic acid adhesion sequence derived from fibronectin. Proc Natl Acad Sci U S A **82**(17):5766-70.

123. Hartman GD, Duggan ME 2000 alpha(v)beta(3) Integrin antagonists as inhibitors of bone resorption. Expert Opin Investig Drugs **9**(6):1281-91.

124. Peyman A, Scheunemann K, Will DW, Knolle J, Wehner V, Breipohl G, Stilz HU, Carniato D, Ruxer J, Gourvest J, Auberval M, Doucet B, Baron R,

Gaillard M, Gadek TR, Bodary S 2001 alpha(v)beta(3) Antagonists based on a central thiophene scaffold. Bioorg Med Chem Lett **11**(15):2011-5.

125.   Lark MW, Stroup GB, Hwang SM, James IE, Rieman DJ, Drake FH, Bradbeer JN, Mathur A, Erhard KF, Newlander KA, Ross ST, Salyers KL, Smith BR, Miller WH, Huffman WF, Gowen M 1999 Design and characterization of orally active Arg-Gly-Asp peptidomimetic vitronectin receptor antagonist SB 265123 for prevention of bone loss in osteoporosis. J Pharmacol Exp Ther **291**(2):612-7.

126.   Horton MA 2001 Integrin antagonists as inhibitors of bone resorption: implications for treatment. Proc Nutr Soc **60**(2):275-81.

127.   Tcheng JE 1996 Glycoprotein IIb/IIIa receptor inhibitors: putting the EPIC, IMPACT II, RESTORE, and EPILOG trials into perspective. Am J Cardiol **78**(3A):35-40.

128.   Coller BS 1997 GPIIb/IIIa antagonists: pathophysiologic and therapeutic insights from studies of c7E3 Fab. Thromb Haemost **78**(1):730-5.

129.   Phillips DR, Scarborough RM 1997 Clinical pharmacology of eptifibatide. Am J Cardiol **80**(4A):11B-20B.

130.   Theroux P 1998 Oral inhibitors of platelet membrane receptor glycoprotein IIb/IIIa in clinical cardiology: issues and opportunities. Am Heart J **135**(5 Pt 2 Su):S107-12.

131.   Farina C, Gagliardi S, Nadler G, Morvan M, Parini C, Belfiore P, Visentin L, Gowen M 2001 Novel bone antiresorptive agents that selectively inhibit the osteoclast V-H+-ATPase. Farmaco **56**(1-2):113-6.

132.   Hall TJ, Chambers TJ 1996 Molecular aspects of osteoclast function. Inflamm Res **45**(1):1-9.

133.   Visentin L, Dodds RA, Valente M, Misiano P, Bradbeer JN, Oneta S, Liang X, Gowen M, Farina C 2000 A selective inhibitor of the osteoclastic V-H(+)-ATPase prevents bone loss in both thyroparathyroidectomized and ovariectomized rats. J Clin Invest **106**(2):309-18.

134.   Li YP, Chen W, Liang Y, Li E, Stashenko P 1999 Atp6i-deficient mice exhibit severe osteopetrosis due to loss of osteoclast-mediated extracellular acidification. Nat Genet **23**(4):447-51.

135.   Li YP, Chen W, Stashenko P 1996 Molecular cloning and characterization of a putative novel human osteoclast-specific 116-kDa vacuolar proton pump subunit. Biochem Biophys Res Commun **218**(3):813-21.

136.   Junge W, Lill H, Engelbrecht S 1997 ATP synthase: an electrochemical transducer with rotatory mechanics. Trends Biochem Sci **22**(11):420-3.

137.   Harrison MA, Finbow ME, Findlay JB 1997 Postulate for the molecular mechanism of the vacuolar H(+)-ATPase (hypothesis). Mol Membr Biol **14**(1):1-3.

138.   Farina C, Gagliardi S 1999 Selective inhibitors of the osteoclast vacuolar proton ATPase as novel bone antiresorptive agents. Drug Discov Today **4**(4):163-172.

139.   Teti A, Blair HC, Teitelbaum SL, Kahn AJ, Koziol C, Konsek J, Zambonin-Zallone A, Schlesinger PH 1989 Cytoplasmic pH regulation and chloride/bicarbonate exchange in avian osteoclasts. J Clin Invest **83**(1):227-33.

140. Ravesloot JH, Eisen T, Baron R, Boron WF 1995 Role of Na-H exchangers and vacuolar H+ pumps in intracellular pH regulation in neonatal rat osteoclasts. J Gen Physiol **105**(2):177-208.

141. Laitala T, Vaananen HK 1994 Inhibition of bone resorption in vitro by antisense RNA and DNA molecules targeted against carbonic anhydrase II or two subunits of vacuolar H(+)-ATPase. J Clin Invest **93**(6):2311-8.

142. Gowen M, Emery J, Kumar S 2000 Emerging therapies for osteoporosis. Emerging Drugs **5**(1):1-43.

143. Finbow ME, Harrison MA 1997 The vacuolar H+-ATPase: a universal proton pump of eukaryotes. Biochem J **324** (**Pt 3**):697-712.

144. Gagliardi S, Nadler G, Consolandi E, Parini C, Morvan M, Legave MN, Belfiore P, Zocchetti A, Clarke GD, James I, Nambi P, Gowen M, Farina C 1998 5-(5,6-Dichloro-2-indolyl)-2-methoxy-2,4-pentadienamides: novel and selective inhibitors of the vacuolar H+-ATPase of osteoclasts with bone antiresorptive activity. J Med Chem **41**(10):1568-73.

145. Manolson M, Landolt-Marticorena C, Yu H, Williams K, Heersche J 1999 Topology and function of the 116 kDa V-ATPase subunit in osteoclasts and yeast. J Bone Miner Res **14**(1):S484.

146. Sobacchi C, Frattini A, Orchard P, Porras O, Tezcan I, Andolina M, Babul-Hirji R, Baric I, Canham N, Chitayat D, Dupuis-Girod S, Ellis I, Etzioni A, Fasth A, Fisher A, Gerritsen B, Gulino V, Horwitz E, Klamroth V, Lanino E, Mirolo M, Musio A, Matthijs G, Nonomaya S, Notarangelo LD, Ochs HD, Superti Furga A, Valiaho J, van Hove JL, Vihinen M, Vujic D, Vezzoni P, Villa A 2001 The mutational spectrum of human malignant autosomal recessive osteopetrosis. Hum Mol Genet **10**(17):1767-73.

147. Blair HC, Teitelbaum SL, Tan HL, Koziol CM, Schlesinger PH 1991 Passive chloride permeability charge coupled to H(+)-ATPase of avian osteoclast ruffled membrane. Am J Physiol **260**(6 Pt 1):C1315-24.

148. Kornak U, Kasper D, Bosl MR, Kaiser E, Schweizer M, Schulz A, Friedrich W, Delling G, Jentsch TJ 2001 Loss of the ClC-7 chloride channel leads to osteopetrosis in mice and man. Cell **104**(2):205-15.

149. Gelb BD, Shi GP, Chapman HA, Desnick RJ 1996 Pycnodysostosis, a lysosomal disease caused by cathepsin K deficiency. Science **273**(5279):1236-8.

150. Saftig P, Hunziker E, Wehmeyer O, Jones S, Boyde A, Rommerskirch W, Moritz JD, Schu P, von Figura K 1998 Impaired osteoclastic bone resorption leads to osteopetrosis in cathepsin-K-deficient mice. Proc Natl Acad Sci U S A **95**(23):13453-8.

151. Hou WS, Bromme D, Zhao Y, Mehler E, Dushey C, Weinstein H, Miranda CS, Fraga C, Greig F, Carey J, Rimoin DL, Desnick RJ, Gelb BD 1999 Characterization of novel cathepsin K mutations in the pro and mature polypeptide regions causing pycnodysostosis. J Clin Invest **103**(5):731-8.

152. Ho N, Punturieri A, Wilkin D, Szabo J, Johnson M, Whaley J, Davis J, Clark A, Weiss S, Francomano C 1999 Mutations of CTSK result in pycnodysostosis via a reduction in cathepsin K protein. J Bone Miner Res **14**(10):1649-53.

153. Fujita Y, Nakata K, Yasui N, Matsui Y, Kataoka E, Hiroshima K, Shiba RI, Ochi T 2000 Novel mutations of the cathepsin K gene in patients with

pycnodysostosis and their characterization. J Clin Endocrinol Metab **85**(1):425-31.

154. Ishikawa T, Kamiyama M, Tani-Ishii N, Suzuki H, Ichikawa Y, Hamaguchi Y, Momiyama N, Shimada H 2001 Inhibition of osteoclast differentiation and bone resorption by cathepsin K antisense oligonucleotides. Mol Carcinog **32**(2):84-91.

155. Inui T, Ishibashi O, Inaoka T, Origane Y, Kumegawa M, Kokubo T, Yamamura T 1997 Cathepsin K antisense oligodeoxynucleotide inhibits osteoclastic bone resorption. J Biol Chem **272**(13):8109-12.

156. Stroup GB, Lark MW, Veber DF, Bhattacharyya A, Blake S, Dare LC, Erhard KF, Hoffman SJ, James IE, Marquis RW, Ru Y, Vasko-Moser JA, Smith BR, Tomaszek T, Gowen M 2001 Potent and selective inhibition of human cathepsin K leads to inhibition of bone resorption in vivo in a nonhuman primate. J Bone Miner Res **16**(10):1739-46.

157. Yamashita DS, Dodds RA 2000 Cathepsin K and the design of inhibitors of cathepsin K. Curr Pharm Des **6**(1):1-24.

158. Rieman DJ, McClung HA, Dodds RA, Hwang SM, Holmes MW, James IE, Drake FH, Gowen M 2001 Biosynthesis and processing of cathepsin K in cultured human osteoclasts. Bone **28**(3):282-9.

159. Yamashita D, Smith W, Zhao Bea 1997 Structure and Design of Potent and Selective Cathepsin K Inhibitors. J Am Chem Soc **119**:11351-11352.

160. Lark MW, Stroup GB, James IE, Dodds RA, Hwang SM, Blake SM, Lechowska BA, Hoffman SJ, Smith BR, Kapadia R, Liang X, Erhard K, Ru Y, Dong X, Marquis RW, Veber D, Gowen M 2002 A potent small molecule, nonpeptide inhibitor of cathepsin K (SB 331750) prevents bone matrix resorption in the ovariectomized rat. Bone **30**(5):746-53.

161. Robichaud J, Oballa R, Prasit P, Falgueyret JP, Percival MD, Wesolowski G, Rodan SB, Kimmel D, Johnson C, Bryant C, Venkatraman S, Setti E, Mendonca R, Palmer JT 2003 A novel class of nonpeptidic biaryl inhibitors of human cathepsin K. J Med Chem **46**(17):3709-27.

162. Tavares FX, Boncek V, Deaton DN, Hassell AM, Long ST, Miller AB, Payne AA, Miller LR, Shewchuk LM, Wells-Knecht K, Willard DH, Jr., Wright LL, Zhou HQ 2004 Design of potent, selective, and orally bioavailable inhibitors of cysteine protease cathepsin k. J Med Chem **47**(3):588-99.

163. Tezuka K, Nemoto K, Tezuka Y, Sato T, Ikeda Y, Kobori M, Kawashima H, Eguchi H, Hakeda Y, Kumegawa M 1994 Identification of matrix metalloproteinase 9 in rabbit osteoclasts. J Biol Chem **269**(21):15006-9.

164. Engsig MT, Chen QJ, Vu TH, Pedersen AC, Therkidsen B, Lund LR, Henriksen K, Lenhard T, Foged NT, Werb Z, Delaisse JM 2000 Matrix metalloproteinase 9 and vascular endothelial growth factor are essential for osteoclast recruitment into developing long bones. J Cell Biol **151**(4):879-89.

165. Fessler LI, Duncan KG, Fessler JH, Salo T, Tryggvason K 1984 Characterization of the procollagen IV cleavage products produced by a specific tumor collagenase. J Biol Chem **259**(15):9783-9.

166. Vu T, Werb Z 1998 Gelatinase B: structure, regulation and function. In Matrix Metalloproteinases. In: Mecham WCPaMP (ed.). Academic Press, San Diego, pp 115-148.

167. Okada Y, Naka K, Kawamura K, Matsumoto T, Nakanishi I, Fujimoto N, Sato H, Seiki M 1995 Localization of matrix metalloproteinase 9 (92-kilodalton gelatinase/type IV collagenase = gelatinase B) in osteoclasts: implications for bone resorption. Lab Invest 72(3):311-22.

168. Inui T, Ishibashi O, Origane Y, Fujimori K, Kokubo T, Nakajima M 1999 Matrix metalloproteinases and lysosomal cysteine proteases in osteoclasts contribute to bone resorption through distinct modes of action. Biochem Biophys Res Commun 258(1):173-8.

169. Shimizu H, Sakamoto M, Sakamoto S 1990 Bone resorption by isolated osteoclasts in living versus devitalized bone: differences in mode and extent and the effects of human recombinant tissue inhibitor of metalloproteinases. J Bone Miner Res 5(4):411-8.

170. Everts V, Delaisse JM, Korper W, Niehof A, Vaes G, Beertsen W 1992 Degradation of collagen in the bone-resorbing compartment underlying the osteoclast involves both cysteine-proteinases and matrix metalloproteinases. J Cell Physiol 150(2):221-31.

171. Everts V, Korper W, Jansen DC, Steinfort J, Lammerse I, Heera S, Docherty AJ, Beertsen W 1999 Functional heterogeneity of osteoclasts: matrix metalloproteinases participate in osteoclastic resorption of calvarial bone but not in resorption of long bone. Faseb J 13(10):1219-30.

172. Bord S, Horner A, Beeton CA, Hembry RM, Compston JE 1999 Tissue inhibitor of matrix metalloproteinase-1 (TIMP-1) distribution in normal and pathological human bone. Bone 24(3):229-35.

CHAPTER 12

MALE OSTEOPOROSIS

Lu Amy Sun, M.D., Ph.D. and Arkadi Chines, M.D.

Procter & Gamble Pharmaceuticals, Inc.
8700 Mason Montgomery Road
Mason, Ohio 45040 USA
E-mail: sun.la@pg.com, chines.aa@pg.com

Male osteoporosis is becoming increasingly recognized as a significant medical issue affecting the older male population. Pande recognized that 25-30% of all hip fractures occur in men.[1] By the age of 90 years, one of every six men will have a hip fracture. Although there is an increase in morbidity and mortality in both male and female after hip fracture, the mortality rate in men is higher.[2,3] This article highlights current understanding of the epidemiology and causes of male osteoporosis, diagnosis, and treatment options.

1. Epidemiology of Male Osteoporosis

In a population based Rochester Epidemiology Project, 348 men aged 20–80 years were assessed by dual energy x-ray absorptiometry (DXA) at lumbar spine, hip, and wrist. Approximately 19% of the men aged 50 years or older were found to have osteoporosis based on the criteria of bone mineral density (BMD) more than 2.5 standard deviations (SD) below the young normal male-specific mean at one or more measurement site. This prevalence rate would translate into an absolute number of approximately 4.5 million males with osteoporosis in the United States.[4]

In the third National Health and Nutrition Examination Survey (NHANES III), a total of 14,636 men (3,090 above the age of 50) were assessed with DXAof the proximal femur.[5] Approximately 3-6% of U.S. men 50 years and older were estimated to have osteoporosis, and an additional 28–47% men to have osteopenia using male-specific hip BMD cutoffs. Using single-energy x-ray absorptiometry, Xu[6] and his colleagues measured calcaneus BMD in 7428 Chinese (4126 women, 3302 men; aged 22-94 years). The incidence of osteoporosis in Chinese men aged 60 years or older was about 6.6%.

Fractures are common in men. It is reported up to 20% of symptomatic vertebral fractures and 30% of hip fractures occur in men.[7] In young men, long bone fractures due to trauma may play a larger role; where in older men (age 70 or above) vertebral and hip fractures predominate, suggesting skeletal fragility is a major risk factor. The increase in fracture incidence in older men is as dramatic as the increase in women, but it begins 5-10 years later in life. The incidence of osteoporotic fracture in women and men is compared in Table 1.

Table 1. Risk of Osteoporotic Hip Fracture in Women and Men[8,9]

Factor	Women	Men
Lifetime risk of hip fracture at age 50	17.5%	6%
US incidence of hip fracture at age 65	8 to 10 per 1,000	4 to 5 per 1,000
Mortality from hip fracture	17%	31%

Although there is an increase in morbidity and mortality in both women and men after hip fracture, the mortality rate in men is higher. Cooper studied 355 individuals with vertebral fractures (79 men, 256 women) who were followed for 5 years.[2] He found the 5-year relative survival after the vertebral fracture was better in women than in men and declined with age at the time of fracture.

There is limited information about mortality after other fractures. Center investigated the mortality associated with all fracture types in elderly women and men in a 5-year prospective cohort study in the semi-urban city of Dubbo, Australia.[10] All residents aged 60 years and older (2413 women and 1898 men) in the area were studied. In women, age-standardized mortality ratios were 2.18 for proximal femur, 1.66 for vertebral, 1.92 for other major, and 0.75 for minor fractures. In men, these ratios were 3.17 for proximal femur, 2.38 for vertebral, 2.22 for other major, and 1.45 for minor fractures. The results indicated men had significantly increased mortality ratio after major fractures. The reasons of increased mortality in male osteoporotic patients include the associated serious comorbid conditions, the onset of osteoporotic fractures at older age, and the increased disability.

2. Causes of Male Osteoporosis

The causes of male osteoporosis are commonly heterogeneous, and can be divided into two major categories; primary (or idiopathic) and secondary. It is important to keep in mind that osteoporosis in men is often a heterogeneous disorder and more than one factor contributes to the disease.

2.1. *Primary Cause of Male Osteoporosis*

Primary or idiopathic osteoporosis can present in men of any age, but is most commonly seen in younger men (60 years or younger). About 40-60% of men with osteoporosis fall into this category. Histomorphometric studies suggest many have decreased bone formation, but some may have increased bone resorption as well.[11,12] These men probably have a genetic predisposition to osteoporosis.

Genetic studies indicate a large component of the variance in BMD is under genetic control, with strong evidence for a major gene locus influencing BMD transmission. Nguyen[13] designed a study to test the hypothesis of a major gene influence on the variation in BMD. BMD and bone mineral content at the lumbar spine and femoral neck were measured in 330 men and 413 women, aged 18-90 years, from 107 nuclear and complex families After adjusting for age and body weight, familial factors accounted for up to 72% of the total variation in BMD. In complex segregation analysis, for all variables examined the best-fitting most parsimonious model consistently suggested the Mendelian transmission of a major gene locus with significant residual correlations among siblings.

Although most studies have been conducted on women, there is evidence to suggest genetic factors and positive family history of fractures are also important determinants of osteoporosis in men.

Kannus studied osteoporotic fracture in twins and found monozygotic twins had a 4-fold higher concordance for fracture than dizygotic twins.[14] Family-based studies have also yielded strong heritability estimates for BMD in males at different skeletal sites and indicated bone mass is significantly lower in relatives of male osteoporotic subjects.[15] Genome-wide linkage studies in men have identified loci on chromosomes 1p36, 1q21, 2p21, 5q33-35, 6p11-12, and 11q12-13 that show definite or probable linkage to BMD, but so far, the causative genes remain to be identified.[16] There are interesting data about some candidate genes with possible implications in male osteoporosis. These data were based on association studies and involve polymorphisms at the vitamin D receptor gene, collagen type I alpha I gene, insulin growth factor I gene, aromatase (CYP 19), insulin growth factor I gene (IGF-I), estrogen receptor alpha unit, and androgen receptor.

2.2. *Secondary Cause of Male Osteoporosis*

The important secondary causes of male osteoporosis are summarized in Table 2.

Table 2 Secondary Causes of Male Osteoporosis

Hypogonadism
Long-term glucocorticoid use
Alcohol and tobacco abuse
Post-transplantation
Gastrointestinal, hepatic, chronic respiratory disease
Chronic renal failure
Endocrinologic disorder (hyperparathyroidism, thyrotoxicosis)
Rheumatoid arthritis
Medications
Neoplastic disease

Hypogonadism is a well-known cause of secondary osteoporosis in men. There is evidenced association of decreased BMD with androgen deficiency. A study from Eastern Europe of men castrated for "sexual delinquency" showed rapid bone loss, particularly in the first 5 years after surgery.[17]   In a study of evaluating side effect of anti-androgen treatment for prostate cancer, it was found that BMD loss is about 3-5% yearly and osteoporotic fracture incidence increases significantly for those patients receiving androgen deprivation therapy.[18]   A recent case-control study of men with hip fractures showed a marked reduction in serum testosterone compared with the control group.[1]   Although low serum testosterone concentrations in men with hip fractures may be due in part to disturbance of the hypothalamic-pituitary-gonadal axis related to the fracture and subsequent surgery, this study suggests hypogonadism is a genuine risk factor for hip fractures in men.[7]

Recent studies indicate an important role of estrogens in the skeletal physiology of men. Higher serum estrogen concentrations are associated with higher BMD in men, independent of their serum androgen concentrations.[19,20,21]   Longitudinal data demonstrate that estrogen is an important determinant of peak bone mass in young men and bone loss in elderly men and that low serum estradiol may be the major cause of bone loss in older men.[22]

As noted above, estrogen is an important determinant of bone density in men and practically all men with hypogonadism have estrogen deficiency. The importance of estrogen was also demonstrated by the finding of osteoporosis in a man with estrogen resistance caused by a loss-of-function mutation in the estrogen receptor gene[23] and in two men with a loss-of-function mutation in the aromatase gene, which resulted in an inability to convert androgen to estrogen.[24,25]   Estrogen therapy in aromatase deficiency resulted in a marked increase in bone mass and a reduction in markers of bone turnover to normal.[25]

Glucocorticoids are widely used in medical practice for their anti-inflammatory and immunosuppressive properties. The systemic chronic use of glucocorticoids is associated with several side effects including osteoporosis. Glucocorticoids have direct and indirect effect on bone. Directly, glucocorticoids inhibit new bone formation, increase bone resorption, and cause aseptic necrosis or avascular necrosis, which all contributes to the accelerated bone loss and increased fracture risk. Indirectly, glucocorticoids induced muscle weakness due to muscle atrophy may augment the risk of fall and fracture.

The effect of glucocorticoids on BMD and fracture is mostly studied in subjects taking oral preparation, as inhaled steroid has minimum effect on suppression of the pituitary-adrenal axis. Among 244,235 glucocorticoids users who had osteoporosis and were involved in a large retrospective cohort study, about 40% of the glucocorticoids users were male. The relative rate of vertebral, non-vertebral, and hip fractures was significantly higher in oral glucocorticoids users compared with topical glucocorticoids users. The fracture risk increased rapidly after the initiation of glucocorticoids therapy as early as 3 months and at a dose as low as 2.5 mg of prednisone a day.[26] Additionally, there was a significant dose response for all fractures (except forearm fracture) with the glucocorticoids.[27]

Transplantation is an established therapy for end-stage disease of the kidney, heart, liver, and lung, and for certain hematologic conditions. The most commonly prescribed immunosuppressive drugs include cyclosporine and azathioprine. *In vitro* studies demonstrated cyclosporine inhibits bone formation in cultured bone. *In vivo* rodent studies suggest cyclosporine has independent adverse effect on bone and mineral metabolism that could contribute to bone loss after organ transplantation.[28] Furthermore, the well-known nephrotoxic effects of cyclosporine result in measurable declines in renal function, decreased synthesis of $1,25(OH)_2D_3$, and inhibition of calcium transport in the intestine. As a result, PTH secretion is increased which in turn increases osteoclast-mediated bone resorption.

The effect of drug on male osteoporosis is best exampled by the long-term antiepileptic drug therapy. To determine whether men who have seizures, but who are otherwise healthy, suffer substantial bone loss in the hip, Andress prospectively examined femoral neck BMD in 81 men aged between 25-54 years old who were on antiepileptic drugs. The results showed long-term antiepileptic drug therapy causes significant bone loss at the hip in the absence of vitamin D deficiency.[29]

Tobacco is linked to an increased prevalence of vertebral fracture in men, likely due to tobacco caused vascular ischemia. The mechanism by which alcohol induces bone loss remains unclear, although bone formation is decreased. The possible mechanism may include calcium and vitamin D deficiencies, alcohol related trauma, and hypogonadism.

3. Evaluation of Male Osteoporosis

There is no published guideline for the evaluation of osteoporosis in men. Nevertheless, evaluation of osteoporosis in men should take into account all risk factors for osteoporosis as discussed earlier.

The initial steps in evaluating osteoporosis in men include a complete medical history, physical examination, and laboratory tests to identify the various risk factors and the underlying diseases that may contribute to male osteoporosis. The recommended laboratory tests are listed in Table 3.

Osteoporosis screening tests should be considered in male patients with significant risk factors for osteoporosis, including long-term glucocorticoid use, hypogonadism, hyperparathyroidism, very low body weight, and immobilization. BMD measurement by DXA scan, heel ultrasonography, or quantitative computed tomography (QCT) should be considered in male patients who have a history of non-traumatic fracture, particularly of the hip, vertebral body, have radiographic osteopenia, and are 75 years of age or older.

Table 3. Laboratory Evaluation of Male Osteoporosis

Complete blood cell count.
Chemistry test including calcium, phosphorus, alkaline phosphatase.
Kidney and liver function test.
Hormonal tests including 25 hydroxyvitamin D level, thyroid-stimulating hormone, testosterone, and parathyroid hormone level.
Additional tests may include serum and/or urine protein electrophoresis and urinary calcium excretion.

The BMD criteria for osteoporosis developed by the World Health Organization are widely used in medical practice and clinical research and are applicable to both genders, although the experience obtained in women is greater than that in men. According to these criteria, patients with BMD at least 2.5 SD below the average value in healthy young adults (T-score <-2.5) have osteoporosis, and those with a T-score between -1 and –2.5 SD are classified as having osteopenia.[30] It should be pointed out that at any given BMD level the risk of fracture is similar between men and women and thus the above classification is applicable to both genders.

4. Prevention and Treatment of Male Osteoporosis

The principles of fracture prevention in men are similar to those in women. Calcium intake should be 1,000 to 1,500 mg per day, and vitamin D intake should be 400 to 800 IU per day. Other prevention strategies include regular weight-bearing exercise and the avoidance of excess alcohol and tobacco use. Table 4 lists the current recommended prevention strategy and the FDA approved drugs used for male osteoporosis indication.

Table 4 Male Osteoporosis Prevention and Treatment

Prevention	Drug Treatment
Risk factor modification.	Testosterone replacement.
Regular exercise to increase muscle strength.	Alendronate 10 mg per day or 70 mg per week.
Avoidance of tobacco and excess alcohol	Risedronate 5 mg per day (glucocoticoid induced osteoporosisin male).
Minimize glucocorticoid intake.	
Calcium 1,000 to 1,500 mg per day.	Teriparatide 20 µg per day.
Vitamin D 400 to 800 IU per day.	

4.1. *Testosterone*

The efficacy of testosterone in treatment of male osteoporosis due to hypogonadism is well supported by clinical practice and controlled clinical trials. An observational study examined the long-term effects of testosterone replacement on bone density in 72 (age 18-74) hypogonadal men; 37 primary hypogonadism and 35 secondary hypogonadism.[31] Patients were on testosterone replacement therapy for up to 16 years, and only 32 patients had baseline bone density measurements. Trabecular BMD of the spine was measured annually using QCT. In patients who had received no previous treatment, testosterone replacement led to a 25% increase in spine BMD. Even in those who had received treatment previously, there was a further increase in BMD of 15%. Similar increases in BMD were seen in men receiving testosterone replacement by transdermal patches and intramuscular injections.

Katznelson compared body composition and bone density in 36 hypogonadism men aged 22–69 years with 44 age-matched eugonadal control subjects.[32] Hypogonadal men had significantly higher body fat and lower spine BMD with QCT measurements compared with the eugonadal control subjects. After 18 month of weekly testosterone enathanate intramuscular injection, subjects with hypogonadism had a significant increase of spine BMD of 5% and trabecular BMD of 14%. Body fat was decreased 13% and muscle mass increased by 17%. Testosterone replacement also decreased bone turnover, as reflected by the reduction in bone-specific alkaline phosphatase and urine deoxypyridinoline excretion.

There are many FDA approved testosterone products for testosterone replacement therapy in men for conditions associated with a deficiency or absence of endogenous testosterone. These androgen products can be delivered through oral (android, Halotestin®), transdermal (Androderm®, AndroGel®), buccal mucosal (Striant® mucoadhesive), or intramuscular injection (testosterone enanthate) route. Androgen products are generally well tolerated. Prostate examination, PSA, and hematocrit levels should be assessed periodically if treatment with testosterone is initiated. Testosterone is the drug of choice in men with osteoporosis due to hypogonadism especially if serum testosterone levels are below 200 ng/dl.[33]

4.2. *Alendronate*

The effect of alendronate in treating male osteoporosis was evaluated in two prospective, controlled clinical trials. The first study was a 2-year, randomized, double-blind, multinational study that enrolled 241 men with osteoporosis.[34] Patients aged 31-87 years were randomized to receive 10 mg daily alendronate or placebo for 2 years. The primary efficacy endpoint was the percent change from baseline in lumbar spine BMD. Alendronate treatment reduced the rate of bone turnover, increased BMD of the spine by 7.1%, reduced the rate of height loss, and decreased significantly the risk of morphometric vertebral fractures. The largest increase occurred during the first 12 months, but BMD continued to increase through 24 months. Changes in BMD at other skeletal sites including femoral neck, trochanter, and hip were all statistically significantly different from placebo.

The second clinical trial that examined the efficacy of alendronate in treating male osteoporosis was an open label, prospective, comparative 2-year study of the use of alendronate 10 mg daily versus alfacalcidol 1 μg daily in 134 men with diagnosed osteoporosis.[35] All men received supplemental calcium (500 mg daily). After 2 years, alfacalcidol-treated patients showed a mean 2.8% increase in lumbar spine BMD (P < 0.01) compared with a mean increase of 10.1% in men receiving alendronate. The corresponding changes in femoral neck BMD were +2.2% and +5.2% for the alfacalcidol and alendronate groups, respectively. The incidence rates of patients with new vertebral fractures were 18.2% and 7.4% for the alfacalcidol and alendronate groups, respectively (P = 0.071). Both therapies were well tolerated. Thus, alendronate produced favorable effects on BMD.[35] Alendronate is approved by the FDA for male osteoporosis indication.

4.3. *Risedronate*

Risedronate is a FDA approved bisphosphonate with indication for glucocorticoid induced osteoporosis in men and women. In two double-blind, placebo-controlled studies, 184 men were enrolled to evaluate the effects of risedronate in patients beginning corticosteroid treatment at a dose of at least 7.5 mg daily prednisone or equivalent (prevention study) or continuing long-term treatment of corticosteroid at that dose (treatment study).[36] The men received either placebo or risedronate (2.5 mg or 5 mg) daily, along with calcium supplementation (500-1000 mg). Endpoints included differences in BMD at the lumbar spine, femoral neck, and femoral trochanter, assessment of vertebral fractures, changes in biochemical markers of bone turnover, and overall safety.

In the prevention study, bone loss was significantly prevented with risedronate 5 mg. In the placebo group, BMD decreased significantly (P < 0.01) by 3.4%, 3.3%, and 3.4% in the lumbar spine, femoral neck, and trochanter, respectively, at 1 year. In the treatment study, risedronate 5 mg significantly ($P < 0.01$) increased BMD by 4.8% at the lumbar spine, 2.1% at the femoral neck, and 2.6% at the femoral trochanter compared with baseline values. When data from the two studies were combined, the incidence of vertebral fractures decreased 82.4% in the pooled risedronate groups compared with placebo ($P = 0.008$). Risedronate was well tolerated in men, with a similar incidence of adverse events in the placebo and treatment groups.[36]

4.4. *Teriparatide*

Teriparatide [rhPTH(1-34)] is the recombinant human 1-34 N-terminal amino acid sequence of parathyroid hormone recently approved in the U.S. for the treatment of men and postmenopausal women at high risk for osteoporotic fracture.

The efficacy of teriparatide [rhPTH(1-34)] in increasing bone mineral density in men was evaluated in a large clinical trial. Four hundred thirty seven men with spine or hip BMD more than 2 SD below the young adult male mean were randomized to daily teriparatide [rhPTH(1-34)] (20 μg or 40 μg) injection or placebo. All subjects also received supplemental calcium and vitamin D. Patients receiving teriparatide [rhPTH(1-34)] 20 or 40 μg a day had statistically significant increase in BMD of lumbar spine and femoral neck from baseline. Teriparatide was well tolerated; the adverse events were similar in the placebo and 20 μg groups, but more frequent in the 40 μg group. This study demonstrated that teriparatide [rhPTH(1-34)] treatment is efficacious in increasing BMD in male osteoporosis patients.[37]

5. Summary

Osteoporosis in men has been recognized as a public health problem. Although 40-60% of male osteoporosis is idiopathic in nature, many factors could lead to and/or contribute to the development of male osteoporosis including age-related bone loss, long-term glucocorticoid use, hypogonadism, and alcohol and tobacco excess. Evaluation of male osteoporosis include thorough medical history, physical examination, laboratory tests, and BMD measurement. Treatment consists of risk factors modification, and adequate calcium and vitamin D intake. Bisphosphonates, and recently approved teriparatide [rhPTH(1-34)], should be considered for men with low BMD, history of vertebral or low trauma non-vertebral fracture, or those patients who are at increased risk for bone loss.

Acknowledgments

The authors appreciably thank Ms. Barbara McCarty-Garcia for her assistance in preparing this manuscript.

REFERENCES

1. Pande, R. M. Francis, Best. Pract. Res. Clin. Rheumatol., 415 (2001).
2. C. Cooper, E. J. Arkinson, S. J. Jacobsen, W. M. O'Fallon, L. J. Melton III, Am. J. Epidemiol., 1001 (1993).
3. O. Johnell, J. Kanis, G. Gullberg, Calcif. Tissue. Int., 182 (2001).
4. L. J. Melton, E. J. Atkinson, M. K. O'Connor, W. M. O'Fallon, B. L. Riggs, J. Bone Miner. Res., 1915 (1998).
5. C. Looker, E. S. Orwoll, C. C. Johnston, R. L. Lindsay, H. W. Wahner, W. L. Dunn, M. S. Calvo, T. B. Harris, S. P. Heyse, J. Bone Miner. Res., 1761 (1997).
6. S. Z. Xu, W. Zhou, X. D. Mao, Osteoporos. Int., 755 (2001).
7. Pande, Ph.D. Thesis, University of London (2000).
8. E. S. Orwoll, Endocrinol. Metab. Clin. North. Am., 349 (1998).
9. S. Amin, D. T. Felson, Rheum. Dis. Clin. North Am., 19 (2001).
10. R. Center, T. V. Nguyen, D. Schneider, P. N. Sambrook, J. A. Eisman, Lancet, 878 (1999).
11. E. Hills, C. R. Dunstan, S. Y. Wong, R. A. Evans, J. Clin. Pathol., 391 (1989).
12. B. E. Nordin, J. Aaron, R. Speed, et al, Scott. Med. J., 171 (1984).

13. T. V. Nguyen, G. Livshits, J. R. Center, K. Yakovenko, J. A. Eisman, J. Clin. Endocrinol. Metab., 3614 (2003).

14. P. Kannus, M. Palvanen, J. Kaprio, J. Parkkari, M. Koskenvuo, BMJ, 1334 (1999).

15. R. A. Evans, G. M. Marel, E. K. Lancaster, S. Kos, M. Evans, S. Y. Wong, Ann. Int. Med., 870 (1988).

16. S. H. Ralston, J. Clin. Endocrinol. Metab., 2460 (2002).

17. J. Stepan, M. Lachman, J. Zverina, V. Pacovsky, D. J. Baylink, J. Clin. Endocrinol. Metab., 523 (1989).

18. R. W. Ross, E. J. Small, J. Urol., 1952 (2002).

19. J. R. Center, T. V. Nguyen, P. N. Sambrook, J. A. Eisman, J. Clin. Endocrinol. Metab., 3626 (1999).

20. G. A. Greendale, S. Edelstein, E. Barrett-Connor, J. Bone Miner. Res., 1833 (1997).

21. S. Khosla, L. J. Melton III, E. J. Atkinson, W. M. O'Fallon, J. Clin. Endocrinol. Metab., 3555 (2001).

22. S. Khosla, L. J. Melton III, E. J. Atkinson, W. M. O'Fallon, G. G. Klee, B. L. Riggs, J. Clin. Endocrinol. Metab., 2266 (1998).

23. E. P. Smith, J. Boyd, G. R. Frank, H. Takahasi, R. M. Cohen, B. Specker, T. C. Williams, D. B. Lubahn, K. S. Korach, N. Engl. J. Med., 1056 (1994).

24. C. Carani, K. Qin, M. Simoni, S. Faustini-Faustini, J. Boyd, K. S. Korach, E. R. Simpson, N. Engl. J. Med., 91 (1997).

25. J. P. Bilezikian, A. Morishima, J. Bell, M. M. Grumbach, N. Engl. J. Med., 599 (1998).

26. T. P. Van Staa, H. G. M. Leufkens, L. Abenhaim, J. Bone Miner. Res., 993 (2000).

27. C. Marcocci, E. Vignali, Osteoporos. Int., S7 (2003).

28. S. Epstein, J. Bone Miner. Res., 1 (1996).

29. D. L. Andress, J. Ozuna, D. Tirschwell, Arch. Neurol., 781 (2002).

30. J. L. Kanis, L. J. Melton, C. Christiansen, C. C. Johnston, N. Khaltaev, J. Bone Miner. Res., 1137 (1994).

31. H. M. Behre, S. Kliesch, E. Leifke, T. M. Link, E. Nieschlag, J. Clin. Endocrinol. Metab., 2386 (1997).

32. Katznelson, J. S. Finkelstein, D. A. Schoenfield, D. I. Rosenthal, E. Anderson, A. Klibanski, J. Clin. Endocrinol. Metab., 4358 (1996).

33. P. J. Snyder, H. Peachey, P. Hannoush, J. A. Berlin, L. Loh, J. H. Holmes, A. Dlewati, J. Staley, J. Santanna, S. C. Kapoor, M. F. Attie, J. G. Haddad, Jr., B. L. Strom, J. Clin. Endocrinol. Metab., 1966 (1999).

34. E. Orwoll, M. Ettinger, S. L. Weiss, N. Engl. J. Med., 604 (2000).

35. J. D. Ringe, H. Faber, A. Dorst, J. Clin. Endocrinol. Metab., 5252 (2001).

36. D. M. Reid, S. Adami, J. P. Devogelaer, A. A. Chines, Calcif. Tissue Int., 242 (2001).

37. E. S. Orwoll, W. H. Scheele, S. Paul, S. Adami, U. Syversen, A. Diez-Perez, J. M. Kaufman, A. D. Clancy, G. A. Gaich, J. Bone Miner. Res., 9 (2003).

CHAPTER 13

OSTEOPOROSIS AND OSTEOARTHRITIS

Yuqing Zhang, DSc, MPH, MB

Clinical Epidemiology Research and Training Unit,
Department of Medicine
Boston University School of Medicine, Boston, Massachusetts
e-mail: yuqing@bu.edu

Osteoarthritis is one of the most common joint disorders in the elderly in China (1, 2) and throughout the world (3). Among adults 60 years of age and older in Beijing, China, prevalence of radiographic osteoarthritis was 34.1% in knee (1) and 46.0% in hand (2), whereas the prevalence of symptomatic osteoarthritis was 11.1% for knee (1) and 4.7% for hand (2). Prevalence of hip and hand osteoarthritis in the United States population is even higher than that observed in Beijing, China (2, 4). Numerous risk factors for osteoarthritis have been studied, and one that has been extensively evaluated is bone mineral density or osteoporosis.

The rarity of co-existence between osteoarthritis and osteoporosis was reported by clinicians four decades ago (5, 6). Two cases series reports indicated a general absence of osteoarthritis in excised femoral head in subjects with femoral fracture (7) or in post mortem skeleton (8). These clinical observations have led numerous investigators to examine the relationship between osteoporosis and osteoarthritis, and to explore the potential role of bone mineral density in the development of osteoarthritis.

Association between osteoporosis or bone mineral density and prevalence of osteoarthritis

In the early 1970's, Foss and Byers compared bone mineral density of patients with hip fracture to those with hip osteoarthritis (9). All participants received anteroposterior radiographs of the pelvis, hips and right hand. The presence of radiographic hip osteoarthritis was determined by changes of specific radiographic features, including joint space narrowing, sclerosis, cysts, or collapse of subchondral bone. Bone mineral density was assessed from measurement of the second metacarpal and expressed as the relative bone areas. The authors reported that among 140 patients with hip fractures, only three of them had suffered from hip osteoarthritis. On the other hand, bone mineral density was much higher among patients with hip osteoarthritis than those with hip fracture. Since then, more than 80 studies have been conducted to explore the association between bone mineral density or osteoporosis and osteoarthritis.

The evidence of an inverse relationship between osteoporosis or low bone mineral density and osteoarthritis, especially osteoarthritis of the knee and hip, comes mainly from cross-sectional epidemiologic studies. In 1991, Copper et al. examined the association between bone mass and prevalence of hip osteoarthritis among 314 men and women aged 50 and over who consecutively attended hospital for hip radiographs for non-skeletal indications (10). Bone mass was assessed using the Singh index grading system of femoral neck trabecular pattern with plain radiographs, and the degree of hip osteoarthritis was graded as normal, mild or marked. There was a statistically significant negative association between osteoporosis and osteoarthritis. However, the analysis did not adjust for weight, a strong confounding variable in the association.

In 1995, Nevitt et al. examined the association between hip osteoarthritis and bone mineral density of the hip, spine, and appendicular skeleton among 4,855 white female participants in the Study of Osteoporotic Fracture (11). Hip osteoarthritis was graded on a summary scale of 0 (no osteoarthritis) to 4 (severe osteoarthritis) based on the number of radiographic features present using pelvic radiographs. Appendicular bone density was measured in all subjects, as well as hip and spine bone mineral density in more than 50% of the participants. Women with grade 3-4 hip osteoarthritis had a higher age-adjusted bone mineral density at the femoral neck and Ward's triangle (9-10%, P < 0.001), trochanter (4%, P < 0.01), lumbar spine (8%; P < 0.01), and distal radius and calcaneus (5%, P < 0.01) compared with those with grade 0-1 osteoarthritis in the worse hip. Elevations in bone mineral density were greatest in the femoral neck of hips with osteoarthritis, in women with bilateral hip osteoarthritis, and in women with hip osteophytes. The findings were essentially unchanged by adjustment for determinants of bone mass. Similar results were also shown from the Rotterdam Study where hip radiographic osteoarthritis was associated with significantly increased bone mineral density (3-8%) in both men and women (12).

High bone mineral density has also been associated with an increased prevalence of knee osteoarthritis. In the Framingham Study (13), investigators assessed bone mineral density of the proximal femur and radius by densitometry. For each subject, a weight-bearing anteroposterior radiograph was also obtained four years previously. Radiographic knee osteoarthritis was graded from 0 to 4 based on Kellgren and Lawrence criteria in 572 women and 360 men with age range from 63 to 91. Individual radiographic features of osteoarthritis, i.e., osteophytes and joint space narrowing, were also assessed separately. Mean femoral bone mineral density at the 3 proximal femur sites was 5-9% higher in men and women with either grade 1, grade 2, or grade 3 knee osteoarthritis, compared with those with no knee osteoarthritis (P<0.001). However, mean femoral bone mineral density in those with severe osteoarthritis (Kellgren and Lawrence grade = 4) was not higher than in those with no osteoarthritis. Women with osteophytes had higher bone mineral density compared with women with no osteophytes. Mean bone mineral density did not differ across levels of joint space narrowing.

The authors hypothesized that relatively stronger association found in women may be due to different risk profiles for knee osteoarthritis between men and women. For instance, knee osteoarthritis in women may be more affected by a metabolic factor while osteoarthritis in men may be more influenced by joint injury. The study did not find an inverse association between radius bone mineral density and prevalence of knee osteoarthritis in subjects of either sex. Similar results were also reported by the investigators in the Rotterdam Study (12) where the inverse relationship between bone mineral density to the prevalence of knee osteoarthritis was much stronger in women, and higher bone mineral density levels were observed with increasing Kellgren and Lawrence scores, except for severe knee osteoarthritis, in women.

Such an inverse relationship also was found in middle-aged (14) young women (15). In 1996, Sowers et al. assessed various mechanical factors in relation to the prevalence of hand and knee osteoarthritis among 573 premenopausal women (age range: 24-45 years). Osteoarthritis was defined using two methods: 1) the presence of Kellgren and Lawrence grade $\geq$ 2, or 2) the highest joint grade in any of the joints of the hand and knee. After adjusting for several potential confounding factors, including age, body mass index, knee injury, smoking, alcohol consumption, hormonal levels and use of hormone replacement therapy, the authors reported that total body bone mineral density was significantly associated with an increased prevalence of knee osteoarthritis.

In contrast to the findings of an inverse association between bone mineral density and knee and hip osteoarthritis, the relation of bone mineral density to the prevalence of hand osteoarthritis from the cross-sectional studies is less clear (14-19). Some studies have shown that subjects with hand osteoarthritis have higher bone mineral density compared to those without such a condition, while others failed to confirm such a relation. Marcelli et al. studied the association between these two conditions among 300 healthy women aged 75 years and above (17). The authors used a hand osteoarthritis combined score, defined as the sum of the grades of joint-space narrowing, ostephytes, erosions and joint misalignment, to define the presence of hand osteoarthritis, and obtained bone mineral density measurement at a number of sites using dual-energy X-ray absorptiometry. Total body bone mineral density, upper limb bone mineral density, lower limb bone mineral density and spine bone mineral density were positively correlated with the hand osteoarthritis combined score; however, no such association was found with femoral neck or Ward's triangle bone mineral density. When the investigators divided the participants into two groups based on their hand osteoarthritis combed score ($\leq$ 20, >20), bone mineral density at all skeletal sites was significantly higher among women with combined score higher than 20 compared to those with score $\leq$ 20.

However, results from other studies failed to confirm such an association. In the middle 1990's, Hochberg and colleagues examined the relation of appendicular bone mass to the prevalence of hand osteoarthritis in 238 white women aged 40 and above (16). Bilateral hand radiographs taken between 1978 and 1991 were read for grade of osteoarthritis using Kellgren-Lawrence scales. Two measures of appendicular bone mass, percent cortical area of the second metacarpal and bone mineral density of the distal radius measured with single photon absorptiometry, were assessed at the same visit. After adjustment for age and body mass index, neither of these measures of appendicular bone mass was associated with the severity of hand osteoarthritis. More recently, Schneider et al. looked at this issue among subjects with clinically diagnosed hand osteoarthritis and community-dwelling, ambulatory white adults (19). Clinically diagnosed hand osteoarthritis was not associated with an increased bone mineral density in either men or women. Contrary to expectations; the only significant difference was that women with hand osteoarthritis had lower bone mineral density at the hip.

Results also varied when different definition was used to define osteoarthritis. For instance, Sowers et al (15) showed that women with the highest grades of hand osteoarthritis had high total body bone mineral density; however, when the hand osteoarthritis was defined as present or absent based on the Kellgren and Lawrence grade (<2 or $\geq$ 2), No difference in total bone mineral density was found between subjects with and without hand osteoarthritis.

Few studies also examined the relationship between osteoarthritis at the lumbar spine and osteoporosis at the spine and other sites of the body, and the results indicated that increased bone mineral density at the spine increases the prevalence of osteoarthritis at the lumbar spine

(20-22). However, some investigators argue that such an inverse association may be attributed to the fact that lumbar osteophytosis and apophyseal osteoarthritis may generate a spuriously increased lumbar bone mineral density.

In summary, results from cross-sectional epidemiologic studies suggested that lower bone mineral density or osteoporosis is associated with a low prevalence of knee or hip osteoarthritis, especially in women. Data also suggest that bone mineral density appears to be more strongly associated with osteophytes than with joint space narrowing. Only a few studies have examined the relationship of these two diseases in men, and the number of male participants, in general, is small; thus, the evidence of an inverse association between osteoporosis and osteoarthritis is not as strong in men as that in women.

Relation of osteoporosis or bone mineral density to the incidence or progression of osteoarthritis

The findings of bone mineral density or osteoporosis in relation to the risk of osteoarthritis or vice versa are complex and intriguing. In the Framingham Osteoarthritis Study, Zhang et al. reported that the effect of bone mineral density and bone mineral density change on the risk of incident knee osteoarthritis is different from that on the risk of progression of knee radiographic osteoarthritis in elderly women (23). The participants in the study received anteroposterior weight bearing knee radiographs at biennial examinations 18 (1983-85) and 22 (1992-93), and femoral neck bone mineral density was assessed using dual photon absorptiometry between 1987-89 and dual x-ray absorptiometry between 1992-93. Two separate indicators were used to define the occurrence and progression of knee osteoarthritis, i.e., the newly developed knee osteoarthritis (incident) and worsening of knee osteoarthritis (progression). Over 8 years of follow-up, the risk of incident radiographic knee osteoarthritis increased from 5.6% among women in the lowest age-specific quartile of bone mineral density at the femoral neck to 14.2, 10.3, and 11.8% among women in the second, third, and highest quartiles, respectively. Multivariable adjusted odds ratios of incident osteoarthritis for each increase quartile of bone mineral density were 1.0, 2.5, 2.0, and 2.3, respectively (p for trend = 0.2). This effect was mainly reflected in an increased risk of osteophytes development. However, risk of progressive osteoarthritis decreased from 34.4 to 22.0, 20.3, and 18.9% as bone mineral density increased. Compared to those in the lowest quartile of bone mineral density, adjusted odds ratios for progressive disease were 0.3, 0.2, and 0.1 among women in the second, third, and highest quartiles (p for trend <0.001), respectively, mainly due to its effect on lowering the risk of joint space loss. Compared to those who lost bone mineral density more than 0.04 g/cm^2 over the followup period, women who gained bone mineral density were at increased risk of incident but at a significantly decreased risk of progressive knee osteoarthritis. Changes in bone mineral density were not associated with osteophyte development, but gain in bone mineral density lowered the risk of joint space loss.

Later, Hart et al reported similar findings using data from the Chingford Study (24). In that study, bone mineral density measurements of the lumbar spine and hip and radiographs of the hands and knees were obtained at baseline, and knee radiographs were repeated 48 months later from 830 white women. Baseline bone mineral density at the lumbar spine and hip was much higher among women with incident knee osteophytes than those without incident disease. In contrast, bone mineral density at the hip was modestly reduced by 2.5% among women whose osteophytes progressed when compared with non-progressors, although the relation was not statistically significant. These findings suggest that bone mineral density may play different roles in the incidence and progression of osteoarthritis.

Several studies also found that individuals with osteoarthritis have an increased rate of bone loss. Sowers et al showed that women who have developed hand osteoarthritis were more likely to have higher baseline bone mass than women who did not develop osteoarthritis, but that these women had a greater likelihood of bone loss over time (25). Later, two other studies also demonstrated that subjects with hip and knee osteoarthritis are at an increased risk of bone loss (12, 26). More recently, Schneider and colleagues (19) indicated that women with clinically diagnosed hand osteoarthritis had significantly lower bone mineral density at the hip than their community dwelling counterparts. No such relation, however, was found among men. Interestingly, in another cohort study, Sowers, et al. showed that women with knee osteoarthritis were less likely than those without radiographic disease to lose bone over 3 years of follow-up; in addition, levels of osteocalcin, a marker of bone turnover, were lower in women with knee and hand osteoarthritis than in women without the disease (27).

A few investigators also assessed the subchondral bone mineral density to the risk of osteoarthritis. For example, Dieppe et al (28) found that patients with increased capitation of the tracer during skeletal scintigraphy, an indication of high risk of progressive cartilage loss, experienced a 10% decrease in tibial subchondral bone mineral density over the five-year study period. However, in another study, Bruyere et al. reported that high subchondral bone mineral density was significantly associated with an increased joint space loss (p = 0.02). And compared to those in the lowest quartile of baseline bone mineral density (<0.73 g/cm^2), subjects in the highest quartile of bone mineral density (>0.96 g/cm^2) experienced more joint space narrowing (p = 0.03). The findings, however, were based on a small number of patients.

In summary, the effect of bone mineral density on the course of the natural history of osteoarthritis and the impact of osteoarthritis on bone loss have only recently been studied in large population samples. Results from cohort studies have shown that the relationship between osteoporosis or bone mineral density and osteoarthritis, or vice versa, is more complex than was recognized from cross-sectional studies. The discrepancies of relationship of bone mineral density to incidence of osteoarthritis from that to progression of osteoarthritis are not fully understood. Osteoarthritis is a process characterized by increased subchondral trabecular thickness and bony sclerosis (29). This increased trabecular thickness might be caused by trabecular microfractures (30). The association between bone mineral density and osteoarthritis can also be explained by local bone remodeling secondary to osteoarthritis, and whether osteoarthritis is able to progress or to stabilize depends on the bone's ability to respond with remodeling (31, 32). Other investigators argued that systematically high bone mineral density might be correlated with the local increased bone thickness and connectivity in the bone plate beneath the cartilage (33), thus, high bone mineral density might contribute to the occurrence of osteoarthritis. To date, no consensus has been reached with regard to the association between these two conditions. And more research work needs to be performed to address this important issue.

Possible mechanisms underlying the relationship between osteoporosis and osteoarthritis

The potential role of bone mineral density in the development of osteoarthritis has been the topic of considerable speculation. This is because the relation between osteoporosis and osteoarthritis is relevant not only for our understanding of the pathogenesis of these two conditions, but also for the development of appropriate management for both osteoarthritis and osteoporosis, especially if treatment for one could theoretically increase the risk for the other.

In the early 1970's, Radin et al (30) suggested that bone stiffness from microtrabecular fractures and their subsequent healing could influence the stiffness of the subchondral bone, and that high subchondral bone mineral density rendered the articular cartilage more susceptible to mechanical stress. However, this hypothesis has been challenged by both animal (34) and human studies (11, 13, 14) in which bone mineral density was strongly associated with osteophytes instead of joint space narrowing, suggesting that high bone mineral density was not directly linked with cartilage loss, a major pathological features of osteoarthritis. More recently, however, osteoarthritis has been relabeled as a whole organ disease because pathological abnormalities are also present in periarticular muscle, ligaments, synovium, the neurosensory system, as well as in bone (35).

Some investigators argue that the inverse association between these two conditions can be attributed to their sharing of similar risk factors. For example, numerous studies have shown that a high body weight is strongly associated with a decreased risk of osteoporosis but associated with an increased risk of osteoarthritis. However, in more recently published studies that have adequately adjusted for body weight (13, 36), the association between these two conditions still exists.

Normal bone metabolism is contingent on the presence of vitamin D. Low tissue levels of vitamin D may impair the ability of bone to respond optimally to processes in osteoarthritis and predispose to progression. Vitamin D may also have different effects on chondrocytes in osteoarthritic cartilage, which has been shown to redevelop vitamin D receptors (37). Observational data from the Framingham Study (38) suggested that the risk for progression of knee osteoarthritis was increased three-fold for individuals in the middle and low tertiles of vitamin D intake and serum levels. However, vitamin D was not associated with risk of incident radiographic knee osteoarthritis. Further evidence of the protective effect of vitamin D on hip osteoarthritis was also shown in the Study of Osteoporotic Fractures (39).

The high incidence of osteoarthritis in women just after menopause has prompted several investigators to examine the role of estrogen in the development of osteoarthritis. Cohort studies have reported that women taking estrogen have a decreased prevalence (40) and incidence (41) of radiographic osteoarthritis. On the other hand, women with high lifetime exposure to endogenous and exogenous estrogens tend to have high bone mineral density. If osteoporosis or low bone mineral density genuinely protects against osteoarthritis, postmenopausal estrogen use might lead to an increased risk of osteoarthritis. The underlying mechanisms for the relation of estrogen levels and osteoarthritis are still not understood. It has been speculated that estrogen exposure could slow the subchondral bone changes and bone turnover that are associated with the progression of knee and hip osteoarthritis (3).

Several lines of evidence also suggest that some growth factors may play a role in linking these two conditions. Autopsy specimens obtained from osteophytes and cartilage of the femoral head in patients with hip osteoarthritis revealed high levels of transforming growth factor beta 1 (TGF-ß1) when compared with control specimens (42). Repeated intra-articular injection of TGF-ß1 into the knees of normal mice results in the development of osteochondral tissue at the margin of the cartilage (43).

In addition, high levels of TGF-ß1 have been found in the synovial fluid of joints with osteoarthritis (44). As other investigators have speculated, TGF-ß1 and other circulating growth factors may provide a bone–forming stimulus that links osteophytes formation in early osteoarthritis with high bone mineral density. Allelic variation at the TGF-ß1 gene have been associated with the development of osteoporosis at the hip (45). However, it is not known whether levels of TGF-ß1 in osteoarthritis joints are related to systemic or periarticular bone metabolism or bone growth factor content. The high levels of TGF-ß1 in synovial fluid in osteoarthritis may be explained by studies that demonstrate that TGF-ß1-receptor messenger RNA levels are dramatically reduced in chondrocytes from osteoarthritic cartilage (46). Loss of receptor responsiveness to TGF-ß1 promotes chondrocytes terminal differentiation and results in the development of degenerative joint disease. This receptor is required for TGF-ß1 to bind and form a complex to transmit a signal, and with a diminished receptor number, there would be excess TGF-ß1 in the joint.

Conclusion

The relation between osteoporosis or bone mineral density and osteoarthritis is complex. An inverse association between osteoporosis and osteoarthritis reported by many cross-sectional epidemiologic studies has been challenged by recent findings from several population-based cohort studies. Further researches should focus on whether, and how, periarticular bone changes contribute to progressive loss of joint function, how this process is influenced by systemic determinants of bone metabolism, and whether medications that electively manipulate bone resumption and bone formation for therapeutic purpose has a role to play in the prevention and treatment of osteoarthritis.

 Y. Q. Zhang

REFERENCES

1. Zhang Y, Xu L, Nevitt MC, et al. Comparison of the prevalence of knee osteoarthritis between the elderly Chinese population in Beijing and whites in the United States: The Beijing Osteoarthritis Study. *Arthritis Rheum.* 2001;44(9):2065-71.

2. Zhang Y, Xu L, Nevitt MC, et al. Lower prevalence of hand osteoarthritis among Chinese subjects in Beijing compared with white subjects in the United States: the Beijing Osteoarthritis Study. *Arthritis Rheum.* 2003;48(4):1034-40.

3. Felson DT, Lawrence RC, Dieppe PA, et al. Osteoarthritis: new insights. Part 1: the disease and its risk factors. *Ann Intern Med.* 2000;133(8):635-46.

4. Nevitt MC, Xu L, Zhang YQ, et al. Very low prevalence of hip osteoarthritis among Chinese elderly in Beijing compared to Caucasians in the U.S.: the Beijing Osteoarthritis Study. *Arthritis Rheum.* 2002;in press.

5. Rechtman AM, Yarrow MW. Osteoporosis. *Am Pract Dig Treat.* 1954;5(9):691-6.

6. de S, Renier JC, Rakic M. [Vertebral arthrosis and osteoporosis. Comparative incidence of discovertebral arthrosis in 2 groups of subjects of comparable age: osteoporotics and non-osteoporotics]. *Rev Rhum Mal Osteoartic.* 1962;29:237-43.

7. Healey JH, Vigorita VJ, Lane JM. The coexistence and characteristics of osteoarthritis and osteoporosis. *J Bone Joint Surg Am.* 1985;67(4):586-92.

8. Byers PD, Contepomi CA, Farkas TA. A post mortem study of the hip joint. Including the prevalence of the features of the right side. *Ann Rheum Dis.* 1970;29(1):15-31.

9. Foss MV, Byers PD. Bone density, osteoarthrosis of the hip, and fracture of the upper end of the femur. *Ann Rheum Dis.* 1972;31(4):259-64.

10. Cooper C, Cook PL, Osmond C, Fisher L, Cawley MI. Osteoarthritis of the hip and osteoporosis of the proximal femur. *Ann Rheum Dis.* 1991;50(8):540-2.

11. Nevitt MC, Lane NE, Scott JC, et al. Radiographic osteoarthritis of the hip and bone mineral density. The Study of Osteoporotic Fractures Research Group. *Arthritis Rheum.* 1995;38(7):907-16.

12. Burger H, van Daele PL, Odding E, et al. Association of radiographically evident osteoarthritis with higher bone mineral density and increased bone loss with age. The Rotterdam Study. *Arthritis Rheum.* 1996;39(1):81-6.

13. Hannan MT, Anderson JJ, Zhang Y, Levy D, Felson DT. Bone mineral density and knee osteoarthritis in elderly men and women. The Framingham Study. *Arthritis Rheum.* 1993;36(12):1671-80.

14.   Hart DJ, Mootoosamy I, Doyle DV, Spector TD. The relationship between osteoarthritis and osteoporosis in the general population: the Chingford Study. *Ann Rheum Dis.* 1994;53(3):158-62.

15.   Sowers MF, Hochberg M, Crabbe JP, Muhich A, Crutchfield M, Updike S. Association of bone mineral density and sex hormone levels with osteoarthritis of the hand and knee in premenopausal women. *Am J Epidemiol.* 1996;143(1):38-47.

16.   Hochberg MC, Lethbridge-Cejku M, Scott WW, Jr., Plato CC, Tobin JD. Appendicular bone mass and osteoarthritis of the hands in women: data from the Baltimore Longitudinal Study of Aging. *J Rheumatol.* 1994;21(8):1532-6.

17.   Marcelli C, Favier F, Kotzki PO, Ferrazzi V, Picot MC, Simon L. The relationship between osteoarthritis of the hands, bone mineral density, and osteoporotic fractures in elderly women. *Osteoporos Int.* 1995;5(5):382-8.

18.   Belmonte-Serrano MA, Bloch DA, Lane NE, Michel BE, Fries JF. The relationship between spinal and peripheral osteoarthritis and bone density measurements. *J Rheumatol.* 1993;20(6):1005-13.

19.   Schneider DL, Barrett-Connor E, Morton DJ, Weisman M. One mineral density and clinical hand osteoarthritis in elderly men and women: the Rancho Bernardo study. *J Rheumatol.* 2002;29(7):1467-72.

20.   Peel NF, Barrington NA, Blumsohn A, Colwell A, Hannon R, Eastell R. Bone mineral density and bone turnover in spinal osteoarthrosis. *Ann Rheum Dis.* 1995;54(11):867-71.

21.   Masud T, Langley S, Wiltshire P, Doyle DV, Spector TD. Effect of spinal osteophytosis on bone mineral density measurements in vertebral osteoporosis. *Bmj.* 1993;307(6897):172-3.

22.   Jones G, Nguyen T, Sambrook PN, Kelly PJ, Eisman JA. A longitudinal study of the effect of spinal degenerative disease on bone density in the elderly. *J Rheumatol.* 1995;22(5):932-6.

23.   Zhang Y, Hannan MT, Chaisson CE, et al. Bone mineral density and risk of incident and progressive radiographic knee osteoarthritis in women: the Framingham Study. *J Rheumatol.* 2000;27(4):1032-7.

24.   Hart DJ, Cronin C, Daniels M, Worthy T, Doyle DV, Spector TD. The relationship of bone density and fracture to incident and progressive radiographic osteoarthritis of the knee: the Chingford Study. *Arthritis Rheum.* 2002;46(1):92-9.

25.   Sowers M, Zobel D, Weissfeld L, Hawthorne VM, Carman W. Progression of osteoarthritis of the hand and metacarpal bone loss. A twenty-year followup of incident cases. *Arthritis Rheum.* 1991;34(1):36-42.

26.   Arden NK, Nevitt MC, Lane NE, et al. Osteoarthritis and risk of falls, rates of bone loss, and osteoporotic fractures. Study of Osteoporotic Fractures Research Group. *Arthritis Rheum.* 1999;42(7):1378-85.

27.   Sowers M, Lachance L, Jamadar D, et al. The associations of bone mineral density and bone turnover markers with osteoarthritis of the hand and knee in pre- and perimenopausal women. *Arthritis Rheum.* 1999;42(3):483-9.

28. Dieppe P, Cushnaghan J, Young P, Kirwan J. Prediction of the progression of joint space narrowing in osteoarthritis of the knee by bone scintigraphy. *Ann Rheum Dis*. 1993;52(8):557-63.

29. Carlson CS, Loeser RF, Purser CB, Gardin JF, Jerome CP. Osteoarthritis in cynomolgus macaques. III: Effects of age, gender, and subchondral bone thickness on the severity of disease. *J Bone Miner Res*. 1996;11(9):1209-17.

30. Radin EL. Mechanical aspects of osteoarthrosis. *Bull Rheum Dis*. 1976;26(7):862-5.

31. Fazzalari NL, Darracott J, Vernon-Roberts B. Histomorphometric changes in the trabecular structure of a selected stress region in the femur in patients with osteoarthritis and fracture of the femoral neck. *Bone*. 1985;6(3):125-33.

32. Gilbertson EM. Development of periarticular osteophytes in experimentally induced osteoarthritis in the dog. A study using microradiographic, microangiographic, and fluorescent bone-labelling techniques. *Ann Rheum Dis*. 1975;34(1):12-25.

33. Buckland-Wright JC, Lynch JA, Macfarlane DG. Fractal signature analysis measures cancellous bone organisation in macroradiographs of patients with knee osteoarthritis. *Ann Rheum Dis*. 1996;55(10):749-55.

34. Dedrick DK, Goldstein SA, Brandt KD, O'Connor BL, Goulet RW, Albrecht M. A longitudinal study of subchondral plate and trabecular bone in cruciate-deficient dogs with osteoarthritis followed up for 54 months. *Arthritis Rheum*. 1993;36(10):1460-7.

35. Brandt KD, Lohmader LS, Doherty M. Pathogenesis of osteoarthritis-Introduction the concept of osteoarthritis as failure of the diarthrodial joint. In: Brandt KD, Doherty M, Lohmader LS, eds. *Osteoarthritis*. New York: Oxford Unversity Press; 1998:70-4.

36. Nevitt MC, lane NE, Scott JC, Genant HK, Hochberg MC. Relationship of hip osteoarthritis to obesity and bone mineral density in older American women:preliminary results from the Study of Osteoporotic Fractures. *Acta Orthop Scand*. 1993;64(suppl):2-5.

37. Bhalla AK, Wojno WC, Goldring MB. Human articular chondrocytes acquire 1,25-(OH)2 vitamin D-3 receptors in culture. *Biochim Biophys Acta*. 1987;931(1):26-32.

38. McAlindon TE, Felson DT, Zhang Y, et al. Relation of dietary intake and serum levels of vitamin D to progression of osteoarthritis of the knee among participants in the Framingham Study. *Ann Intern Med*. 1996;125(5):353-9.

39. Lane NE, Gore LR, Cummings SR, et al. Serum vitamin D levels and incident changes of radiographic hip osteoarthritis: a longitudinal study. Study of Osteoporotic Fractures Research Group. *Arthritis Rheum*. 1999;42(5):854-60.

40. Nevitt MC, Cummings SR, Lane NE, et al. Association of estrogen replacement therapy with the risk of osteoarthritis of the hip in elderly white women. Study of Osteoporotic Fractures Research Group. *Arch Intern Med*. 1996;156(18):2073-80.

41. Zhang Y, McAlindon TE, Hannan MT, et al. Estrogen replacement therapy and worsening of radiographic knee osteoarthritis: the Framingham Study. *Arthritis Rheum.* 1998;41(10):1867-73.

42. Uchino M, Izumi T, Tominaga T, et al. Growth factor expression in the osteophytes of the human femoral head in osteoarthritis. *Clin Orthop.* 2000(377):119-25.

43. van Beuningen HM, Glansbeek HL, van der Kraan PM, van den Berg WB. Osteoarthritis-like changes in the murine knee joint resulting from intra-articular transforming growth factor-beta injections. *Osteoarthritis Cartilage.* 2000;8(1):25-33.

44. Pujol JP. TGF-beta and osteoarthritis: in vivo veritas? *Osteoarthritis Cartilage.* 1999;7(5):439-40.

45. Keen RW, Snieder H, Molloy H, et al. Evidence of association and linkage disequilibrium between a novel polymorphism in the transforming growth factor beta 1 gene and hip bone mineral density: a study of female twins. *Rheumatology (Oxford).* 2001;40(1):48-54.

46. Serra R, Johnson M, Filvaroff EH, et al. Expression of a truncated, kinase-defective TGF-beta type II receptor in mouse skeletal tissue promotes terminal chondrocyte differentiation and osteoarthritis. *J Cell Biol.* 1997;139(2):541-52.

CHAPTER 14

OSTEOPOROSIS IN PEDIATRICS

Horacio Plotkin, M.D. and Richard Lutz, M.D.
Inherited Metabolic Diseases Section,
Department of Pediatrics
University of Nebraska Medical Center and
Children's Hospital, Omaha, Nebraska
E-mail: hplotkin@unmc.edu
rlutz@unmc.edu

1. Introduction

There has been no consensus about a definition for "osteoporosis" in pediatrics. Furthermore, to our knowledge there are no large studies published showing the relationship of bone density (areal or volumetric) and occurrence of fractures in the pediatric population. For example, children with mild osteogenesis imperfecta (OI), who may not suffer fractures, usually have bone mineral densities (as measured by DEXA) that are several standard deviations below the mean for their ages. The WHO definition of "osteopenia" and "osteoporosis" in adults, certainly does not apply to the pediatric population, particularly because T scores can not be used as reference [1]. Among pediatric bone specialists, bone density by DEXA is considered "abnormal" when it is more than 2 standard deviations above or below the mean value for age. Reference values for different devices have been published [2-8], although accurate reference data for infants is lacking. Weight, height and bone age influence the bone density results [9-13], and they should be taken into consideration when interpreting results. Today, DEXA is the method most commonly used to assess bone density in pediatrics. The technique has several drawbacks and technical issues that makes it sometimes difficult to diagnose osteoporosis with certainty [14]. DEXA is a two-dimensional measurement of a three-dimensional object. Rotation of the vertebrae in the case of scoliosis, vertebral deformities in the case of spina bifida, presence of hardware (e.g. a shunt, metallic rods, etc.) and vertebral fractures can make interpretation of the results difficult. Also, bone density should be measured in at least two different regions. Patients with cerebral palsy, for example, spend most of the time in the sitting position, which creates a mechanical stimulation to their spines, whereas their hips do not support any weight. Measuring only the lumbar spine can give a falsely normal or near-normal result. For these reasons, bone density should not be used as the sole outcome of clinical research studies in children. Recently, some publications have reported results of "volumetric" vertebral bone density based on the 2-dimentional bone density reported by DEXA [15]. The formula for vBMD is vBMD = BMC/(projection area)$^{1.5}$. This approach assumes a perfectly cubic vertebra, and should be used with caution in the case of patients with vertebral fractures, in whom the result of vBMD will be artificially higher. There are other methods to measure bone density (e.g. QCT, ultrasound, pQCT; see chapter 6) but their use has not been generalized to pediatrics.

Bone mass acquisition during childhood and adolescence has been regarded as an important risk factor for osteoporosis in adult age [16, 17]. It is well known that peak bone mass accretion is attained around puberty [3, 18]. Some authors have even suggested that postmenopausal osteoporosis may have its basis during childhood [19, 20]. Adequate calcium intake during growth may influence peak bone density, and may be a very important step in preventing subsequent postmenopausal and senile osteoporosis. Calcium intake during adolescence appears to affect skeletal calcium retention directly, and a daily calcium intake of up to 1600 mg may be required. [21]. Dietary habits can influence bone acquisition during adolescence. Interestingly, the components of soda beverages (e.g. sugar, caffeine, phosphate) could not be linked to decrease bone mass in teenagers [22]. Particularly, phosphate intake does not appear to affect calcium absorption [23]. Effects of consuming soda beverages appear to have an effect on bone related to milk displacement [24]. Calcium supplements may be necessary in children that consume low amounts of dairy products. Calcium carbonate, calcium lactate, calcium sulfate and calcium citrate appear to have similar absorption rates when administered as supplements [25, 26]. Gastric acid is not necessary for absorption of even poorly soluble preparations, as long as they are taken with meals [27].

It has been noted that health professionals working in almost any pediatric specialty will eventually come across cases of children with metabolic bone disease, either primary or secondary. Growing bones are particularly sensitive to injury; therefore there are many conditions that cause osteoporosis in children, including primary bone conditions and osteoporosis secondary to systemic diseases (Table 1).

Table 1. Causes of osteoporosis in pediatric patients

Primary
- Osteogenesis imperfecta (brittle bones disease)
- Syndromes resembling osteogenesis imperfecta
- Idiopathic Juvenile Osteoporosis
- Rickets
    - Nutritional
    - Prematurity
    - Genetic
    - Neoplastic
- Hypophosphatasia
- Hyperphosphatasia
- Parathyroid Disorders
- Primary hypomagnesemia
- Ehlers-Danlos Syndrome
- Marfan syndrome

Secondary
- Endocrine causes
    - Type I diabetes mellitus
    - Cushing syndrome
    - Anorexia Nervosa
    - Turner Syndrome
    - Hypogonadism
    - Hyperprolactinemia

Table 1. (cont'd)

- Gastroenterologic causes
  - Malabsorption
  - chronic liver disease
  - Total parenteral nutrition
  - Cystic fibrosis

- Inborn errors of metabolism
  - Galactosemia
  - Lysinuric protein intolerance
  - Glycogen storage diseases
  - Gaucher disease
  - Phenylketonuria

- Neurological causes
  - Cerebral palsy
  - Spina bifida
  - Muscular dystrophy

- Renal causes
  - Renal osteodystrophy
  - Fanconi Syndrome
  - Renal Tubular Acidosis

- Drugs/toxics
  - Corticosteroids
  - Anticonvulsants
  - Aluminum-containing antacids
  - Rifampicin
  - Cadmium, Lead
  - Heparin
  - Methotrexate, cyclosporine
  - Medroxyprogesterone acetate, GnRH agonists

- Other causes
  - Prolonged immobilization
  - Transplant
  - Malignancy

2. Primary osteoporosis in pediatrics

2.1. Nutritional Rickets

Rickets is caused by a defective mineralization of cartilage in the growth plate. Therefore, only children can have rickets, whereas osteomalacia (defective mineralization in bone) can occur in both children and adults [28]. There are different causes for rickets, namely nutritional, genetic, drug-induced and rickets of prematurity. Pettifor [29] has classified the causes of rickets in "calciopenic" (e.g. alterations of vitamin D metabolism and dietary calcium deficiency), "phosphopenic" (e.g. dietary phosphorus deficiency, impaired intestinal phosphate absorption, increased renal phosphate loss), and "inhibition of mineralization" (e.g. hereditary hypophosphatasia, aluminum toxicity, fluoride toxicity and first generation bisphosphonates).

Vitamin D is absorbed primarily in the jejunum. Absorption of oral doses ranges from 55% to 99%. There are two main sources of vitamin D for humans: vitamin D3 (cholecalciferol), produced by the skin after UV radiation (290-320 nm), and vitamin D2, (ergosterol), provided by vegetal sources. Both have identical biological actions. Vitamins D2 and D3 are concentrated in the liver, where hydroxylation in position 25 occurs by a microsomal and mitochondrial enzyme, generating 25 (OH) vitamin D3 [30]. Measurements in serum of 25 (OH) vitamin D3 give an indication of the nutritional vitamin D status of the patient. 25 (OH) vitamin D3 is hydroxylated again in the kidneys. Hydroxylation in position 1 in the mitochondria yields 1,25 (OH)2 vitamin D3 (calcitriol), that is at least 10 times more potent than 25 (OH) vitamin D3. Although calcitriol is considered to be the most active form of the vitamin, at least 30 other metabolites are generated by the kidney [31], and their biological significance is not clear. Particularly, 24,25 (OH)2 vitamin D3 may have biological role, or may regulate the production of 1,25 (OH)2 vitamin D3.

Nutritional rickets can be the product of low vitamin D content in breast milk in the case of infants feed exclusively with mother's milk. Breast milk vitamin D content of breast milk varies from 4-100 IU/L

[32]. This means that an infant would have to drink at least four liters of breast milk/day to receive 400 IU of vitamin D. Vitamin D reserve of the neonate is dependent on mother's vitamin D status. As vitamin D is produced by the skin after exposure to UV light, low or no sun exposure of infants can cause rickets, particularly if the infant has dark skin.

Hypovitaminosis D in the mother can cause congenital rickets [33]. Also, chronic anticonvulsant therapy may cause rickets, regardless of good vitamin D intake. This is more common with Phenobarbital and Phenytoin. The main mechanism is related to induction of hepatic cytochrome P-450 hydroxylation, generating inactive metabolites [34]. 25-hyidroxy vitamin D levels were reported to be low in children on chronic anticonvulsant therapy [35] and the number of fractures found to be associated with the use of anticonvulsants in patients with cerebral palsy in an institution [36]. A different study did not find a relationship between serum 25 (OH) vitamin D levels and use of anticonvulsants in patients with cerebral palsy [37] On the other hand, calcitriol levels in plasma are reportedly not low in patients taking medication for seizures [38, 39]. Different medications may affect bone in different ways. It is not clear what dose of vitamin D is required to prevent this type of rickets, or even if any supplementation is needed at all [39]. Possibly 800-1,000 IU/day, plus good calcium intake, would be sufficient.

The pathophysiology of rickets is not completely understood, as the role of the many vitamin D metabolites is not clear. Interestingly, calcitriol levels can be normal in patients with rickets, suggesting that it is not the only active form of the vitamin [40, 41]. It has even been suggested that calcidiol might function as an agonist for calcitriol [42].

Clinical features of patients with rickets are summarized in Table 2, and a typical radiograph can be seen in Figure 1.

There are different treatment modalities for rickets. It has been estimated that a young adult exposed to sunlight in the whole body, at a dose causing minimal erythema, generates an amount of vitamin D equivalent to 10,000 IU of vitamin D3 [43]. Rickets can be treated orally with 5,000 to 15,000 IU/day of vitamin D for 3-4 weeks [44]. In cases when compliance can not be assured, 100,000-500,000 IU can be given PO or IM every 6 months, although 600,000 IU in a single dose may be sufficient [45]. Calcium intake must be optimized at the same time.

 H. Plotkin and R. Lutz

Calcium, phosphorus and PTH should normalize in 1 to 3 weeks, whereas alkaline phosphatase remains elevated for several months. Radiological lesions and clinical symptoms improve rapidly with treatment.

Table 2. Clinical features of rickets

• Infant: seizures, apnea, tetany
• Delay in motor milestones
• Hypotonia
• Enlargement of wrists
• Progressive bowing of long bones
• Rachitic rosary
• Harrison's sulcus
• "Violin case" deformity of the chest
• Late closure of anterior fontanelle
• Parietal and frontal bossing
• Craniotabes
• Craniosynostosis
• Delay in teeth eruption
• Enamel hypoplasia
• Osteoporosis
• Myopathy with N deep tendon reflexes
• Prone to infections (impaired fagocytosis and neutrophil motility)
• X-rays:
• Widening of ephyphisial plate
• Cupping
• Deformities in shaft of long bones
• X-rays of the costochondral junction are not useful in the diagnosis of rickets.
• Healing: broadened bands of increased density

2.2. *Vitamin D pseudodeficiency (PDDR)*

Albright et al. [46] were the first to publish the concept of hormonal resistance when they described rickets resistant to vitamin D therapy in 1937. This was probably a case of X-linked hypophosphatemic rickets. Prader et al. [47] later described a form of vitamin D resistant rickets. The physiopathology of this genetic disease has been elucidated, and it is now known that it is caused by a defect in the conversion of calcidiol (25 (OH) vitamin D3) to calcitriol by the 1αhydroxylase in the kidney

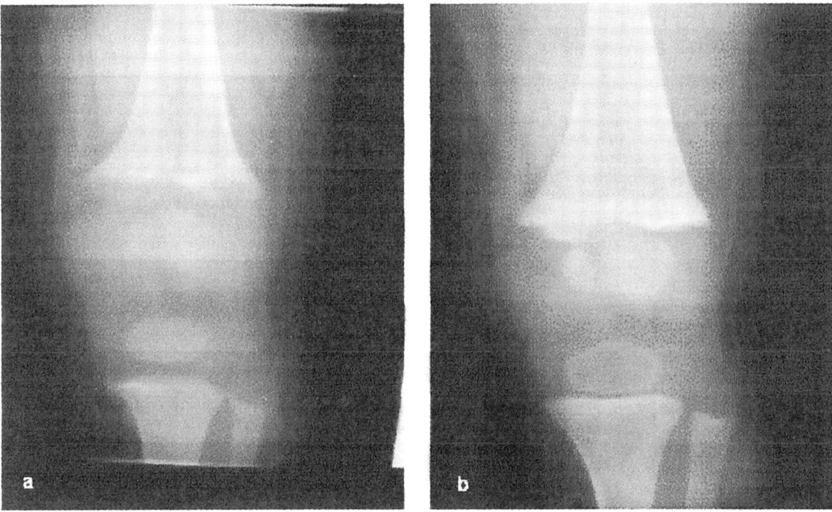

Figure 1. X-rays showing typical features of vitamin D deficiency rickets in an 8 mo. old boy (a), and the changes after 3 months of treatment (b).

[48, 49]. For this reason, patients have low levels of 1,25 (OH)2 vitamin D in serum, clinical signs of rickets, and they respond to treatment with calcitriol.Furthermore, an injection of PTH extract will fail to increase the serum levels of 1,25 (OH)2 vitamin D in these patients [50]. This condition is autosomal recessive [51], and is particularly common in northeastern Quebec, Canada [52]. Reconstruction of the genealogy showed most of the obligate carriers of the mutated VDD1 gene to be related to a small set of founders who settled in New France in the 17th century [52]. The genetic defect has been mapped to chromosome 12q14 by linkage analysis [53]. These patients usually have no clinical manifestations at birth, but during the first two years of life, muscle weakness, poor gross motor development, irritability or growth retardation become evident [54]. Physical and radiological signs are similar to those of nutritional rickets (Figure 2). Biochemical studies will show that calcium, phosphate and 1,25 (OH)2 vitamin D levels are low,

and serum alkaline phosphatase activity and PTH are above normal, while 25 (OH) vitamin D levels are usually within normal limits [55-57]. It is of note that levels of 1,25 (OH)2 vitamin D can be inadequately low for the levels of calcium, phosphorus and PTH [58]. Calcitriol treatment [59] rapidly restores biochemical parameters to normality and dramatically improves signs and symptoms of rickets. During pregnancy there is normally an increase of calcitriol circulating levels [60], therefore calcitriol doses should be increased, usually doubled, during the second half of pregnancy [61].

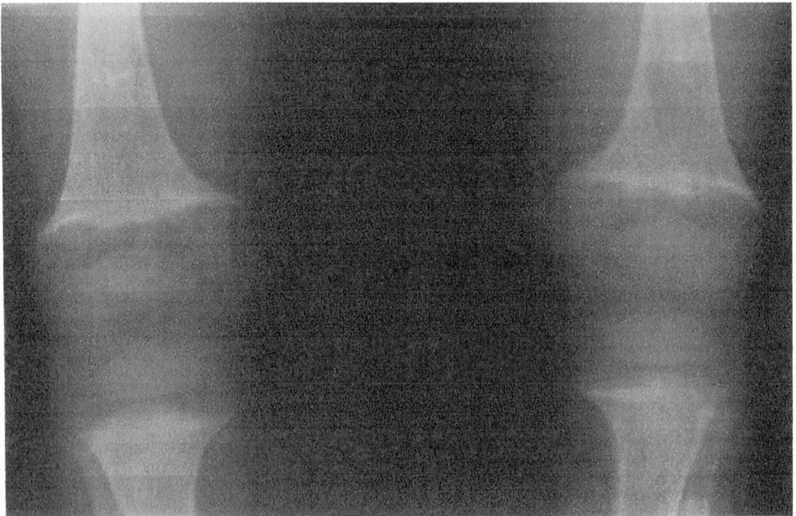

Figure 2. knee x-ray of a girl with PDDR.

2.3. *Hereditary 1,25-dihydroxyvitamin D resistant rickets (HVDRR)*

This condition has been also known as vitamin D-dependent rickets type II. It was first described in the literature in 1978 by two different groups [62, 63]. It is inherited in an autosomal recessive fashion. The defect in target cells of these patients is heterogenous and commonly appears to be a mutation in the gene encoding the vitamin D receptor (VDR) [64], causing an end-organ resistance to the vitamin [65]. Serum levels of

1,25 (OH)$_2$ D3 are elevated, and the clinical picture is of rickets with severe hypocalcemia and alopecia. Very large doses of IV calcium are necessary to treat this condition. This condition can be lethal in the perinatal period [66, 67].

Two different phenotypes have been described. In the "receptor-negative" (or "ligand-binding negative") phenotype, ^{3H}-1,25(OH)2D3 binding is negative in cultured fibroblasts [68]. In the "receptor-positive" (or "ligand-binding positive") phenotype ^{3H}-1,25(OH)2D3 binding is normal in cells, but VDR binding to DNA is defective [69, 70].At least 10 different mutations causing this phenotype has been described [54]

In a mice model of HVDRR, the maternal VDR-dependent intestinal Ca absorption was replaced by passive Ca absorption entrained by a higher Ca intake to ensure normal fetal mineralization [71].

A variant of this disease occurs with typical clinical and biochemical features of HVDRR but without alopecia [66]. The presence of alopecia has been regarded as a sign of severity [72], but it has also been suggested that its absence is not a predictive sign of a lesser resistance and of responsiveness to Vitamin D treatment [66]. .Recently, a novel mutation in helix H12 in the ligand-binding domain of the vitamin D receptor was described to be associated with this variant [73].

2.4. *Osteogenesis imperfecta (brittle bones disease)*

Osteogenesis imperfecta (OI) [74] is a group of heterogeneous disorders with the common feature of bone fragility secondary to mutations in the genes codifying for pro-collagen type I (COL1A1 and COL1A2). The clinical picture of OI is the product of numerous different mutations, and it has been suggested that there are at least twelve different clinical forms [74, 75]. In fact, severity varies in a continuum throughout the OI population, and it is very hard to categorize patients in definite categories. The prevalence of OI is estimated to be 1 in 20,000 infants [76], but the incidence is probably higher, because being a heterogeneous condition, misdiagnosis is frequent. The prevalence of OI appears to be similar throughout the world and in all races [77-80]. In the majority of cases mutations within the COL1A1 or COL1A2 genes can be identified. A comprehensive listing of the mutations within type I collagen genes resulting in OI [81] is now maintained in the internet (http://www.le.ac.uk/genetics/collagen).

Besides brittle bones (Figure 3), all other clinical characteristics of OI are variable, and even different members of the same family may present with a different degree of severity [82]. Wormian bones are present in skull in about 60% of the cases of OI [83], but they can be present in other genetic conditions. Individuals affected with moderate and severe OI have osteoporosis due to the basic bone defect, which is often worsened by immobilization secondary to fractures or surgery, and decreased physical activity. It is of note that metaphyseal fractures (often considered as being pathognomonic of non-accidental injury), can be present in children with OI [84].   Other clinical features are joint hyperlaxity, muscle weakness, chronic unremitting bone pain, and skull deformities (e.g. posterior flattening) due to bone fragility in infants with severe OI. Fractures may still occur after puberty [85], and bone fragility persists throughout life.

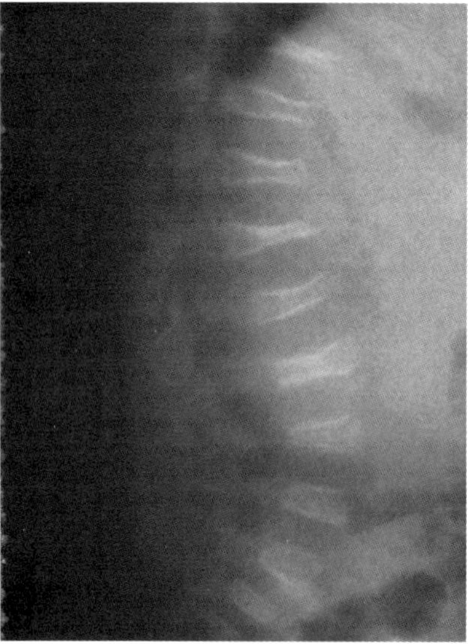

Figure 3. Severe vertebral fractures in an infant with osteogenesis imperfecta.

On the other hand, individuals with mild forms of the disease may have normal stature, no deformities and no fractures at all, and the condition be diagnosed when an x-ray is obtained for other reasons.

People with OI have a high tolerance for pain, and fractures can be discovered in infants only after x-rays are taken for other reasons, and they can occur without any signs of pain. Infants with mild OI can suffer unexplained fractures in the first months of life, with the fracture rate decreasing dramatically thereafter.

Several organs and systems can be affected in individuals with OI. Basilar invagination is an uncommon but potentially fatal occurrence in OI. The prevalence of this complication in patients with OI is not known [86]. Treatment of basilar invagination is difficult, and it tends to progress despite fusion surgery in 80% of the cases [86]. On the other hand, prolonged external orthotic immobilization may stabilize symptoms and halt further invagination [86]. Paraplegia in an adolescent with OI after chiropractic manipulation has been reported [87]. Other rare neurological manifestations of OI include macrocephaly, benign communicating hydrocephalus and cerebral atrophy, Dandy-Walker malformation and idiopathic seizures [88]. Usually, there is no alteration of the intellectual status. Hypoaccusis is said to be present in about 50% of the individuals with mild forms of OI after the third decade of life [89]. Hearing screening in children with OI is warranted. The incidence of congenital malformations of the heart in children with OI is probably similar to that of the normal population [83, 90]. The prevalence of mitral valve prolapse varies from 3.4% [91] to 6.9% [90] in different series. These lesions rarely have clinical significance [92]. Hypercalciuria is present in about 36% of affected individuals [93, 94]. This hypercalciuria does not appear to affect renal function [94]. Some patients with OI have a hypermetabolic state, typically reflected by excessive diaphoresis, associated with increased oxygen consumption and elevated thyroxine levels [95]. This has generated a misconception regarding malignant hyperthermia in subjects with OI. Patients with OI may develop hyperthermia during surgery, but it is rarely malignant. Still, patients with OI should be considered as high risk for anesthesia [96] because they are prone to fracture, may have neck and jaw deformities that will make intubation difficult, and sometimes severe thoracic deformities and kyphoscoliosis may cause restrictive problems [97]. Also, dentinogenesis imperfecta and valvular heart disease must also to be taken into account when evaluating the anesthetic risk of these patients.

Individuals with OI may develop respiratory complications, secondary to kyphoscoliosis. Spine deformities are associated with restrictive complications [98]. The skin in a patient with OI has a tendency to bruise. This may be related to an increase in capillary fragility caused by the underlying collagen defect. Decreased platelet retention and reduced factor VIII R:Ag have also been described in OI [99]. Joint hyperlaxity is common [100], and can lead to dislocation of hips and radial heads. Constipation, sprains, flat feet and hernias are also common in people with OI [101]. Dentinogenesis imperfecta (DI) is caused by an abnormal dentin, with normal enamel [102, 103]. The prevalence of DI in the OI population is of about 28% [104]. For unknown reasons, the permanent dentition is usually less affected than the primary dentition. Interestingly, subjects with OI do not have an increased susceptibility to cavities and do not always have more dental pain. Class III malocclusion (the cusp of the posterior mandibular teeth interdigitate a tooth or more ahead of their opposing maxillary counterparts [105]) is a common finding in patients with OI, with a prevalence of 60-80% [106, 107]. Patients may require surgical correction of the malocclusion [108].

Life expectancy in subjects with non-lethal OI appears to be the same as the normal population [109], except in cases of severe OI with respiratory or neurological complications [110].

Mode of inheritance in OI is almost always dominant or a new dominant mutation, regardless of the clinical form of OI. In cases of families with healthy parents that have more than one child with OI, the possibility of a germ cell mosaicism [111] has been proposed as an explanation [112, 113]. These cases were previously thought to have been transmitted in a recessive fashion. It is thought that in at least 6% of the cases of lethal OI, one of the parents is carrier of a germ cell line mosaicism [114].

Severity of OI ranges from mild cases with no deformity, normal stature and no fractures, to forms that are lethal in the perinatal period. In a first attempt to classify OI, in 1906 Looser divided it in two forms [115]: "congenita" (Vrolik) and "tarda" (Lobstein), depending on the severity of the presentation. In OI congenital. multiple fractures may occur *in-utero*, whereas in OI tarda, fractures occur at the time of birth or later. OI tarda has also been sub-divided in "gravis" and "levis" [115]. This classification is no longer current because it is considered as an over-simplification of the complex clinical picture of OI.

Sillence proposed a classification reflecting the spectrum of clinical presentation of OI [79, 116]. While there is no consistency in the literature about the characteristics of the different types and members of the same family (that should have the same OI type) may differ dramatically in severity and clinical presentation [117], the classification has received general acceptance. In their original report [79] Sillence et al. defined four groups. "Type I" individuals have a mild presentation, with bone fragility, blue sclera and pre-senile deafness. These patients have their first fracture in the preschool period, and fractures may be present at birth. This is a very important issue when evaluating cases of suspected child abuse. Inheritance is dominant in all cases.

Type II includes patients with lethal perinatal OI. Radiological features include radiographically crumpled ("accordion-like") femora and beaded ribs. Sclera is in most cases blue, but white in some individuals. There have been cases of "type II survivors" that are still alive after twelve   years of birth, therefore lethality in this form is the most common outcome, but not the rule (data not published). Type III patients have progressive deformity, short stature, triangular face and white sclera. All cases in this group were sporadic in the original publication

Type IV includes a more heterogeneous group of patients with white sclera and dominant inheritance. Clinical features are variable. Paterson et al. made a more exhaustive description of type IV OI [118], suggesting that there is a wide range for the age at first fracture and for total number of fractures in this group.

This classification has several drawbacks, the main one being the overlap among different types. Blue sclera has been proposed as a sign that differentiate type I from type IV individuals. In clinical practice, scleral hue has very little significance for the diagnosis and classification of OI unless is very dark blue, as blue sclera may be present in normal children and in genetic diseases, and has no relation to clinical severity. The numeric classification of OI should be used with caution, and clinical form and severity must always be referred in each individual case. Lately, more types have been added to the "classic four" described by Sillence. Following previous publications on the subject [74, 92], we propose that the individuals should be described in reference to their clinical presentation and severity. Clinical forms described in the literature are summarized in Table 3.

There have also been attempts to classify OI according to radiological characteristics [119]. Some of the features suggested for classification are not present until age 5 or 10 years, and children of early ages cannot be classified using this scheme. This approach appears to be practical in terms of therapeutic decisions, and should be developed in more detail. There have also been attempts to classify OI according to severity [85, 120].

2.4.1. *Mild OI with normal stature*

The hallmark of this form of OI is normal stature. Affected individuals are fully ambulatory, and do not have bowing of the long bones. This condition is transmitted with an autosomal dominant trait. Despite absence of fractures, bone density can be very low, with no relation with clinical severity. Bone density is often normal during the first months of life, and individuals fail to increase bone mineral density when compared to normal controls. Fractures may occur during the first months of life, even at birth [121], and their incidence decrease dramatically after puberty. In some cases the diagnosis is an incidental finding after a fracture [122]. Dentinogenesis imperfecta can be present even in very mild cases, and it has been suggested that this characteristic is useful to distinguish two forms of mild OI [123]. Early hypoacusis [124, 125] and cardiovascular problems, particularly aortic valvular disease [121] can be present in these patients.

The most common mutation causing mild OI causes a reduction in the production of otherwise normal type I collagen. Mutations causing production of a severely affected RNA will also promote its intra-cellular destruction by a process called "nonsense mediated RNA decay" [126-128] and therefore cause a clinical picture of mild OI with less, albeit normal, collagen.

There are other less common mechanisms for underproduction of collagen (e.g. mutations that lead to retention of an intron within the mature transcript [129], mutations within the 3' untranslated region affecting polyadenylation, or synthesis of a pro-collagen chain which is unable to incorporate within the triple helical molecule). Frameshift mutations within the terminal exon of either collagen gene can lead to synthesis of a full sized pro-collagen chain which is rapidly degraded intracellularly after it fails to incorporate into the collagen molecule [130].

2.4.2. Moderate OI with short stature

These individuals typically have short stature, bowing of long bones, and vertebral fractures, but no triangular face. Scoliosis and joint laxity may be present. Patients with this form of OI are generally ambulatory, but they may need aids for ambulation. Based in the presence of DI, moderate OI has been sub-divided in two forms [123].

2.4.3. Severe OI with triangular face

These patients have a characteristic triangular face, caused by a larger head in conjunction with under-development of the facial bones. Other characteristics are short stature, chest deformities, severe bowing of the long bones, vertebral fractures and severe scoliosis. They are frequently wheelchair-bound, although some are able to walk with aids. Altered structure of the growth plates lead to a particular appearance of the metaphyses and epihpyses described as "popcorn".

2.4.4. Lethal OI

In this form of OI, affected newborns do not survive the perinatal period. Possible causes of death are malformations or hemorrhages of the central nervous system [131], extreme fragility of the ribs, or pulmonary hypoplasia [132]. The infants present with multiple intrauterine fractures, including skull, long bones and vertebrae, beaded ribs, and severe deformity of the long bones [133]. Prenatal differential diagnosis between severe and lethal OI is not possible. Extremely severe cases can be born dismembered [134]. The vast majority of cases are autosomal dominant new mutations [114, 135, 136]. It has been suggested that there may be different clinical forms of lethal OI [137].

2.4.5. Congenital brittle bones with dense areas in bones

Described in only one infant [138] who died shortly after birth and presented with an OI phenotype that differed from the usual lethal form in that the skeleton had regions of increased bone density. This girl had dysmorphic facial features, including loss of mandibular angle, low set ears, soft skull, and large anterior and posterior fontanelles. Multiple fractures in the long bones and ribs where present at birth, together with bilateral upper and lower limb contractures. The ends of the long bones were radiographically dense. The patient died after a few hours and histopathological studies identified extramedullary hematopoiesis in the liver, little lamellar bone formation, decreased number of osteoclasts, abnormally thickened bony trabeculae with retained cartilage in long bones, and diminished marrow spaces similar to those seen in dense bone diseases such as osteopetrosis and pycnodysostosis. Genetic testing showed that the child was heterozygous for a COL1A14321G$\rightarrow$T transversion in exon 52 that changed a conserved aspartic acid to tyrosine (D1441Y). Abnormal proA1(I) chains were slow to assemble into dimers and trimers, and abnormal molecules were retained intracellularly for an extended period [138].

2.5. Syndromes resembling osteogenesis imperfecta (SROI) [139]

This diseases share the common phenotype of congenital brittle bones, although they differ in other characteristics. Particularly, they are not caused by mutations in the pro-collagen genes. In some the mutation has been identified, in others it is yet to be detected.

2.5.1. *Congenital brittle bones with hyperplastic callus formation*

Some patients with congenital brittle bones develop hyperplastic calluses in long bones after a fracture or use of intramedullary rod surgery [121]. Inflammation or osteosarcoma may be suggested by hard, painful and warm swellings over long bones. The size and shape of the callus may remain stable for many years after a initial rapid growth period [140]. Histology shows increased production of abnormal, poorly organized and incompletely mineralized extracellular matrix [141], the bone lamellae are arranged in a mesh-like fashion, as opposed to a parallel arrangement in patients with OI [142]. A series of case reports of hyperplastic callus formation can be found in the literature [115, 140, 143-148]. Calcification of the interosseous membrane between radius and ulna may be present, determining a clinical sign, as patients are unable to pronate and supinate the forearm. Sclera is white in this form of SROI and no dentinogenesis imperfecta is present. Mutations in the pro-collagen genes have not been identified so far. Inheritance appears to be autosomal dominant, with variable penetrance.

2.5.2. *Osteoporosis pseudoglioma syndrome [149, 150]*

This SROI was first described in three families in 1972 [151]. Other report described a South African family of Indian origin with the condition [152]. Inheritance is autosomal recessive. Individuals with Osteoporosis-pseudoglioma syndrome have mild to moderate brittle bones with blindness due to hyperplasia of the vitreous, corneal opacity and secondary glaucoma. The ocular pathology may be secondary to failed regression of the primary vitreal vasculature during fetal growth [153]. The genetic defect has been mapped to chromosome region 11q12-13 [154]. The defect is specifically in the LRP5 gene, that encodes for the low-density lipoprotein receptor-related protein 5 [153]. Treatment with pamidronate has shown promising results in this group of patients [155].

2.5.3. *Other ocular forms of SROI*

At least two other forms of SROI with ocular involvement have been described: one with retinopathy, optic atrophy and severe psychomotor retardation [156], and another with cataracts and microcephaly [157].

2.5.4. *Congenital brittle bones with craniosynostosis (Cole-Carpenter syndrome)*

Two boys [158] and a girl [159] have been described in the literature with this particular SROI. The two boys appeared to be normal at birth, but developed multiple metaphyseal fractures, associated with low bone density in the entire skeleton and craniosynostosis, hydrocephalus, ocular proptosis, and facial dysmorphism after several months. One of the patients had also hypercalciuria. Neurological development is normal. Both boys where wheelchair-bound at adult age, with very short stature, severe bone involvement and normal intellectual and neurological development (unpublished data).

2.5.5. *Congenital brittle bones with congenital joint contractures*

First described by Bruck et al in 1897 in an adult patient [160], in this SROI patients are born with brittle bones, leading to multiple fractures and joint contractures and pterygia (arthrogryposis multiplex congenita) [161, 162]. Wormian bones are present, and inheritance appears to be recessive [163, 164]. The basic defect was mapped to locus 17p12 (18 cM interval), where a bone telopeptidyl hydroxylase is located [165]. The mutation leads to under-hydroxilated lysine residues within the telopeptides of collagen type I, with aberrant cross-linking in bone, but not in cartilage or ligaments. The lysine residues in the triple helix are normally modified, suggesting that collagen crosslinking is regulated primarily by tissue-specific enzymes that hydroxylate only telopeptide lysine residues, but not those in the helical portion of the molecule [165].

2.5.6. *Congenital brittle bones with mineralization defect*

Undistinguishable from moderate to severe OI on a clinical basis, this rare SROI [166], has a prevalence of about 6% of the OI population. A mineralization defect affecting the bone matrix and sparing growth cartilage is evident in bone biopsies. These patients have normal teeth and no wormian bones. There are no radiological signs of growth plate involvement, despite the mineralization defect evident in histology. The case of two siblings from healthy consanguineous parents suggested gonadal mosaicism or a somatic recessive trait [166], but the pattern of inheritance is not known. No mutations of COL1A1 and COL1A2 genes have been found in these patients, and collagen structure appears to be normal. This could be a form of fibrogenesis imperfecta ossium [167, 168], that presents with similar characteristics in bone biopsy.

2.5.7. *Congenital brittle bones with rhizomelia*

This particular SROI with short humeri and femora and recessive inheritance was described in an indigenous Quebec tribe [169]. Severity is moderate. Fractures may be present at birth, and the condition progresses with early lower limb deformities, coxa vara and low bone density. By histomorphometry, the bone in congenital brittle bones with rhizomielia is not different to that of mild OI. The genetic defect has been mapped to the short arm of chromosome 3 by linkage studies [170], where there are no genes that code for type I pro-collagen.

2.6. Idiopathic Juvenile Osteoporosis

This condition was first described by Dent and Friedman in 1965 [171], as a syndrome with onset of osteoporosis prior to puberty, back and appendicular pain, gait abnormalities, and that resolves spontaneously after puberty. Initial symptoms may be related to long bone fractures, gait problems [172] or back pain [173].

The mean age of onset was 7 years in a group of 21 patients followed by R. Smith [174], with a range of 1 to 13 years. This highlights the fact that IJO may start at a very early age. Other causes of osteoporosis must be ruled out, particularly those related to malignancy [175]. "Neo-osseous porosis" (metaphyseal osteopenia) has been described as a radiological lesion pathognomonic of IJO [176], but it has been observed also in polyglandular autoimmune syndrome [177].

Table 3. Osteogenesis imperfecta and Syndromes resembling OI

Osteogenesis Imperfecta

- Mild OI with normal stature
- Moderate OI with short stature
- Severe OI
- Lethal OI
- Congenital brittle bones with dense areas in bones

Syndromes resembling OI (SROI)

- Congenital brittle bones with craniosynostosis and ocular proptosis
- Congenital brittle bones with congenital joint contractures
- Osteoporosis-pseudoglioma syndrome
- Congenital brittle bones with optic atrophy, retinopathy and severe psychomotor retardation
- Congenital brittle bones with microcephaly and cataracts
- Congenital brittle bones with redundant callus
- Congenital brittle bones with mineralization defect
- Congenital brittle bones with rhizomelia

The etiology is obscure and the diagnosis is based both on the exclusion of other diseases and on the clinical evolution of the patients. [178]. Histomorphometric analysis of bone biopsies of patients with IJO showed that it is characterized by a decreased cancellous bone volume and a very low bone formation rate on cancellous surfaces [179]. The disturbance of bone remodeling in IJO is limited to cancellous bone, but there may also be a modeling defect affecting the internal cortex. The process causing IJO appears to mainly affect bone surfaces that are in contact with the bone marrow cavity [180].

Treatment with calcitonin [181], sodium fluoride [182], calcitriol [183] and bisphosphonates [184] has been attempted. Since spontaneous recovery occurs it remains impossible to assess the efficacy of treatments. Despite this, without treatment vertebral fractures may not recover completely.

2.7. *Hypophosphatasia*

Hypophosphatasia is a rare inborn error of metabolism, with an estimated incidence of 1 per 100,000 births [185]. It is characterized by rickets or osteomalacia secondary to low activity of the tissue non-specific isoenzyme of alkaline phosphatase (TNSALP) [186-188]. Biochemically it is characterized by reduced activity of the TNSALP, and increased levels of TNSALP substrates, namely pyridoxal-5'-phosphate (PLP), inorganic pyrophosphate (PPi) and phosphoethanolamine (PEA) in serum and urine [189, 190]. There is no animal model for this disease [185].

Clinical severity is extremely variable, ranging from death *in utero* [191] to pathologic fractures first presenting in adulthood. Severe forms of the disease are inherited in an autosomal recessive fashion [192]; the pattern of transmission of mild forms is uncertain [193]. Prenatal genetic diagnosis has been accomplished [194].

Clinically, six forms of hypophosphatasia can be distinguished, although individual case assignment may be challenging. The classification is based on the age when skeletal lesions are discovered: perinatal (lethal), infantile, childhood and adult. Two particular forms include odontohypohposphatasia, and "pseudohypophosphatasia". In the former only biochemical and dental manifestations are present, with no clinical changes in bones. The later is clinically indistinguishable from infantile hypophosphatasia, but serum ALP activity is normal [195]. It has been postulated that in these cases there is a mutant TNSALP that still has activity in vitro, but not in vivo [185]. As a consequence of this, PEA, PPi and PLP are elevated in serum and urine, despite normal, or elevated, alkaline phosphatase activity levels [196].

Shohat et al. [191] have further characterized perinatal hypophosphatasia. Affected subjects have lethal short limb dwarfism with very soft calvaria, polyhydramnios, blue sclerae and spurs in the mid-portion of the forearms and lower legs. They found considerable variability in the skeletal radiographs. In addition to the well known radiographic features such as generalized decrease in the size of ossified bones with some bones not ossified at all, other changes observed include marked variability in the amount of bone ossification, variability between patients as to which bones were most severely affected, unusually dense, round, flattened, butterfly shaped; and sagittally clefted vertebral bodies, variability in femoral shape including "chromosome" like, "campomelic" like, and shortening with or without metaphyseal cupping or irregularities, and osteochondral projections (Bowdler spurs) of the midshaft of the fibula and ulna. Affected newborns may survive briefly, but die of severe respiratory compromise, accompanied by fever of unknown origin, anemia, irritability, bradycardia, seizures and intracranial hemorrhage [186].

The mutation has been mapped to chromosome 1p36.1-34 in the case of infantile form [197]. Compound heterozygosity in the TNSALP gene can be responsible for childhood and adult hypophosphatasia [193].

Treatment was attempted with non-steroidal anti-inflammatory drugs in patients with childhood hypophosphatasia with some clinical improvement [198], but more experience is needed before this therapy can be recommended.

2.8. Hyperphosphatasia

Hyperphosphatasia is a rare autosomal recessive disease affecting bone remodeling. Affected children present an accelerated bone turnover and elevation in alkaline phosphatase activity in serum. Clinically it resembles adult Paget disease, but with a characteristic symmetrical involvement of long bones. There is severe osteopenia, focal areas of radiolucency and the vertebral bodies are either biconcave or flat. The skull is enlarged with widening of the diploeic space. The appearance is called "cotton wool". Widening of the diaphyses and lack of cortico-medullary separation in the long bones can be present. There is also progressive loss of muscular strength with delayed walking. The diaphyses are widened, the femurs and tibias are bowed and there is an increased head size. Mental and endocrine development is normal. So far, no mutation has been described for this disease.

One patient treated with pamidronate showed significant radiological improvement after one year of treatment [199]. Treatment with very high doses of bisphosphonates (10 times the usual dose) in a case of possible idiopathic hyperphosphatasia led to osteopetrosis [200].

2.9. Primary hypomagnesemia

Hypomagnesemia in childhood is relatively frequently noted in the neonatal period due to maternal causes, such as decreased intake due to vomiting, overuse of laxatives and neonatal causes such as intrauterine growth retardation, birth asphyxia and exchange transfusion [201].

Pathogenesis of hypocalcemia can be related to impaired parathyroid gland function [202], or an end-organ dysfunction [203]. Therefore, primary hypomagnesemia will always present with hypocalcemia, but PTH levels can be low, normal or elevated.

Seizures and persistent hypocalcemia is a typical presentation. Hypomagnesemia is first managed by parenteral treatment with magnesium and by oral administration of magnesium supplements once serum magnesium levels are normalized. A burst in circulating parathyroid hormone levels to well above the physiological range may be observed at the start of therapy. The serum magnesium levels of the mother and father may be just below the normal range, with normal serum calcium. This type of infantile primary hypomagnesemia appears to be a hereditary disease with autosomal recessive characteristics, although a partially penetrant X-linked or autosomal dominant trait cannot be excluded [204].

3. Secondary osteoporosis in pediatrics

Growing bones are at risk for osteoporosis under many pathologic circumstances (Table 1). Mechanical stimulation is paramount for bone strengthening at any age [205], and immobilization is a common cause of osteoporosis [206, 207] . Prolonged therapeutic bed rest, immobilization due to motor paralysis from injury of the central nervous system or peripheral nerves, application of cast to treat fractures, are common causes of disuse osteoporosis. Moreover, bone mass has been found to be closely related to muscle mass in normal individuals [208]. Children who require prolonged total parenteral nutrition (TPN) in early life are at risk for abnormalities in growth and nutritional status in later childhood; requiring long-term dietary, growth, and nutritional monitoring [209-211]. Prematurity and genetic diseases are some of the causes of low bone density in the pediatric population. Children with short bowel syndrome had decreased bone mineral content compared with control subjects; however, this difference does not appear to be significant when adjusted for differences in weight and height [212]. This underscores the importance of analyzing bone density results in light of the whole clinical picture. Generally speaking, it is fair to say that every pediatric specialist will eventually evaluate a child with secondary osteoporosis, regardless of their sub-specialty. A description of some causes of secondary osteoporosis in pediatrics follows.

3.1. Immobilization

The molecular mechanism of mechanical stress-induced bone formation remains to be fully elucidated. The 'mechanostat' theory of bone enunciated by Harold Frost [213, 214] views the skeleton from a biomechanical perspective. From such point of view, the skeleton can be conceived as 'a biomechanically-regulated structure that can be systemically disturbed (in the cybernetic sense), the strength of which depends on the intrinsic stiffness (material properties) and the spatial distribution (architectural properties) of the mineralized tissue'[215]. The biomechanical feedback system involved (bone 'mechanostat') would not control bone mass to optimize bone strength; it would rather control bone material quality and architecture (through a modulation of bone modeling and remodeling) in order to optimize bone stiffness. The natural stimuli for the bone mechanostat would be the customary strains of bone tissue (sensed by osteocytes) that are induced by gravitational forces and, more importantly, the contractions of regional muscles [215]. Mechanical stimulation is paramount for bone strengthening [216]. Immobilization is a well-known cause of osteoporosis [206, 207]. Reduction of mechanical stress on bone inhibits osteoblast-mediated bone formation and accelerates osteoclast-mediated bone resorption, and leads to the so-called 'disuse osteoporosis'.

Gravity influence for short periods of time is not enough to keep bone mass stable, as suggested by occurrence of severe osteoporosis in patients with cerebral palsy [37]. Although they are obviously subjected to gravity, the fact that there is no mechanical stimulation to the bones in the lower body makes them a suitable model to test the effects of mechanical stimulation in bones that are not otherwise subject to impact. Non-ambulatory patients with spina bifida, who have not sensation or strength in the lower limbs, may present with similar problems. Fractures are a consequence of decreased bone density, although their occurrence depends on multiple factors. It is therefore a weak outcome parameter for research studies. Bone mineral density, although not a true "density" in the physics sense, is a good follow-up parameter for treatment dealing with osteoporosis. Measurement of the bone mineral content is also possible with DEXA, with low radiation dose. The in-vivo coefficient of variation of the method (CV = % SD/mean) has been estimated in 0.7% for femoral neck measurements [3]. The entrance radiation dose is less than 8.8 rem for one hip.

3.2. Neuromuscular diseases

Individuals with cerebral palsy (CP) typically suffer progressive loss of bone mineral density due to immobilization [37]. In children with CP, the age when the child first walked, fracture history, use of anticonvulsant medication, and serum vitamin-D levels do not correlate with bone-mineral density after adjustment for walking status and the nutritional status [37]. This suggests that the main cause of osteoporosis in these children is the lack of weight bearing and activity. Extra mechanical stimulation of their bones, provided that nutritional factors are controlled, is warranted. Weight bearing for short periods of time is not enough to keep bone mass stable, as suggested by occurrence of severe osteoporosis in patients with CP despite being placed in the vertical position for 1-2 hours per day [37]. Children with CP are unable to increase bone mass, and even lose bone mass progressively as shown in Figure 4. Cerebral palsy is the most common physical disability of childhood, with an incidence of 2-3 per 1000 live births [205]. It has been estimated that over 100,000 children in the United States have some degree of neurological impairment attributable to CP [217]. The severity of the condition varies widely. Most children with CP are ambulatory and are not cognitively impaired. The most profoundly involved subgroup has spastic quadriplegia, comprising roughly 20%

of all children with CP [218, 219]. This subgroup is characterized by severe physical and cognitive impairments, and a high prevalence of poor growth and/or malnutrition. This subgroup is non-ambulatory, and often has multiple other problems including seizure disorder, swallowing difficulties and gastric reflux that necessitate feeding tubes, and osteopenia that results in fractures. Decreased bone mineral density is also present in patients with advanced Duchenne's muscular dystrophy (DMD). It is often worsened by corticosteroid therapy [220], but it may be present even in ambulatory patients [221, 222]. As a consequence, the incidence of vertebral fractures is increased in this population, particularly after initiation of corticosteroid therapy [223].

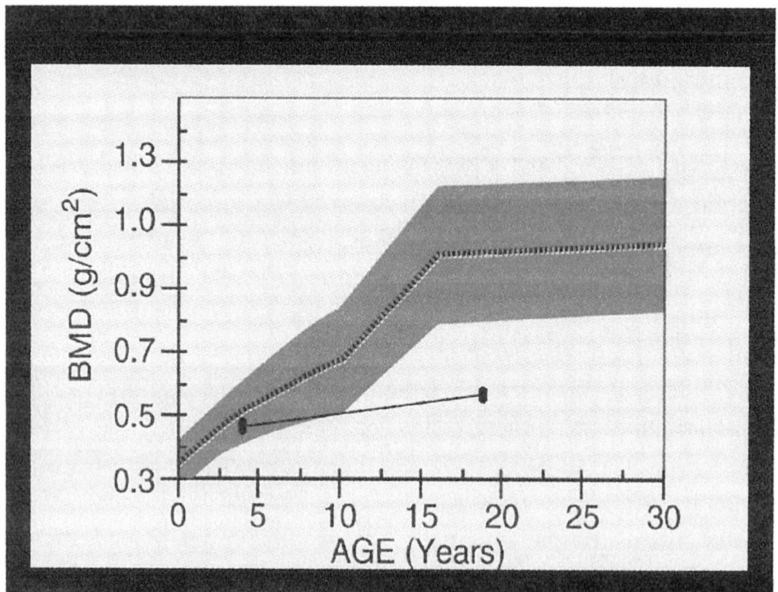

Figure 4. Bone mineral density progression in children with cerebral palsy. Reference values for age are shown in gray (based on data from Henderson, R.C. Dev Med Child Neurol, 39:224-227, 1997).

Vertebral fractures appear after about three years under steroid treatment, and after about 8 years under treatment, 75% of the patients may have vertebral fractures [223].

3.3. Type I diabetes mellitus

Although type I diabetes of recent onset may not have an impact on BMD and growth parameters in children [224], poor metabolic control may expose adolescents with long-standing type 1 diabetes to the risk of developing osteopenia in adult age [225]. In fact, adult patients with IDDM show a reduced bone mineral density [226]. Using peripheral quantitative computed tomography (pQCT), a group [227] concluded that there is a decrease of trabecular bone density, total bone density, and cortical bone density in children and adolescents with type I diabetes. Trabecular bone density appears to be inversely correlated with the duration of the disease and the concentration of glycosylated hemoglobin (HbA1), whereas total BMD correlates inversely with serum levels of HbA1 [227]. On the other hand, a different study using QCT found that cortical bone density is slightly but significantly lower in diabetic children than in controls; but there is no difference between patients and controls regarding trabecular bone density [228]. The decrease in cortical bone density in the diabetic group did not correlate with age, sex, duration of diabetes, or glycosylated hemoglobin levels in this case [228]. There are no current recommendations about prevention of osteoporosis in this particular group of patients. Maximizing calcium and vitamin D intake is warranted.

3.4. Renal causes

Chronic metabolic acidosis may increase alkali mobilization from the bone and thus promote the development of osteoporosis [229]. Children with idiopathic nephrotic syndrome are at risk for low bone mass, probably related to high doses of steroids [230]. Decreased lumbar spine bone mineral density in kidney transplant patients is related to height and repeated transplants, but interestingly, it does not appear to be influenced by weight, pre-existing renal disease, gender, or rejection events [231]. The factors that affect bone mineral density and the long term effects of transplantation on bone mineral density in children is still unknown [232].

3.5. *Hypogonadism*

Osteoporosis is a common feature of different hypo-estrogenic states [233]. The syndrome of "athletic amenorrhea" causes bone demineralization in girls participating in strenuous training. This results in the "female athlete triad": disordered eating, amenorrhea, and osteoporosis [234] with increased risk of skeletal fragility, fractures and vertebral instability [235]. Menstrual abnormalities in the female athlete result from hypothalamic suppression of the spontaneous pulsatile secretion of gonadotropin releasing hormone [235]. Patients with anorexia nervosa are also at risk of osteoporosis. The occurrence of low bone mass in this particular group is so common, that it has been suggested that an eating disorder should be suspected in severely underweight young individuals (primarily girls) presenting with low impact fractures [236]. Multiple factors contribute to the bone loss experienced by patients with anorexia nervosa, and the associated estrogen deficiency may not be the major contributor [237], as bone density abnormalities are present before any alteration in estrogen levels can be detected.

Turner syndrome causes reduced areal [238] and volumetric [239] bone mineral density. This effect is not only seen in adults but also in affected girls [240]. Bone density measured by DPA (dual photon absorptiometry) or DEXA appeared to be normal after being corrected for height or bone age [241-243], but trabecular lumbar spine vBMD was reduced when measured with QCT [244]. Fracture risk appears to be increased in this group [241 , 245]. It has been suggested that estrogen replacement may optimize bone mass acquisition in girls with Turner syndrome [233, 246, 247]. It has been suggested that optimizing bone mass in patients with Turner syndrome may require earlier induction of puberty than currently recommended [248], although the ideal timing for start of hormonal replacement therapy is not clear [242, 243].

3.6. *Malabsorption*

Celiac disease, inflammatory bowel diseases, gastrectomy, cholestatic liver diseases, liver transplantation, and hepatitis C can affect bone mineralization and remodeling [249]. Children with celiac disease are at risk for lower bone mineral density, and it has been suggested that a strict gluten-free diet may improve bone mineralization [250, 251]. Despite lower bone density, these children may not be at greater risk of fracture [252]. Patients with end stage liver disease are prone to develop osteopenia and osteoporosis [253]. Prevalence ranges from 10 to 56%, depending on the nature of liver disease [254]. Children with cholestatic liver disease may develop the so-called "hepatic osteodystrophy" [255]. Those who undergo liver transplant are at even higher risk of bone fractures secondary to osteoporosis. The role of cholestatic liver disease is well recognized, but as of yet, the underlying etiology is unknown [256]. Immunosuppression protocols that use lower doses of prednisone administration over shorter time intervals may help prevent bone loss after orthotopic liver transplant [253]. Osteoporosis is a frequent complication in children with cystic fibrosis (CF) regardless of their age [257, 258], but it is more common in children with poor nutritional status. Osteoporosis appears to be more prevalent in patients with greater disease severity [259]. Levels of calcidiol and calcitriol were found to be lower in patients with CF than in controls. Although low calcidiol levels are related to malabsorption, it is not clear why these patients have low levels of calcitriol. Older patients with CF with progressively diminishing sunlight exposure may be at increased risk for development of osteopenia [260]. Osteoporosis in patients with CF probably is related to nutritional factors [261] and respiratory complications (e.g., decreased forced expiratory volume in 1 second [262]) and is therefore not related to a primary defect in bone mineral metabolism. This has a significant impact in therapeutic decisions, and suggests that prevention of osteoporosis with adequate vitamin D supplementation in children with CF is warranted.

3.7. Inborn errors of metabolism

Lysosomal storage disorders are caused by genetic defects of lysosomal enzymes that lead to accumulation of different substrates in the lysosome, with consequent impairment in cellular function. There are more than 40 different diseases caused by this mechanism. It is a misconception that all lysosomal storage diseases cause skeletal changes [263]. The vast majority of them affect predominantly the central nervous system. The radiological manifestations of lysosomal storage diseases are grouped as "dysostosis multiplex" [264, 265]. Shafts of bones are widened with thin cortices, and pathological fractures can be present. Epiphyseal centers are poorly developed; the mid-shafts are enlarged, and limbs are short. Metacarpals are broadened distally and taper at their proximal ends (Figure 5). Phalanges are bullet-shaped. Coxa valga, small femoral heads and poorly developed pelvis is often seen. Lower ribs are broad and the lateral part of the clavicle is hypoplastic. Vertebrae are hypoplastic, and patients have pectus carinatum, short stature and kyphosis, hypoplasia of the odontoid, vertebral fractures, macrocephaly and hydrocephalus.

Gaucher's disease is a multisystemic lipidosis characterized by organomagaly (hepatosplenomegaly), bone-marrow infiltration leading to hematologic problems, and bone involvement (osteonecrosis and bone thinning) [266], associated with the presence of pathological cells of the reticuloendothelial system, which contain undegraded glycosphingolipids, particularly glucosylceramide [267]. There are three clinical forms of the disease. Type 1, the most common, is the adult, non-neuronopathic form and is common among Ashkenazi Jews [268]. Type 2 is the infantile form, and type 3 is the juvenile form. Severity and age of onset vary widely. All types are autosomal recessive. The mutation is located in chromosome 1 (q21-q31), where a gene encoding for acid beta-glucosidase is located [269]. Recently it has been suggested that there may be more types of Gaucher disease [270, 271]. Infiltration of the medullary space by Gaucher cells, erosion of bone, osteonecrosis in the area of the fracture, and disuse osteoporosis are the main etiological factors for fractures in this group [272]. Bone lesions in patients with Gaucher's disease may be secondary to high concentrations of IL-6 in serum [273].

Lysinuric protein intolerance is an autosomal recessive disorder which first appears in the infant, after weaning from mother's milk, as failure to thrive, vomiting and diarrhea. Later signs are; failure to grow, hepatomegaly, muscular weakness and osteoporosis, associated with aversion to animal protein and mental retardation in some [274]. Skeletal manifestations may include fractures after minor trauma, severe osteoporosis, abnormal thickening of cortex of the metacarpals, thin cortices of the long bones, endplate impression of vertebrae, rickets-like metaphyses, or early destruction of cartilage, and delayed bone age [275]. The disease is characterized by marked lysinuria, and hyperammonemia after protein intake. There is an impaired transport of cationic amino acids at the basolateral membrane of intestinal and renal epithelia, characterized chemically by renal hyperdiaminoaciduria, especially lysinuria, and by impaired formation of urea with hyperammonemia after protein ingestion [276]. The presence of the transport defect of diaminoacids into the hepatocytes distinguishes LPI from other hyperdibasicaminoacidurias [277]. Skin fibroblast can be used to study a corresponding transport defect in intestinal and renal membranes [278]. Citrulline [279] and lysine [280] supplements have been used for treatment of LPI. They have been found to correct the deficiency of the urea cycle intermediates and to protect the patients from hyperammonemia and its consequences.

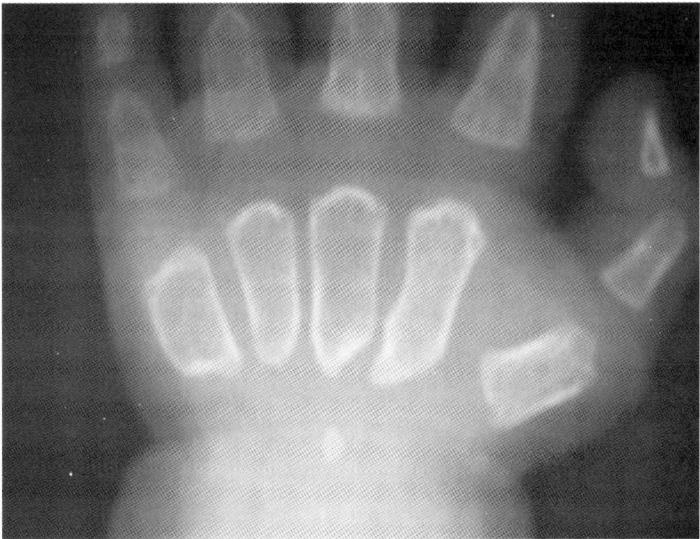

Figure 5. Metacarpal bones in a case of mucopolysaccharidosis.

Children affected with phenylketonuria (PKU) may have lower bone density, despite an adequate diet as per current recommendations [281]. Furthermore, long-lasting dietary restriction in patients with PKU may increase the risk of late complications of dietary therapy, such as osteoporosis [282].The changes noted could not be related after age correction to serum phenylalanine levels, protein intake, or mineral intakes. It is unclear whether deficits in bone mineralization in this population are a consequence of the disease itself or its treatment [283].

3.8. Malignancy and steroid induced osteoporosis

Impaired development of bone mineral density is a recognized complication in pediatric patients with cancer [284, 285]. Osteoporosis of the femoral neck can be evident as early as one year after initiation of chemotherapy, independently of the type of tumor. This decreased bone density is independent of the well-known effects of chemotherapy on growth [285-287]. On the other hand, eleven years after diagnosis of childhood Hodgkin disease or non-Hodgkin lymphoma, the whole-body bone mass of a group of survivors was only slightly reduced and the size-adjusted bone mass was normal [288]. The deleterious effects of glucocorticoids have been known for many years [289], but only recently the precise cellular and molecular basis of these effects have begun to be elucidated. Glucocorticoid induced bone disease is characterized by a decrease in bone formation [290] and in-situ death of isolated segments of bone (osteonecrosis) [291]. A study in pigs showed that ischemic necrosis is actually caused not only by necrosis but also by apoptosis [292]. It has been shown that prednisolone stimulate apoptosis in osteoblasts and osteocytes in mice and humans [293, 294], and that glucocorticoids promote osteoclast survival [295].

3.9. Prematurity

Infants with osteopenia of prematurity (OOP) have decreased bone mineral content as a result of inadequate Ca and P intake after birth. Eighty percent of bone mineralization in the fetus occurs during the third trimester.[296] in normal circumstances. The intrauterine accretion of Ca and P is much higher in the fetus compared to extrauterine life. For example, a fetus who weighs 1 kg and is at 27 weeks gestation incorporates daily approximately 110 mg/kg of Ca and 76 mg/kg of P into the body from placental transfer.[297] This accretion rate of the "reference fetus" corresponds to intake of 12.2 mL/kg/d of 10 % Ca gluconate and 3.6 mEq/kg/d of potassium phosphate in parenteral nutrition (PN) solutions. However, this comparison may not be valid. The "reference fetus" usually develops in a normal metabolic environment and has sustained weight gain and growth. In contrast, VLBW infants, especially micro-premies, are usually very sick, are growing in an unstable metabolic environment, and usually do not achieve sustained weight gain for at least several weeks postnatally.

The best approach to OOP is prevention. To prevent OOP, an adequate amount and ratio of Ca and P intake is needed together with an adequate caloric intake, and particularly an adequate intake of vitamin D. Increased parenteral intakes of calcium and phosphorus result in greater retention of these minerals during parenteral nutrition therapy and in greater bone mineral content after therapy [298]. The proportion between Ca and P in parenteral nutrition of premature babies should be 1.7:1 [297, 299].

3.10. Juvenile rheumatoid arthritis

Osteoporosis is a serious problem in patients with chronic juvenile arthritis (JCA). The available data suggest that bone loss results from multifactorial processes which lead to bone degradation through the activation of osteoclasts [300]. : Glucocorticoids are obviously involved in the development of osteoporosis in JCA, but the role of other factors affecting bone mineralization remains unclear. Data suggest that early onset disease is also an important factor in the development of osteoporosis in JCA [301]. Also, the role of calcium and vitamin D supplementation for the prevention and treatment of osteoporosis associated with pediatric rheumatic diseases remains to be established [302].

Methotrexate is the gold standard for management of moderate to severe polyarthritis [303], although other "disease-modifying antirheumatic drugs" (DMARDs) such as sulfasalazine and cyclosporine are being used in combination with methotrexate in certain cases. These drugs provide major steroid sparing effect in many children with severe JRA with the hope that osteoporosis and growth failure will be reduced [303]. One study suggested that most young adults with JA attain a normal bone mineral density if the disease goes into remission, while young adults with active disease have increased risk for osteopenia and osteoporosis [304]. If a patient with rheumatic disease experiences sudden and unexplained pain localized in the forefoot, above the ankle, below the knee, or in the pelvis, a stress fracture should be suspected [305].

3.11. Drugs and toxics

Chronic therapy with heparin can cause osteoporosis. Low molecular weight (LMW) heparins potentially have significant advantages over unfractionated heparin and oral anticoagulants for both the prevention and treatment of thromboembolic events in children [306]. The advantages of LMW heparins over unfractionated heparin include a longer half-life (allowing once-daily or twice-daily subcutaneous dosing), high bioavailability and predictable anticoagulant response (avoiding the need for dose adjustment or laboratory monitoring in most patients), and a low risk of heparin-induced thrombocytopenia and osteoporosis [307]. Long-term exposure to treatment and prophylaxis of venous thromboembolism cause a modest but progressive decrease in BMD, more evident in patients on low-molecular-weight heparins (LMWH) than on acenocoumarol. [308].

Methotrexate osteopathy was first reported in children with leukemia treated with high doses of the drug, but it can also occur in patients treated with low doses [309]. Bone problems are characterized by severe lower extremity pain and osteoporosis involving the lower extremities, as well as thick dense provisional zones of calcification and growth arrest lines resembling scurvy. [310]. This can lead to fractures [311]. Patients with ALL may not have long-term effects on their bones after remission despite high doses of steroids (dexamethasone) and methotrexate (without cranial irradiation) [312]. In those who have low bone mineral density, it appears to be related to low physical activity levels [313]. The mechanism is multifactorial including previous chemotherapy, limited exercise capacity, and relative physical inactivity [314].

4. Work-up

Although work-up will vary depending on the suspected cause of osteoporosis, basic phospho-calcic biochemical tests should be always performed when evaluating a pediatric patient for osteoporosis. This includes; serum calcium, phosphorus, magnesium, alkaline phosphatase, creatinine, PTH, 25 vitamin D, 1,25 vitamin D, and urinary calcium, phosphorus, and creatinine.

Other tests may be requested in specific situations, including cAMP, biochemical markers of bone formation (Osteocalcin, Procollagen Type I C-Terminal Propeptide, Procollagen Type I N- Terminal Propeptide), and biochemical markers of bone resorption (Serum: Tartrate Resistant Acid Phosphatase, Type I Collagen Telopeptide, Urine: Collagen Crosslinks – Pyridinoline, Deoxypyridinoline, NTx- Hydroxyproline, and Galactosyl-hydroxylysine). It is of note that the interpretation of these markers in the pediatric population may be difficult [315], and are mostly used as markers to follow-up treatments.

Bone mineral density tests can be used to aid in the diagnosis and as a useful follow-up tool. In most cases measured by dual energy X-ray absorptiometry (DEXA), it can also be measured by QCT, pQCT and ultrasound.

Specific x-rays may be obtained, including wrists and/or knee x-rays for rickets, bone age, spine x-rays to rule out vertebral fractures, skull x-rays to assess the presence of wormian bones, long bones x-rays to assess bone deformity and bone quality, as well as cortical thickness.

5. Treatment

Prevention of metabolic bone diseases is often possible, particularly in the case of nutritional rickets and many secondary forms. Once established, and apart from treating the primary cause in children with secondary osteoporosis, the use of bisphosphonates in the pediatric population to treat osteoporosis has increased recently [316]. Children with cerebral palsy may benefit from standing programs, although the benefits of this therapy are yet to be demonstrated [317].

Pamidronate is a second-generation bisphosphonate with a chemical structure based on pyrophosphate, the one naturally occurring inhibitor of bone resorption [318]. The exact mechanism of action of the bisphosphonates remains unclear, although effects on both osteoblasts [319, 320] and osteoclasts [321-323] have been documented. Several non-controlled studies using pamidronate for pediatric populations have been published for treatment of osteogenesis imperfecta [184, 324-333] and secondary osteoporosis [334-338], all showing promising results.

Treatment of OI was classically focused on fracture and pain management and surgical correction of deformity (whenever possible). Several medical therapies had failed to increase bone density and decrease the incidence of fractures in this population [339], including vitamin C [340, 341], sodium fluoride [85, 342, 343], magnesium [344, 345], anabolic steroids [346, 347], and calcitonin [348, 349].

In children with OI over three years of age receiving treatment with pamidronate, there is a mean annualized increase of about 40 percent in bone mineral density, in infants this change can be as high as 200% per year [327]. The deviation of bone mineral density from normal, as indicated by the Z score, improves in several points. The cortical width of the metacarpals increases significantly, as well as the vertebral heights. The mean incidence of radiologically confirmed fractures decreases as well, but there is concern about the long term effects of pamidronate on fracture healing in children [350]. All the children treated report substantial relief of chronic pain and fatigue. In younger children, the results are even more remarkable, with signs of pain practically disappearing soon after start of treatment [327].

The drug is administered intravenously, in a dose calculated per body weight, in cycles of two or three consecutive days every four months. Evidence suggests that it can also be administered in one day monthly or every three months, with a dose calculated per body surface or at a fixed dose, depending on the protocol used [332, 351]. Patients usually receive an annual dose of 9-12 mg/kg, although lower doses may also be effective [352]. There are usually no adverse side effects, except for an acute phase reaction (a flu-like syndrome) the first time the drug is administered.

Despite higher risk of injury due to increased mobility a marked decrease in fracture rate is noted, suggesting a direct effect of the therapy. The disappearance of bone pain and decreased fracture incidence may contribute to greater mobility [353]. It is well known that physical activity is an essential factor for the development of the skeletal system [354]. Thus, increased mobility may synergize with the direct inhibitory effect of pamidronate on bone resorption to increase bone mass [333].

In young patients, pamidronate does not have a detrimental effect on growth. Instead, the height Z score increases in patients that have started treatment before three years of age [327]. Height z-scores increase significantly in patients with type III OI and do not change in patients with type I and IV OI after one year of pamidronate therapy [355]. After four years of pamidronate therapy, mean height z-scores increased significantly in children with moderate OI, whereas non-significant trends to increase are characteristic of patients with mild and severe OI in a published study [355]. Biopsy size (taken form the iliac crest) does not change significantly with pamidronate treatment in children with OI, but cortical width increases by about 90% and cancellous bone volume increases by about 45% due to higher trabecular number, whereas trabecular thickness remains stable [323]. In the growing skeleton pamidronate appears to have a two-fold effect. On one side, both bone resorption and formation are inhibited. However, osteoclasts and osteoblasts are active on different surfaces (and are thus uncoupled) during modeling of cortical bone. This causes a selective targeting of resorption while continuing bone formation can increase cortical width. There is no evidence for a mineralization defect in children with OI treated with pamidronate [323].

Serum levels of ionized calcium drop and serum PTH levels almost double after the first pamidronate infusion [356]. At the same time, urinary excretion of the bone resorption marker type I collagen N-telopeptide (related to creatinine - uNTX/uCr) decreases by about 60 to 70% during the first infusion cycle, and when expressed as a percentage of the age and sex-specific mean value in healthy children, decreases from a mean of about 130 at baseline to a mean of 50 after four years of therapy. On the other hand, parathyroid hormone levels increase by about 30% in the same period.

Oral bisphosphonates (Pamidronate, Alendronate, Risedronate) can be used in children with OI that are able to swallow pills and have no gastro-esophagic reflux. Patients taking oral bisphosphonates have the theoretical risk of gastric discomfort or even severe burning of the esophagus if the drug is not taken properly.

An adequate calcium and vitamin D intake is warranted, particularly in regions with low sun exposure. Daily vitamin D requirements are of 400 IU, and calcium requirements vary with age.

Long-term effects and ideal dose scheme of bisphosphonate treatment are not well characterized; therefore this therapy should be administered only under strict protocols.

Growth hormone (GH), IGF-1 and PTH have the potential to increase bone mass in children. Except for a treatment protocol with growth hormone in children with severe OI [357], the experience in children with these agents has been anecdotal. Children with OI treated with GH can be responders or non-responders in terms of linear growth [357]. Treatment determines an increase in cancellous bone volume and trabecular number in "responders", but cortical bone does not change at all, even in those responding in terms of growth. Furthermore, bone resorption is increased in "non-responders". PICP appears to be higher at baseline for responders, but response to GH in children with OI can not be accurately predicted. An increase of fracture rate during GH therapy has been reported [358, 359]. In a controlled study, comparing 7 children with mild OI with 7 receiving no treatment, fracture rate was not different between the groups [360]. GH should not be used as a first-line therapy in OI [361].

Only limited experience has been achieved on the use of bisphosphonates in children receiving pharmacologic doses of glucocorticoids. A prospective multicenter, open study of oral pamidronate (5 or 10 mg/day) in 38 children with rheumatologic diseases aged 9 to 16 years, with low BMD and receiving glucocorticoid treatment for at least 6 months, or with a history of bone fragility fractures showed a significant increase in lumbar spine BMD in all subjects after 1 year of treatment [362, 363]. In the only double-blind study of IV pamidronate in children published so far, Henderson et al. showed promising results in the treatment of children with cerebral palsy [337]. In a case of a child with normal bone density that received very high doses of pamidronate, osteopetrosis developed [200]. Lower doses of pamidronate will possibly prevent development of osteopetrosis and delayed fracture healing. More research is warranted on these aspects.

REFERENCES

1. Plotkin, H, Sawyer, A and Bachrach, L, Journal of Bone and Joint Surgery Am, 85 (2003).
2. Glastre, C, Braillon, P, David, L, Cochat, P, Meunier, PJ and Delmas, PD, J Clin Endocrinol Metab, 70 (1990).
3. Zanchetta, JR, Plotkin, H and Alvarez Filgueira, ML, Bone, 16 (1995).
4. Braillon, PM and Cochat, P, Appl Radiat Isot, 49 (1998).
5. Bailey, DA, Int J Sports Med, 18 Suppl 3 (1997).
6. Molgaard, C, Thomsen, BL, Prentice, A, Cole, TJ and Michaelsen, KF, Arch Dis Child, 76 (1997).
7. Faulkner, RA, Bailey, DA, Drinkwater, DT, McKay, HA, Arnold, C and Wilkinson, AA, Calcif Tissue Int, 59 (1996).
8. Nguyen, TV, Maynard, LM, Towne, B, Roche, AF, Wisemandle, W, Li, J, Guo, SS, Chumlea, WC and Siervogel, RM, Journal of Clinical Densitometry, 4 (2001).
9. Mazess, RB, Journal of Pediatrics, 113 (1988).
10. DePriester, JA, Cole, TJ and Bishop, NJ, Bone and Mineral, 12 (1991).
11. Trouerbach, WT, de Man, SA, Gommers, D, Zwamborn, AW and Grobbee, DE, Bone Miner, 13 (1991).
12. Plotkin, H, Nunez, M, Alvarez Filgueira, ML and Zanchetta, JR, Calcif Tissue Int, 58 (1996).
13. Plotkin, H, Nuñez, M, Alvarez Filgueira, ML and Zanchetta, JR, Archivos Argentinos de Pediatría, 94 (1996).
14. Schonau, E, Pediatric Nephrology, 12 (1998).
15. Carter, DR, Bouxsein, ML and Marcus, R, J Bone Miner Res, 7 (1992).
16. Seeman, E, Young, N, Szmukler, G, Tsalamandris, C and Hopper, JL, Osteoporosis International, Suppl 1 (1993).
17. Kelly, PJ, Eisman, JA and Sambrook, PN, Osteoporosis International, 1 (1990).
18. Heaney, RP, Abrams, S, Dawson-Hughes, B, Looker, A, Marcus, R, Matkovic, V and Weaver, C, Osteoporosis International, 11 (2000).
19. Matkovic, V, Jelic, T, Wardlaw, GM, Ilich, JZ, Goel, PK, Wright, JK, Andon, MB, Smith, KT and Heaney, RP, J Clin Invest, 93 (1994).
20. Matkovic, V, Journal of Rheumatology, 19 (1992).
21. Matkovic, V, J Intern Med, 231 (1992).

22. Fitzpatrick, LA and Heaney, RP, Journal of Bone and Mineral Research, 18 (2003).
23. Heaney, RP, Am J Clin Nutr, 72 (2000).
24. Fitzpatrick, LA, Mayo Clinic Proceedings, 77 (2002).
25. Heaney, RP, Dowell, S, Bierman, J, Hale, CA and Bendich, A, Journal of the American College of Nutrition, 20 (2001).
26. Martin, BR, Weaver, CM, Heaney, RP, Packard, PT and Smith, DL, J Agric Food Chem, 50 (2002).
27. Heaney, RP, Osteoporosis International, 1 (1991).
28. Frame, B and Parfitt, AM, Ann Int Med, 89 (1978).
29. Pettifor, J, in: Pediatric bone: Biology and diseases, Ed. Glorieux, FH, Pettifor, JM and Jueppner, H (Academic Press, San Diego,2003), p. 541
30. Norman, AW, Roth, J and Orci, L, Endocrine Reviews, 3 (1982).
31. Horst, RL and Reinhardt, TA, in: Vitamin d, Ed. Feldman, D, Glorieux, FH and Pike, JW (Academic Press, San Diego,1997), p. 13
32. Curran, JS and Barness, LA, in: Nelson's textbook of pediatrics, Ed. Behrman, RE, Kliegman, RM and Jenson, HB (W.B. Saunders, Philadelphia,2000), p. 155
33. Anatoliotaki, M, Tsilimigaki, A, Tsekoura, T, Schinaki, A, Stefanaki, S and Nikolaidou, P, Acta Paediatrica, 92 (2003).
34. Hahn, TJ, Hendin, BA, Scharp, CR and Haddad, JGJ, New England Journal of Medicine, 287 (1972).
35. Hahn, TJ, Hendin, BA, Scharp, CR, Boisseau, VC and Haddad, JGJ, New England Journal of Medicine, 292 (1975).
36. Bischoff, F, Basu, D and Pettifor, JM, Dev Med Child Neurol., 44 (2002).
37. Henderson, RC, Lin, PP and Greene, WB, J Bone Joint Surg Am, 77 (1995).
38. Jubiz, W, Haussler, MR, McCain, TA and Tolman, KG, Journal of Clinical Endocrinology and Metabolism, 44 (1977).
39. Ala-Houhala, M, Korpela, R, Koivikko, M, Koskinen, T, Koskinen, M and Koivula, T, Neuropediatrics, 17 (1986).
40. Chesney, RW, Zimmerman, J, Hamstra, A, DeLuca, HF and Mazees, RB, Am J Dis Child, 135 (1981).
41. Compston, JE, Vedi, S, Merrett, AL, Clemens, TL, O'Riordan, JL and Woodhead, JS, Metab Bone Dis Relat Res, 3 (1981).
42. Parfitt, AM, in: Vitamin d, Ed. Feldman, D, Glorieux, F, H, and Pike, JW (Academic Press, San Diego,1997), p. 645
43. Holick, MF, in: Rickets, Ed. Glorieux, FH (Raven Press, New York,1991), p. 1
44. Kruse, K, Journal of Pediatrics, 126 (1995).
45. Shah, BR and Finberg, L, Journal of Pediatrics, 125 (1994).
46. Albright, F, Butler, AM and Bloomberg, E, American Journal of Diseases in Children, 54 (1937).
47. Prader, VA, Illig, R and Heierli, E, Helv Paediatr Acta, 16 (1961).
48. Fraser, D, Kooh, SW, Kind, HP, Hollick, MF, Tanaka, Y and DeLuca, HF, New England Journal of Medicine, 289 (1973).

49. Fu, GK, Lin, D, Zhang, MY, Bikle, DD, Shackleton, CH, Miller, WL and Portale, AA, Mol Endocrinol, 11 (1997).

50. Aarskog, D, Aksnes, L and Markestad, T, Pediatrics, 71 (1983).

51. Scriver, CR, Pediatrics, 45 (1970).

52. De Braekeleer, M and Larochelle, J, Ann Hum Genet, 55 (1991).

53. Labuda, M, Morgan, K and Glorieux, FH, American Journal of Human Genetics, 47 (1990).

54. Portale, AA and Miller, WL, in: Pediatric bones: Biology and diseases, Ed. Glorieux, FH, Pettifor, J and Jueppner, H (Academic Press, San Diego,2003), p. 583

55. Stoop, JW, Schraagen, MJ and Tiddens, HA, Acta Paediatrica Scandinava, 56 (1967).

56. Arnaud, C, Maijer, R, Reade, t, Scriver, CR and Whelan, DT, Pediatrics, 46 (1970).

57. Scriver, CR, Reade, TM, DeLuca, HF and Hamstra, AJ, New England Journal of Medicine, 299. (1978).

58. Wang, JT, Lin, CJ, Burridge, SM, Fu, GK, Labuda, M, Portale, AA and Miller, WL, Am J Hum Genet, 63 (1998).

59. Delvin, EE, Glorieux, FH, Marie, PJ and Pettifor, JM, Journal of Pediatrics, 99 (1981).

60. Delvin, EE, Salle, BL, Glorieux, FH, Adeleine, P and David, LS, Journal of Pediatrics, 109 (1986).

61. Glorieux, FH and St-Arnaud, R, in: Vitamin d, Ed. Feldman, D, Glorieux, FH and Pike, JW (Academic Press, San DIego,1997), p. 755

62. Brooks, MH, Bell, NH, Love, L, Stern, PH, Orfei, E, Queener, SF, Hamstra, AJ and DeLuca, HF, New England Journal of Medicine, 298 (1978).

63. Marx, SJ, Spiegel, AM, Brown, EM, Gardner, DG, Downs, RW, Attie, M, Hamstra, AJ and DeLuca, HF, Journal of Clinical Endocrinology and Metabolism, 47 (1978).

64. Malloy, PJ, Hochberg, Z, Tiosano, D, Pike, JW, Hughes, MR and Feldman, D, J Clin Invest, 86 (1990).

65. Liberman, UA, Eil, C and Marx, SJ, Journal of Clinical Investigation, 71 (1983).

66. Fraher, LJ, Karmali, R, Hinde, FR, Hendy, GN, Jani, H, Nicholson, L, Grant, D and O'Riordan, JL, Eur J Pediatr, 145 (1986).

67. Liberman, UA, Samuel, R, Halabe, A, Kauli, R, Edelstein, S, Weisman, Y, Papapoulos, SE, Clemens, TL, Fraher, LJ and O'Riordan, JL, Lancet, 1 (1980).

68. Chen, TL, Hirst, MA, Cone, CM, Hochberg, Z, Tietze, HU and Feldman, D, J Clin Endocrinol Metab, 59 (1984).

69. Hughes, MR, Malloy, PJ, Kieback, DG, Kesterson, RA, Pike, JW, Feldman, D and O'Malley, BW, Science, 242 (1988).

70. Malloy, PJ, Hochberg, Z, Pike, JW and Feldman, D, J Clin Endocrinol Metab, (1989).

71. Rummens, K, Van Cromphaut, SJ, Carmeliet, G, Van Herck, E, Van Bree, R, Stockmans, I, Bouillon, R and Verhaeghe, J, Pediatr Res, (2003).

72.   Marx, SJ, Bliziotes, MM and Nanes, M, Clin Endocrinol (Oxf), 25 (1986).
73.   Malloy, PJ, Xu, R, Peng, L, Clark, PA and Feldman, D, Mol Endocrinol, 16 (2002).
74.   Plotkin, H, Primorac, D and Rowe, D, in: Pediatric bone - biology and disease, Ed. Glorieux, F, Pettifor, J and Juppner, J (Elsevier Science, San Diego, CA,2003), p. 443
75.   Sillence, D, Bone, 27 (2000).
76.   Orioli, IM, Castilla, EE and Barbosa-Neto, JG, J Med Genet, 23 (1986).
77.   Komai, T, Kunii, H and Ozaki, Y, American Journal of Human Genetics, 8 (1956).
78.   Heiberg, A, Clinical Genetics, 23 (1983).
79.   Sillence, DO, Senn, A and Danks, DM, J Med Genet, 16 (1979).
80.   Andersen, PE and Hauge, M, Clin Genet, 36 (1989).
81.   Dalgleish, R, Nucleic Acids Research, 25 (1997).
82.   Smith, R, Int J Exp Pathol, 75 (1994).
83.   Vetter, U, Pontz, B, Zauner, E, Brenner, RE and Spranger, J, Calcif Tissue Int, 50 (1992).
84.   Dent, JA and Paterson, CR, J Pediatr Orthop, 11 (1991).
85.   Albright, JA and Grunt, JA, J Bone Joint Surg [Am], 53 (1971).
86.   Sawin, PD and Menezes, AH, J Neurosurg, 86 (1997).
87.   Ziv, I, Rang, M and Hoffman, HJ, J Bone Joint Surg [Br], 65 (1983).
88.   Brooks, ML, Gall, C, Wang, AM, Schick, R and Rumbaugh, CL, Comput Med Imaging Graph, 13 (1989).
89.   Garretsen, AJ, Cremers, CW and Huygen, PL, Ann Otol Rhinol Laryngol, 106 (1997).
90.   Hortrop, J, Tsipouras, P, Hanley, JA, Maron, BJ and Shapiro, JR, Circulation, 73 (1986).
91.   Vetter, U, Maierhofer, B, Muller, M, Lang, D, Teller, WM, Brenner, R, Frohneberg, D and Worsdorfer, O, Eur J Pediatr, 149 (1989).
92.   Rowe, DW and Shapiro, JR, in: Metabolic bone disease and clinically related disorders, Ed. Avioli, LV and Krane, SM (Academic Press, San Diego,1998), p. 651
93.   Chines, A, Petersen, DJ, Schranck, FW and Whyte, MP, Journal of Pediatrics, 119 (1991).
94.   Chines, A, Boniface, A, McAlister, W and Whyte, M, Bone, 16 (1995).
95.   Cropp, GJ and Myers, DN, Pediatrics, 49 (1972).
96.   Paily, BT, in: Preanesthetic assessment, Ed. Frost, EAM 1996), p. 301
97.   Cho, E, Dayan, SS and Marx, GF, Br J Anaesth, 68 (1992).
98.   Falvo, KA, Klain, DB, Krauss, AN, Root, L and Auld, PA, American Review of Respiratory Disease, 108 (1973).
99.   Evensen, SA, Myhre, L and Stormorken, H, Scand J Haematol, 33 (1984).
100. Wordsworth, P, Ogilvie, D, Smith, R and Sykes, B, Br J Rheumatol, 26 (1987).
101. Spence, PA, Cohen, Z and Salerno, TA, Can Med Assoc J, 131 (1984).
102. Lukinmaa, PL, Ranta, H, Ranta, K and Kaitila, I, J Craniofac Genet Dev Biol, 7 (1987).

103. Lindau, BM, Dietz, W, Hoyer, I, Lundgren, T, Storhaug, K and Noren, JG, Int J Pediatr Dent, 9 (1999).
104. Lund, AM, Jensen, BL, Nielsen, LA and Skovby, F, Journal of Craniofacial Genetics & Developmental Biology, 18 (1998).
105. Johnsen, D and Tinanoff, N, in: Nelson textbook of pediatrics, Ed. Behrman, RE, Kliegman, RM and H.B., J (W.B. Saunders, Philadelphia,2000), p. 1110
106. Schwartz, S and Tsipouras, P, Oral Surg Oral Med Oral Pathol, 57 (1984).
107. O'Connell, AC and Marini, JC, Oral Surgery, Oral Medicine, Oral Pathology, Oral Radiology, & Endodontics, 87 (1999).
108. Whitestone, BW and Chapnick, P, J Can Dent Assoc, 52 (1986).
109. Paterson, CR, Ogston, SA and Henry, RM, Bmj, 312 (1996).
110. McAllion, SJ and Paterson, CR, J Clin Pathol, 49 (1996).
111. Zlotogora, J, Human Genetics, 102 (1998).
112. Constantinou-Deltas, CD, Ladda, RL and Prockop, DJ, Am J Med Genet, 45 (1993).
113. Wallis, GA, Starman, BJ, Zinn, AB and Byers, PH, Am J Hum Genet, 46 (1990).
114. Byers, PH, Tsipouras, P, Bonadio, JF, Starman, BJ and Schwartz, RC, American Journal of Human Genetics, 42 (1988).
115. King, JD and Boblechko, WP, The Journal of Bone and Joint Surgery, 53B (1971).
116. Sillence, D, Clin Orthop, (1981).
117. Constantinou, CD, Pack, M, Young, SB and Prockop, DJ, Am J Hum Genet, 47 (1990).
118. Paterson, CR, McAllion, S and Miller, R, J Bone Joint Surg [Br], 65 (1983).
119. Hanscom, DA, Winter, RB, Lutter, L, Lonstein, JE, Bloom, BA, Bradford, DS and Aldred, MJ, J Bone Joint Surg [Am], 74 (1992).
120. Bauze, RJ, Smith, R and Francis, MJ, J Bone Joint Surg [Br], 57 (1975).
121. Smith, R, Clinics in Rheumatic Diseases, 12 (1986).
122. Match, RM and Corrylos, EV, American Journal of Sports Medicine, 11 (1983).
123. Levin, LS, Salinas, CF and Jorgenson, RJ, Lancet, 1 (1978).
124. Shapiro, JR, Pikus, A, Weiss, G and Rowe, DW, JAMA, 247 (1982).
125. Pedersen, U, Scand Audiol, 13 (1984).
126. Serin, G, Gersappe, A, Black, JD, Aronoff, R and Maquat, LE, Mol Cell Biol, 21 (2001).
127. Frischmeyer, PA, van Hoof, A, O'Donnell, K, Guerrerio, AL, Parker, R and Dietz, HC, Science, 295 (2002).
128. Maquat, LE, Curr Biol, 12 (2002).
129. Johnson, C, Primorac, D, McKinstry, M, McNeil, J, Rowe, D and Lawrence, JB, J Cell Biol, 150 (2000).
130. Willing, MC, Pruchno, CJ and Byers, PH, Am J Med Genet, 45 (1993).
131. Pauli, RM and Gilbert, EF, J Pediatr, 108 (1986).
132. Shapiro, JR, Burn, VE, Chipman, SD, Jacobs, JB, Schloo, B, Reid, L, Larsen, N and Louis, F, Bone, 10 (1989).

133. Andrews, M and Amparo, EG, AJR Am J Roentgenol, 160 (1993).

134. Heller, RH, Winn, KJ and Heller, RM, Am J Obstet Gynecol, 121 (1975).

135. Prockop, DJ, J Clin Invest, 75 (1985).

136. Cole, WG and Dalgleish, R, J Med Genet, 32 (1995).

137. Sillence, DO, Barlow, KK, Garber, AP, Hall, JG and Rimoin, DL, Am J Med Genet, 17 (1984).

138. Pace, JM, Chitayat, D, Atkinson, M, Wilcox, WR, Schwarze, U and Byers, PH, J Med Genet, 39 (2002).

139. Plotkin, H, BioMed Central Pediatrics, in press (2004).

140. Banta, JV, Schreiber, RR and Kulik, WJ, J Bone Joint Surg [Am], 53 (1971).

141. Morike, M, Windsheimer, E, Brenner, R, Nerlich, A, Bushart, G, Teller, W and Vetter, U, J Orthop Res, 11 (1993).

142. Glorieux, FH, Rauch, F, Plotkin, H, Wart, L, Travers, R, Roughley, P, Lalic, L, Glorieux, DF, Fassier, F and Bishop, NJ, J Bone Miner Res, 15 (2000).

143. Roberts, JB, J Bone Joint Surg [Am], 58 (1976).

144. Burke, TE, Crerand, SJ and Dowling, F, J Pediatr Orthop, 8 (1988).

145. Burchardt, AJ, Wagner, AA and Basse, P, Acta Radiol, 35 (1994).

146. Azouz, EM and Fassier, F, Skeletal Radiol, 26 (1997).

147. Kutsumi, K, Nojima, T, Yamashiro, K, Hatae, Y, Isu, K, Ubayama, Y and Yamawaki, S, Skeletal Radiol, 25 (1996).

148. Nakamura, K, Kurokawa, T, Nagano, A and Umeyama, T, Arch Orthop Trauma Surg, 116 (1997).

149. Beighton, P, Clin Genet, 29 (1986).

150. Capoen, J, De Paepe, A and Lauwers, H, J Belge Radiol, 76 (1993).

151. Bianchine, JW, Briard-Guillemot, ML, Maroteaux, P, Frezal, J and Harrison, HE, Am. J. Hum. Genet., 24 (1972).

152. Beighton, P, Winship, I and Behari, D, Clin Genet, 28 (1985).

153. Gong, Y, Slee, RB, Fukai, N, Rawadi, G, Roman-Roman, S, Reginato, AM, Wang, H, Cundy, T, Glorieux, FH, Lev, D, Zacharin, M, Oexle, K, Marcelino, J, Suwairi, W and Heeger, S, Cell, 107 (2001).

154. Gong, Y, Vikkula, M, Boon, L, Beighton, P, Ramesar, R, Peltonen, L, Somer, H, Hirose, T, Dallapiccola, B, De Paepe, A, Swoboda, W, Zabel, B, Superti-Furga, A, Steinmann, B, Brunner, HG, Jans, A, Boles, RG, Adkins, W, van den Boogaard, M-J, Olsen, BR and Warman, ML, American Journal of Human Genetics, 59 (1996).

155. Zacharin, M and Cundy, T, The Journal of Pediatrics, 137 (1999).

156. 156. al Gazali, LI, Sabrinathan, K and Nair, KG, Clin Dysmorphol, 3 (1994).

157. Buyse, M and Bull, MJ, Birth Defects Orig Artic Ser, 14 (1978).

158. Cole, DE and Carpenter, TO, J Pediatr, 110 (1987).

159. Amor, DJ, Savarirayan, R, Schneider, AS and Bankier, A, American Journal of Medical Genetics, 92 (2000).

160. Blacksin, MF, Pletcher, BA and David, M, Pediatr Radiol, 28 (1998).

161. McPherson, E and Clemens, M, Am J Med Genet, 70 (1997).

162. Leroy, JG, Nuytinck, L, De Paepe, A, De Rammelaere, M, Gillerot, Y, Verloes, A, Loeys, B and De Groote, W, Pediatric Radiology, 28 (1998).

163. Viljoen, D, Versfeld, G and Beighton, P, Clin Genet, 36 (1989).
164. Brady, AF and Patton, MA, Clin Dysmorphol, 6 (1997).
165. Bank, RA, Robins, SP, Wijmenga, C, Breslau-Siderius, LJ, Bardoel, AFJ, Van der Sluijs, HA, Pruijs, HEH and TeKoppele, JM, Proc Natl Acad Sci USA, 96 (1999).
166. Glorieux, FH, Wart, L, Rauch, F, Lalic, L, Roughley, P and Travers, R, Journal of Bone and Mineral Research, 17 (2002).
167. Baker, SL, Dent, CE, Friedman, M and Watson, L, Journal of Bone and Joint Surgery Br, 48 (1966).
168. Lang, R, Vignery, AM and Jensen, PS, Bone, 7 (1986).
169. Ward, L, Rauch, F, Travers, R, Chabot, G, Azouz, E, Lalic, L, Roughley, PJ and Glorieux, FH, Bone, 31 (2002).
170. Labuda, M, Morissette, J, Wart, LM, Rauch, F, Lalic, L, Roughley, PJ and Glorieux, FH, Bone, 31 (2002).
171. Dent, CE and Friedman, M, QJM, 134 (1965).
172. Villaverde, V, De Inocencio, J, Merino, R and Garcia-Consuegra, J, Journal of Rheumatology, 25 (1998).
173. Dimar, JRn, Campbell, M, Glassman, SD, Puno, RM and Johnson, JR, American Journal of Orthopedics, 24 (1995).
174. Smith, R, Br J Rheumatol, 34 (1995).
175. Child, JA and Smith, IE, British Medical Journal, 29 (1975).
176. Dent, CE, Postgrad Med J, 53 (1977).
177. Vela, BS, Dorin, RI and Hartshorne, MF, Skeletal Radiology, 19 (1990).
178. Krassas, GE, Annals of the New York Academy of Sciences, 900 (2000).
179. Rauch, F, Travers, R, Norman, ME, Taylor, A, Parfitt, AM and Glorieux, FH, Journal of Bone and Mineral Research, 15 (2000).
180. Rauch, F, Travers, R, Norman, ME, Taylor, A, Parfitt, AM and Glorieux, FH, Bone, 31 (2002).
181. Jackson, EC, Strife, CF, Tsang, RC and Marder, HK, Am J Dis Child, 142 (1988).
182. 182.
183. Saggese, G, Bertelloni, S, Baroncelli, GI, Perri, G and Calderazzi, A, Am J Dis Child, 145 (1991).
184. Papapoulos, SE, in: Osteoporosis, Ed. Marcus, R, Feldman, D and Kelsey, J 1996), p. 1209
185. Whyte, MP, in: The metabolic & molecular bases of inherited disease, Ed. Scriver, CH, Beaudet, AL, Sly, WS and Valle, D (McGraw-Hill, New York,2001), p. 5313
186. Caswell, AM, Whyte, MP and Russell, RGG, Crit Rev Clin Lab Sci, 28 (1992).
187. Orimo, H, Hayashi, Z, Watanabe, A, Hirayama, T, Hirayama, T and Shimada, T, Human Molecular Genetics, 3 (1994).
188. Orimo, H, Goseki-Sone, M, Sato, S and Shimada, T, Genomics, 42 (1997).
189. Whyte, MP, Mahuren, JD, Vrabel, LA and Coburn, SP, J Clin Invest., 76 (1985).

190. Whyte, MP, in: Primer on the metabolic bine diseases and disorders of mineral metabolism, Ed. Favus, MJ (American Society for Bone and Mineral Research, Washington,2003), p. 423

191. Shohat, M, Rimoin, DL, Gruber, HE and Lachman, RS, Pediatric Radiology, 21 (1991).

192. Moore, CA, Ward, JC, Rivas, ML, Magill, HL and Whyte, MP, American Journal of Medical Genetics, 36 (1990).

193. Henthorn, PS and Whyte, MP, Clin Chem, 38 (1992).

194. Henthorn, PS and Whyte, MP, Prenatal Diagnosis, 15 (1995).

195. Scriver, CR and Cameron, D, New England Journal of Medicine, 281 (1969).

196. Cole, DE, Salisbury, SR, Stinson, RA, Coburn, SP, Ryan, LM and Whyte, MP, New England Journal of Medicine, 314 (1986).

197. Greenberg, CR, Evans, JA, McKendry-SMith, S, Redekopp, S, Haworth, JC, Mulivor, R and Chodricker, BN, American Journal of Human Genetics, 46 (1990).

198. Girschick, HJ, Seyberth, HW and Huppertz, HI, Bone, 25 (1999).

199. Cassinelli, HR, Mautalen, CA, Heinrich, JJ, Miglietta, A and Bergada, C, Bone and Mineral, 19 (1992).

200. Whyte, MP, Wenkert, D, Clements, KL, McAlister, WH and Mumm, S, New England Journal of Medicine, 349 (2003).

201. Geven, WB, Monnens, LA and Willems, JL, Miner Electrolyte Metab, 19 (1993).

202. Suh, SM, Tashjian, AHJ, Matsuo, N, Parkinson, DK and Fraser, D, J Clin Invest, 52 (1973).

203. Woodard, JC, Webster, PD and Carr, AA, Am J Dig Dis, 17 (1972).

204. Challa, A, Papaefstathiou, I, Lapatsanis, D and Tsolas, O, Acta Paediatr, 84 (1995).

205. Rosen, MG and Dickinson, JC, Am J Obstet Gynecol, 167 (1992).

206. Chapchal, G, J Int Coll Surg, 44 (1965).

207. Takata, S and Yasui, N, J Med Invest, 48 (2001).

208. Schiessl, H, Frost, HM and Jee, WS, Bone, 22 (1998).

209. Klein, G, Nutrition, 14 (1998).

210. 210. Leonberg, BL, Chuang, E, Eicher, P, Tershakovec, AM, Leonard, L and Stallings, VA, J Pediatr, 132 (1998).

211. Buchman, AL and Moukarzel, A, Clinical Nutrition, 19 (2000).

212. Dellert, SF, Farrell, MK, Specker, BL and Heubi, JE, J Pediatr, 132 (1998).

213. Frost, HM, Anat Rec, 219 (1987).

214. Frost, HM, Ferretti, JL and Jee, WSS, Calcif Tissue Int, 62 (1998).

215. Ferretti, JL, Cointry, GR, Capozza, RF and Frost, HM, Mech Ageing Dev, 124 (2003).

216. Sugiyama, T, Yamaguchi, A and Kawai, S, J Bone Miner Metab, 20 (2002).

217. Newacheck, P and Taylor, WR, Am J Public Health, 82 (1992).

218. Cans, C, Dev Med Child Neurol, 42 (2000).

219. Bottos, M, Granato, T, Allibrio, G, Gioachin, C and Puata, ML, Dev Med Child Neurol, 41 (1999).

220. Bianchi, ML, Mazzanti, A, Galbiati, E, Saraifoger, S, Dubini, A, Cornelio, F and Morandi, L, Osteoporos Int., 14 (2003).
221. Larson, CM and Henderson, RC, J Pediatr Orthop, (2000).
222. Aparicio, LF, Jurkovic, M and DeLullo, J, J Pediatr Orthop, 22 (2002).
223. Bothwell, JE, Gordon, KE, Dooley, JM, MacSween, J, Cummings, EA and Salisbury, S, Clin Pediatr (Phila), 42 (2003).
224. Pascual, J, Argente, J, Lopez, MB, Munoz, M, Martinez, G, Vazquez, MA, Jodar, E, Perez-Cano, R and Hawkins, F, Calcif Tissue Int, 62 (1998).
225. Valerioa, G, del Puente, A, Esposito-del Puente, A, Buonoc, P, Mozzilloc, E and Franzese, A, Hormone Research, 58 (2002).
226. Piepkorn, B, Kann, P, Forst, T, Andreas, J, Pfutzner, A and Beyer, J, Horm Metab Res, 29 (1997).
227. Lettgen, B, Hauffa, B, Mohlmann, C, Jeken, C and Reiners, C, Horm Res, 43 (1995).
228. Roe, TF, Mora, S, Costin, G, Kaufman, F, Carlson, ME and Gilsanz, V, Metabolism, 40 (1991).
229. Weger, W, Kotanko, P, Weger, M, Deutschmann, H and Skrabal, F, Nephrol Dial Transplant, 15 (2000).
230. Gulati, S, Godbole, M, Singh, U, Gulati, K and Srivastava, A, Am J Kidney Dis, 41 (2003).
231. Acott, PD, Crocker, JF and Wong, JA, Pediatr Transplant, 7 (2003).
232. el-Husseini, AA, el-Agroudy, AE, Sobh, MA and Ghoneim, MA, Nefrologia, 23 (2003).
233. Davies, MC, Gulekli, B and Jacobs, HS, Clin Endocrinol (Oxf), 43 (1995).
234. Kazis, K and Iglesias, E, Adolesc Med, 14 (2003).
235. Eliakim, A and Beyth, Y, J Pediatr Adolesc Gynecol, 16 (2003).
236. Vestergaard, P, Emborg, C, Stoving, RK, Hagen, C, Mosekilde, L and Brixen, K, Orthop Nurs, 22 (2003).
237. Gordon, CM and Nelson, LM, Curr Opin Obstet Gynecol, 15 (2003).
238. Rubin, K, Pediatrics, 102 (1998).
239. Gravholt, CH, Lauridsen, AL, Brixen, K, Mosekilde, L, Heickendorff, L and Christiansen, JS, J Clin Endocrinol Metab, 87 (2002).
240. Shore, RM, Chesney, RW, Mazess, RB, Rose, PG and Bargman, GJ, Calcif Tissue Int, 34 (1982).
241. Ross, JL, Long, LM, Feuillan, P, Cassorla, F and Cutler, GB, Jr., J Clin Endocrinol Metab, 73 (1991).
242. Neely, EK, Marcus, R, Rosenfeld, RG and Bachrach, LK, J Clin Endocrinol Metab, 76 (1993).
243. Shaw, NJ, Rehan, VK, Husain, S, Marshall, T and Smith, CS, Clin Endocrinol (Oxf), 47 (1997).
244. Nanao, K, Tsuchiya, Y, Kotoh, S and Hasegawa, Y, J Pediatr Endocrinol Metab, 15 (2002).
245. Gravholt, CH, Vestergaard, P, Hermann, AP, Mosekilde, L, Brixen, K and Christiansen, JS, Clin Endocrinol (Oxf), 59 (2003).
246. Stepan, JJ, Musilova, J and Pacovsky, V, J Bone Miner Res, 4 (1989).

247.	Naeraa, RW, Brixen, K, Hansen, RM, Hasling, C, Mosekilde, L, Andresen, JH, Charles, P and Nielsen. J, Calcif Tissue Int, 49 (1991).

248.	Hogler, W, Briody, J, Moore, B, Garnett, S, Lu, PW and Cowell, CT, J Clin Endocrinol Metab, 89 (2004).

249.	Sylvester, FA, Curr Opin Pediatr, 11 (1999).

250.	Mora, S, Barera, G, Ricotti, A, Weber, G, Bianchi, C and Chiumello, G, Am J Clin Nutr, 67 (1998).

251.	Kavak, US, Yuce, A, Kocak, N, Demir, H, Saltik, IN, Gurakan, F and Ozen, H, J Pediatr Gastroenterol Nutr, 37 (2003).

252.	West, J, Logan, RF, Card, TR, Smith, C and Hubbard, R, Gastroenterology, 125 (2003).

253.	Scolapio, JS, DeArment, J, Hurley, DL, Romano, M, Harnois, D and Weigand, SD, JPEN J Parenter Enteral Nutr, 27 (2003).

254.	Isaia, G, Di Stefano, M, Roggia, C, Ardissone, P and Rosina, F, Forum (Genova), 8 (1998).

255.	Klein, GL, Soriano, H, Shulman, RJ, Levy, M, Jones, G and Langman, CB, Pediatr Transplant, 6 (2002).

256.	Ng, TMH and Bajjoka, IE, Ann Pharmacother, 33 (1999).

257.	Grey, AB, Ames, RW, Matthews, RD and Reid, IR, Thorax, 48 (1993).

258.	Bhudhikanok, GS, Lim, J, Marcus, R, Harkins, A, Moss, RB and Bachrach, LK, Pediatrics, 97 (1996).

259.	Gibbens, DT, Gilsanz, V, Boechat, MI, Dufer, D, Carlson, ME and Wang, CI, J Pediatr, 113 (1988).

260.	Reiter, EO, Brugman, SM, Pike, JW, Pitt, M, Dokoh, S, Haussler, MR, Gerstle, RS and Taussig, LM, J Pediatr, 106 (1985).

261.	Salamoni, F, Roulet, M, Gudinchet, F, Pilet, M, Thiebaud, D and Burckhardt, P, Arch Dis Child, 74 (1996).

262.	Henderson, RC and Madsen, CD, J Pediatr, 128 (1996).

263.	Hoffmann, GF, Nyhan, W, Zschocke, J, Kahler, SG and Mayatepek, E, in: Inherited metabolic diseases, (Lippincot Williams & Wilkins, Philadelphia,2002), p. 344

264.	Lee, FA, Donnell, GN and Gwinn, JL, Pediatr Radiol, 5 (1977).

265.	Crandall, BF, Philippart, M, Brown, WJ and Bluestone, DA, Am J Med Genet, 12 (1982).

266.	Groen, JJ, Isr J Med Sci, 1 (1965).

267.	Beutler, E, Blood Rev, 2 (1988).

268.	Brautbar, A, Elstein, D, Abrahamov, A, Zeigler, M, Chicco, G, Beutler, E, Scott, CR and Zimran, A, Blood Cells Mol Dis, 31 (2003).

269.	Ginns, EI, Choudary, PV, Tsuji, S, Martin, B, Stubblefield, B, Sawyer, J, Hozier, J and Barranger, JA, Proc Natl Acad Sci U S A, 82 (1985).

270.	Goker-Alpan, O, Schiffmann, R, Park, JK, Stubblefield, BK, Tayebi, N and Sidransky, E, J Pediatr, 143 (2003).

271.	Mignot, C, Gelot, A, Bessieres, B, Daffos, F, Voyer, M, Menez, F, Fallet Bianco, C, Odent, S, Le Duff, D, Loget, P, Fargier, P, Costil, J, Josset, P,

Roume, J, Vanier, MT, Maire, I and Billette de Villemeur, T, Am J Med Genet, 120A (2003).

272. Katz, K, Cohen, IJ, Ziv, N, Grunebaum, M, Zaizov, R and Yosipovitch , Z, J Bone Joint Surg Am, 69 (1987).

273. Allen, MJ, Myer, BJ, Khokher, AM, Rushton, N and Cox, TM, QJM, 90 (1997).

274. Perheentupa, J and Simell, O, Birth Defects Orig Artic Ser, 10 (1974).

275. Svedstrom, E, Parto, K, Marttinen, M, Virtama, P and Simell, O, Skeletal Radiol, 22 (1993).

276. Simell, O, Perheentupa, J, Rapola, J, Visakorpi, JK and Eskelin, LE, Am J Med, 59 (1975).

277. Simell, O, Pediatr Res, 9 (1975).

278. Smith, DW, Scriver, CR, Tenenhouse, HS and Simell, O, Proc Natl Acad Sci USA, 84 (1987).

279. Rajantie, J, Simell, O, Rapola, J and Perheentupa, J, J Pediatr, 97 (1980).

280. Lukkarinen, M, Nanto-Salonen, K, Pulkki, K, Aalto, M and Simell, O, Metabolism, 52 (2003).

281. Allen, JR, Humphries, IR, Waters, DL, Roberts, DC, Lipson, AH, Howman-Giles, RG and Gaskin, KJ, Am J Clin Nutr, 59 (1994).

282. 282. Zeman, J, Bayer, M and Stepan, J, Acta Paediatr, 88 (1999).

283. Hillman, L, Schlotzhauer, C, Lee, D, Grasela, J, Witter, S, Allen, S and Hillman, R, Eur J Pediatr, 155 (1996).

284. Arikoski, P, Komulainen, J, Voutilainen, R, Riikonen, P, Parviainen, M, Tapanainen, P, Knip, M and Kroger, H, J Pediatr Hematol Oncol, 20 (1998).

285. Arikoski, P, Komulainen, J, Riikonen, P, Voutilainen, R, Knip, M and Kroger, H, Journal of CLinical Endocrinology and Metabolism, 84 (1999).

286. Shalet, SM, Archives of Disease in Childhood, 64 (1989).

287. Leiper, A, Pediatric Haematology and Oncology, 7 (1990).

288. Nysom, K, Holm, K, Michaelsen, KF, Hertz, H, Muller, J and Molgaard, C, Med Pediatr Oncol, 37 (2001).

289. Cushing, H, Bull Johns Hospinks Hosp, 50 (1932).

290. Dempster, D, Journal of Bone and Mineral Research, 4 (1989).

291. Mankin, HJ, New England Journal of Medicine, 326 (1992).

292. Kim, HKW, Popp, DJ and Hunter, DD, Journal of Bone and Mineral Research, 16 (2001).

293. Weinstein, RS, Jilka, RL, Parfitt, AM and Manolagas, SC, J Clinic Invest, 102 (1998).

294. Weinstein, RS, Bone, 23 (1998).

295. Weinstein, RS, Chen, JR, Powers, CC, Stewart, SA, Landes, RD, Bellido, T, Jilka, RL, A.M., P and Manolagas, SC, Journal of Clinical Investigation, 109 (2002).

296. Heaney, RP and Skillman, TG, Journal of Clinical Endocrinology and Metabolism, 33 (1971).

297. Ziegler, EE, O'Donnell, AM, Nelson, SE and Fomon, SJ, Growth, 40 (1976).

298.   Prestridge, LL, Schanler, RJ, Shulman, RJ, Burns, PA and Laine, LL, J Pediatr, 122 (1993).

299.   Pelegano, JF, Rowe, JC, Carey, DE, LaBarre, DJ, Raye, JR, Edgren, KW and Horak, E, Journal of Pediatrics, 114 (1989).

300.   Lepore, L, Pennesi, M, Barbi, E and Pozzi, R, Clin Exp Rheumatol, 9 Suppl 6 (1991).

301.   Celiker, R, Bal, S, Bakkaloglu, A, Ozaydin, E, Coskun, T, Cetin, A and Dincer, F, Rheumatol Int, (2003).

302.   Cimaz, R, Best Pract Res Clin Rheumatol, 16 (2002).

303.   Murray, KJ and Lovell, DJ, Best Pract Res Clin Rheumatol, 16 (2002).

304.   Haugen, M, Lien, G, Flato, B, Kvammen, J, Vinje, O, Sorskaar, D and Forre, O, Arthritis Rheum, (2000).

305.   Maenpaa, HM, Soini, I, Lehto, MU and Belt, EA, Clin Exp Rheumatol, 20 (2002).

306.   Albisetti, M and Andrew, M, Eur J Pediatr, 161 (2002).

307.   Eikelboom, JW and Hankey, GJ, Med J Aust, 177 (2002).

308.   Wawrzynska, L, Tomkowski, WZ, Przedlacki, J, Hajduk, B and Torbicki, A, Pathophysiol Haemost Thromb, 33 (2003).

309.   Zonneveld, IM, Bakker, WK, Dijkstra, PF, Bos, JD, van Soesbergen, RM and Dinant, HJ, Arch Dermatol, 132 (1996).

310.   Schwartz, AM and Leonidas, JC, Skeletal Radiol, 13-16 (1984).

311.   Stanisavljevic, S and Babcock, AL, Clin Orthop, 125 (1977).

312.   Lequin, MH, van der Shuis, IM, Van Rijn, RR, Hop, WC, van ven Huevel-Eibrink, MM, MuinckKeizer-Schrama, SM and van Kuijk, C, J Clin Densitom, 5 (2002).

313.   Tillmann, V, Darlington, AS, Eiser, C, Bishop, NJ and Davies, HA, J Bone Miner Res, 17 (2002).

314.   Warner, JT, Evans, WD, Webb, DK, Bell, W and Gregory, JW, Pediatr Res, 45 (1999).

315.   Schonau, E and Rauch, F, Hormone Research, 48 (suppl) (1997).

316.   Orcel, P and Beaudreuil, J, Joint Bone Spine, 69 (2002).

317.   Caulton, JM, Ward, KA, Alsop, CW, Dunn, G, Adams, JE and Mughal, MZ, Arch Dis Child, 89 (2004).

318.   Rodan, GA and Balena, R, Annals of Medicine, 25 (1993).

319.   Plotkin, LI, Parfitt, AM, Manolagas, SC and Bellido, T, JCI, 104 (1999).

320.   Mathov, I, Plotkin, LI, Sgarlata, CL, Leoni, J and Bellido, T, Journal of Bone and Mineral Research, 16 (2001).

321.   Hughes, DE, Wright, KR, Uy, HL, Sasaki, A, Yoneda, T, Roodman, GD, Mundy, GR and Boyce, BF, Journal of Bone & Mineral Research, 10 (1995).

322.   Halasy-Nagy, JM, Rodan, GA and Reszka, AA, Bone, 29 (2001).

323.   Rauch, F, Travers, R, Plotkin, H and Glorieux, FH, Journal of Clinical Investigation, 110 (2002).

324.   Bembi, B, Parma, A, Bottega, M, Ceschel, S, Zanatta, M, Martini, C and Ciana, G, J Pediatr, 131 (1997).

325.   Astrom, E and Soderhall, S, Acta Paediatrica, 87 (1998).

326. Glorieux, FH, Bishop, NJ, Plotkin, H, Chabot, G, Lanoue, G and Travers, R, New England Journal of Medicine, 339 (1998).

327. Plotkin, H, Rauch, F, Bishop, N, Montpetit, K, Ruck-Gibbis, J, Travers, R and Glorieux, FH, Journal of Clinical Endocrinology and Metabolism, 85 (2000).

328. Plotkin, H, Montpetit, K, Cloutier, S, Bilodeau, N, Gervais, N, Rabzel, M, Travers, R and Glorieux, FH, Journal of Bone and Mineral Research, S1 (2000).

329. Plotkin, H and Glorieux, FH, Drug Development Research, 49 (2000).

330. Gonzalez, E, Pavia, C, Ros, J, Villaronga, M, Valls, C and Escola, J, J Pediatr Endocrinol Metab, 14 (2001).

331. Lee, YS, Low, SL, Lim, LA and Loke, KY, Eur J Pediatr, 160 (2001).

332. Astrom, E and Soderhall, S, Arch Dis Child, 86 (2002).

333. Montpetit, K, Plotkin, H, Rauch, F, Bilodeau, N, Cloutier, S, Rabzel, M and Glorieux, FH, Pediatrics, 111 (2003).

334. Profumo, RJ, Reese, JC, Foy, TM, Garibaldi, LR and Kane, RE, Transplantation, 57 (1994).

335. Samuel, R, Katz, K, Papapoulos, S, Yosipovitch, Z, Zaizov, R and Liberman, U, Pediatrics, 94 (1994).

336. Shaw, NJ, Boivin, CM and Crabtree, NJ, Archives of Disease in Childhood, 83 (2000).

337. Henderson, RC, Lark, RK, Kecskemethy, H, Miller, F, Harcke, T and Bachrach, S, Journal of Pediatrics, 141 (2002).

338. Barr, RD, Guo, CH, Wiernikowski, J, Webber, C, Wright, M and Atkinson, S, Med Pediatr Oncol, 39 (2002).

339. Albright, JA, Clin Orthop, (1981).

340. Winterfeldt, EA, Eyring, EJ and Vivian, VM, Lancet, 760 (1970).

341. Kurz, D and Eyring, EJ, Pediatrics, 54 (1974).

342. Bilginturan, N and Ozsoylu, S, Turk J Pediatr, 8 (1966).

343. Aeschlimann, MI, Grunt, JA and Crigler, JF, Jr., Metabolism, 15 (1966).

344. Solomons, CC and Styner, J, Calcif Tissue Res, 3 (1969).

345. Granda, JL, Falvo, KA and Bullough, PG, Clin Orthop, (1977).

346. Cattell, HS and Clayton, B, J Bone Joint Surg Am, 50 (1968).

347. Castells, S, Clin Orthop, 93 (1973).

348. August, GP, Shapiro, J and Hung, W, J Pediatr, 91 (1977).

349. Pedersen, U, Charles, P, Hansen, HH and Elbrond, O, Acta Orthop Scand, 56 (1985).

350. Munns, CFJ, Rauch, F, Zeitlin, L, Fassier, F and Glorieux., FH, Journal of Bone and Mineral Research, 18 (2003).

351. Steelman, J and Zeitler, P, J Pediatr, 142 (2003).

352. Gandrud, LM, Cheung, JC, Daniels, MW and Bachrach, LK, J Pediatr Endocrinol Metab, 16 (2003).

353. Plotkin, H, Gibis, J and Glorieux, FH, Bone, 28 (2001).

354. Frost, HM, Calcif Tissue Int, 42 (1988).

355. Zeitlin, L, Rauch, F, Plotkin, H and Glorieux, FH, Pediatrics, 111 (2003).

356.   Rauch, F, Plotkin, H, Travers, R, Zeitlin, L and Glorieux, FH, Journal of Clinical Endocrinology and Metabolism, 88 (2003).
357.   Marini, JC, Hopkins, E, Glorieux, FH, Chrousos, GP, Reynolds, JC, Gundberg, CM and Reing, CM, Journal of Bone and Mineral Research, 18 (2003).
358.   Kinugasa, A, Fujita, K, Inoue, F, Kodo, N and Sawada, T, Acta Pediatrica Scandinava, 379 (1991).
359.   Kodama, H, Kubota, K and Abe, T, J Pediatr, 132 (1998).
360.   Antoniazzi, F, Bertoldo, F, Mottes, M, Valli, M, Sirpresi, S, Zamboni, G, Valentini, R and Tato, L, J Pediatr, 129 (1996).
361.   Wright, NM, Journal of Pediatric Endocrinology & Metabolism, 13 (2000).
362.   Falcini, F, Trapani, S, Civinini, R, Capone, A, Ermini, M and Bartolozzi, G, J Endocrinol Invest, 19 (1996).
363.   Bianchi, ML, Cimaz, R, Bardare, M, Zulian, F, Lepore, L, Boncompagni, A, Galbiati, E, Corona, F, Luisetto, G, Giuntini, D, Picco, P, Brandi, ML and Falcini, F, Arthritis & Rheumatism, 43 (2000).

s

CHAPTER 15

GENETICS OF OSTEOPOROSIS

Volodymyr Dvornyk[1], Yao-Zhong Liu[1,2], Hui Shen, Yong-Jun Liu[1,2],
Hong-Wen Deng[1,2]

[1]*Osteoporosis Research Center and Department of Biomedical Sciences
Creighton University, 601 N. 30th St., Suite 6787, Omaha, NE 68131*

[2]*Laboratory of Molecular and Statistical Genetics, College of Life Sciences
Hunan Normal University, ChangSha, Hunan 410081, P. R. China*

1. Introduction

Osteoporosis is a systemic skeletal disease characterized by low bone mineral density (BMD) and microarchitectural deterioration of bone tissue, with a consequent increase in bone fragility and susceptibility to fracture.[1,2] It is well known that BMD and other determinants of osteoporotic fracture are under strong genetic control. Identification and characterization of specific loci or genes involved in determining osteoporosis and associated phenotypes not only contribute to a greater understanding of the pathogenesis of osteoporosis, but also lead to the development of better diagnosis, prevention and treatment strategies of the disease. Genetic determination of osteoporosis may be monogenic or polygenic. In this review, we are mainly concerned with the polygenic form, although a limited few monogenic forms will also be briefly mentioned. Genetics research of osteoporosis represents one of the most active areas for bone biology research. Several reviews have nicely summarized the results of the candidate genes research.[3-6] In this chapter, we first give an overview of the evidence that osteoporosis and associated traits have a genetic basis, then briefly summarize the main findings that come from linkage and association studies, with a focus on some promising chromosomal regions, and finally discuss the future challenges and directions.

2. Evidence for Genetic Basis of Osteoporosis and Associated Traits

Fracture is the ultimate consequence of osteoporosis. Ideally, scientists would perform genetic studies with fracture as an endpoint, and search for genes underlying the differential susceptibility to fracture. Genetic epidemiological studies have shown that a family history of fracture is a significant risk factor for fracture.[7,8] However, prospective 25-year follow up of a nationwide cohort of elderly Finnish twins showed that susceptibility to osteoporotic fracture (OF) is not strongly influenced by genetic factors. In women, the pairwise concordance rate for fracture was 9.5% in monozygotic pairs and 7.9% in dizygotic pairs. In men, the figures were 9.9% and 2.3%, respectively.[9] Deng and colleagues[10] estimated that the narrow-sense heritability of Colles' fracture was approximately 0.25 in a cohort of white American women, thus accounting for approximately one-quarter of the variation in total Colles' fracture risk observed. Genetic factors, at most, account for about one third of the variance in the liability to fracture [11] Two formal and direct studies recently performed by us[10] demonstrated a significant and moderately high genetic determination for OF, with heritability ranging from 25% to 53%. Importantly, although both BMD and OF have high degrees of genetic determination and the phenotypic correlation between them is high, the genetic correlation between them is very low and not significant; and only about 1% of additive genetic variance is shared between BMD and OF.[10] Fractures are relatively rare and tend to occur late in life. Although vertebral fractures are relatively common compared with hip and wrist fractures, they do not always come to clinical attention and their diagnosis may prove uncertain.[12] The relatively low OF heritability and difficulty in recruitment of an adequate sample in which to perform mapping studies of fracture in humans lead investigators to adopt alternative strategies using surrogate traits.

Bone strength is an ultimate measurement of resistance to fracture. It is mainly determined by BMD, bone size, and bone quality.[3,13] However, bone strength cannot be directly measured *in vivo* in human. The most powerful, measurable determinant of fracture risk is the amount of bone in the skeleton,[14,15] and the most powerful predictor of future fracture is low bone mass as measured by BMD.[16-20] Consequently, the vast majority of genetic studies of osteoporosis to date have used BMD as a surrogate phenotype. BMD is a complex phenotype because it results from remodeling processes affecting bone compartments (endosteal and periosteal), and therefore bone size, and the process differ according to age and gender.[21] BMD in both sons and daughters correlates most closely with the average parental BMD.[22] Twin studies have shown that the heritability estimates of BMD ranged from 0.5-0.9.[23-27] Since environmental influences can differ considerably between generations, heritability estimates of BMD in inter-generational studies have generally been lower than those reported in twin studies, ranging from 0.46-0.67.[22,28-31] Most of the segregation analyses[28,32-34] suggest that at least one major gene for population BMD variation exists. The genetic correlation between lumbar spine and femoral neck BMD is 0.64, and approximately one-third of the genetic influence on variance of femoral neck BMD is mediated through the same gene or genes that influence the lumbar spine.[35] Therefore, there are some common and specific genetic factors underlying the determination of BMD in various skeletal sites. However, a recent study indicated that genetic correlation between fracture and BMD is not significant despite a high phenotypic correlation between fracture and BMD.[36] Thus, all important fracture risk factors need to be studied in order to find genes for this trait. In addition, there are obvious gender differences in the genetic components of BMD.[37] Men generally have larger bone size and greater cortical mass,[38] which is associated with considerable fracture risk reduction. Whether the genetic determinants of BMD in humans also would be influenced by gender remains to be elucidated.

Bone size is also an important determinant of OFs. A longer hip axis length is associated with increased hip fracture risk independent of BMD.[39] However, there have been few reports on the estimation of heritability of variation in bone size.[40-42] In 49 pedigrees with 703 subjects, after adjusting for sex, age, weight, height, lifestyle factors, and the significant interactions among these factors, heritability estimates were, respectively, 0.48, 0.64, and 0.6 for bone size at the hip, spine, and wrist.[42] In addition, forearm width and hip axis length are also highly heritable with heritability estimates of greater than 0.5.[23,43]

Quantitative ultrasound (QUS) measurements, including broadband ultrasound attenuation (BUA) and speed of sound (SOS), reflect quality of bone. Subjects with lower BUA at baseline have a higher risk of hip and vertebral fractures, possibly independent of BMD.[44] Estimates of heritability based on twin studies for age- and weight-adjusted BUA and SOS are 0.74 and 0.82, respectively.[23,45] Bivariate genetic analysis indicated that the genetic correlation between BUA and BMD ranged between 0.43 and 0.51, whereas the environmental correlation ranged between 0.2 and 0.28.[45]

Bone formation and resorption markers may predict hip fracture in elderly white women.[46] Each standard deviation higher in bone specific alkaline phosphatase values was associated with a 4% lower level of BMD in both lumbar spine and femoral neck.[47] The genetic contribution to variation in bone turnover after attainment of peak bone mass is established,[48-50] although the genetic effects on bone turnover are smaller than those on BMD and bone size. However, the genetic contribution to variation in rate of bone loss has not been shown consistently.

In order to understand the genetic basis for decreased bone strength, and ultimately osteoporotic fractures, one needs to assess the inheritance of, and identify the specific genes associated with, a multitude of skeletal traits, such as BMD, bone size, QUS, and bone turnover. If osteoporotic fractures are not studied as the phenotype, the genes identified need to be tested for relevance to osteoporotic fracture. Above results consistently support the hypothesis that genetic factors are a major determinant of BMD and, possibly, variance in bone size, bone turnover, and QUS measurements. This hypothesis has fueled most osteoporosis genetics investigations over the last decade.

3. Searching for Osteoporosis Genes

There are several approaches to identifying genes for osteoporosis: animal models, genome-wide linkage scans, the candidate gene approach (association studies)[44], gene expression studies. The first two are comprehensively reviewed in the other chapters of this book. One major advantage of using an animal model is that it is possible to control for the heterogeneity of environmental factors in animals, which is otherwise impossible in human studies. Genome-wide scans test only linkage and are robust to population admixture/stratification. A disadvantage is that they have relatively low statistical power to detect genes with modest effects unless the sample size as reflected by the informative relative pairs is sufficiently large. Genome scan not only guides candidate gene research by according greater priority to candidates that are located within regions of linkage, but also identifies novel chromosomal regions within which no known candidates have been recognized.

The candidate gene approach tests for the association between a particular gene variant and osteoporosis (BMD variation), and depends on linkage disequilibrium of markers with functional mutations. It is generally prone to population admixture/stratification in yielding false positive or negative results.[51,52] To overcome this problem, the transmission disequilibrium test (TDT) is commonly employed to test specific candidate genes for both association and linkage.[53]

3.1. *Candidate Gene Association Studies*

There are three types of candidate genes: functional candidate genes, positional candidate genes, and expressional candidate genes. Functional candidate genes are based upon a priori knowledge of the phenotype and the potential function of the gene involved. Such knowledge may come from clinical observation or physiological studies of affected individuals, from studies of known disease-related process, from animal models of disease, and from pharmacogenetic studies. Positional candidate genes are genes targeted because of their location within regions identified through genetic linkage analyses. Expressional candidate genes are identified through differences in gene expression using cDNA or protein microarrays. Candidate genes are commonly examined by association studies, using a case-control design. Since the first report of an association study between the α2-HS-glycoprotein (ASHG) gene and bone mass,[54] the list of candidate genes investigated for linkage and association with osteoporosis and associated traits has been constantly updated and expanded. Currently, there are more than 200 genes that have been proposed as potential candidates for osteoporosis and associated traits.[55]

3.1.1. Functional candidate genes

Among the multiple candidate genes harboring polymorphic loci so far investigated in relation to BMD and fracture, the vitamin D receptor (VDR) gene has received greatest attention. The relationship between the VDR genotype and BMD has been studied in Caucasians, East Asians, and Africans. A meta-analysis combining the results of 75 articles and abstracts published between 1994 and 1998 which examined the relationship between the VDR polymorphisms (BsmI, ApaI, TaqI, EcoRV, and FokI) and osteoporosis-related phenotypes (BMD, fracture, and QUS) have shown a highly significant association between VDR polymorphisms and BMD. Positive results were significantly more common in studies that included premenopausal rather than postmenopausal women, and the association may have been missed in some studies because of small sample size and other confounding factors.[56]

Collagen type I α1 (COL1A1) is the most abundant protein in bone, and mutations in the genes encoding collagen type Iα1 and collagen type Iα2 are estimated to be responsible for up to 90% of cases of the Mendelian disease osteogenesis imperfecta. Polymorphisms affecting the coding regions of the collagen type I genes are rare and do not appear to be associated with osteoporosis.[57] Grant et al.[58] described a G→T polymorphism in intron 1 of the COLIA1 gene at a binding site for the Sp1 transcription factor, and reported decreased BMD and increased fracture risk for carriers of the s allele in an analysis of 205 predominantly postmenopausal British women. Since that time, numerous studies have been performed in both Caucasians and Asians. The unfavorable effect of the s allele has not been seen consistently across different studies, and a G→T polymorphism in intron 1 of the COLIA1 gene at a binding site for the Sp1 transcription factor does not appear to exist in Asians.[59,60] Recently performed meta-analyses about association of COL1A1 Sp1 polymorphism with BMD and/or the risk of prevalent fractures concluded that the COLIA1 Sp1 polymorphism showed a dose-response relationship to prevalence of fractures (increases stepwise from *SS* homozygotes to *Ss* heterozygotes and further to *ss* homozygotes).[61-63] Further, the association with fracture was stronger than expected on the basis of the observed differences in BMD. Because a large part of the inherited predisposition to fracture is due to inherited factors in bone density, and/or material quality of bone etc, authors concluded that the Sp1 effect on fractures may be mediated in part by its influence on bone quality other than BMD.

Since the recognition of the VDR gene polymorphism as one of the important parameters predictive of bone variables, candidate gene approach has become the mainstay of the methodology for genetic study of osteoporosis. A series of novel polymorphisms have been identified as related to bone mass variation and risk for osteoporotic fractures. Most of the polymorphisms are from the genes encoding the important pathways of bone and mineral homeostasis and metabolism. The most notable genes include TGF-β1 (transforming growth factor-β1), IL-6 (interleukin-6), IGF-I (insulin-like growth factor-I), CT (calcitonin), and CTR (calcitonin receptor).

TGF-β1 is a potential mediator of coupling between bone resorption and formation. The TGF-β1 gene has seven exons, of which exons 5 to 7 encode the active TGF-β1. In vitro, TGF-β1 inhibits mature osteoclasts and the proliferation of mononuclear osteoclast precursors and stimulates the proliferation or differentiation of preosteoblasts. Bone matrix is the tissue with the highest concentration of TGF-β1. The commonly employed markers for the TGF-β1 gene are the DNA sequence variations detectable by allele specific PCR assays. In a study of a large sample involving 1,706 female dizygotic twins, the T→C polymorphism of intron 5 was associated with femoral neck BMD.[64] Another study on the C509→T polymorphism in 625 postmenopausal Japanese women detected its relationship with lumbar spine and total body BMD.[65] Two independent studies on the T→C polymorphism of signal sequence region yielded different results in terms of the polymorphism's effect on BMD. While the study on the Japanese population identified that the *CC* genotype was associated with higher BMD and lower frequency of vertebral fracture as compared to the *TT* genotype,[66] another one on the

German population detected that the *TT* genotype instead had higher BMD and less bone loss.[67] Two other polymorphisms, the 713-8delC and the T→C of exon 1, were also related to BMD, bone turnover, bone loss, and response to VD and HRT treatment.[68-70]

IL-6, as a pleiotropic cytokine, has important effects on osteoclast differentiation and function. It was found to mediate estrogen deficiency related bone loss in rodents.[71] Its expression was up-regulated in the bone tissue from osteoporotic patients.[72] A few studies have demonstrated the relationship of several polymorphisms of the IL-6 gene with bone phenotypes, including the variable number tandem repeat (VNTR) polymorphism in the gene's 3'-flank region,[73] the CA repeat polymorphism,[74] the *Bsr*BI endonuclease C/G polymorphism at (nt)-634 of the promoter region,[75] and the −174 G→C polymorphism.[76]

IGF-1 is produced by osteoblasts and stimulates skeletal growth through its regulation of cell proliferation, differentiation, DNA synthesis, and collagen and non-collagen protein.[77,78] It also functions as a mediator of a series of hormones in bone metabolism, such as growth hormone, estrogen, and parathyroid hormone.[79,80] A CA repeat polymorphism upstream of the transcriptional initiation site of the gene has been investigated in several studies.[81,82] Association of the polymorphism with both BMD and serum IGF-1 levels was identified. As serum IGF-1 levels correlated with bone mass in both inbred strains of mice[83] and humans[84,85] and corresponded to skeletal content of IGF-1,[83] the difference in BMD between IGF-1 genotypes may be mediated via serum IGF-1 variation. But the causative relationship between serum IGF-1 and bone mass needs further investigation.

CT is a polypeptide hormone secreted by parafollicular cells of the thyroid gland. It inhibits osteoclastic bone resorption and stimulates urinary calcium excretion. Polymorphisms of both the CT and the CTR genes were studied for their relationship with bone mass. CTR gene's *Alu*I restriction enzyme polymorphism was associated with spine and femoral neck BMD,[86,87] This association was higher in the younger subset of the sample,[86] suggesting the polymorphism may have more influence on the peak bone mass than age-related bone loss. Two other polymorphisms of the CTR gene, the *Taq*I polymorphism and the T→C polymorphism, were also found to be related to lumbar and femoral neck

BMD.[88,89] The CT gene's CA repeat polymorphism was correlated with lumbar BMD in a group of Japanese postmenopausal women, with the 10-repeat allele being associated with lower BMD values.[90]

Other candidate genes investigated include, but are not limited to, those encoding parathyroid hormone (PTH),[91-93] calcium-sensing receptor,[94,95] osteocalcin,[93,96-98] interleukin-6 binding proteins,[99] apolipoprotein E,[100-103] AHSG,[104] interleukin-1 receptor antagonist,[105] androgen receptor (ADR),[106-108] peroxisome proliferator-activated receptor gamma [109], tumor necrosis factor receptor 2,[110] P57,[111] methylenetetrahydrofolate reductase (MTHFR),[112-114] aromatase (CYP19),[115-117] Werner helicase (WRN),[118] CC chemokine receptor-2 (CCR2),[119] *klotho*,[120] and runt-related gene 2 (RUNX2)/core binding factor A1 (Cbfa1).[121]

Despite considerable efforts, it is still premature to draw conclusions about the potential influence of these genes on BMD, osteoporosis, and fracture. Results from association studies of candidate genes are often inconsistent. Reasons for false positive or negative results include population admixture,[52] small sample sizes and low statistical power, different sets of genes operating in different populations, variable linkage disequilibrium among populations,[122] or low prior probability of the involvement of the gene in question in the overall risk of the disease.[123] In response to these problems, some guidelines have been suggested to ensure robust results. These include (1) significantly increased sample sizes; (2) incorporation of diverse study designs including case-control, family-based association studies and intermediate phenotype data sets;[124] (3) replication of findings in additional study groups of similar ethnic origin.[125]

3.1.2. Gene-by-gene and gene-by-non-genetic factor interactions

Gene-by-gene or gene-by-non-genetic factor interactions were identified in many studies, reflecting multi-factor determination of bone mass and complexities of the genetic basis underlying BMD.

Relationships between the estrogen receptor α (ER-α) gene polymorphisms (TA, CA, *Pvu*II, and *Xba*I) and BMD/fracture have been extensively investigated and yielded contrasting results. A recent meta-analysis indicated that *XX* homozygotes (women carrying two copies of the gene variant without an *Xba*I restriction site) have higher BMD and also a decreased risk of fractures when compared with carriers of the *x* allele, whereas the *Pvu*II polymorphism is not associated with either BMD or fracture risk.[126] Notably, a significant gene-gene interaction between VDR and ER-α gene polymorphisms has been suggested by several authors.[127-130] In addition, several studies assessed whether genotypes of ER-α are associated with bone changes in women with and without hormone replacement therapy.[131-133] Although results are inconsistent, the information obtained should turn out to be helpful in choosing optimum therapy for osteoporosis for these different genotypes (genotype-specific treatment).

In postmenopausal women, the fracture risk was found to depend on the VDR gene's *baT* haplotype in only the COL1A1 *GT* and *TT*, but not the *GG* genotype group.[134] The interaction could exist not only between different genes, but also among different loci of the same gene; the two haplotype groups, *AABBtt* and *aabbTT*, formed by the combination of the three polymorphismic sites of the VDR gene, significantly differed in lumbar BMD.[128]

Non-genetic factors, including age,[135-138] race,[139,140] calcium intake,[135,141-143] vitamin D supplementation,[144] hormone replacement therapy (HRT),[100,145,146] years since menopause,[147] smoking,[31,148,149] birthweight [150], BMI,[151] testosterone levels,[151] and exercise[152,153] may also interact with genetic factors in determination of bone mass.

As an example for gene-environment interaction in bone metabolism, the effect of calcium or vitamin D intake on BMD accrual or retention was analyzed in several independent studies.[135,141,143,144] That effect was observed in only the VDR gene's *Bb*, and possibly *BB*, but not *bb* subjects.[135,144] In contrast, the study by Kiel et al.[141] showed that only the *bb*, rather the *BB* and *Bb*, subjects had BMD increase in response to calcium intake. The observed inconsistency may be related to age differences of subjects between the studies.

The above inconsistency underscores the importance of another factor, age, for its pivotal role to interact with other factors in determination of BMD. According to Riggs et al.,[154] the VDR genotypic difference in BMD tended to blur with advancing age and eventually disappeared by the age of 70, implying erosion of genotypic differentiation of BMD by environmental effects accumulated with time. Such a result is generally confirmed by another study, where BMD was associated with VDR polymorphisms only before puberty,[135] but contradicted by the study of postmenopausal Dutch women, whose BMD genotypic differentiation was sharpened by advancing age.[155]

Gene-age interaction was also suggested to influence weight, where subjects with the genotype ER-α-*PP* tended to gain weight and *Pp* and *pp* lost weight with advancing age.[156] Since weight and bone mass are highly correlated,[157,158] the finding implies that the effect of gene-age interaction on BMD might be mediated through weight. In addition, weight, or probably height, itself may also potentially interact with the VDR polymorphism to influence BMD variation. Vandevyver et al.[159] found in a group of elderly women that BMD differentiation among the *Bsm*I genotypes could be detected only in non-obese women with BMI < 30 kg/m^2. Similarly, it was also reported that association of the *f* and *b* alleles of the VDR gene with lower BMD could be determined in postmenopausal female subjects only with BMI < 25 kg/m^2.[160] The findings are consistent with the previously reported data that covariates, such as weight and height, may obscure associations of the VDR and ER-α genotypes with BMD.[129]

Hormone replacement therapy (HRT) is another important environment factor modulating genetic effects on bone. It was showed that the ER-α genotype-related difference in BMD was eliminated by long-term HRT.[146] HRT could also remove the difference in BMD change between the subjects with the apolipoprotein E4 allele and those without.[100] Another study identified those with the VDR-*bb*/ER-*PP* genotype as a group who might benefit most from long term HRT since, according to the study, only the subjects with the genotype *bbPP* had increased heel stiffness index in response to long term HRT.[145]

Studies on race (Caucasian vs. African American) by VDR genotype interaction have not yielded positive results.[139,140] This may be unexpected given that the association between the VDR polymorphism and BMD is much more often detected in American Caucasians than in African Americans.[161].

3.2. *Linkage Studies*

3.2.1. *Linkage approach*

Linkage studies test whether a phenotypic locus is transmitted with genetic markers of known chromosomal position. Linkage approach does not rely on the linkage disequilibrium among genes or markers in adjacent genomic regions, therefore, can be used to search for any genomic region contributing relatively large variation in complex traits without any prior knowledge. In contrast to population association approach, the linkage one is robust to population admixture/stratification. However, genomic region detected by linkage study is generally large (~30 cM), which is not feasible for physical mapping. Hence, fine-mapping efforts are needed to narrow a QTL to a small region to eventually identify a specific gene.[156,162] The linkage approach has been successfully used to locate gene(s) underlying genetic traits with Mendelian inheritance, but its application to complex traits can be complicated.[163] In this case, very large samples are necessary to be screened and/or genotyped,[53,164,165] otherwise, the power to detect linkage would be limited.

3.2.2. *Linkage studies in humans*

In recent years, the linkage approach has been widely applied to search for osteoporosis genes. Some linkage studies were performed in candidate genomic loci or targeted chromosomal regions. In a sibpair linkage study of 23 candidate genes, Duncan et al.[166] genotyped 64 microsatellite markers in a sample of 115 probands identified from patients with primary osteoporosis and 499 of their relatives. Suggestive linkage was found between BMD and the PTHR1 gene (LOD>2.7). Suggestive evidence of linkage was also observed with the genes for epidermal growth factor (EGF), COLIA1, COLIA2, VDR, ER-α, IL-α, IL-4, and IL-6. In the studies of genetic linkage between osteopenia and allelic variants of five candidate genes (IL-6, IL-6R, CaSR, and MGP) in adult Japanese women, a significant linkage of the IL-6 locus and allelic variants at the TNF-α locus to osteopenia and low BMD was observed.[167,168] In contrast, no evidence of linkage between spine or hip BMD and the polymorphisms at the IGF-I and IL-6 genes was found in a sample of healthy premenopausal Caucasian and African-American sibling pairs.[169,170]

Deng et al.[171] simultaneously tested linkage and/or association (via TDT) for three candidate genes (VDR, BGP, and PTH) as putative QTLs underlying spine or hip BMD variation. The obtained results support the VDR gene as a QTL underlying spine BMD variation and BGP as a QTL underlying hip or spine BMD variation. Using similar statistical methods, Andrew et al.[172] found a strong pleiotropic linkage between broadband ultrasound attenuation and BMD in postmenpausal women.

Human chromosomal region 11q12-13 has been of great interest for many investigators in the field of bone genetics during the past few years. Three distinct Mendelian traits that are BMD related, including osteoporosis-pseudoglioma,[173] autosomal recessive osteopetrosis,[174] and an autosomal dominant trait characterized by high bone mass (HBM),[175] have been linked to this region. Little et al.[176] refined this region with the expanded HBM pedigrees. A systematic search for mutations that segregated with the HBM phenotype revealed that a mutation in the low-density lipoprotein receptor-related protein 5 gene results in the HBM phenotype. A study in 374 sib pairs for 7 microsatellite markers typed in 11q12-13 reported linkage to normal femoral neck BMD variation (LOD=3.50 with marker D11S987).[177] However, a subsequent study with an expanded sample size (595 sib pairs) revealed much reduced signals for linkage, with a LOD score less than 2.2 achieved at D11S987.[178] Deng et al.[179] genotyped five markers in this region (~27 cM centering on D11S987) for 635 individuals from 53 extended pedigrees (including 1,249 sib pairs), but did not find linkage involving BMD at the spine, hip, wrist, or total body BMC.

3.2.3. Replications

Several genomic regions candidate for BMD variation have been replicated across different studies. The genomic region 2p23-24 linked to spine BMD in Caucasians[180] overlaps the region 2p21.1-24 revealed for both proximal and distal forearm BMD in Chinese sib pairs.[181] A number of candidate genes, such as CALM2 (calmodulin 2), STK (serine/threonine kinase), as well as POMC (pro-opiomelanocortin) reside in this region. A genome scan of a large sample of female UK twin pairs[182] confirmed the presence of QTLs for BMD variation at 1p36 and 3p21 reported previously.[166,181] These regions contain important candidate genes for BMD, including TNFR2 and PTHR1. There is also potential evidence for replication on chromosomal region 4q31 and 13q34 in three different studies.[166,171,181] Two candidate genes (COL4A1 and COL4A2) are located at 13q34.

Several groups have made extensive efforts in either independent or expanded samples (partially overlapped with initial samples) to confirm the findings in their initial stage studies. To confirm the QTLs influencing BMD revealed by Deng et al.,[171] Huang et al.[183] conducted a second-stage linkage study with denser markers within the initial localized regions in expanded pedigrees. Evidence of potential replication (LOD>1.0) was found at several regions, such as 10q26, 7p22, 12q13, and 13q33-34. A study by the same group[184] also replicated a QTL at 17q23 influencing wrist bone size variation revealed earlier.[185] Another group reported replications of their initial stage results on chromosome 1q for spine BMD,[186] on chromosomes 14 and 15 for hip BMD,[187] and at chromosomes 3 and 9 for femoral structure.[188]

3.3. *Gene Expression Studies*

In the last 20 years, extensive research has been devoted to studying the expression of genes involved in bone metabolism in order to identify those contributing to osteoporosis. A large number of expressional candidate genes have been determined by studies in two principal areas: (1) finding differences in gene expression between normal and diseased tissues and (2) determining effects of various inherent regulators (hormones, receptors, etc.) on bone tissues or cells. The list of some expressional candidate genes is given in Table 1.

Table 1. Candidate expressional genes for BMD and osteoporosis regulated by various factors.

Gene	Factor(s)	Tissue	Expression	Ref.
ALP	estrogen + PTH	Human osteoblastic cells	+	190
	inhibitors of phosphodiesterases	Mouse osteoblastic / bone marrow stromal cells	n.a./+	195
	IL-4	Mouse osteoblastic cells	-	197
CollαI	bFGF	Ovariectomized rat lumbar vertebrae	+	209
	inhibitors of phosphodiesterases	Mouse osteoblastic / bone marrow stromal cells	n.a./+	195
	glucose	Mouse osteoblastic cells	+	210
α1(I) procollagen	estrogen + PTH	Human osteoblastic SaOS-2 cells	+	190
	PPARγ2	Prototypic cell line with mixed phenotype	-	211
Best5	IFNα	Rat osteoblasts culture	+	194
	IFNγ	Rat osteoblasts culture	+	194
c-jun	PTH	Mouse distal femur metaphyses	+	193
	glucose	Mouse osteoblastic cells	+	210
IL-6	androgens	Murine bone-marrow derived stromal cells	-	191
	PTH	Rat stromal cells	+	212
	LIF/dexamethasone	Rat stromal cells	+/-	213
	IL-1β + TNFα	Human cultured osteoblasts and bone marrow stromal cells	+	214
LIF	LIF/dexamethasone	Rat calvaria	+/-	213
	IL-1β + TNFα	Human cultured osteoblasts and bone marrow stromal cells	+	214
OCN	bFGF	Ovariectomized rat lumbar vertebrae	+	209
	PPARγ2	Prototypic cell line with mixed phenotype	-	211
	glucose	Mouse osteoblastic cells	-	210

OPG	estrogen	Human fetal osteoblastic cells	+	206
	estrogen via ER-α	Mouse bone marrow stromal cell	+	208
	vitamin D_3	Human osteoblastic cells	+	207
	IL-1β	Human fetal osteoblastic cells	+	207
	TNFα	Human fetal osteoblastic cells	+	207
	BMP2	Human fetal osteoblastic cells	+	207
	dexamethasone	Human osteoblastic cells	-	204
		Human primary marrow stromal cells	-	204
OPG-L	IL-1β	Human osteoblasts	+	205
		Human primary marrow stromal cells	+	205
	TNFα	Human osteoblasts	+	205
		Human primary marrow stromal cells	+	205
	dexamethasone	Human fetal osteoblastic cells	+	204
		Human primary marrow stromal cells	+	204
	IL-6	Human osteoblasts	-	205
OPN	inhibitors of phosphodiesterases	Mouse osteoblastic / bone marrow stromal cells	n.a./+	195
	PGE_2	Isolated rabbit osteoclasts	-	215
OSM	LIF/dexamethasone	Rat calvaria	n.a./-	213
	IL-1β + TNFα	Human cultured osteoblasts and bone marrow stromal cells	-	214
11β-HSD1	TNFα	Human adipose stromal cells	+	216
	IGF-1	Human adipose stromal cells	-	216
IGF	bFGF	Ovariectomized rat lumbar vertebrae	+	209
OSM-R	LIF/dexamethasone	Rat calvaria	+/-	213

IL-11-R	LIF/dexamethasone	Rat calvaria	/-	213
LIF-R	LIF/dexamethasone	Rat calvaria	+	213
M-CSF	estrogen	Mouse bone marrow stromal cells	-	217
IGF-BP	estrogen + PTH	Human osteoblastic cells	+	190
junB	PTH	Mouse distal femur metaphyses	+	193
c-fos	PTH	Mouse distal femur metaphyses	+	193
fra-2	PTH	Mouse distal femur metaphyses	+	193
IL-4R	vitamin D_3	Mouse osteoblastic cells	+	197
Tob	BMP2	Mouse calvaria-derived osteoblast precursor cells	+	196
COX2	BMP2	Mouse osteoblastic cells	+	218
PGE_2	BMP2	Mouse osteoblastic cells	+	218
Osf2/Cbfa1	PPARγ2	Prototypic cell line with mixed phenotype	-	211
Adipsin	PPARγ2	Prototypic cell line with mixed phenotype	-	211
aP2	PPARγ2	Prototypic cell line with mixed phenotype	-	211
IL-11	IL-1β + TNFα	Human cultured osteoblasts and bone marrow stromal cells	+	214
EP_4	PGE_2	Rat osteoblastic cell lines	+	219
aP1	glucose	Mouse osteoblastic cells	+	210

Abbreviations: n.a., not affected; +, upregulated; -, downregulated; ALP, alkaline phosphatase; bFGF, basic fibroblast growth factor; BMP, bone morphogenetic protein; Cbfa1, core-binding factor α1; COX, cyclo-oxygenase; CT-1, cardiotrophin-1; EP_4, prostaglandin E_2 receptor subtype EP_4; ER, estrogen receptor; IFN, interferon; IGF, insulin-like growth factor; IGF-BP, IGF-binding protein; IL, interleukin; LIF, leukemia inhibitory factor; M-CSF, macrophage colony-stimulating factor; OCN, osteocalcin; OPG, osteoprotegerin; OPG-L, osteoprotegerin ligand; OPN, osteopontin; OSM, oncostatin M; PG, prostaglandin; PPARγ2, peroxisome proliferator-activated receptor γ2; PTH, parathyroid hormone; R, receptor; TGF, transforming growth factor; TNF, tumor necrosis factor; 17β-E_2, 17β-estradiol 2; 11β-HSD1, hydroxysteroid dehydrogenase type 1.

3.3.1. Comparative gene expression studies of healthy and diseased tissues

The first focus is rather straightforward, because it provides immediate information about the regulation of genes known to be related to the disease. Surprisingly, there are only a few such studies of osteoporotic vs normal bone tissues. For example, a comparative study of biopsies from healthy and osteoporotic patients indicated that cytokines IL-1α, IL-1β, and IL-6 mRNAs were expressed significantly more often in bone samples from postmenopausal women with osteoporotic fractures than in postmenopausal women with normal bone density or postmenopausal women on hormone replacement therapy.[72]

A similar study, but made using the primary cultures of human osteoblasts, produced somewhat different results.[189] In particular, no expression of IL-1α was detected as compared to the bone marrow biopsies.[72] These differences in expression profiles might be due to various factors, such as different origin or heterogeneity of the tissues, their physiological conditions, etc. Importantly, expression of some genes was inconsistent in the subjects of the same group under study. The reason for such variation may be that expression of these genes has a complex mode of regulation and depends on multiple factors. In such a case, a "snapshot" of a genome-wide expression profile might shed light on what genes may be actually responsible for this variation.

3.3.2. Effects of various inherent regulators on gene expression profiles of bone-related tissues

These studies have been done using mainly various animal models and cell cultures that allows for the control of experimental conditions. Due to major bone effects of corticosteroids, a number of studies have been done to elucidate their effects on bone development. In particular, estrogen was reported to modulate osteoblast proliferation and function regulated by parathyroid hormone in osteoblastic SaOS-2 cells.[190] Androgens were shown to inhibit the expression of the interleukin-6 gene.[191] Natural and synthetic human parathyroid hormones have an effect on the expression of multiple genes of bone metabolism.[192,193]

In rats, a novel cDNA (best5), which is important for the response of osteoblasts to stimuli that modulate proliferation/differentiation, was recently demonstrated by differential display PCR to be regulated during osteoblast differentiation and bone formation in vitro and in vivo. Expression of best5 mRNA is induced in cultures of osteoblasts by both interferon-α and interferon-γ.[194]

The selective inhibitors for a respective phosphodiesterase isozyme were shown to have a different effect on bone morphogenetic protein 4 (BMP-4)-induced alkaline phosphatase activity, a cellular differentiation marker, and expression of osteopontin and collagen type I in different cell lines with osteogenetic potential.[195] On the other hand, Tob, a member of the emerging family of antiproliferative proteins, is a negative regulator of BMP/Smad signaling in osteoblasts.[196] Treatment of MC3T3 cells with interleukin-4 resulted in increased cellular proliferation (10-20%) and inhibition of alkaline phosphatase levels (20-40%); in turn, interleukin-4 was upregulated by 1,25-dihydroxyvitamin D_3.[197]

One of the latest breakthroughs in the field of bone molecular biology is discovery of osteoprotegerin (OPG), which is a member of the tumor necrosis factor receptor family, and a potent inhibitor of osteoclastogenesis.[198,199] Mice in which this protein gene is knocked out exhibit dramatic reduction of bone mass and rapid development of osteoporosis.[200] OPG-deficient mice also exhibit medial calcification of the aorta and renal arteries, suggesting that regulation of OPG, its signaling pathway or its ligand(s) may play a role in the long observed association between osteoporosis and vascular calcification.[201] Further studies have revealed that the level of osteoprotegerin expression is regulated by multiple factors, including vitamin D, cytokines, BMP-2, glucocorticoids, and estrogen.[202-208]

Acknowledgment

This project was partially supported by grants from the Health Future Foundation of the USA, from the National Institute of Health (K01 AR02170-01, R01 GM60402-01A1), from the State of Nebraska Cancer and Smoking Related Disease Research Program, the State of

Nebraska Tobacco Settlement Fund, and the US department of Energy (DE-FG03-00ER63000/A00). The project has also benefited from projects supported by the Hunan Province Special Professor Start-up Fund (25000612), grants (30025025), (30170504), and (30230210) from the Chinese National Science Foundation (CNSF), a seed grant (25000106), a key project grant from the Ministry of Education of P. R. China, and a young scientist development grant from the Huo Ying Dong Education Foundation of Hong-Kong. We thank Fuhua Xu and Hui Shen for their computer simulation work on statistical power calculation for linkage studies. We thank an anonymous reviewer for constructive comments that helped to improve the manuscript.

REFERENCES

1. S.R. Cummings, S.M. Rubin and D. Black, Clin. Orthop., 163 (1990).
2. L.J. Melton, III, S.H. Kan, M.A. Frye, H.W. Wahner, W.M. O'Fallon and B.L. Riggs, Am. J. Epidemiol., 1000 (1989).
3. J.A. Eisman, Endocr. Rev., 788 (1999).
4. Y.Z. Liu, Y.J. Liu, R.R. Recker and H.W. Deng, J. Endocrinol., 147 (2003).
5. S.H. Ralston, Rev. Endocr. Metab. Disord., 13 (2001).
6. R.R. Recker and H.W. Deng, Endocrine, 55 (2002).
7. S.R. Cummings, M.C. Nevitt, W.S. Browner, K. Stone, K.M. Fox, K.E. Ensrud, J.A. Cauley, D. Black and T.M. Vogt, N. Engl. J. Med., 767 (1995).
8. R.W. Keen, D.J. Hart, N.K. Arden, D.V. Doyle and T.D. Spector, Osteoporos. Int., 161 (1999).
9. P. Kannus, M. Palvanen, J. Kaprio, J. Parkkari and M. Koskenvuo, BMJ, 1334 (1999).
10. H.W. Deng, W.M. Chen, S. Recker, M.R. Stegman, J.L. Li, K.M. Davies, Y. Zhou, H.W. Deng, R.P. Heaney and R.R. Recker, J. Bone Miner. Res., 1243 (2000).
11. A. MacGregor, H. Snieder and T.D. Spector, BMJ, 1669 (2000).
12. R.D. Blank, J. Bone Miner. Res., 1207 (2001).

13. X. Li, G. Masinde, W. Gu, J. Wergedal, S. Mohan and D.J. Baylink, Genomics, 734 (2002).
14. C.C. Johnston, S.L. Hui and P.S. Wiske, in Osteoporosis: Recent Advances in Pathogenesis and Treatment, Ed. H.F.DeLuca, (University Park Press, Baltimore, 1981)
15. D.M. Black, S.R. Cummings, H.K. Genant, M.C. Nevitt, L. Palermo and W. Browner, J. Bone Miner. Res., 633 (1992).
16. S.L. Hui, C.W. Slemenda and C.C. Johnston, J. Clin. Invest., 1804 (1988).
17. S.L. Hui, C.W. Slemenda and C.C. Johnston, Ann. Intern. Med., 355 (1989).
18. S.R. Cummings, D.M. Black, M.C. Nevitt, W. Browner, J.A. Cauley, K. Ensrud, H.K. Genant, L. Palermo, J. Scott and T.M. Vogt, Lancet, 72 (1993).
19. L.J. Melton, III, E.J. Atkinson, W.M. O'Fallon, H.W. Wahner and B.L. Riggs, J. Bone Miner. Res., 1227 (1993).
20. P.D. Ross, C. Huang, J. Davis, K. Imose, J. Yates, J. Vogel and R. Wasnich, Bone, 325 (1995).
21. Y. Duan, E. Seeman and C.H. Turner, J. Bone Miner. Res., 2276 (2001).
22. E.A. Krall and B. Dawson-Hughes, J. Bone Miner. Res., 1 (1993).
23. N.K. Arden, J. Baker, C. Hogg, K. Baan and T.D. Spector, J. Bone Miner. Res., 530 (1996).
24. J.C. Christian, P.L. Yu, C.W. Slemenda and C.C. Johnston, Am. J. Hum. Genet., 429 (1989).
25. J. Dequeker, J. Nijs, A. Verstraeten, P. Geusens and G. Gevers, Bone, 207 (1987).
26. N.A. Pocock, J.A. Eisman, J.L. Hopper, M.G. Yeates, P.N. Sambrook and S. Eberl, J. Clin. Invest., 706 (1987).
27. C.W. Slemenda, J.C. Christian, C.J. Williams, J.A. Norton and C.C. Johnston, J. Bone Miner. Res., 561 (1991).
28. R. Gueguen, P. Jouanny, F. Guillemin, C. Kuntz, J. Pourel and G. Siest, J. Bone Miner. Res., 2017 (1995).
29. M.R. Sowers, M. Boehnke, M.L. Jannausch, M. Crutchfield, G. Corton and T.L. Burns, Calcif. Tissue Int., 110 (1992).
30. H.W. Deng, M.R. Stegman, K.M. Davies, T. Conway and R.R. Recker, J. Clin. Densitom., 251 (1999).
31. H.W. Deng, W.M. Chen, T. Conway, Y. Zhou, K.M. Davies, M.R. Stegman, H. Deng and R.R. Recker, Genet. Epidemiol., 160 (2000).
32. H.W. Deng, G. Livshits, K. Yakovenko, F.H. Xu, T. Conway, K.M. Davies, H.W. Deng and R.R. Recker, Ann. Hum. Genet., 61 (2002).
33. G. Livshits, D. Karasik, O. Pavlovsky and E. Kobyliansky, Hum. Biol., 155 (1999).
34. L.R. Cardon, C. Garner, S.T. Bennett, I.J. Mackay, R.M. Edwards, J. Cornish, M. Hegde, M.A. Murray, I.R. Reid and T. Cundy, J. Bone Miner. Res., 1132 (2000).
35. T.V. Nguyen, G.M. Howard, P.J. Kelly and J.A. Eisman, Am. J. Epidemiol., 3 (1998).

36.   H.W. Deng, M.C. Mahaney, J.T. Williams, J. Li, T. Conway, K.M. Davies, J.L. Li, H. Deng and R.R. Recker, Genet. Epidemiol., 12 (2002).

37.   E.S. Orwoll, J.K. Belknap and R.F. Klein, J. Bone Miner. Res., 1962 (2001).

38.   P.W. Lu, C.T. Cowell, S.A. LLoyd-Jones, J.N. Briody and R. Howman-Giles, J. Clin. Endocrinol. Metab, 1586 (1996).

39.   K.G. Faulkner, S.R. Cummings, D. Black, L. Palermo, C.C. Gluer and H.K. Genant, J. Bone Miner. Res., 1211 (1993).

40.   M. Moller, A. Horsman, B. Harvald, M. Hauge, K. Henningsen and B.E. Nordin, Calcif. Tissue Res., 197 (1978).

41.   S.L. Ferrari, R. Rizzoli, D. Slosman and J.P. Bonjour, J. Clin. Endocrinol. Metab., 358 (1998).

42.   H.W. Deng, X.T. Deng, T. Conway, F.H. Xu, R.P. Heaney and R.R. Recker, J. Clin. Densitom., 45 (2002).

43.   D.M. Smith, W.E. Nance, K.W. Kang, J.C. Christian and C.C. Johnston, J. Clin. Invest., 2800 (1973).

44.   T.V. Nguyen, J. Blangero and J.A. Eisman, J. Bone Miner. Res., 392 (2000).

45.   G.M. Howard, T.V. Nguyen, M. Harris, P.J. Kelly and J.A. Eisman, J. Bone Miner. Res., 1318 (1998).

46.   P. Garnero, Osteoporos. Int., S55-S65 (2000).

47.   M. Harris, T.V. Nguyen, G.M. Howard, P.J. Kelly and J.A. Eisman, Bone, 141 (1998).

48.   P.J. Kelly, J.L. Hopper, G.T. Macaskill, N.A. Pocock, P.N. Sambrook and J.A. Eisman, J. Clin. Endocrinol. Metab., 808 (1991).

49.   A. Tokita, P.J. Kelly, T.V. Nguyen, J.C. Qi, N.A. Morrison, L. Risteli, J. Risteli, P.N. Sambrook and J.A. Eisman, J. Clin. Endocrinol. Metab., 1461 (1994).

50.   P. Garnero, N.K. Arden, G. Griffiths, P.D. Delmas and T.D. Spector, J. Clin. Endocrinol. Metab, 140 (1996).

51.   H.W. Deng, W.M. Chen and R.R. Recker, Genetics, 885 (2001).

52.   H.W. Deng, Genetics, 1319 (2001).

53.   D.B. Allison, Am. J. Hum. Genet., 676 (1997).

54.   J.E. Eichner, C.A. Friedrich, J.A. Cauley, M.I. Kamboh, J.P. Gutai, L.H. Kuller and R.E. Ferrell, Calcif. Tissue Int., 345 (1990).

55.   L. Jia, N.C. Ho, S.S. Park, J. Powell and C.A. Francomano, Am. J. Med. Genet., 275 (2001).

56.   G. Gong, H.S. Stern, S.C. Cheng, N. Fong, J. Mordeson, H.W. Deng and R.R. Recker, Osteoporos. Int., 55 (1999).

57.   L.D. Spotila, A. Colige, L. Sereda, C.D. Constantinou-Deltas, M.P. Whyte, B.L. Riggs, J.L. Shaker, T.D. Spector, E. Hume and N. Olsen, J. Bone Miner. Res., 923 (1994).

58.   S.F. Grant, D.M. Reid, G. Blake, R. Herd, I. Fogelman and S.H. Ralston, Nat. Genet., 203 (1996).

59.   K.O. Han, I.G. Moon, C.S. Hwang, J.T. Choi, H.K. Yoon, H.K. Min and I.K. Han, Bone, 135 (1999).

60. S.F. Lei, F.Y. Deng, X.H. Liu, Q.R. Huang, Y. Qin, Q. Zhou, D.K. Jiang, Y.M. Li, X.Y. Mo, M.Y. Liu, X.D. Chen, X.S. Wu, H. Shen, V. Dvornyk, L. Zhao, R.R. Recker and H.W. Deng, J. Bone Miner. Metab., 34 (2003).

61. Z. Efstathiadou, A. Tsatsoulis and J.P. Ioannidis, J. Bone Miner. Res., 1586 (2001).

62. V. Mann, E.E. Hobson, B. Li, T.L. Stewart, S.F. Grant, S.P. Robins, R.M. Aspden and S.H. Ralston, J. Clin. Invest, 899 (2001).

63. V. Mann and S.H. Ralston, Bone, 711 (2003).

64. R.W. Keen, H. Snieder, H. Molloy, J. Daniels, M. Chiano, F. Gibson, L. Fairbairn, P. Smith, A.J. MacGregor, D. Gewert and T.D. Spector, Rheumatology, 48 (2001).

65. Y. Yamada, A. Miyauchi, Y. Takagi, M. Tanaka, M. Mizuno and A. Harada, J. Mol. Med., 149 (2001).

66. Y. Yamada, A. Miyauchi, J. Goto, Y. Takagi, H. Okuizumi, M. Kanematsu, M. Hase, H. Takai, A. Harada and K. Ikeda, J. Bone Miner. Res., 1569 (1998).

67. V. Hinke, T. Seck, C. Clanget, C. Scheidt-Nave, R. Ziegler and J. Pfeilschifter, Calcif. Tissue Int., 315 (2001).

68. B.L. Langdahl, J.Y. Knudsen, H.K. Jensen, N. Gregersen and E.F. Eriksen, Bone, 289 (1997).

69. Y. Yamada, Mech. Ageing Dev., 113 (2000).

70. F. Bertoldo, L. D'Agruma, F. Furlan, F. Colapietro, M.T. Lorenzi, N. Maiorano, A. Iolascon, L. Zelante, V. Locascio and P. Gasparini, J. Bone Miner. Res., 634 (2000).

71. S.C. Manolagas and R.L. Jilka, N. Engl. J. Med., 305 (1995).

72. S.H. Ralston, J. Bone Miner. Res., 883 (1994).

73. R.E. Murray, F. McGuigan, S.F. Grant, D.M. Reid and S.H. Ralston, Bone, 89 (1997).

74. K. Tsukamoto, H. Yoshida, S. Watanabe, T. Suzuki, M. Miyao, T. Hosoi, H. Orimo and M. Emi, J. Hum. Genet., 148 (1999).

75. N. Ota, T. Nakajima, I. Nakazawa, T. Suzuki, T. Hosoi, H. Orimo, S. Inoue, Y. Shirai and M. Emi, J. Hum. Genet., 267 (2001).

76. S.L. Ferrari, P. Garnero, S. Emond, H. Montgomery, S.E. Humphries and S.L. Greenspan, Arthritis Rheum., 196 (2001).

77. E. Canalis, J. Clin. Invest, 709 (1980).

78. E. Canalis, T. McCarthy and M. Centrella, J. Clin. Invest, 277 (1988).

79. T.L. McCarthy, M. Centrella and E. Canalis, Endocrinology, 1569 (1990).

80. S.E. Inzucchi and R.J. Robbins, J. Clin. Endocrinol. Metab, 691 (1994).

81. C.J. Rosen, E.S. Kurland, D. Vereault, R.A. Adler, P.J. Rackoff, W.Y. Craig, S. Witte, J. Rogers and J.P. Bilezikian, J. Clin. Endocrinol. Metab., 2286 (1998).

82. F. Rivadeneira, J.J. Houwing-Duistermaat, N. Vaessen, J.M. Vergeer-Drop, A. Hofman, H.A. Pols, C.M. van Duijn and A.G. Uitterlinden, J. Clin. Endocrinol. Metab, 3878 (2003).

83. C.J. Rosen, H.P. Dimai, D. Vereault, L.R. Donahue, W.G. Beamer, J. Farley, S. Linkhart, T. Linkhart, S. Mohan and D.J. Baylink, Bone, 217 (1997).

84.   E.S. Kurland, F.K. Chan, C.J. Rosen and J.P. Bilezikian, J. Clin. Endocrinol. Metab, 2576 (1998).

85.   E.S. Kurland, C.J. Rosen, F. Cosman, D. McMahon, F. Chan, E. Shane, R. Lindsay, D. Dempster and J.P. Bilezikian, J. Clin. Endocrinol. Metab, 2799 (1997).

86.   V. Braga, M. Mottes, S. Mirandola, V. Lisi, G. Malerba, L. Sartori, G. Bianchi, D. Gatti, M. Rossini, D. Bianchini and S. Adami, Calcif. Tissue Int., 361 (2000).

87.   F.J. Tsai, W.C. Chen, H.Y. Chen and C.H. Tsai, Gynecol. Obstet. Invest, 82 (2003).

88.   L. Masi, L. Becherini, E. Colli, L. Gennari, R. Mansani, A. Falchetti, A.M. Becorpi, C. Cepollaro, S. Gonnelli, A. Tanini and M.L. Brandi, Biochem. Biophys. Res. Commun., 190 (1998).

89.   J. Taboulet, M. Frenkian, J.L. Frendo, N. Feingold, A. Jullienne and M.C. de Vernejoul, Hum. Mol. Genet., 2129 (1998).

90.   M. Miyao, T. Hosoi, M. Emi, T. Nakajima, S. Inoue, S. Hoshino, M. Shiraki, H. Orimo and Y. Ouchi, J. Hum. Genet., 346 (2000).

91.   G. Gong, M.L. Johnson, M.J. Barger-Lux and R.P. Heaney, Osteoporos. Int., 307 (1999).

92.   T. Hosoi, M. Miyao, S. Inoue, S. Hoshino, M. Shiraki, H. Orimo and Y. Ouchi, Calcif. Tissue Int., 205 (1999).

93.   H.W. Deng, H. Shen, F.H. Xu, H.Y. Deng, T. Conway, H.T. Zhang and R.R. Recker, J. Bone Miner. Res., 678 (2002).

94.   I. Takacs, G. Speer, E. Bajnok, A. Tabak, Z. Nagy, C. Horvath, K. Kovacs and P. Lakatos, Bone, 849 (2002).

95.   K. Tsukamoto, H. Orimo, T. Hosoi, M. Miyao, N. Ota, T. Nakajima, H. Yoshida, S. Watanabe, T. Suzuki and M. Emi, Calcif. Tissue Int., 181 (2000).

96.   Y. Dohi, M. Iki, H. Ohgushi, S. Gojo, S. Tabata, E. Kajita, H. Nishino and K. Yonemasu, J. Bone Miner. Res., 1633 (1998).

97.   A. Gustavsson, P. Nordstrom, R. Lorentzon, U.H. Lerner and M. Lorentzon, Osteoporos. Int., 847 (2000).

98.   M.R. Sowers, M. Willing, T.L. Burns, S. Deschenes, B. Hollis, M. Crutchfield and M. Jannausch, J. Bone Miner. Res., 1411 (1999).

99.   D. Karasik, C.J. Rosen, M.T. Hannan, K.E. Broe, B. Dawson-Hughes, D.R. Gagnon, P.W. Wilson, M. Visser, J.A. Langlois, S. Mohan and D.P. Kiel, Calcif. Tissue Int., 323 (2002).

100. L.M. Salamone, J.A. Cauley, J. Zmuda, A. Pasagian-Macaulay, R.S. Epstein, R.E. Ferrell, D.M. Black and L.H. Kuller, J. Bone Miner. Res., 308 (2000).

101. H.P. Sennels, J.C. Sand, B. Madsen, J.B. Lauritzen, M. Fenger and H.L. Jorgensen, Scand. J. Clin. Lab Invest, 247 (2003).

102. M. Shiraki, Y. Shiraki, C. Aoki, T. Hosoi, S. Inoue, M. Kaneki and Y. Ouchi, J. Bone Miner. Res., 1438 (1997).

103. K. Zajickova, I. Zofkova, M. Hill, A. Horinek and A. Novakova, J. Endocrinol. Invest, 312 (2003).

104. J.M. Zmuda, J.E. Eichner, R.E. Ferrell, D.C. Bauer, L.H. Kuller and J.A. Cauley, Calcif. Tissue Int., 5 (1998).

105. R.W. Keen, K.L. Woodford-Richens, J.S. Lanchbury and T.D. Spector, Bone, 367 (1998).

106. B.L. Langdahl, L. Stenkjaer, M. Carstens, C.L. Tofteng and E.F. Eriksen, Calcif. Tissue Int., 237 (2003).

107. H.Y. Chen, W.C. Chen, M.C. Wu, F.J. Tsai and C.H. Tsai, Eur. J. Obstet. Gynecol. Reprod. Biol., 52 (2003).

108. T. Salmen, A.M. Heikkinen, A. Mahonen, H. Kroger, M. Komulainen, H. Pallonen, S. Saarikoski, R. Honkanen and P.H. Maenpaa, J. Bone Miner. Res., 319 (2003).

109. S. Ogawa, T. Urano, T. Hosoi, M. Miyao, S. Hoshino, M. Fujita, M. Shiraki, H. Orimo, Y. Ouchi and S. Inoue, Biochem. Biophys. Res. Commun., 122 (1999).

110. L.D. Spotila, H. Rodriguez, M. Koch, K. Adams, J. Caminis, H.S. Tenenhouse and A. Tenenhouse, J. Bone Miner. Res., 1376 (2000).

111. T. Urano, T. Hosoi, M. Shiraki, H. Toyoshima, Y. Ouchi and S. Inoue, Biochem. Biophys. Res. Commun., 422 (2000).

112. R.R. McLean, D. Karasik, J. Selhub, K.L. Tucker, J.M. Ordovas, G.T. Russo, L.A. Cupples, P.F. Jacques and D.P. Kiel, J. Bone Miner. Res., 410 (2004).

113. B. Abrahamsen, J.S. Madsen, C.L. Tofteng, L. Stilgren, E.M. Bladbjerg, S.R. Kristensen, K. Brixen and L. Mosekilde, J. Bone Miner. Res., 723 (2003).

114. M. Miyao, H. Morita, T. Hosoi, H. Kurihara, S. Inoue, S. Hoshino, M. Shiraki, Y. Yazaki and Y. Ouchi, Calcif. Tissue Int., 190 (2000).

115. L. Masi, L. Becherini, L. Gennari, A. Amedei, E. Colli, A. Falchetti, M. Farci, S. Silvestri, S. Gonnelli and M.L. Brandi, J. Clin. Endocrinol. Metab, 2263 (2001).

116. J. Somner, S. McLellan, J. Cheung, Y.T. Mak, M.L. Frost, K.M. Knapp, A.S. Wierzbicki, M. Wheeler, I. Fogelman, S.H. Ralston and G.N. Hampson, J. Clin. Endocrinol. Metab, 344 (2004).

117. J.M. Zmuda, J.A. Cauley, M.E. Danielson and R.E. Ferrell, Metabolism, 521 (2003).

118. N. Ogata, M. Shiraki, T. Hosoi, Y. Koshizuka, K. Nakamura and H. Kawaguchi, J. Bone Miner. Metab, 296 (2001).

119. Y. Yamada, F. Ando, N. Niino and H. Shimokata, Genomics, 8 (2002).

120. N. Ogata, Y. Matsumura, M. Shiraki, K. Kawano, Y. Koshizuka, T. Hosoi, K. Nakamura, Kuro-o M and H. Kawaguchi, Bone, 37 (2002).

121. T. Vaughan, J.A. Pasco, M.A. Kotowicz, G.C. Nicholson and N.A. Morrison, J. Bone Miner. Res., 1527 (2002).

122. J.N. Hirschhorn, K. Lohmueller, E. Byrne and K. Hirschhorn, Genet. Med., 45 (2002).

123. N.J. Risch, Nature, 847 (2000).

124. L.R. Cardon and J.I. Bell, Nat. Rev. Genet., 91 (2001).

125. D.N. Cooper, R.L. Nussbaum and M. Krawczak, Hum. Genet., 207 (2002).

126. J.P. Ioannidis, I. Stavrou, T.A. Trikalinos, C. Zois, M.L. Brandi, L. Gennari, O. Albagha, S.H. Ralston and A. Tsatsoulis, J. Bone Miner. Res., 2048 (2002).

127. M. Willing, M.R. Sowers, D. Aron, M.K. Clark, T.L. Burns, C. Bunten, M. Crutchfield, D. D'Agostino and M. Jannausch, J. Bone Miner. Res., 695 (1998).

128. L. Gennari, L. Becherini, L. Masi, R. Mansani, S. Gonnelli, C. Cepollaro, S. Martini, A. Montagnani, G. Lentini, A.M. Becorpi and M.L. Brandi, J. Clin. Endocrinol. Metab., 939 (1998).

129. H.W. Deng, J. Li, J.L. Li, M.L. Johnson, G. Gong and R.R. Recker, Osteoporos. Int., 499 (1999).

130. J. Long, P. Liu, Y. Zhang, H. Shen, Y. Liu, V. Dvornyk and H.W. Deng, J. Hum. Genet., 514 (2003).

131. H. Mizunuma, T. Hosoi, H. Okano, M. Soda, T. Tokizawa, I. Kagami, S. Miyamoto, Y. Ibuki, S. Inoue, M. Shiraki and Y. Ouchi, Bone, 379 (1997).

132. K.O. Han, J.T. Choi, I. Moon, H. Yoon, I.K. Han, H. Min, Y. Kim and Y. Choi, Osteoporos. Int., 290 (1999).

133. H.W. Deng, J.L. Li, J.L. Li, M.L. Johnson, G. Gong, K.M. Davis and R.R. Recker, Hum. Genet., 576 (1998).

134. A.G. Uitterlinden, A.E. Weel, H. Burger, Y. Fang, C.M. van Duijn, A. Hofman, J.P. van Leeuwen and H.A. Pols, J. Bone Miner. Res., 379 (2001).

135. S.L. Ferrari, J.P. Bonjour and R. Rizzoli. The vitamin D receptor gene and calcium metabolism. Trends Endocrinol.Metab., 9, 259 (1998).

136. S.L. Hui, P.S. Wiske, J.A. Norton and C.C. Johnston, J. Chronic. Dis., 715 (1982).

137. P. Steiger, S.R. Cummings, D.M. Black, N.E. Spencer and H.K. Genant, J. Bone Miner. Res., 625 (1992).

138. K.E. Ensrud, L. Palermo, D.M. Black, J.A. Cauley, M. Jergas, E.S. Orwoll, M.C. Nevitt, K.M. Fox and S.R. Cummings, J. Bone Miner. Res., 1778 (1995).

139. J.C. Fleet, S.S. Harris, R.J. Wood and B. Dawson-Hughes, J. Bone Miner. Res., 985 (1995).

140. S.S. Harris, T.R. Eccleshall, C. Gross, B. Dawson-Hughes and D. Feldman, J. Bone Miner. Res., 1043 (1997).

141. D.P. Kiel, R.H. Myers, L.A. Cupples, X.F. Kong, X.H. Zhu, J. Ordovas, E.J. Schaefer, D.T. Felson, D. Rush, P.W. Wilson, J.A. Eisman and M.F. Holick, J. Bone Miner. Res., 1049 (1997).

142. L.A. Rubin, G.A. Hawker, V.D. Peltekova, L.J. Fielding, R. Ridout and D.E. Cole, J. Bone Miner. Res., 633 (1999).

143. M.A. Brown, M.A. Haughton, S.F. Grant, A.S. Gunnell, N.K. Henderson and J.A. Eisman, J. Bone Miner. Res., 758 (2001).

144. W.C. Graafmans, P. Lips, M.E. Ooms, J.P. van Leeuwen, H.A. Pols and A.G. Uitterlinden, J. Bone Miner. Res., 1241 (1997).

145. Y. Giguere, S. Dodin, C. Blanchet, K. Morgan and F. Rousseau, J. Bone Miner. Res., 1076 (2000).

146. T. Salmen, A.M. Heikkinen, A. Mahonen, H. Kroger, M. Komulainen, S. Saarikoski, R. Honkanen and P.H. Maenpaa, J. Bone Miner. Res., 315 (2000).

147. L. Gennari, L. Becherini, R. Mansani, L. Masi, A. Falchetti, A. Morelli, E. Colli, S. Gonnelli, C. Cepollaro and M.L. Brandi, J. Bone Miner. Res., 1379 (1999).

148.   K.A. Hollenbach, E. Barrett-Connor, S.L. Edelstein and T. Holbrook, Am. J. Public Health, 1265 (1993).

149.   D.P. Kiel, Y. Zhang, M.T. Hannan, J.J. Anderson, J.A. Baron and D.T. Felson, Osteoporos. Int., 240 (1996).

150.   E.M. Dennison, N.K. Arden, R.W. Keen, H. Syddall, I.N. Day, T.D. Spector and C. Cooper, Paediatr. Perinat. Epidemiol., 211 (2001).

151.   L. Gennari, L. Becherini, A. Falchetti, L. Masi, F. Massart and M.L. Brandi, J. Steroid Biochem. Mol. Biol., 1 (2002).

152.   J.S. Lindberg, W.B. Fears, M.M. Hunt, M.R. Powell, D. Boll and C.E. Wade, Ann. Intern. Med., 647 (1984).

153.   A.M. Davee, C.J. Rosen and R.A. Adler, J. Bone Miner. Res., 245 (1990).

154.   B.L. Riggs, T.V. Nguyen, L.J. Melton, III, N.A. Morrison, W.M. O'Fallon, P.J. Kelly, K.S. Egan, P.N. Sambrook, J.M. Muhs and J.A. Eisman, J. Bone Miner. Res., 991 (1995).

155.   A.G. Uitterlinden, H. Burger, Q. Huang, F. Yue, F.E. McGuigan, S.F. Grant, A. Hofman, J.P. van Leeuwen, H.A. Pols and S.H. Ralston, N. Engl. J. Med., 1016 (1998).

156.   H.W. Deng, W.M. Chen and R.R. Recker, Am. J. Hum. Genet., 1027 (2000).

157.   Y. Liel, J. Edwards, J. Shary, K.M. Spicer, L. Gordon and N.H. Bell, J. Clin. Endocrinol. Metab., 1247 (1988).

158.   P. Jouanny, F. Guillemin, C. Kuntz, C. Jeandel and J. Pourel, Arthritis Rheum., 61 (1995).

159.   C. Vandevyver, T. Wylin, J.J. Cassiman, J. Raus and P. Geusens, J. Bone Miner. Res., 241 (1997).

160.   C.L. Tofteng, J.E. Jensen, B. Abrahamsen, L. Odum and C. Brot, J. Bone Miner. Res., 1535 (2002).

161.   J.M. Zmuda, J.A. Cauley, M.E. Danielson, R.L. Wolf and R.E. Ferrell, J. Bone Miner. Res., 1446 (1997).

162.   H.W. Deng, J. Li, J.L. Li, R. Dowd, K.M. Davies, M.L. Johnson, G. Gong, H.W. Deng and R.R. Recker, J. Clin. Endocrinol. Metab., 2748 (2000).

163.   E.S. Lander and N.J. Schork, Science, 2037 (1994).

164.   N. Risch and K. Merikangas, Science, 1516 (1996).

165.   M.M. Xiong, J. Krushkal and E. Boerwinkle, Ann. Hum. Genet., 431 (1998).

166.   E.L. Duncan, M.A. Brown, J. Sinsheimer, J. Bell, A.J. Carr, B.P. Wordsworth and J.A. Wass, J. Bone Miner. Res., 1993 (1999).

167.   N. Ota, S.C. Hunt, T. Nakajima, T. Suzuki, T. Hosoi, H. Orimo, Y. Shirai and M. Emi, Hum. Genet., 253 (1999).

168.   N. Ota, S.C. Hunt, T. Nakajima, T. Suzuki, T. Hosoi, H. Orimo, Y. Shirai and M. Emi, Genes Immun., 260 (2000).

169.   I. Takacs, D.L. Koller, M. Peacock, J.C. Christian, S.L. Hui, P.M. Conneally, C.C. Johnston, Jr., T. Foroud and M.J. Econs, J. Clin. Endocrinol. Metab, 4467 (1999).

170.   I. Takacs, D.L. Koller, M. Peacock, J.C. Christian, W.E. Evans, S.L. Hui, P.M. Conneally, C.C. Johnston, Jr., T. Foroud and M.J. Econs, Bone, 169 (2000).

171.   H.W. Deng, F.H. Xu, Q.Y. Huang, H. Shen, H.Y. Deng, T. Conway, Y.J. Liu,
        Y.Z. Liu, J.L. Li, H.T. Zhang, K.M. Davies and R.R. Recker, J. Clin.
        Endocrinol. Metab., 5151 (2002).

172.   T. Andrew, Y.T. Mak, P. Reed, A.J. MacGregor and T.D. Spector, Osteoporos.
        Int., 745 (2002).

173.   Y. Gong, M. Vikkula, L. Boon, J. Liu, P. Beighton, R. Ramesar, L. Peltonen,
        H. Somer, T. Hirose, B. Dallapiccola, A. De Paepe, W. Swoboda, B. Zabel, A.
        Superti-Furga, B. Steinmann, H.G. Brunner, A. Jans, R.G. Boles, W. Adkins,
        M.J. van den Boogaard, B.R. Olsen and M.L. Warman, Am. J. Hum. Genet.,
        146 (1996).

174.   R.P. Heaney, M.J. Barger-Lux, K.M. Davies, R.A. Ryan, M.L. Johnson and G.
        Gong, Osteoporos. Int., 426 (1997).

175.   M.L. Johnson, G. Gong, W. Kimberling, S.M. Recker, D.B. Kimmel and R.R.
        Recker, Am. J. Hum. Genet., 1326 (1997).

176.   R.D. Little, J.P. Carulli, R.G. Del Mastro, J. Dupuis, M. Osborne, C. Folz, S.P.
        Manning, P.M. Swain, S.C. Zhao, B. Eustace, M.M. Lappe, L. Spitzer, S.
        Zweier, K. Braunschweiger, Y. Benchekroun, X. Hu, R. Adair, L. Chee, M.G.
        FitzGerald, C. Tulig, A. Caruso, N. Tzellas, A. Bawa, B. Franklin, S. McGuire,
        X. Nogues, G. Gong, K.M. Allen, A. Anisowicz, A.J. Morales, P.T. Lomedico,
        S.M. Recker, P. Van Eerdewegh, R.R. Recker and M.L. Johnson, Am. J. Hum.
        Genet., 11 (2002).

177.   D.L. Koller, L.A. Rodriguez, J.C. Christian, C.W. Slemenda, M.J. Econs, S.L.
        Hui, P. Morin, P.M. Conneally, G. Joslyn, M.E. Curran, M. Peacock, C.C.
        Johnston and T. Foroud, J. Bone Miner. Res., 1903 (1998).

178.   D.L. Koller, M.J. Econs, P.A. Morin, J.C. Christian, S.L. Hui, P. Parry, M.E.
        Curran, L.A. Rodriguez, P.M. Conneally, G. Joslyn, M. Peacock, C.C. Johnston
        and T. Foroud, J. Clin. Endocrinol. Metab., 3116 (2000).

179.   H.W. Deng, F.H. Xu, T. Conway, X.T. Deng, J.L. Li, K.M. Davies, H.W.
        Deng, M.L. Johnson and R.R. Recker, J. Clin. Endocrinol. Metab., 3735
        (2001).

180.   M. Devoto, K. Shimoya, J. Caminis, J. Ott, A. Tenenhouse, M.P. Whyte, L.
        Sereda, S. Hall, E. Considine, C.J. Williams, G. Tromp, H. Kuivaniemi, L. Ala-
        Kokko, D.J. Prockop and L.D. Spotila, Eur. J. Hum. Genet., 151 (1998).

181.   T. Niu, C.K. Chen, H. Cordell, J. Yang, B. Wang, Z. Wang, Z. Fang, N.J.
        Schork, C.J. Rosen and X. Xu, Hum. Genet., 226 (1999).

182.   S.G. Wilson, P.W. Reed, A. Bansal, M. Chiano, M. Lindersson, M. Langdown,
        R.L. Prince, D. Thompson, E. Thompson, M. Bailey, P.W. Kleyn, P.
        Sambrook, M.M. Shi and T.D. Spector, Am. J. Hum. Genet., 144 (2003).

183.   Q.Y. Huang, F.H. Xu, H. Shen, L.J. Zhao, H.Y. Deng, Y.J. Liu, V. Dvornyk, T.
        Conway, K.M. Davies, J.L. Li, Y.Z. Liu, R.R. Recker and H.W. Deng. A
        second stage genome scan for QTLs influencing BMD variation. Calcif.Tissue
        Int., (2004).

184.   H.W. Deng, H. Shen, F.H. Xu, H. Deng, T. Conway, Y.J. Liu, Y.Z. Liu, J.L. Li,
        Q.Y. Huang, K.M. Davies and R.R. Recker, Am. J. Med. Genet., 121 (2003).

185. H.W. Deng, F.H. Xu, Y.Z. Liu, H. Shen, H. Deng, Q.Y. Huang, Y.J. Liu, T. Conway, J.L. Li, K.M. Davies and R.R. Recker, Am. J. Med. Genet., 29 (2002).

186. M.J. Econs, D.L. Koller, S.L. Hui, P.M. Conneally, C.C. Johnston, M. Peacock and T. Foroud, J. Bone Miner. Res., S189 (2002).

187. M. Peacock, D.L. Koller, S.L. Hui, C.C. Johnston, P.M. Conneally, T. Foroud and M.J. Econs, J. Bone Miner. Res., S176 (2002).

188. D.L. Koller, K.E. White, G. Liu, S.L. Hui, P.M. Conneally, C.C. Johnston, M.J. Econs, T. Foroud and M. Peacock, J. Bone Miner. Res., S236 (2002).

189. C.A. Walsh, M.A. Birch, W.D. Fraser, A.F. Ginty and J.A. Gallagher, Int. J. Exp. Pathol., 159 (2000).

190. M. Nasu, T. Sugimoto, H. Kaji and K. Chihara, J. Endocrinol., 305 (2000).

191. T. Bellido, R.L. Jilka, B.F. Boyce, G. Girasole, H. Broxmeyer, S.A. Dalrymple, R. Murray and S.C. Manolagas, J. Clin. Invest., 2886 (1995).

192. D. Stanislaus, X. Yang, J.D. Liang, J. Wolfe, R.L. Cain, J.E. Onyia, N. Falla, P. Marder, J.P. Bidwell, S.W. Queener and J.M. Hock, Bone, 209 (2000).

193. D. Stanislaus, V. Devanarayan and J.M. Hock, Bone, 819 (2000).

194. T.S. Grewal, P.G. Genever, A.C. Brabbs, M. Birch and T.M. Skerry, FASEB J., 523 (2000).

195. S. Wakabayashi, T. Tsutsumimoto, S. Kawasaki, T. Kinoshita, H. Horiuchi and K. Takaoka, J. Bone Miner. Res., 249 (2002).

196. Y. Yoshida, S. Tanaka, H. Umemori, O. Minowa, M. Usui, N. Ikematsu, E. Hosoda, T. Imamura, J. Kuno, T. Yamashita, K. Miyazono, M. Noda, T. Noda and T. Yamamoto, Cell, 1085 (2000).

197. D.L. Lacey, J.M. Erdmann, H.L. Tan and J. Ohara, J. Cell. Biochem., 122 (1993).

198. L.C. Hofbauer, S. Khosla, C.R. Dunstan, D.L. Lacey, W.J. Boyle and B.L. Riggs, J. Bone Miner. Res., 2 (2000).

199. W.S. Simonet, D.L. Lacey, C.R. Dunstan, M. Kelley, M.S. Chang, R. Luthy, H.Q. Nguyen, S. Wooden, L. Bennett, T. Boone, G. Shimamoto, M. DeRose, R. Elliott, A. Colombero, H.L. Tan, G. Trail, J. Sullivan, E. Davy, N. Bucay, L. Renshaw-Gegg, T.M. Hughes, D. Hill, W. Pattison, P. Campbell and W.J. Boyle, Cell, 309 (1997).

200. A. Mizuno, N. Amizuka, K. Irie, A. Murakami, N. Fujise, T. Kanno, Y. Sato, N. Nakagawa, H. Yasuda, S. Mochizuki, T. Gomibuchi, K. Yano, N. Shima, N. Washida, E. Tsuda, T. Morinaga, K. Higashio and H. Ozawa, Biochem. Biophys. Res. Commun., 610 (1998).

201. N. Bucay, I. Sarosi, C.R. Dunstan, S. Morony, J. Tarpley, C. Capparelli, S. Scully, H.L. Tan, W. Xu, D.L. Lacey, W.J. Boyle and W.S. Simonet, Genes Dev., 1260 (1998).

202. F. Gori, L.C. Hofbauer, C.R. Dunstan, T.C. Spelsberg, S. Khosla and B.L. Riggs, Endocrinology, 4768 (2000).

203. L.C. Hofbauer, C. Shui, B.L. Riggs, C.R. Dunstan, T.C. Spelsberg, T. O'Brien and S. Khosla, Biochem. Biophys. Res. Commun., 334 (2001).

204. L.C. Hofbauer, F. Gori, B.L. Riggs, D.L. Lacey, C.R. Dunstan, T.C. Spelsberg and S. Khosla, Endocrinology, 4382 (1999).

205. L.C. Hofbauer, D.L. Lacey, C.R. Dunstan, T.C. Spelsberg, B.L. Riggs and S. Khosla, Bone, 255 (1999).
206. L.C. Hofbauer, S. Khosla, C.R. Dunstan, D.L. Lacey, T.C. Spelsberg and B.L. Riggs, Endocrinology, 4367 (1999).
207. L.C. Hofbauer, C.R. Dunstan, T.C. Spelsberg, B.L. Riggs and S. Khosla, Biochem. Biophys. Res. Commun., 776 (1998).
208. M. Saika, D. Inoue, S. Kido and T. Matsumoto, Endocrinology, 2205 (2001).
209. R.A. Power, U.T. Iwaniec and T.J. Wronski, Bone, 143 (2002).
210. M. Zayzafoon, C. Stell, R. Irwin and L.R. McCabe, J. Cell. Biochem., 301 (2000).
211. B. Lecka-Czernik, I. Gubrij, E.J. Moerman, O. Kajkenova, D.A. Lipschitz, S.C. Manolagas and R.L. Jilka, J. Cell. Biochem., 357 (1999).
212. S. Chiba, M. Un-No, R.M. Neer, K. Okada, G.V. Serge and K. Lee, J. Vet. Med. Sci., 641 (2002).
213. F. Liu, J.E. Aubin and L. Malaval, Bone, 212 (2002).
214. G. Lisignoli, A. Piacentini, S. Toneguzzi, F. Grassi, B. Cocchini, A. Ferruzzi, G. Gualtieri and A. Facchini, Clin. Exp. Immunol., 346 (2000).
215. H. Kaji, T. Sugimoto, M. Kanatani, M. Fukase, M. Kumegawa and K. Chihara, J. Bone Miner. Res., 62 (1996).
216. J.W. Tomlinson, I. Bujalska, P.M. Stewart and M.S. Cooper, Endocr. Res., 711 (2000).
217. S. Srivastava, M.N. Weitzmann, R.B. Kimble, M. Rizzo, M. Zahner, J. Milbrandt, F.P. Ross and R. Pacifici, J. Clin. Invest., 1850 (1998).
218. D. Chikazu, X. Li, H. Kawaguchi, Y. Sakuma, O.S. Voznesensky, D.J. Adams, M. Xu, K. Hoshio, V. Katavic, H.R. Herschman, L.G. Raisz and C.C. Pilbeam, J. Bone Miner. Res., 1430 (2002).
219. M. Weinreb, M. Machwate, N. Shir, M. Abramovitz, G.A. Rodan and S. Harada, Bone, 275 (2001).

CHAPTER 16

PHARMACOGENETICS AND PHARMACOGENOMICS OF OSTEOPOROSIS

Dong-Hai Xiong[1,2,3], Ji-Rong Long[2], Sun Xiao[1], Hong-Wen Deng[1,2,3]

[1]*Laboratory of Molecular and Statistical Genetics, College of Life Sciences, Hunan Normal University, Changsha, Hunan 410081, P. R. China*

[2]*Osteoporosis Research Center, Creighton University Medical Center, Omaha, NE 68131*

[3]*Department of Biomedical Sciences, Creighton University, Omaha, NE 68131*

Osteoporosis, a common complex disease determined by multiple genetic, environmental and lifestyle factors, is mainly characterized by low bone density, leading to increased risk of low trauma fracture. Current genetics studies have shown that genetic factors play an important role not only in the etiopathogenesis but also in the treatment of osteoporosis. This fact has great implication in terms of anti-osteoporosis clinical therapeutics. Several potential ways to use genetic information for the prevention and treatment of osteoporosis are reviewed and discussed in this article. The first application is identification of novel genes or genetic variants of candidate genes that are associated with osteoporosis, which could be used either as drug targets or as reagents for drug development. Second, genetic approaches could furnish genetic profiling for drug efficacy or toxicity assessment. Finally, the knowledge gained through genetic studies can be applied to anti-osteoporosis gene therapy and personalized treatment. Genomics is also fostering new strategies in osteoporosis research and prevention. Pharmacogenomics, functional genomics, proteomics and modern bioinformatics will greatly contribute to optimizing osteoporosis drug development and therapeutics.

Keywords: Osteoporosis, Genetics, Etiopathogenesis, Drug discovery, Treatment , New strategies

Introduction

Osteoporosis is mainly characterized by the unbalanced loss of bone mass with decreased density and deteriorated bone microarchitecture that results in osteoporotic fracture. It is a common bone disease inflicting up to 40% of women and 12% of men at some point during life[1]. The social economic burden of osteoporosis is so large that its etiology, prevention and treatment have become the most urgent issues that need to be coped with worldwide.

Ideal anti-osteoporosis drugs should inhibit osteoclastic bone resorption and stimulate new bone formation with little or no side effects. However, no known medications convincingly meet all the above expectations. Current therapeutic agents are mainly bone resorption inhibitors such as estrogen and related compounds like SERMs (selective estrogen receptor modulators), bisphosphonates, and calcitonin. In addition, enough calcium and vitamin D supplementation is often required for most anti-osteoporosis treatments[2]. No acceptable bone formation stimulator is widely available now[3].

Like the disease *per se*, prevention and treatment of osteoporosis were also influenced by genetic factors. For example, the efficacy of calcium supplementation with or without vitamin D intake on preventing osteoporosis was associated with specific genotypes of both VDR (vitamin D receptor) and TGF-β1 (transformation growth factor beta1) genes[4-10]. The anti-osteoporosis effects of hormone replacement therapy (HRT) were reported to be dependent on different genotypes of ER-α (estrogen receptor alpha) gene[11-15]. Moreover, the Sp1 polymorphism of COLIA1 gene was shown to influence BMD response to the etidronate therapy[16]. These studies suggested that the personalized anti-osteoporosis therapies according to specific genetic background of individuals may be necessary to reduce both the unnecessary medical expense and unwanted side effects and increase therapeutic efficiency at the same time[2].

Pharmacogenetics Approaches

Previous Studies

By means of the population-based association method, several major candidate genes, such as vitamin D receptor (VDR), estrogen receptor alpha (ER-α) and collagen I alpha 1 (COLIA1) genes, have been investigated with regard to anti-osteoporosis drug responses. We outlined the related previous studies as follows.

The major biological function of VDR is to mediate the multiple and complex actions of 1,25-(OH)2 vitamin D including its effect on calcium transport and homeostasis and bone resorption. Many association studies have been conducted on the relationship between various bone phenotypes with VDR gene polymorphisms, such as the VDR Bsm I and Taq I polymorphisms. Based on the summarized data, Liu et al[17] tentatively concluded that bb or TT genotypes were more advantageous in terms of bone metabolism, calcium homeostasis, bone accrual during childhood and bone retention later in life while BB or tt individuals might be more likely to develop osteoporosis. Data from some pharmacogenetic studies provided some support. In the Framingham study cohort, dietary calcium intake was positively associated with BMD only among those with the bb genotype[7]. In a sample of 60 postmenopausal women the calcium absorption efficiency on low calcium intake was significantly lower in subjects with BB genotype than those with bb genotype[4]. Matsuyama et al[8] also reported that the bb genotype was associated with a greater increase in BMD in response to the vitamin D supplementation in Japanese. Furthermore, it was reported in a Japanese study that the TT homozygotes benefited from HRT more than the Tt heterozygotes[18]. However, the opposite or 'no association' conclusions were made in other studies[5,6,19-21]. These discrepancies may be accounted for by many confounding variables such as population admixture, epistasis, gene × environment interaction, linkage disequilibrium and allele or locus heterogeneity across different populations. Further studies with robust study designs are needed for a better understanding of the relationship between the VDR polymorphisms and the efficacy of anti-osteoporotic therapies.

Pharmacogenetic studies of the ER-α gene mainly involve two marker loci, the Xba I and Pvu II polymorphisms. Deng et al[11] reported a positive association between the XX homozygotes and the increase of spine BMD in response to HRT treatment in postmenopausal Caucasian women. As for the Pvu II polymorphism, the study of a cohort of Finnish perimenopausal women showed that P allele was significantly associated with the reduction in the incidence of new fractures in the group treated with HRT. But in the non-HRT group, the Pvu II polymorphism was not significantly associated with fracture risk[12]. This result suggests that the gene × drug interaction may have influence on the results of association studies, which might be one of the confounding factors underlying the outcome of osteoporosis research. Ongphiphadhanakul et al[14] also found that the increase in vertebral BMD responding to estrogen therapy was significantly lower in Thai postmenopausal women without the P allele compared to those with the P allele, which partially supported Salmen et al's conclusion[12]. In addition, BMD changes after HRT were reported to be associated with another polymorphism in the ER-α gene, a T262C transition in exon 1, which may be in linkage disequilibrium with the Pvu II polymorphism[15]. However, no significant difference in BMD change was observed between different genotypes of either Pvu II or Xba I polymorphisms after treatment with selective estrogen receptor modulators[22].

For the COLIA1 gene, the Sp1 polymorphism was often studied. Cultured osteoblasts from "Ss" heterozygotes produced increased amount of the collagen α1(I) chain because the s allele had greater affinity for transcription factor Sp1 than did the S allele. The resulted overproduction of α1(I)3 in collagen may be responsible for impaired bone strength[16]. In agreement with this theory, many studies showed the association between the Sp1 polymorphism and the risk for osteoporosis or fractures[17]. Although inconsistent association results exist, two meta-analyses[23,24] supported that the presence of s allele was significantly associated with low BMD and fracture prevalence though such effect on bone metabolism was moderate and could be easily modified by environmental factors. In keeping with this, one pharmacogenetic research demonstrated that the s allele negatively influence BMD response to the etidronate therapy since femoral neck BMD obviously increased in the SS group while decreased in the Ss/ss group[16]. This finding also implied the possible clinical value of using COLIA1 Sp1 polymorphism in targeting etidronate therapy to patients who are most likely to respond, with potential advantages in terms of cost and clinical outcome.

Although there is clear evidence for association between genetic polymorphisms in candidate genes and variable therapeutic effects, the results from multiple pharmacogenetic studies in bone field are largely inconsistent as indicated above. The most likely explanation for this inconsistency is a lack of power given the small sample sizes involved (often less than 100 in each comparison group). For instance, meta-analyses suggest a weak but positive association between BMD and BsmI[25], but the main effect of the VDR genotypes can hardly be detected rightly if a study is inadequately powered. Many other reasons may also apply, such as population stratification, difficulty in precisely measuring drug response phenotype, subtlety of functional effects of polymorphisms, focusing on single SNPs instead of haplotypes or ignoring genetic heterogeneity, gene × gene (G × G) and gene × environment (G × E) interactions[26]. Yet, it seems a little bit premature to speculate about these factors if the studies lack enough power. Therefore, pharmacogenetic studies employing sound experimental designs and robust statistical methods, and most importantly, sufficient power, are needed to track down causal genetic variants influencing drug response variability and devise genotype-specific interventions to reduce osteoporosis incidence in normal populations[27]. Such issues were briefly discussed in the following.

Experimental Design

Compared with studies of complex diseases where multiple approaches can be utilized, choices for pharmacogenetic studies are limited. In most cases it is impossible to administer a drug to multiple family members, which precludes the use of other methods like linkage analyses and TDT (transmission disequilibrium test)[28]. Therefore, the population-based association method is the most feasible and frequently used approach in pharmacogenetics.

Three designs are prevalent in population-based association studies: cohort, randomized control and case-control designs. Currently, cohort or randomized control studies dominate the osteoporosis pharmacogenetic field and almost all these studies did not differentiate 'case' and 'control' in the pharmacogenetic context. Such practice is reasonable because longitudinal BMD change in response to a specific treatment is the predominant phenotype studied, which is a quantitative trait. However, extreme discordant phenotype (EDP) methodology, which belongs to the category of case-control design, is a promising approach to clinical osteoporosis pharmacogenetics, although it has not been used in the filed until now. EDP method aims at teasing apart the complex trait of drug efficacy or toxicity by identifying groups with extreme responses to a drug ('sensitivity' versus 'resistance' to drug efficacy or toxicity), while ignoring the group with intermediate drug response, which has the majority of individuals[29,30]. In bone field, for example, the "resistant outlier" could represent a patient with little BMD accretion in response to a large dose of anti-osteoporosis drug, whereas the "sensitive outlier" could be a patient exhibiting an exaggerated BMD accretion to a low dose of drug. Such statistically significant outliers, who should harbor genetic variants causing the extreme pharmacogenetic phenotypes, may be more useful than minor inter-individual differences in the general population in dissecting the causal genetic variants of relatively big pharmaceutical effects[30], which could serve as drug targets or reagents to facilitate novel anti-osteoporosis drug development.

Factors Influencing the Power of Genetic Association Study

Sample size is one of the most important issues influencing the power of a study, which depends upon the hypothesis being tested and the study design required to adequately address the problem. For a cohort or randomized control design, where BMD changes are often used as phenotypic data, statistical power analyses [Fig. (1)] using the program at http://statgen.iop.kcl.ac.uk/gpc/qtlassoc.html[31] showed the following results under the assumption of complete LD (D'=1), the exactly matched QTL : Marker allele frequencies, and the lack of allelic heterogeneity. First, to achieve ~80% statistical power (α=0.001) ~600 subjects are needed to detect a QTL accounting for ~ 5% of phenotypic variation due to genotypic effects. Second, assuming that both a candidate gene and treatments account for 5% of the variation in a phenotype, ~950 subjects are needed to detect such a G×T interaction with ~80% statistical power (α=0.001) (Figure 1).

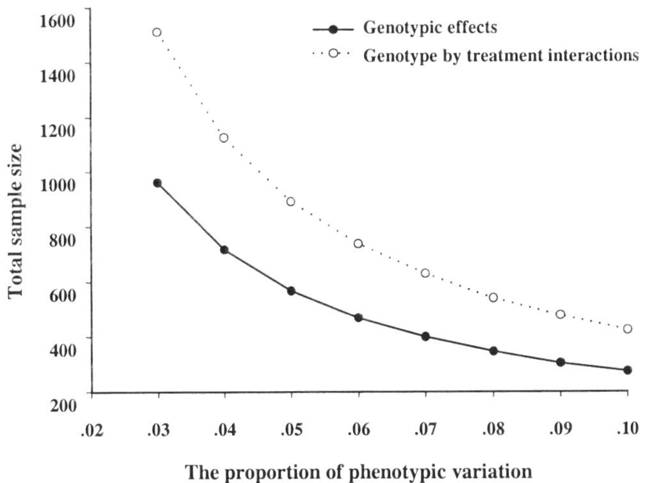

Figure 1 Total sample size for ANOVA analyses to achieve 80% power under differential phenotypic variations due to genotypic effects or genotype by treatment interactions.

The other key issues for any genetic association study affecting power are LD patterns, allele frequency difference and allelic heterogeneity. The reasons include: 1) LD is highly variable across the human genome[32,33], so if the genetic marker is in close proximity to a QTL of large effect, but LD=0, then this functional variant will still be missed no matter how big the sample size is (i.e. power will equal zero); 2) the degree of LD between functional variant and genetic marker will fall rapidly if the allelic frequencies of each are not closely matched, leading to a great loss of power[34]; On the other hand, the power of an association study is greatest when the allele frequencies of the marker and the causal variant match exactly[35]; 3) the allelic heterogeneity for the gene can drastically reduce the power of the study. In the presence of such problem, the omnibus tests or collective testing of alleles can be substantially more powerful than separate testing of individual allelic variants[36].

Still using the program at http://statgen.iop.kcl.ac.uk/gpc/qtlassoc.html[31], the impact of the above issues on the design of association studies can be exemplified. Suppose the lack of allelic heterogeneity, if LD is not complete (e.g. D'=0.8) and there is moderate QTL : marker mismatch (say 0.10:0.20), the study would require 1200 subjects to achieve ~80% statistical power (α=0.001) for the detection of a QTL main effect that accounts for ~ 5% of the total phenotypic variation (and 3000 if D'=0.5). Thus, the sample sizes under nonideal situations should be significantly larger than that under ideal situations (600 as mentioned above) to achieve the same statistical power.

Pathway Approaches

Current pharmacogenetic studies in the osteoporosis field only studied several prominent candidate genes such as the VDR, TGF-β1, ER-α and COLIA1 genes. However, panels of genes underlying the pathways through which certain anti-osteoporosis drugs play their role have not been investigated systematically. Pharmacogenetic studies in other fields have provided substantial evidence that genetic polymorphisms in pathway genes, i.e., those that encode drug metabolizing enzymes, drug transporters and drug targets, contribute to interpatient variability in drug response or toxicity risk[37]. Therefore, it is natural for us to apply the same principle to the osteoporosis field. For example, a panel of genes underlying calcium homeostasis and vitamin D metabolism, transport and action merit investigation regarding whether they are associated with the efficacy of calcium and vitamin D supplementation on preventing postmenopausal osteoporosis. Such practice, combined with the optimum study design and robust analysis approaches, would markedly increase the statistical power to find the real genetic loci underlying anti-osteoporosis drug response or toxicity and detect the important interaction terms like $G \times G$ interaction[30].

Haplotype Analysis and Tagging SNPs

Typically, only one or a few SNPs from candidate genes are genotyped for association with osteoporotic drug effects. The results obtained were often different and may not represent the true situation regarding the association between the candidate genes and the efficacy of certain anti-osteoporosis drugs. With the ever decreasing cost of high-throughput genotyping and the ever increasing density of SNP maps, it could be expected that the traditional univariate (one locus) pharmacogenetic studies will give way to candidate gene studies adopting haplotype analyses where patterns of LD throughout the gene region are determined [38].

The human genome has been portrayed as a series of high LD regions separated by short discrete segments of very low LD[39]. Those high LD regions usually exhibit limited haplotype diversity, so that a small number of distinct haplotypes account for most of the chromosomes in such genomic regions ("haplotype blocks") in a population[40-42]. Haplotype blocks may extend from a few to >100 kb[40,42]. Within haplotype blocks, allelic dependence yields redundancy among markers and improves the chances of detecting association when only a fraction of the markers is tested[39]. Therefore, it is feasible to identify a parsimonious set of htSNPs (haplotype-tagging SNPs) that could distinguish the haplotypic variations in a population and cover the majority of genetic information contained in the candidate genes[43]. Such tagging approaches are hoped to reduce the genotyping efforts with only a modest reduction in statistical power relative to direct assays of all common SNPs in block regions[44]. In some cases, such haplotype approaches might offer more power to detect associations than simply measuring individual SNPs[45]. Therefore, it can be expected that haplotype analysis and tagging approaches will help identify many more pharmacogenetic variants efficiently and accelerate the development of novel anti-osteoporosis drugs.

However, the concept of "haplotype blocks" arising from early LD mapping using human genomic data[40-42,46,47], has subsequently been recognized to be largely artifactual since "block" definitions are arbitrary[41] and boundaries vary with marker density[39]. In such context, currently there is no consensus about the best methods to tag most informative SNPs[44]. In addition, the possibility of effectively tagging rare (<5%) SNPs, without having to resort to genotyping all identified SNPs, is still uncertain. Therefore, the idea of using tagging SNPs for large genomic regions, or even genome wide association studies, is premature before proper LD maps have been developed. Just as we now have genetic linkage maps, we also require reliable LD maps before identifying which subsets of markers will be sufficient for LD marker sets[48]. Otherwise, tagging strategy may prove to be a false economy for LD mapping over large regions.

Population Admixture/Stratification

The pharmacogenetic association approach is prone to population admixture/stratification in yielding false positive or false negative results[49,50]. Spurious associations between genotype and intervention outcomes could arise if the population under study consists of a mixture of two or more subpopulations that have different allele frequencies and disease risks (for environmental or genetic reasons unrelated to the allele under study)[51]. Recently developed association methods for unrelated population samples, such as genomic control and structured association[52-54] are robust to population admixture but have not been used in pharmacogenetic studies of osteoporosis. Under some necessary assumptions, these methods may obviate many (but not every) concerns about population structure by using the features of the genome present in the sample to correct for stratification. The genome control method exploits the fact that population stratification generates "over dispersion" of the statistics that are used to assess association. By testing multiple markers throughout the genome, the degree of overdispersion can be estimated and accounted for in association analyses. The structured association method assumes that the study population is composed of homogeneous sub-populations, which may be classified using data from multiple marker loci and then association analyses can be conducted within homogeneous subpopulations. Both these methods need to assume, e.g., that differentiation of marker loci across the whole human genome is constant, which awaits data for justification.

Pharmacogenomic Strategies for Osteoporosis

Genome-wide Association Approach

Taking advantage of LD widely existent across the human genome, the genome-wide association approach can detect association between a particular genomic region and a disease or relevant drug response no matter whether the markers are functional variants per se[55]. Such strategy is not constrained by the current knowledge of the proteins involved in the disease etiology or drug response variability[26] and could limit the search for the causative variants within the regions showing association with the disease or drug response[55].

The International HapMap Project just aims to greatly facilitate the genome-wide association studies by identifying the common patterns of DNA sequence variation in the human genome[55]. The haplotypes thus characterized could then be tested for association with variable drug response, to provide a genome-wide perspective on the genetic contributors to drug efficacy or toxicity[26]. However, since HapMap relies on LD across the genome and does not focus on polymorphisms of potential functional significance, such important functional variants will be missed if they are not in LD or only in weak LD with SNPs in the haplotype map. This fact suggests that, in addition to haplotypes identified by HapMap, inclusion of documented functional SNPs and SNPs in non-block regions (which may harbor functional variants) is necessary to completely survey genetic contributors to drug response variability[26].

Genome-wide Mapping in the Mouse to Identify Drug Response Genes

The laboratory mouse is an ideal model system for pharmacogenomic research. The advantages include: a) the content and structure of the human and mouse genomes are closely related; b) the easiness to create large 'family pedigrees' in a relatively short period; c) the easiness to administer a drug to all the family members so that family-based approaches like linkage analysis and TDT (transmission disequilibrium test) can be employed; d) non-genetic factors such as diet and environment can be carefully controlled. Most importantly, well-defined mouse strains are available in which genetic factors have been fixed through inbreeding[56]. Genetic complexity could be significantly reduced and the 'informativeness' of breeding fully ensured by the wise use of such mouse strains.

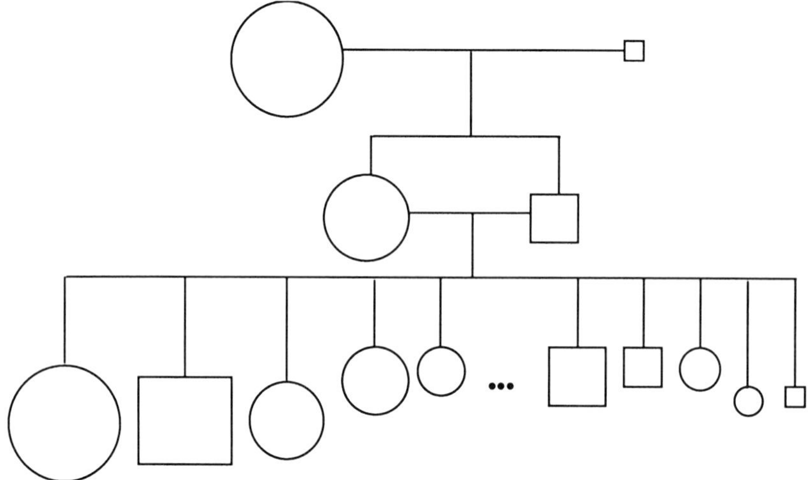

Figure 2 QTL mapping in mice based on F2 design. (The size of the symbols represent different individual osteoporosis drug response values).

Mapping 'osteoporosis drug response genes' can be productive in F2 mice because of the independent segregation of genes for this polygenic phenotype in the F2 generation. The design of such experiment is given in Fig. (2). The strategy behind is to map QTLs influencing drug efficacy by crossing the parental strains that differ significantly in drug phenotype and then intercrossing the F1 progeny to generate a large number of F2 mice (range 250-1000)[57,58]. Then the genome-wide linkage analysis can be conducted within such a large pedigree to find loci influencing drug response. The power of linkage studies to detect drug response loci in mice may be much greater than that in humans[56,57]. The loci identified may serve as basis for finding drug response genes in human populations. However, we still have to take caution when applying achievement in mouse genomics to pharmacogenomic studies of human osteoporosis because of species differences in drug metabolism and action mechanisms[56]. Several reviews have pointed out the difficulty of using animal models to understand human diseases[59,60]. The inherent genomic difference between human and mouse species, the polygenic nature and the complex G × G and G × E interactions influencing osteoporosis and its treatment, all mean that underlying causes and drug targets for human osteoporosis could be different from those identified by mouse genetics. Thus, new drugs targeting the pathway of mouse bone metabolism may not pass Phase II clinical trial[59,60]. This suggested that some research emphasis should be placed on testing bone phenotypes in human populations for the genes identified in animal models at an early stage of drug development.

Functional Genomics and Bioinformatics

The aforementioned pharmacogenomic approaches to osteoporosis are just in their infancy. They should be further developed and combined with other functional genomic approaches to be more powerful in the genetic dissection of osteoporosis. Functional genomics broadly includes a set of technologies and strategies focused on finding the function of genes and understanding how the genome works together to generate whole patterns of biological function[61]. Currently, DNA microarrays may be the most powerful of the techniques that address global functional genomics questions. The goal of analyzing the expression of thousands of genes can be achieved in a single experiment using DNA microarrays. Thus the study of global gene expression patterns that are affected in symphony by specific diseases and drug treatments can be greatly facilitated. Moreover, DNA microarrays can be used for drug target validation and disease diagnoses[62]. In a recent review, it was also shown that microarrays could be employed to identify molecular subtypes of given disease traits to help find the genetic loci specific to each subtype[63]. Such an application may provide an alternative way to identify genes underlying osteoporosis[64]. Yet, the DNA microarrays approach is not perfect since it only aims at the level of RNA alterations. A complementary approach is proteomics, which is the analysis of global changes in protein expression. It deals with changes that DNA microarrays cannot, which include protein abundance, protein-protein interactions and post-translational modifications[61]. Now the proteomics approach is being applied to the discovery of new drug targets and the study of drug response, thus leading to the birth of pharmacoproteomics. The judicious use of DNA microarrays and/or proteomics techniques with advanced bioinformatics tools in the osteoporosis research can complement pharmacogenomic methods for the better understanding and treatment of osteoporosis. In addition, the ever-expanding Pharmacogenetics and Pharmacogenomics Knowledge Base (PharmGKB, http://www.pharmgkb.org), which is a public repository of genotype and phenotype information relevant to pharmacogenetics, will greatly catalyze research in the osteoporosis field[65].

Significance of Genetic/Genomic Approaches to Anti-Osteoporosis Treatment

Integrating the achievement in osteoporosis genetics, pharmaco-genetics/-genomics, functional genomics and bioinformatics into the treatment of this disease is the end goal of such studies. Several potential applications are illustrated in Fig. (3). First, novel osteoporosis drug discovery and design can benefit from the progress in the genetic research regarding its etiology. The identified osteoporosis susceptibility genes can serve as the starting point for the development of osteoporosis drug. Pharmaco-genetics/-genomics studies can also suggest novel drug targets to pursue, which could lead to entirely new types of anti-osteoporosis drugs[66]. Another important application of pharmacogenetics/-genomics is to furnish genetic profiling for drug efficacy or toxicity assessment[67], which holds the promise for the optimal anti-osteoporosis treatment, personalized medicine and molecular prognosis and diagnosis. This will greatly promote the development of pharmaceutical industry in terms of administering the appropriate types of drugs to the corresponding types of patient population according to the genetic tests, thus improving the therapeutic efficacy and reducing unwanted side effects of commercial osteoporosis drugs. Finally, modern functional genomics and bioinformatics approaches could provide differential gene expression or protein profiles for osteoporosis patients with/without treatment versus healthy controls. Such approaches, combined with traditional methods or other functional studies, will promote the application of genetics into osteoporosis research and treatment in every aspect.

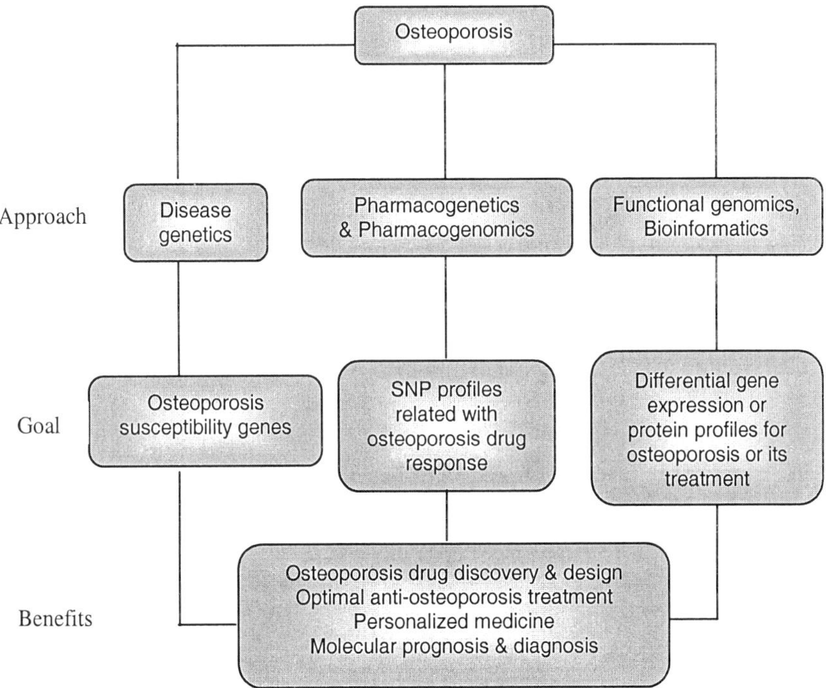

Figure 3 Influence of genetics/genomics on anti-osteoporosis clinical therapeutics.

Acknowledgments

The study was partially supported by grants from Health Future Foundation, National Institute of Health, the State of Nebraska. It also benefited from grants by National Science Foundation of China, Huo Ying Dong Foundation and Ministry of Education of P.R. China.

REFERENCES

1.   S. H. Ralston, QJM., 247 (1997).

2.   D. H. Xiong, J. R. Long, R. R. Recker and H. W. Deng, Pharmacogenomics. J., 261 (2003).

3.   G. R. Mundy, Annu. Rev. Med., 337 (2002).

4.   B. Dawson-Hughes, S. S. Harris and S. Finneran, J. Clin. Endocrinol. Metab, 3657 (1995).

5.   S. L. Ferrari, R. Rizzoli, D. O. Slosman and J. P. Bonjour, J. Bone Miner. Res., 363 (1998).

6.   W. C. Graafmans, P. Lips, M. E. Ooms, J. P. van Leeuwen, H. A. Pols and A. G. Uitterlinden, J. Bone Miner. Res., 1241 (1997).

7.   D. P. Kiel, R. H. Myers, L. A. Cupples, X. F. Kong, X. H. Zhu, J. Ordovas, E. J. Schaefer, D. T. Felson, D. Rush, P. W. Wilson, J. A. Eisman and M. F. Holick, J. Bone Miner. Res., 1049 (1997).

8.   T. Matsuyama, S. Ishii, A. Tokita, K. Yabuta, S. Yamamori, N. A. Morrison and J. A. Eisman, Lancet, 1238 (1995).

9.   Y. Yamada, A. Harada, T. Hosoi, A. Miyauchi, K. Ikeda, H. Ohta and M. Shiraki, J. Bone Miner. Res., 415 (2000).

10. R. Young, F. Wu, W. N. Van de, R. Ames, G. Gamble and I. R. Reid, J. Clin. Endocrinol. Metab, 697 (2003).

11. H. W. Deng, J. Li, J. L. Li, M. Johnson, G. Gong, K. M. Davis and R. R. Recker, Hum. Genet., 576 (1998).

12. T. Salmen, A. M. Heikkinen, A. Mahonen, H. Kroger, M. Komulainen, S. Saarikoski, R. Honkanen and P. H. Maenpaa, J. Bone Miner. Res., 2479 (2000).

13. T. Salmen, A. M. Heikkinen, A. Mahonen, H. Kroger, M. Komulainen, S. Saarikoski, R. Honkanen and P. H. Maenpaa, J. Bone Miner. Res., 315 (2000).

14. B. Ongphiphadhanakul, S. Chanprasertyothin, P. Payatikul, S. S. Tung, N. Piaseu, L. Chailurkit, S. Chansirikarn, G. Puavilai and R. Rajatanavin, Clin. Endocrinol. (Oxf), 581 (2000).

15. B. Ongphiphadhanakul, S. Chanprasertyothin, P. Payattikul, S. Saetung, N. Piaseu, L. Chailurkit, S. Chansirikarn, G. Puavilai and R. Rajatanavin, J. Endocrinol. Invest, 749 (2001).

16. A. M. Qureshi, R. J. Herd, G. M. Blake, I. Fogelman and S. H. Ralston, Calcif. Tissue Int., 158 (2002).

17. Y. Z. Liu, Y. J. Liu, R. R. Recker and H. W. Deng, J. Endocrinol., 147 (2003).

18. T. Kurabayashi, M. Tomita, H. Matsushita, T. Yahata, A. Honda, K. Takakuwa and K. Tanaka, Am. J. Obstet. Gynecol., 1115 (1999).

19. J. Marc, J. Prezelj, R. Komel and A. Kocijancic, Osteoporos. Int., 303 (1999).

20. S. Palomba, F. G. Numis, G. Mossetti, D. Rendina, P. Vuotto, T. Russo, F. Zullo, C. Nappi and V. Nunziata, Hum. Reprod., 192 (2003).

21. C. L. Tofteng, J. E. Jensen, B. Abrahamsen, L. Odum and C. Brot, J. Bone Miner. Res., 1535 (2002).

22. K. Yoneda, Y. Tanji, N. Ikeda, Y. Miyoshi, T. Taguchi, Y. Tamaki and S. Noguchi, Cancer Lett., 223 (2002).

23. Z. Efstathiadou, A. Tsatsoulis and J. P. Ioannidis, J. Bone Miner. Res., 1586 (2001).

24. V. Mann, E. E. Hobson, B. Li, T. L. Stewart, S. F. Grant, S. P. Robins, R. M. Aspden and S. H. Ralston, J. Clin. Invest, 899 (2001).

25. A. Thakkinstian, C. D'Este, J. Eisman, T. Nguyen and J. Attia, J. Bone Miner. Res., 419 (2004).

26. J. A. Johnson and J. J. Lima, Pharmacogenetics, 525 (2003).

27. D. B. Goldstein, S. K. Tate and S. M. Sisodiya, Nat. Rev. Genet., 937 (2003).

28. J. J. McCarthy and R. Hilfiker, Nat. Biotechnol., 505 (2000).

29. D. W. Nebert, Clin. Genet., 247 (1999).

30. D. W. Nebert, Eur. J. Pharmacol., 107 (2000).

31. S. Purcell, S. S. Cherny and P. C. Sham, Bioinformatics., 149 (2003).

32. D. E. Reich, S. F. Schaffner, M. J. Daly, G. McVean, J. C. Mullikin, J. M. Higgins, D. J. Richter, E. S. Lander and D. Altshuler, Nat. Genet., 135 (2002).

33. L. Kruglyak, Nat. Genet., 139 (1999).

34. I. P. Tu and A. S. Whittemore, Am. J. Hum. Genet., 641 (1999).

35. B. Muller-Myhsok and L. Abel, Science, 1328 (1997).

36.   J. A. Longmate, Am. J. Hum. Genet., 1229 (2001).

37.   J. A. Johnson, Trends Genet., 660 (2003).

38.   D. B. Goldstein, K. R. Ahmadi, M. E. Weale and N. W. Wood, Trends Genet., 615 (2003).

39.   L. R. Cardon and G. R. Abecasis, Trends Genet, 135 (2003).

40.   M. J. Daly, J. D. Rioux, S. F. Schaffner, T. J. Hudson and E. S. Lander, Nat. Genet., 229 (2001).

41.   S. B. Gabriel, S. F. Schaffner, H. Nguyen, J. M. Moore, J. Roy, B. Blumenstiel, J. Higgins, M. DeFelice, A. Lochner, M. Faggart, S. N. Liu-Cordero, C. Rotimi, A. Adeyemo, R. Cooper, R. Ward, E. S. Lander, M. J. Daly and D. Altshuler, Science, 2225 (2002).

42.   N. Patil, A. J. Berno, D. A. Hinds, W. A. Barrett, J. M. Doshi, C. R. Hacker, C. R. Kautzer, D. H. Lee, C. Marjoribanks, D. P. McDonough, B. T. Nguyen, M. C. Norris, J. B. Sheehan, N. Shen, D. Stern, R. P. Stokowski, D. J. Thomas, M. O. Trulson, K. R. Vyas, K. A. Frazer, S. P. Fodor and D. R. Cox, Science, 1719 (2001).

43.   P. Sebastiani, R. Lazarus, S. T. Weiss, L. M. Kunkel, I. S. Kohane and M. F. Ramoni, Proc. Natl. Acad. Sci. U. S. A, 9900 (2003).

44.   M. E. Weale, C. Depondt, S. J. Macdonald, A. Smith, P. S. Lai, S. D. Shorvon, N. W. Wood and D. B. Goldstein, Am. J Hum. Genet, 551 (2003).

45.   H. K. Tabor, N. J. Risch and R. M. Myers, Nat. Rev. Genet., 391 (2002).

46.   E. Dawson, G. R. Abecasis, S. Bumpstead, Y. Chen, S. Hunt, D. M. Beare, J. Pabial, T. Dibling, E. Tinsley, S. Kirby, D. Carter, M. Papaspyridonos, S. Livingstone, R. Ganske, E. Lohmussaar, J. Zernant, N. Tonisson, M. Remm, R. Magi, T. Puurand, J. Vilo, A. Kurg, K. Rice, P. Deloukas, R. Mott, A. Metspalu, D. R. Bentley, L. R. Cardon and I. Dunham, Nature, 544 (2002).

47.   G. C. Johnson, L. Esposito, B. J. Barratt, A. N. Smith, J. Heward, G. Di Genova, H. Ueda, H. J. Cordell, I. A. Eaves, F. Dudbridge, R. C. Twells, F. Payne, W. Hughes, S. Nutland, H. Stevens, P. Carr, E. Tuomilehto-Wolf, J. Tuomilehto, S. C. Gough, D. G. Clayton and J. A. Todd, Nat. Genet., 233 (2001).

48.   N. Maniatis, A. Collins, J. Gibson, W. Zhang, W. Tapper and N. E. Morton, Am. J. Hum. Genet., 846 (2004).

49.   H. W. Deng, W. M. Chen and R. R. Recker, Genetics, 885 (2001).

50.   H. W. Deng, Genetics, 1319 (2001).

51.   H. M. Colhoun, P. M. McKeigue and S. G. Davey, Lancet, 865 (2003).

52.   B. Devlin, K. Roeder and S. A. Bacanu, Genet. Epidemiol., 273 (2001).

53.   B. Devlin and K. Roeder, Biometrics, 997 (1999).

54.   J. K. Pritchard, M. Stephens, N. A. Rosenberg and P. Donnelly, Am. J. Hum. Genet., 170 (2000).

55.   Nature, 789 (2003).

56. J. W. Watters and H. L. McLeod, Trends Pharmacol. Sci., 55 (2003).
57. R. R. Recker and H. W. Deng, Endocrine., 55 (2002).
58. C. J. Rosen, W. G. Beamer and L. R. Donahue, Osteoporos. Int., 803 (2001).
59. M. A. Lindsay, Nat. Rev. Drug Discov., 831 (2003).
60. D. F. Horrobin, Nat. Rev. Drug Discov., 151 (2003).
61. P. D. Shilling and J. R. Kelsoe, Pharmacogenomics., 31 (2002).
62. W. E. Evans and M. V. Relling, Science, 487 (1999).
63. E. E. Schadt, S. A. Monks and S. H. Friend, Biochem. Soc. Trans., 437 (2003).
64. V. Dvornyk, R. R. Recker and H. W. Deng, Osteoporos. Int, 451 (2003).
65. T. E. Klein and R. B. Altman, Pharmacogenomics. J., 1 (2004).
66. A. E. Ferentz, Pharmacogenomics., 453 (2002).
67. G. A. Rodan and T. J. Martin, Science, 1508 (2000).

CHAPTER 17

STUDYING OSTEOPOROSIS AT THE WHOLE-GENOME LEVEL: PROBLEMS AND PROSPECTS

Volodymyr Dvornyk[1], Peng Xiao[1], Yong-Jun Liu[1], Hui Shen[1],
Hong-Wen Deng[1,2,3]

[1]Osteoporosis Research Center and
[2]Department of Biomedical Sciences,
Creighton University, Omaha, NE 68131, USA

[3]Laboratory of Molecular and Statistical Genetics, College of Life Sciences,
Hunan Normal University, ChangSha, Hunan 410081, P. R. China

1. Introduction

Osteoporosis is one of the greatest challenges in the modern medicine and genetics. This is not only because of its large prevalence in human populations and constantly increasing costs for treatment, but also due to the complex mode of its determination. During the last few decades, immense efforts have been made to unravel the etiology of this disorder in order to find a cure. It was found that onset and development of this highly heritable disease are determined by many genetic and environmental factors.[1-4] The extensive studies in the bone field have produced large amount of valuable data, but further progress has been hampered by the inherent limitations of the conventional methods commonly used in this research. A complex and polygenic basis of osteoporosis called for methods and techniques able to utilize a whole-genome approach to study molecular and genetic mechanisms of the disorder.

2. Whole-Genome Linkage and Association Studies

2.1. *Whole-Genome Linkage Scan*

The whole-genome linkage scan (WGS) has now become one of the major tools to decipher genetic basis of complex traits. In the genome scan, linkage analysis is carried out using panels of microsatellite markers, spaced uniformly throughout the entire human genome to identify quantitative trait loci (QTLs) underlying the studied phenotypes. In contrast to candidate gene association studies, the genome-wide linkage scan does not rely on the linkage disequilibrium (LD) among genes or markers in adjacent genomic regions. It can be used to search for any genomic region contributing relatively large variation in complex traits without any prior knowledge about the potential importance of specific genes or genomic regions. Thus, this approach offers the potential of identifying genes previously unsuspected of having an effect on the phenotype of interest.

A number of WGS studies have been conducted to search for genes underlying osteoporosis.[5] Most studies focused on bone mineral density (BMD), a strong and well-established risk factor for osteoporotic fracture. Some other intermediate phenotypes, such as bone size, serum osteocalcin concentration, and quantitative ultrasound of the calcaneus bone, have also been employed in a few WGS studies. Within the past decade, at least eleven WGS for population normal BMD variation have been published (including conference abstracts), with the major findings summarized in Table 1.

The first WGS for BMD was performed in 149 individuals from seven pedigrees (74 sib pairs) having low BMD.[6] A WGS for 218 individuals from 96 Chinese nuclear families (153 sib pairs) revealed several regions for wrist BMD.[7] A study in a total of 595 healthy premenopausal sister pairs suggested linkage for peak BMD at the spine and hip.[8] A WGS study in 53 extended pedigrees (1,249 sib pairs) and identified several QTLs for BMD at the hip, spine, and wrist.[9] The Framingham Study of 33 pedigrees with 1,164 subjects (691 sib pairs) suggested the importance of 6p21 and 21qter for BMD.[10] A WGS in

1,094 nonidentical twins and 444 concordant and discordant sib pairs reported linkage of BMD to 3p21 and 1p36.[11] A recent study using 664 subjects from 29 Mexican-American families, linkage was detected at 4p for forearm BMD.[12] Most recently, a WGS in 207 osteoporotic families in Iceland, using phenotypes that combine osteoporotic fractures and BMD, showed linkage to 20p12.3.[13] Their subsequent fine mapping and positional cloning efforts revealed BMP2 as a gene contributing to BMD variation and osteoporotic fractures.[13]

Putative genomic regions have been identified on every human chromosome except Y, as we summarized elsewhere.[5] Several genomic regions have been replicated by at least two studies and may deserve intensive follow-up analyses. Chromosome 11q12-13 is of particular interest due to the fact that variation in bone density in the general population was linked to the chromosome region containing the LRP5 gene,[8,14] chromosome 1p36,[6,7,11,15,16] harbors a strong candidate gene, TNFR2 mapped to this region. Other promising regions include chromosomes 2p23-p24,[6,7] 4q25-q32,[9,17] 6p21,[8,10,18] 12q13,[9,17] and 12q23-24.[9,10,19] However, except a few limited replications, the significant genomic regions are largely different across various studies. Lack of replication for linkage findings reflects the complexity of genetic inheritance of osteoporosis. Other possible reasons may lie in the diversity of study designs, sample sizes, ascertainment schemes, and statistical analyses employed. From the statistical genetics standpoint, insufficient power in linkage analysis is conceivably one of the major factors contributing to the inconsistent results. It is likely that the robust and powerful linkage testing requires sample sizes far larger than most of those currently employed in the linkage studies in the field of bone genetics.

2.2. Fine Mapping

Genome-wide linkage scans have suggested several genomic regions, which may harbor genes underlying BMD variation as well as other bone related phenotypes. Through extension and replication studies based on these initial results, confirmed evidence for linkage may be found at one or more regions. However, the regions normally are very large, encompassing ~30 cM and containing more than 20 megabases of DNA sequences,[20] which is not feasible for physical mapping. Therefore, "fine mapping" those regions to a small interval (~1 cM) is an essential step to identify the causal gene(s). It has been shown that linkage studies with saturation markers of a candidate region contribute very little to this effort.[21,22] Empirical data suggested that, in linkage-based experiments, increasing map density up to the 2.5-5 cM level efficiently extracts valuable additional information; beyond this level, little benefit could be gained from typing additional markers due to an accumulation of the confounding effects of mapping and genotyping errors.[21] A simulation study performed by Atwood and Heard-Costa[22] also indicated that a linkage study with dense markers could be useful in narrowing the region to 1-2 cM only when the QTL accounts for nearly all the variation in the trait. If the QTL accounts for a small proportion of the total variation, as in complex traits, this method may have a limited value.

An alternative approach for further narrowing those candidate regions is regional LD mapping. There are two commonly used regional LD mapping strategies: a positional candidate approach, in which specific genes or variants are examined on the basis of proposed relationships with the phenotype; and a positional cloning approach, in which markers are selected for evaluation purely on the basis of their proximity to one another in a chromosome region.[23] By examining allelic variations across a region of known linkage, it should be possible to see variations in the strength of associations between these markers and the phenotype, enabling the trait-associated locus and causative mutation to be mapped.[23] Both case-control strategy and transmission disequilibrium test can be applied under these conditions. In some circumstances, additional information could be obtained by examining the degree of deviation from Hardy-Weinberg equilibrium at a series of closely linked marker loci.[24] Although such strategies were successful in identifying genes involved in monogenic gene disorders, such as cystic fibrosis and Huntington disease,[25,26] this has proved to be more difficult to achieve in complex traits and has relied on the characterization of large numbers of polymorphisms within a region.[27,28]

Due to higher abundance, lower mutation rate, and the accessibility of automated high-throughput genotyping, single nucleotide polymorphism

(SNP) markers are preferred over microsatellite markers for LD mapping.[29] Compared to usage of individual SNP markers, greater power can be achieved by using haplotype analysis.[23] One of the major limitations of LD mapping is poor understanding of the patterns of LD throughout human genome. It has been widely assumed that LD declines as markers become more distant from disease polymorphisms. However, recent studies of LD at various locations of the human genome have suggested that this belief is a significant oversimplification of the real situation.[30-33] Consistent with the complex evolutionary history of any set of haplotypes, there is marked genomic variability in LD across the genome. The genome has been portrayed as a series of high LD regions separated by short discrete segments of very low LD.[34] Those high LD regions also exhibit limited haplotype diversity, so that a small number of distinct haplotypes account for most of the chromosomes in the population, and they are now termed as "haplotype blocks".[32,35,36] Experimental data have shown that haplotype blocks could range from a few kb to more than 100 kb.[32,35] Within haplotype blocks, allelic dependence yields redundancy among markers and improves the chances of detecting association when only a fraction of the markers is tested.[34] By contrast, in low LD regions, low correlation between markers means these regions can only be characterized adequately by typing many, or even all, markers. A recent empirical study suggested that the number and diversity of haplotypes varied greatly from gene to gene, making generalities about haplotypes across candidate genes in the human genome difficult to identify. In addition, the complete resolution of common haplotypes and block structure was dependent on SNP density, with complete SNP discovery leading to different inferences of haplotype structure than incomplete SNP discovery.[37]

The long range LD may be useful for initial whole genome association scans (see below), but is potentially a problem for high-resolution fine mapping, because strong associations might be observed far from the causative site, and these could lead to effort being spent on the wrong location. This issue has been reflected by a fine mapping study on Crohn's disease,[27] in which a 250 kb region shows strong association with the disease and the strong LD across the region results in multiple SNPs having equivalent genetic information. Consequently, genetic evidence alone is not sufficient to identify the causal mutation within this region.

A successful example using LD mapping to refine genomic regions is seen in a recent study,[13] in which the BMP2 was identified as a gene contributing to BMD variation and osteoporotic fractures. LD mapping has also been successfully applied to refine genomic regions underlying several other complex diseases.[27,38,39] It is worthwhile to remember that, whatever genomic evidence has been shown, definitive biological evidence of a role for a mutation or polymorphism will require functional studies.

2.3. *Whole-Genome Association Mapping*

With recent progress on SNP identification and high throughput genotyping technology, the whole genome association mapping now seems applicable and has attracted recent interest. Genome-wide association mapping in a case-control or family-based study using haplotypes generated from SNPs may be much more powerful than linkage analysis and also yield a finer map resolution.[40-42]

However, the practical aspects of whole genome association mapping are currently daunting. The major obstruct is how to choose the marker density and select the appropriate SNPs. This issue largely depends on the patterns of LD across the human genome. LD varies not only across different genomic regions, but also in different ethnic groups.[30,36,43] For example, LD extended for about 60 kb in the US population of North-European descent; in contrast, the same loci showed much shorter regions of LD in a Nigerian population.[30] Therefore, in order to decide the marker density and to select the appropriate SNPs for a genome-wide association study, LD patterns must be detailed in specific ethnic populations. Suitable markers are identified in different populations through international collaborative efforts such as the SNP Consortium (http://snp.cshl.org/) and the Haplotype Mapping project ("HapMap", http://hapmap.cshl.org/) – a genome-wide catalogue of common haplotype blocks in multiple human populations.[44] However, recent studies suggest that because haplotype blocks can arise from several causes, simply identifying them does not ensure either their conservation within or between populations or their utility for mapping genes associated with a disease.[45] Another potential problem for whole genome association study is multiple testing. Because massive statistical tests will be performed for very large numbers of markers on many subjects, the expected frequency of false positive results will be very high. The most appropriate mechanism for preventing this problem has been a matter of debate.[46,47] Unfortunately, unlike linkage tests in which the LOD score threshold (LOD$\geq$3.3) has been widely accepted,[48] there is no international consensus for the interpretation of genetic association studies. Risch and Merikangas[40] suggested that under some simplifying assumptions, a significance threshold of $p = 5 \times 10^{-8}$ would produce a genome-wide false-positive rate of 5%. However, this guideline was based on a Bonferroni correction which, given the correlations between adjacent SNPs, is too conservative and may lead to decreased statistical power. Developing a widely accepted method with realistic calculations of false-positive rates for highly correlated genomic data is vital for the success of genome-wide association studies.[23]

It is also worth to briefly note that the use of LD for mapping relies on the assumption that common genetic variants are responsible for susceptibility to common diseases, and this assumption is still being debated.[49,50]

3. High-Throughput Methods for Analysis of Differential Gene Expression

Although the methods for genome-wide linkage and association studies give valuable data about genes, which may contribute to a trait, they provide no information about how the genes contribute to the trait. Such information may be of particular importance for the development of efficient therapy for these disorders. Methods for the study of gene expression are complementary to the methods of linkage and association mapping. They are efficient in unraveling molecular and genetic mechanisms of disease onset and development and give important information about the regulation of gene function under various conditions.

3.1. *Limitations of the Traditional Gene Expression Studies of Osteoporosis*

Conventional gene expression studies (Northern and Southern blots) have substantially contributed to unraveling possible mechanisms of the onset and development of osteoporosis. Using these methods, a large number of candidate genes have been determined to contribute to the disease (see ref. 51 for review).

However, these methods have significant inherent limitations. The main drawback is that by using these methods only a relatively small number of genes can be surveyed at a time. Hence, while these methods may provide information about gene expression of already known genes, they have a limited power to discover the large number of genes potentially contributing to the trait. Given that there are at least about 200 genes known to be related to bone metabolism[52] and probably more yet unknown genes, this limitation of the traditional methods seems to be severe. Furthermore, the development of bone disorders is a multistage process, and each stage in the various cell types involved is probably regulated differently and by a different set of genes and factors.

Another major limitation is that the conventional methods of studying gene expression demand a relatively large amount of RNA. This amount increases proportionally to the number of the studied genes. Although this issue is perhaps not so important for the cell culture research, it becomes critical when human fresh tissues, e.g., bone biopsies, are studied due to their usually small amount, limited availability, and high cost. All of the above limiting factors make the traditional methods hardly appropriate for studying gene expression at the whole-genome level.

Attempts to overcome these limitations and to approach studying gene expression at the whole-genome scale resulted in the development of more powerful, high-throughput methods for the analysis of differential gene expression. At present, there are five commonly used high-throughput differential gene expression methods: expressed sequence tag (EST) sequencing, subtractive cloning, differential display, serial analysis of gene expression (SAGE), and cDNA microarray hybridization. Below we provide a brief overview of these methods with particular reference to their advantages and drawbacks, which are summarized in Table 2.

3.2. *EST Sequencing*

This method was firstly proposed in 1991.[53] It is based on creating cDNA libraries from the tissues of interest, random sampling clones from these libraries, followed by a single sequencing reaction from a large number of clones. Although the method is technically simple, it requires relatively large amounts of polyA+ RNA for the cDNA library construction (up to 5.0 µg), and is laborious due to extensive cloning and high sequencing requirements in order to generate a statistically sufficient amount of data. For example, to compare gene expression profiles during differentiation of rat osteoblasts, in total 9,281 ESTs were sequenced from the day-8 and day-17 cell cultures.[54]

EST sequencing was used to obtain a gene expression profile of human bone marrow stromal cells.[55] In this study, sequencing data analysis of 4,258 ESTs showed 60 novel genes in the human bone marrow stromal cells cDNA library, which were not found in nonredundant human mRNA and protein databases. The high-throughput EST sequencing was one of the key methods used to compile a Skeletal Gene Database.[52,56]

3.3. *Subtractive Cloning*

Subtractive cloning has been extensively used since the 1980's (e.g., ref. [57,58]). Later it was modified to employ reverse transcription and PCR techniques (reverse transcription representational difference analysis, RT-RDA).[59] In this method, RNA is isolated from two tissues or cells of interest and double-stranded cDNA is synthesized and amplified by PCR. The cDNA from the experimental tissue is then referred to as a "tester", and cDNA from the control tissue is designated as a "driver". The latter is then used to subtract shared transcripts. After first-round amplification, the tester is hybridized to an excess of driver DNA, and sequences that are distinctive to the tester are amplified by PCR.

Subtractive cloning has been successfully used for studying various aspects of bone development and metabolism, including discovery of novel genes involved in these processes.[60-65]

Although being a relatively inexpensive and flexible technique, subtractive cloning suffers from important limitations. First, it lacks sensitivity, i.e., is unable to determine small differences in gene expression levels. Second, it allows only direct comparison and only two samples at a time. Third, the method involves a series of various biochemical and molecular biology procedures that makes it laborious.

3.4. *Differential Display*

This PCR-based technique was introduced in 1992 and is also known as RNA fingerprinting.[66,67] It is somewhat similar to the randomly amplified polymorphic DNA technique (RAPD). The difference is that, in differential display, arbitrary primers are used in conjunction with a reverse transcription primer to amplify cDNA from previously isolated RNA. The obtained cDNA fragments are then separated and visualized on a polyacrylamide gel. Bands, which are differentially visualized in the compared samples, are then isolated, cloned and sequenced, and obtained sequences are compared against databases to identify respective genes. Likewise, DNA fingerprinting and RAPD, throughput and resolution of this method can be significantly increased by using fluorescent labeled primers and automated sequencers.

Major advantages of differential display are its simplicity as compared to the other high-throughput differential gene expression methods and the requirement of minute amounts (5-10 ng) of RNA. It also enables investigators to analyze many samples simultaneously. It is particularly suitable for the analysis of small samples, such as bone biopsies, minor populations of cells, etc. RNA differential display has been widely used to study various aspects of osteogenesis and bone disorders (e.g., ref. [68-75]).

However, the mRNA differential display has a number of important limitations. A principal one is that aberrant priming at both the 5' and 3' ends results in competition in the PCR, precluding detection of messages other than those which are abundantly expressed.[76] It leads to generating false-positive results, especially when small amounts of RNA are analyzed.[77] Other limitations include: 1) generally low reproducibility; 2) under-representation and redundancy of mRNA signals;[78] 3) frequent priming by the G/C rich 5' primer at both ends;[79,80] and 4) a bias for high copy number mRNAs.[78,81]

3.5. *Serial Analysis of Gene Expression (SAGE)*

SAGE is another DNA sequence-based method. It is essentially an enhanced version of EST sequencing.[82] Double stranded cDNA prepared from the tissue(s) of interest is cleaved with a restriction endonuclease (anchoring enzyme) which is predicted to cut every transcript at least once. The 3' ends of the resulting cDNA fragments are then purified using streptavidin-coated magnetic beads and divided into two populations, each of which is ligated to a different linker containing a type IIS restriction endonuclease (tagging enzyme) recognition sequence. Such enzymes cleave DNA at a distance of up to 20 bp away from their recognition site. Digestion of the two cDNA populations thus results in the generation of a short sequence consisting of the linker and a short portion of its adjacent cDNA. Following the creation of blunt ends, the two populations are ligated to each other and total cDNA is amplified by PCR, resulting in the generation of products with two tags (a ditag) orientated tail to tail with an anchoring enzyme recognition site at either end. Following cleavage at each anchoring enzyme recognition sequence and concatenation of ditags via this site, products are cloned and individual clones consisting of at least 25 tags (25-75) are selected for sequencing.

SAGE has recently been used to characterize the coordinate regulation of gene expression during osteoblast differentiation and maturation of murine osteoblast-like MC3T3-E1 cells,[83,84] to study the patterns of gene expression associated with osteoblast and adipocyte differentiation of murine mesenchymal progenitor cell 3T3-F442A induced by bone morphogenetic protein-2,[85] and to characterize the involvement of Ets transcription factors in osteoblast differentiation and matrix mineralization.[86] The results obtained from these studies demonstrate the ability of SAGE to not only identify large numbers of transcripts at once, but also to quantify their presence. However, generating good SAGE libraries is a technical challenge. This process involves a number of biochemical procedures; any inconsistency or incompleteness of the reactions eventually affects the quality of the sequence tags and results in misleading artifacts and false data.

3.6. cDNA Microarrays

The microarrays are the most recently developed technique for high throughput analysis of differential gene expression. It provides a means to overcome many of the above limitations and to identify bone-associated genes, which may contribute to BMD variation and osteoporosis.

Briefly, microarrays represent a miniaturized Northern blot procedure, in which cDNA or oligonucleotide probes are spotted or directly synthesized on a synthetic base (glass slide or plastic membrane). Total or messenger RNA of interest is reverse transcribed and labeled with radioactive, fluorescent or other markers. The obtained cDNA or cRNA is then hybridized to the microarray. After the hybridization, the data are acquired with an image reader or laser scanner and analyzed with respective applied software. The different microarray technology platforms, their merits and shortcomings are comprehensively described in a number of reviews (e.g., [87-89]).

Microarrays allow simultaneous monitoring of gene expression for tens of thousands of genes. Microarrays are, therefore, useful when one wants to survey a large number of genes quickly or when the sample available for studying is small.

In the field of bone-related disorders, microarrays have been used since 1997, when Heller and co-workers[90] applied this technique to discover genes involved in rheumatoid arthritis. Since then, microarrays have been applied to study various aspects of osteogenesis as well as gene expression profiles in osteoporotic tissues.

Using the microarray approach, researchers have performed extensive studies on the orchestrated gene expression during the process of osteoblast differentiation.[91-98] These studies have provided novel insights into the mechanisms of bone formation and mineralization. The microarray technique has proved to be powerful in finding genes of interest. For example, using this approach, researchers have successfully identified genes relevant to osteogenesis, among other genes related to myoblastic and adipocytic pathways.[99]

3.7. *What to Use: Cell Cultures or Fresh Tissue Samples?*

Until now, most of the high-throughput gene expression studies of bone-related diseases have been performed on cultured cell lines of humans and model organisms, such as rats and mice. Using cell cultures has certain advantages, such as virtually no limit for tissue supply, high purity and homogeneity of desired cell populations, possibility to easily modify experimental conditions, etc. On the other hand, it brings up a potential problem that may introduce a significant bias into the results obtained. Serial passage was shown to have an effect on the expression level of 27 out of the 2,000 selected genes in MC3T3-E1 preosteoblastic cells.[100] Even primary cultures of stromal cells from human bone marrow gradually lose their osteogenic potential[101,102] that may suggest changes in gene expression profiles. Furthermore, cultured cells lack relationships with other tissues. In terms of studying such a complex disorder as osteoporosis, it is a significant shortcoming, because it eliminates the influence of many genes and/or other local or systemic factors (e.g., hormones, inflammatory cytokines, etc.), which are not expressed in the analyzed tissues, but influence their development. These multiple factors may interact in vivo thereby changing a magnitude of their effect. Such conditions may hardly be reproduced in vitro and therefore may result in a significant bias of gene expression profiles of cultured cells as compared to freshly isolated ones. For example, it was shown that expression profiles of in vitro replicative senescence model of human fibroblasts and the cells isolated from an elderly donor are different.[103] Given that, studying fresh tissue samples may be a promising approach to obtain closer to reality data on expression profiles for genes that are tissue specific and differentially expressed locally.

On the other hand, using freshly isolated cells is challenging due to the morphological and physiological properties of tissues. For example, bone marrow is very heterogeneous in terms of cell composition, and consists of many cell types, which are able to differentiate into various cell lineages. Some cell types of interest, such as bone marrow mesenchymal stem cells, which are osteoblast precursors, or various subsets of other cells involved in bone remodeling (e.g., monocytes, B and T cells) comprise only a minor portion of the whole bone marrow cell population. It makes difficult to isolate sufficiently large number of intact cells and to obtain homogeneous cell sample. Accordingly, the yield of RNA for the analysis is low. However, continuous advances in the methods of immunomagnetic cell isolation and linear RNA amplification[104] provide solutions for these problems.

Another concern is inter-individual variations in the data due to differences in age, sex, physiological status, and other characteristics of subjects. It may be largely reduced by close matching subjects by phenotype. One more way is pre-profile mixing of patient cRNA samples.[105] Appropriate RNA pooling can provide equivalent power and improve efficiency and cost-effectiveness for microarray experiments with a modest increase in total number of subjects.[106,107] However, this pooling should be done with caution, because it can suggest differences between populations where there are none (i.e. when one individual's mRNA level is sufficiently different to affect the average represented by the pool). This problem can be compounded further when relatively few individuals are used in the construction of mRNA pools[108] and when many small changes are taken into consideration, as was the case in the study by Kyng *et al.* who used a cut-off value of 1.5-fold change.[109]

In terms of limited availability of fresh bone biopsies, some of the reviewed high-throughput methods of differential gene expression become hardly applicable, because they demand relatively large amounts of RNA.

All above considerations are equally applicable to the methods of proteomic analysis reviewed further in this chapter.

3.8. *The High-Throughput Methods of Differential Gene Expression Analysis in Study of Osteoporosis: the Prospects*

The methods of high-throughput analysis of differential gene expression have a relatively short history of their application to the field of bone biology and metabolism, and more significant results from their use for study of osteoporosis are yet to come. These methods seem to be a powerful tool in designing effective new drugs, as they may provide important information about regulation of multiple gene expression in various tissues by therapeutic agents. Since blood often mediates between drugs and target tissues, studying gene expression profiles in peripheral blood cells may give important insights into the mechanisms of drug effect. For example, specific "gene signatures" can predict therapeutic outcome of chemoagents.[110,111] A number of studies suggest that monocytes of peripheral blood may be a potential target for drugs,[112-114] and microarray gene expression profiles of these cells may provide important information about the efficiency of drug administration or/and other therapeutic means.[115]

The high-throughput gene expression methods are a powerful tool for research in pharmacogenomics and discovering genes which represent new targets for drug development.[51,54] The potential implication of genomics and pharmacogenomics in clinical research and clinical medicine is that disease could be treated according to genetic and specific individual markers, selecting medications and dosages that are optimized for individual patients.

Another application of the high-throughput gene expression methods in the field of bone biology is testing various hypotheses about an effect of various environmental, lifestyle or inherent regulating factors on the BMD variation, risk of osteoporotic fractures, onset and development of osteoporosis. For example, smoking is suggested as one of the major lifestyle factors increasing bone resorption and a risk of osteoporotic fractures.[116,117] However, molecular mechanisms of this effect are largely unknown. Are they similar to the modulation of bone resorption by cytokines or other inborn factors? What constituents of tobacco smoke are the primary stimulators? How do they interact with genes involved in bone metabolism? These are only a few of the many problems in bone biology, which can be solved with the aid of the high-throughput methods of gene expression profiling. Recent advances in functional genomics and the development of the computer methods make it possible to analyze the gene expression changes in the context of known biological pathways.[118-120]

Modern technologies in cell and molecular biology make it possible to obtain a genome-wide expression profile of a single cell.[121] Single-cell gene expression analysis is currently used to generate data within the fundamental unit, the single cell, thereby avoiding assumptions or questions about cell population homogeneity, whether cell-type or temporal. The data obtained with this approach suggest that even morphologically identical cells may have quite distinct transcriptomes, which gives deeper insights into cell differentiation and functional assignment.[122,123] Given that the processes of osteogenesis and bone metabolism are multistage and involve many cell types (osteogenic precursors, various bone cellular components, T and B cells, etc.), including those, which are able to transdifferentiate (e.g., bone marrow mesenchymal stem cells, hemopoietic stem cells), this approach is very promising for fine characterization of the distinct bone related cell types. Single-cell expression profiling also offers a highly parallel view of the workings of a gene regulatory network at one specific point in time, and will hopefully provide insights that could lead to an improved ability to interpret gene expression patterns.

Another promising methodology for identification of genes and their mechanisms is a combined approach of genetic epidemiology (for gene mapping) and microarray studies in humans. Recent identification of the lipoxygenase gene Alox15 as a regulator of BMD in mice[124] may serve as a nice example of a high potential of this approach in osteoporosis studies.

4. Proteomics

Although DNA microarray technology has been widely applied to gene expression assay of diverse complex disease at mRNA level, including complex bone disorders, it has an important limitation in terms that many studies have indicated a poor correlation between mRNA and protein expression level.[125-128] Undergoing alternative mRNA splicing and complicated posttranslational modification, mature translational protein products are definitely different from mRNA expression. Presumably, this is the major reason of the little mutual confirmation between results of DNA microarray technology and proteomics assay. Since it was firstly defined,[129,130] proteomics, a variety of approaches unveiling the large-scale gene expression and functions at the protein level, has burgeoned in the biological research at the systemic level. Proteome indicates all the proteins and protein complexes of a cell line, tissue or organism at a specific time and environment.[131] Proteomics analyzes the characteristics of proteins at the proteome level. In the post-genome era, proteins and important metabolites becomes the focus of research.[132] Proteomics clearly is an important component for functional genomics research.

There are three major types of proteomics: protein expression proteomics, structural proteomics, and functional proteomics.[133] Different but pertinent experimental methods are bestowed on each one.

For protein expression proteomics, which focuses on the quantitative comparison of protein expression between samples of different variables, such as case and control, two-dimensional polyacrylamide gel electrophoresis (2-DE)[134] is the prevailing method for protein separation. Considering the deficiencies, less sensitivity and only one gel for one sample, in 2-DE, two improved 2-DE technologies have been invented recently, which are immobilized pH gradients 2-DE[135] and differential in-gel electrophoresis (DIGE),[136] respectively. In DIGE, particularly, two protein samples are tagged with two different fluorescent dyes and run on the same environment, which reduces the discords caused by different gels. Some alternative approaches without electrophoresis, such as liquid chromatography (LC),[137-139] capillary electrophoresis,[140,141] also have been developed because of time-consuming and nonautomatic limitations of 2-DE. Among those approaches, isotope-coded affinity tags (ICAT)[142] is one of the most promising alternatives to electrophoresis. Further structural information of different expressed proteins will be acquired to identify those proteins. Obviously, there is no better way to substitute mass spectrometry (MS)–based techniques at present. Electrospray ionization (ESI) and matrix-assisted laser desorption/ionization (MALDI) are the two techniques most commonly used to volatize and ionize the proteins or peptides for mass spectrometric analysis.[143,144] Tandem mass spectra (MS/MS) sequences the given peptide ion by using inert energetic gas to randomly collide with it and then get the tandem spectrum to induce the sequence. To specifically identify proteins, the trend towards the combination of liquid chromatography with ESI- or

MALDI-MS/MS will continue.[145] Antibody arrays also have been newly developed in protein expression profiling.[146] The basic principle is similar to DNA microarray. But antibodies, instead of cDNAs or oligonucleotides, are arrayed on a solid support for antibody microarray.

Structural proteomics aims at mapping out the structure of protein complexes or the proteins in a specific cellular organelle.[147] X-ray crystallography, nuclear magnetic resonance (NMR) spectroscopy and electron crystallography are the three predominant techniques in protein structural analysis [148]. Using these techniques, structural data of ribosomal subunits,[149-151] complete ribosome and its functional complexes[152] as well as the actin networks of *Dictyostelium* cells,[153] have been unraveled.

Biological functions are mainly carried out by the interaction between proteins. Another important goal for proteomics is system-wide understanding of protein-protein interactions. Clarifying the protein-protein interactions and posttranslational modifications, functional proteomics most likely will reach the goal. Currently, there are two genetic ways of identifying protein interactions, glutathione *S*-transferase (GST)-fusion technique[154] and yeast two-hybrid system.[155] Particularly, the yeast two-hybrid method is one of the best-established *in vivo* approaches to map protein-protein interactions.[156] In this method, proteins of interest are fused to a DNA-binding domain as baits. Other proteins are fused to a transcription-activating domain as preys. Baits screen preys via activating the reporter gene when there are interactions between them. Protein microarray is another encouraging technology providing a well-controlled, *in vitro* way to study function on a system-wide or genome-wide basis.[157] Not only proteins, but also DNA, ligands and drugs can be arrayed on a solid support to test protein-protein, protein-ligand as well as protein-drug interactions. Protein microarrays have been successfully utilized n studies of yeast protein kinases [158] and yeast calmodulin- and phospholipid-interacting proteins.[159] The advantages and disadvantages of various methods in proteomics are summarized in Table 3.

Proteomics is a promising and rapidly developing approach and somewhat exploited in complex trait diseases, such as cardiovascular disease,[160,161] kidney disease[162] and cancer.[163,164] Reports on proteomics studies of complex bone disorders are relatively scarce. 2-DE combined with MALDI-TOF (time of flight)-MS approach was used to study synovial fluids and plasmas from patients suffering from rheumatoid arthritis, reactive arthritis and osteoarthritis, and several proteins have been found expressed differently.[165] In a study on the metastasized prostate cancer cells causing a predominantly osteosclerotic response, applying the same method, galectin-1 modulated osteoblastic proliferation and differentiation.[166] A proteomics-based analysis of *Bmp1*[-/-] *Tll1*[-/-] doubly null mouse embryo fibroblasts identified type XI collagen as a novel substrate for mammalian bone morphogenetic protein 1-like proteases.[167] These examples showed that proteomics may be successfully applied to both hypothesis-free and hypothesis-driven studies of complex bone disorders. In the first example,[165] the research compared the protein expressing profiles among different disease samples without any assumption on the biochemical pathway. In the second and third examples,[166,167] however, specific hypotheses had been made before the studies, research just limited on the presumed proteins or protein group and the proteomics approach was used to prove those hypotheses. Employing proteomics approach on cultured cells, pioneering studies identified some novel proteins important for the development of bone marrow hematopoietic cells,[168] mesenchymal chondroblasts,[169] and osteoclasts.[170] These studies provide novel insights into the mechanisms of bone formation and mineralization. The proteomics technology has been proven powerful in finding proteins (and thus the genes involved) of interest. Proteomics approach is efficient for analyzing complex and chronic bone diseases. Further study can be done on different expressed proteins in complex bone disorders. Combined with structural and functional proteomics, the specific effects and positions of those proteins in the pathway leading to the disorders will be identified. On the other hand, altered expressed proteins in complex bone disorders may also contribute to potential targets for drugs. Recently, a proteomics approach has been incorporated into seeking inhibitors of osteoclast-mediated bone resorption and is currently screening for bone anabolic agents.[171]

Table 1. Evidence for the presence of linkage with osteoporosis-related phenotypes

Location	Markers	Candidate Genes	Phenotypes	*P* or LOD (Z) value	Reference
1p36	D1S450	TNFRSF1B; PLOD	Hip BMD	LOD=2.29	[6]
	D1S214	MTHFR	Femoral neck BMD	LOD=3.53	[16]
	D1S468		Quantitative ultrasound	LOD=2.74	[15]
			Whole-body BMD	LOD=2.4	[11]
1q21-23	D1S484	BGP; IL-6R	Spine BMD	LOD=3.11	[8]
2p25			Spine bone size	LOD=1.54	[172]
2p23-24	D2S149		Hip BMD	LOD=2.25	[6]
2p21-24	D2S2976-D2S405	CALM2; STK; POMC	Proximal forearm BMD	LOD=2.15	[7]
			Distal forarm BMD	LOD=2.14	
2p21	D2S305	COL6A3	Spine bone size	LOD=2.15	[172]
2q23	D2S160	IL-1α	Femoral neck BMD	LOD=1.4	[17]
2q37	D2S125		Wrist bone size	LOD=2.28	[172]
3p21	D3S1289-D3S3559	PTHR1	Femoral neck BMD	LOD=2.7~3.5	[17]
			Spine BMD	LOD=2.1~2.7	[11]
3p26	D3S1297		Wrist BMD	LOD=1.82	[9]
3q12-26	D3S1271-D3S1614	COL8A1; PLOD2	Pelvis axis width	LOD=3.1	[173]
			Midfemur width	LOD=2.8	
			Femur head width	LOD=2.8	
			Femur head width	LOD=5.0	[174]
			Femur shift width	LOD=3.6	

4p16	D4S412	FGFR3	Wrist bone size	LOD=2.00	[172]
			Hip BMD	LOD=2.2	
4p15	D4S2639	BMP-3	Radius midpoint BMD	LOD=4.05	[175]
4q11	D4S428		Femur neck axis length	LOD=3.9	[173]
			Midfemur width	LOD=3.5	
4q26	D4S429	EGF	Femoral neck BMD	LOD=1.8	[17]
4q31			Spine BMD	LOD=3.08	[9]
4q32	D4S413		Wrist BMD	LOD=2.26	[9]
4q34	D4S1539		Hip BMD	LOD=2.95	[6]
5p15.2	D5S817		Quantitative ultrasound	LOD=2.69	[15]
5p14	D5S2845		Trochanter BMD	LOD=1.75	[10]
5q12	D5S647-D5S644	CRTL1	Femur neck axis length	LOD=4.3	[173]
5q23	D5S2017	IL-4	Femora neck BMD	LOD=1.2	[17]
5q33-35	D5S422	ON; PDGFRB	Femoral neck BMD	LOD=1.87	[8]
6p21	D6S2427	TNF-α	Femoral neck BMD	LOD=2.93	[10]
			Lumbar spine BMD	LOD=1.88	
			Osteoporosis and osteopenia defined by radial bone BMD	P=0.001	[18]
6p11-12	D6S462	BMP-6	Spine BMD	LOD=1.94	[8]
6q25	D6S1577	ER-α	Lumbar spine BMD	LOD=1.4	[17]
7p22	D7S531		Spine BMD	LOD=1.93	[9]
7p21	D7S503	IL-6	Lumbar spine BMD	LOD=1.2	[17]
7q32	D7S1805		Femoral head width	LOD=5.0	[174]

8q21	D8S2324		Femoral head width	LOD=6.0	[174]
8q24.3	D8S373	TNFRSF11B	Ward's BMD	LOD=2.13	[10]
9p24			Wrist BMD	LOD=1.87	[9]
9q11-12			Wrist bone size	LOD=2.23	[172]
9q21	D9S175	COL15A1	Wrist bone size	LOD=1.56	[172]
10q26	D10S1651	FGFR2	Hip BMD	LOD=2.29	[9]
11p15	D11S4046	IGF-2	Spine bone size	LOD=2.78	[172]
11q12-13	D11S987	LRP5	Spine BMD	LOD=5.74	[176]
	D11S1313		Spine BMD	LOD=1.97	[8]
11q24	CD3D		Spine BMD	LOD=2.08	[6]
12q13	D12S83	VDR; COLA2A1	Lumbar spine BMD	LOD=1.7	[17]
	D12S368		HipBMD	Lob=1.69	[9]
12q23			Lumbar spine BMD	LOD=2.08	[10]
12q24.2	D12S1723	IGF1	Lumbar spine BMD	LOD=2.08	[9]
13q21	D13S800		Hip BMD	LOD=3.1	[175]
13q34		COL4A1; COL4A2	Distal forearm BMD	LOD=1.67	[7]
	D13S285		Spine BMD	LOD=1.77	[9]
14q11			Hip bone size	LOD=1.65	[172]
14q21.3	D14S587	BMP-4	Lumbar spine BMD	LOD=1.92	[10]
14q31-32			Trochanter BMD	LOD=1.99	[8]
15p11	D15S165		Spine BMD	LOD=1.6	[9]
16q11.1-13	D16S753-D16S771		Serum osteocalcin level	LOD=3.35	[177]
17p13	D17S1852		Wrist BMD	LOD=1.99	[9]
17p11	D17S1857		Hip BMD	LOD=1.58	[9]
17q21	D17S791	COL1A1; CHAD; HOX	Femur head width	LOD=3.6	[173]

17q23	D17S787	TBX2	Wrist bone size	LOD=3.98	[172]
	D17S807		Femoral neck BMD	LOD=1.7	[17]
19p13	D19S226	COMP; PRTN3	Femur neck axis length	LOD=2.8	[173]
			Femur head width	LOD=2.8	
			Femur head width	LOD=3.2	[174]
			Hip bone size	LOD=2.83	[172]
20p11.1-13.12	D20S447-D20S107	CDMP1	Serum osteocalcin level	LOD=2.78	[177]
21q22-qter	D21S2055	COL6A1; COL6A2	Trochanter BMD	LOD=2.39	[10]
	D21S1446		Trochanter BMD	LOD=3.14	
22q12-13	D22S423		Spine BMD	LOD=2.13	[8]

Abbreviations: BGP, osteocalcin; BMP-3, bone morphogenic protein-3; BMP-4, bone morphogenic protein-4; BMP-6, bone morphogenic protein-6; CALM2, calmodulin 2; CHAD, chondroadherin; CDMP1, cartilage-derived morphogenetic protein 1; COL1A1, type 1 collagen A1; COL2A1, type 2 collagen A1; COL4A1, type IV collagen A1; COL4A2, type IV collagen A2; COL15A1, collagen type V A5; COL6A1; collagen type VI A1; COL6A2, collagen type VI A2; COL6A3, collagen type VI A3; COL8A1, type VIII collagen A1; COMP, cartilage oligomeric matrix protein; CRTL1, cartilage linking protein 1; EGF, epidermal growth factor; ER-α, estrogen receptor α; FGFR2, fibroblast growth factor 2; FGFR3, fibroblast growth factor 3; HOX: homeobox genes; IGF1, insulin-like growth factor 1; IGF-2, insulin-like growth factor 2; IL-1 α, Interleukin-1 α; IL-4, interleukin-4; IL-6, interlukin-6; IL-6R, interleukin-6 receptor; LRP5, low density lipoprotein receptor-related protein 5; MTHFR, methylenetetrahydrofolate reductase; ON, osteonectin; PDGFRB, platelet-derived growth factor receptor-β; PLOD, lysyl hydroxylase; POMC, pro-opiomelanocortin; PRTN3, proteinase 3; PTHR1, PTH receptor type 1; STK, serine/threonine kinase; TBX2, T-box 2; TNF-α, tumor necrosis factor alpha; TNFRSF1B, Tumor necrosis factor receptor subfamily 1B; TNFRSF11B, Osteoporotegerin; VDR, vitamin D receptor.

Table 2. Comparison of the high-throughput methods for differential gene expression analysis.

Method	Minimum polyA RNA required	Throughput	Sequencing requirements	Sensitivity	Analysis of many samples in a single experiment	Applicability to studying small tissue samples
EST sequencing	1.0-5.0 µg	Low	High	High	+	+
Subtractive cloning	10-100 ng	Medium	Low	Low	−	++
Differential display	10-100 ng	High	Medium	Low	+++	+++
SAGE	1.0-5.0 µg	High	High	High	+	++
Microarray hybridization	100+ ng[*]	High	−	High	+++	+++

Linear amplification of RNA is required prior to RNA labeling, if the amount is < 1 µg.

Table 3. A summary of the features of the methods in proteomics.

Types of Proteomics	Methods	Advantages	Disadvantages
Protein Expression Proteomics	**Protein isolation**		
	2-DE	Distinguishing phosphorylated and nonphosphorylated proteins	Inability to detect large or hydrophobic proteins
	DIGE	Resolving two protein samples	The same as the above
	ICAT	Independent of gel	At least one cysteine residue in one protein
	Protein identification		
	MALDI-TOF MS	Generating peptide mass fingerprinting	Dependent on specific enzymes and the mass accuracy
	ESI-MS/MS	Producing amino acid sequence of a peptide	Not allowing to analyzing compounds outside of the target list
	Antibody microarray	Simple and convenient	Lacking enough specific antibodies
Structural Proteomics	X-ray crystallography	Detecting proteins from a large size range	Only suitable for crystal proteins
	NMR	Determining proteins in solution	Protein size no more than 300 amino acid residues
	Electron crystallography	Providing both an image and the corresponding diffraction pattern of a crystalline protein	Not an atomic structure
Functional Proteomics	GST-fusion technique	Identifying protein-protein interactions and purifying proteins	Several steps affecting protein activities
	Yeast two-hybrid system	Specially powerful for protein-protein interactions from known genome	Inability to measure membrane proteins and transcription factors
	Protein microarray	Directly identifying biochemical activities and various interactions	Limited to available chips from vendors

5. Conclusions

The molecular mechanism determining a quantitative trait has three levels of regulation, which correspond to DNA, mRNA, and protein. Each of the three groups of methods reviewed in this article represents, in fact, a certain level of the regulation. Whole-genome linkage and association methods search for candidate genes at the DNA level, high-throughput gene expression profiling helps to determine these genes at the mRNA level, proteomics identifies candidate loci at the protein level. Eventually, a combined approach with protein and high-throughput gene expression analyses and genetic epidemiology studies (linkage, association, and mapping studies) should be powerful in our struggle for identifying genes and their interaction in underlying bone related phenotypes and diseases.

Acknowledgments

The investigators were partially supported by grants from Health Future Foundation of the USA, the National Institutes of Health (K01 AR02170-01, R01 GM60402-01A1), the State of Nebraska Cancer and Smoking Related Disease Research Program, and US Department of Energy (DE-FG03-00ER63000/A00). The study also benefited from support (to HWD) of Hunan Province Special Professor Start-up Fund (25000612), Chinese National Science Foundation (CNSF) Outstanding Young Scientist Award (30025025), CNSF Grant (30170504), Seed Fund from the Ministry of Education of P. R. China (25000106), and a key project grant from the Ministry of Education of P. R. China.

REFERENCES

1. P. Jouanny, F. Guillemin, C. Kuntz, C. Jeandel and J. Pourel, Arthritis Rheum., 61 (1995).
2. H.W. Deng, W.M. Chen, T. Conway, Y. Zhou, K.M. Davies, M.R. Stegman, H. Deng and R.R. Recker, Genet. Epidemiol., 160 (2000).
3. M.M. Hla, J.W. Davis, P.D. Ross, A.J. Yates and R.D. Wasnich, Calcif. Tissue Int., 291 (2001).
4. A. Prentice, Proc. Nutr. Soc., 45 (2001).
5. Y.Z. Liu, Y.J. Liu, R.R. Recker and H.W. Deng, J. Endocrinol., 147 (2003).
6. M. Devoto, K. Shimoya, J. Caminis, J. Ott, A. Tenenhouse, M.P. Whyte, L. Sereda, S. Hall, E. Considine, C.J. Williams, G. Tromp, H. Kuivaniemi, L. Ala-Kokko, D.J. Prockop and L.D. Spotila, Eur. J. Hum. Genet., 151 (1998).
7. T. Niu, C.K. Chen, H. Cordell, J. Yang, B. Wang, Z. Wang, Z. Fang, N.J. Schork, C.J. Rosen and X. Xu, Hum. Genet., 226 (1999).
8. D.L. Koller, M.J. Econs, P.A. Morin, J.C. Christian, S.L. Hui, P. Parry, M.E. Curran, L.A. Rodriguez, P.M. Conneally, G. Joslyn, M. Peacock, C.C. Johnston and T. Foroud, J. Clin. Endocrinol. Metab., 3116 (2000).
9. H.W. Deng, F.H. Xu, Q.Y. Huang, H. Shen, H.Y. Deng, T. Conway, Y.J. Liu, Y.Z. Liu, J.L. Li, H.T. Zhang, K.M. Davies and R.R. Recker, J. Clin. Endocrinol. Metab., 5151 (2002).
10. D. Karasik, R.H. Myers, L.A. Cupples, M.T. Hannan, D.R. Gagnon, A. Herbert and D.P. Kiel, J. Bone Miner. Res., 1718 (2002).
11. S.G. Wilson, P.W. Reed, A. Bansal, M. Chiano, M. Lindersson, M. Langdown, R.L. Prince, D. Thompson, E. Thompson, M. Bailey, P.W. Kleyn, P. Sambrook, M.M. Shi and T.D. Spector, Am. J. Hum. Genet., 144 (2003).
12. C.M. Kammerer, J.L. Schneider, S.A. Cole, J.E. Hixson, P.B. Samollow, J.R. O'Connell, R. Perez, T.D. Dyer, L. Almasy, J. Blangero, R.L. Bauer and B.D. Mitchell, J. Bone Miner. Res., 2245 (2003).
13. U. Styrkarsdottir, J.B. Cazier, A. Kong, O. Rolfsson, H. Larsen, E. Bjarnadottir, V.D. Johannsdottir, M.S. Sigurdardottir, Y. Bagger, C. Christiansen, I. Reynisdottir, S.F. Grant, K. Jonasson, M.L. Frigge, J.R. Gulcher, G. Sigurdsson and K. Stefansson, PLoS Biol., E69 (2003).
14. D.L. Koller, L.A. Rodriguez, J.C. Christian, C.W. Slemenda, M.J. Econs, S.L. Hui, P. Morin, P.M. Conneally, G. Joslyn, M.E. Curran, M. Peacock, C.C. Johnston and T. Foroud, J. Bone Miner. Res., 1903 (1998).
15. D. Karasik, R.H. Myers, M.T. Hannan, D. Gagnon, R.R. McLean, L.A. Cupples and D.P. Kiel, Osteoporos. Int., 796 (2002).
16. M. Devoto, C. Specchia, H.H. Li, J. Caminis, A. Tenenhouse, H. Rodriguez and L.D. Spotila, Hum. Mol. Genet., 2447 (2001).

17. E.L. Duncan, M.A. Brown, J. Sinsheimer, J. Bell, A.J. Carr, B.P. Wordsworth and J.A. Wass, J. Bone Miner. Res., 1993 (1999).

18. N. Ota, S.C. Hunt, T. Nakajima, T. Suzuki, T. Hosoi, H. Orimo, Y. Shirai and M. Emi, Genes Immun., 260 (2000).

19. B.D. Mitchell, R.L. Bauer, R. Perez, J.E. Hixson, S.A. Cole and C.M. Kammerer. Genome-wide scan for loci influencing bone density in Mexican Americans. Am.J.Hum.Genet., 63 (1998).

20. R.R. Recker and H.W. Deng, Endocrine, 55 (2002).

21. R. Feakes, S. Sawcer, J. Chataway, F. Coraddu, S. Broadley, J. Gray, H.B. Jones, D. Clayton, P.N. Goodfellow and A. Compston, Genet. Epidemiol., 51 (1999).

22. L.D. Atwood and N.L. Heard-Costa, Genet. Epidemiol., 99 (2003).

23. L.R. Cardon and J.I. Bell, Nat. Rev. Genet., 91 (2001).

24. H.W. Deng, W.M. Chen and R.R. Recker, Am. J. Hum. Genet., 1027 (2000).

25. B. Kerem, J.M. Rommens, J.A. Buchanan, D. Markiewicz, T.K. Cox, A. Chakravarti, M. Buchwald and L.C. Tsui, Science, 1073 (1989).

26. Anonymous, Cell, 971 (1993).

27. J.D. Rioux, M.J. Daly, M.S. Silverberg, K. Lindblad, H. Steinhart, Z. Cohen, T. Delmonte, K. Kocher, K. Miller, S. Guschwan, E.J. Kulbokas, S. O'Leary, E. Winchester, K. Dewar, T. Green, V. Stone, C. Chow, A. Cohen, D. Langelier, G. Lapointe, D. Gaudet, J. Faith, N. Branco, S.B. Bull, R.S. McLeod, A.M. Griffiths, A. Bitton, G.R. Greenberg, E.S. Lander, K.A. Siminovitch and T.J. Hudson, Nat. Genet., 223 (2001).

28. D.A. van Heel, D.P. McGovern, L.R. Cardon, B.M. Dechairo, N.J. Lench, A.H. Carey and D.P. Jewell, Am. J. Med. Genet., 253 (2002).

29. I.C. Gray, D.A. Campbell and N.K. Spurr, Hum. Mol. Genet., 2403 (2000).

30. D.E. Reich, M. Cargill, S. Bolk, J. Ireland, P.C. Sabeti, D.J. Richter, T. Lavery, R. Kouyoumjian, S.F. Farhadian, R. Ward and E.S. Lander, Nature, 199 (2001).

31. J.K. Pritchard and M. Przeworski, Am. J. Hum. Genet., 1 (2001).

32. M.J. Daly, J.D. Rioux, S.F. Schaffner, T.J. Hudson and E.S. Lander, Nat. Genet., 229 (2001).

33. E. Dawson, G. Abecasis, S. Bumpstead, Y. Chen, S. Hunt, D.M. Beare, J. Pabial, T. Dibling, E. Tinsley, S. Kirby, D. Carter, M. Papaspyridonos, S. Livingstone, R. Ganske, E. Lohmussaar, J. Zernant, N. Tonisson, M. Remm, R. Magi, T. Puurand, J. Vilo, A. Kurg, K. Rice, P. Deloukas, R. Mott, A. Metspalu, D.R. Bentley, L.R. Cardon and I. Dunham, Nature, 544 (2002).

34. L.R. Cardon and G.R. Abecasis, Trends Genet., 135 (2003).

35. N. Patil, A.J. Berno, D.A. Hinds, W.A. Barrett, J.M. Doshi, C.R. Hacker, C.R. Kautzer, D.H. Lee, C. Marjoribanks, D.P. McDonough, B.T. Nguyen, M.C. Norris, J.B. Sheehan, N. Shen, D. Stern, R.P. Stokowski, D.J. Thomas, M.O. Trulson, K.R. Vyas, K.A. Frazer, S.P. Fodor and D.R. Cox, Science, 1719 (2001).

36. S.B. Gabriel, S.F. Schaffner, H. Nguyen, J.M. Moore, J. Roy, B. Blumenstiel, J. Higgins, M. DeFelice, A. Lochner, M. Faggart, S.N. Liu-Cordero, C. Rotimi, A. Adeyemo, R. Cooper, R. Ward, E.S. Lander, M.J. Daly and D. Altshuler, Science, 2225 (2002).

37. D.C. Crawford, C.S. Carlson, M.J. Rieder, D.P. Carrington, Q. Yi, J.D. Smith, M.A. Eberle, L. Kruglyak and D.A. Nickerson, Am. J. Hum. Genet., 610 (2004).

38. Y. Horikawa, N. Oda, N.J. Cox, X. Li, M. Orho-Melander, M. Hara, Y. Hinokio, T.H. Lindner, H. Mashima, P.E. Schwarz, L. Bosque-Plata, Y. Horikawa, Y. Oda, I. Yoshiuchi, S. Colilla, K.S. Polonsky, S. Wei, P. Concannon, N. Iwasaki, J. Schulze, L.J. Baier, C. Bogardus, L. Groop, E. Boerwinkle, C.L. Hanis and G.I. Bell, Nat. Genet., 163 (2000).

39. Y. Zhang, N.I. Leaves, G.G. Anderson, C.P. Ponting, J. Broxholme, R. Holt, P. Edser, S. Bhattacharyya, A. Dunham, I.M. Adcock, L. Pulleyn, P.J. Barnes, J.I. Harper, G. Abecasis, L. Cardon, M. White, J. Burton, L. Matthews, R. Mott, M. Ross, R. Cox, M.F. Moffatt and W.O. Cookson, Nat. Genet., 181 (2003).

40. N. Risch and K. Merikangas, Science, 1516 (1996).

41. L.B. Jorde, Genome Res., 1435 (2000).

42. K.M. Weiss and A.G. Clark, Trends Genet., 19 (2002).

43. S. Shifman, J. Kuypers, M. Kokoris, B. Yakir and A. Darvasi, Hum. Mol. Genet., 771 (2003).

44. J. Couzin, Science, 941 (2002).

45. M.S. Phillips, R. Lawrence, R. Sachidanandam, A.P. Morris, D.J. Balding, M.A. Donaldson, J.F. Studebaker, W.M. Ankener, S.V. Alfisi, F.S. Kuo, A.L. Camisa, V. Pazorov, K.E. Scott, B.J. Carey, J. Faith, G. Katari, H.A. Bhatti, J.M. Cyr, V. Derohannessian, C. Elosua, A.M. Forman, N.M. Grecco, C.R. Hock, J.M. Kuebler, J.A. Lathrop, M.A. Mockler, E.P. Nachtman, S.L. Restine, S.A. Varde, M.J. Hozza, C.A. Gelfand, J. Broxholme, G.R. Abecasis, M.T. Boyce-Jacino and L.R. Cardon, Nat. Genet., 382 (2003).

46. N.E. Morton, Am. J Hum. Genet., 690 (1998).

47. H. Campbell and I. Rudan, Pharmacogenomics J, 349 (2002).

48. E.S. Lander and L. Kruglyak, Nat. Genet., 241 (1995).

49. K.M. Weiss and J.D. Terwilliger, Nat. Genet., 151 (2000).

50. J.K. Pritchard, Am. J. Hum. Genet., 124 (2001).

51. V. Dvornyk, R. Recker and H.W. Deng, Osteoporos. Int., 451 (2003).

52. L. Jia, N.C. Ho, S.S. Park, J. Powell and C.A. Francomano, Am. J. Med. Genet., 275 (2001).

53. M.D. Adams, J.M. Kelley, J.D. Gocayne, M. Dubnick, M.H. Polymeropoulos, H. Xiao, C.R. Merril, A. Wu, B. Olde and R.F. Moreno, Science, 1651 (1991).

54. J.P. Carulli, M. Artinger, P.M. Swain, C.D. Root, L. Chee, C. Tulig, J. Guerin, M. Osborne, G. Stein, J. Lian and P.T. Lomedico, J. Cell. Biochem. Suppl., 286 (1998).

55. L. Jia, M.F. Young, J. Powell, L. Yang, N.C. Ho, R. Hotchkiss, P.G. Robey and C.A. Francomano, Genomics, 7 (2002).

56. N.C. Ho, L. Jia, C.C. Driscoll, E.M. Gutter and C.A. Francomano, J. Bone Miner. Res., 2095 (2000).

57. Y. Chien, D.M. Becker, T. Lindsten, M. Okamura, D.I. Cohen and M.M. Davis, Nature, 31 (1984).

58. G.H. Travis and J.G. Sutcliffe, Proc. Natl. Acad. Sci. USA, 1696 (1988).

59. N. Lisitsyn, N. Lisitsyn and M. Wigler, Science, 946 (1993).

60. A.A. Culbert, G.A. Wallis and K.E. Kadler, Am. J. Med. Genet., 167 (1996).

61. D. Bachner, D. Schroder, N. Betat, M. Ahrens and G. Gross, Biofactors, 11 (1999).

62. D.N. Petersen, G.T. Tkalcevic, A.L. Mansolf, R. Rivera-Gonzalez and T.A. Brown, J. Biol. Chem., 36172 (2000).

63. H. Ito, H. Akiyama, H. Iguchi, K. Iyama, M. Miyamoto, K. Ohsawa and T. Nakamura, J. Biol. Chem., 24023 (2001).

64. T. Maeda, M. Abe, K. Kurisu, A. Jikko and S. Furukawa, J. Biol. Chem., 3628 (2001).

65. K. Roundy, R. Smith, J.J. Weis and J.H. Weis, J. Bone Miner. Res., 278 (2003).

66. P. Liang and A.B. Pardee, Science, 967 (1992).

67. J. Welsh, K. Chada, S.S. Dalal, R. Cheng, D. Ralph and M. McClelland, Nucleic Acids Res., 4965 (1992).

68. F. Gori, P. Divieti and M.B. Demay, J. Biol. Chem., 46515 (2001).

69. M. Hadjiargyrou, E.P. Rightmire, T. Ando and F.T. Lombardo, Bone, 149 (2001).

70. A.H. Jheon, B. Ganss, S. Cheifetz and J. Sodek, J. Biol. Chem., 18282 (2001).

71. A.E. Kearns, M.M. Donohue, B. Sanyal and M.B. Demay, J. Biol. Chem., 42213 (2001).

72. F.F. Safadi, J. Xu, S.L. Smock, M.C. Rico, T.A. Owen and S.N. Popoff, J. Cell. Biochem., 12 (2001).

73. J. Zhi, D.W. Sommerfeldt, C.T. Rubin and M. Hadjiargyrou, J. Bone Miner. Res., 1994 (2001).

74. C.H. Gouveia, J.J. Schultz, D.J. Jackson, G.R. Williams and G.A. Brent, Thyroid, 663 (2002).

75. H. Ohishi, K. Furukawa, K. Iwasaki, K. Ueyama, A. Okada, S. Motomura, S. Harata and S. Toh, J. Pharmacol. Exp. Ther., 818 (2003).

76. 76. P. Ledakis, H. Tanimura and T. Fojo, Biochem. Biophys. Res. Commun., 653 (1998).

77. X. Yang, Y. Nakao, M.M. Pater and A. Pater, Carcinogenesis, 563 (1996).

78. M.H. Linskens, J. Feng, W.H. Andrews, B.E. Enlow, S.M. Saati, L.A. Tonkin, W.D. Funk and B. Villeponteau, Nucleic Acids Res., 3244 (1995).

79. M. Hadman, B.L. Adam, G.L. Wright, Jr. and T.J. Bos, Anal. Biochem., 383 (1995).

80.　　D. Graf, A.G. Fisher and M. Merkenschlager, Nucleic Acids Res., 2239 (1997).

81.　　D.J. Bertioli, U.H. Schlichter, M.J. Adams, P.R. Burrows, H.H. Steinbiss and J.F. Antoniw, Nucleic Acids Res., 4520 (1995).

82.　　V.E. Velculescu, L. Zhang, B. Vogelstein and K.W. Kinzler, Science, 484 (1995).

83.　　A. Seth, B.K. Lee, S. Qi and C.P. Vary, J. Bone Miner. Res., 1683 (2000).

84.　　R. Kitching, S. Qi, V. Li, A. Raouf, C.P. Vary and A. Seth, J. Bone Miner. Metab., 269 (2002).

85.　　X. Ji, D. Chen, C. Xu, S.E. Harris, G.R. Mundy and T. Yoneda, J. Bone Miner. Metab., 132 (2000).

86.　　C.P. Vary, V. Li, A. Raouf, R. Kitching, I. Kola, C. Franceschi, M. Venanzoni and A. Seth, Exp. Cell Res., 213 (2000).

87.　　M. Schena, R.A. Heller, T.P. Theriault, K. Konrad, E. Lachenmeier and R.W. Davis, Trends Biotechnol., 301 (1998).

88.　　C.B. Epstein and R.A. Butow, Curr. Opin. Biotechnol., 36 (2000).

89.　　L.W. Hal-Nicole, O. Vorst, M.-M.L. Houwelingen-Adele, E.J. Kok, A. Peijnenburg, A. Aharoni, A.J. van Tunen and J. Keijer, J. Biotechnol., 271 (2000).

90.　　R.A. Heller, M. Schena, A. Chai, D. Shalon, T. Bedilion, J. Gilmore, D.E. Woolley and R.W. Davis, Proc. Natl. Acad. Sci. USA, 2150 (1997).

91.　　G.R. Beck, Jr., B. Zerler and E. Moran, Cell Growth Differ., 61 (2001).

92.　　J. Chen, Q. Zhong, J. Wang, R.S. Cameron, J.L. Borke, C.M. Isales and R.J. Bollag, Mol. Cell. Endocrinol., 43 (2001).

93.　　D.S. de Jong, E.J. van Zoelen, S. Bauerschmidt, W. Olijve and W.T. Steegenga, J. Bone Miner. Res., 2119 (2002).

94.　　M. Doi, A. Nagano and Y. Nakamura, Biochem. Biophys. Res. Commun., 381 (2002).

95.　　R.M. Locklin, B.L. Riggs, K.C. Hicok, H.F. Horton, M.C. Byrne and S. Khosla, J. Bone Miner. Res., 2192 (2001).

96.　　A. Raouf and A. Seth, Bone, 463 (2002).

97.　　B.L. Vaes, K.J. Dechering, A. Feijen, J.M. Hendriks, C. Lefevre, C.L. Mummery, W. Olijve, E.J. van Zoelen and W.T. Steegenga, J. Bone Miner. Res., 2106 (2002).

98.　　H. Qi, D.J. Aguiar, S.M. Williams, A. La Pean, W. Pan and C.M. Verfaillie, Proc. Natl. Acad. Sci. USA, 3305 (2003).

99.　　J. Theilhaber, T. Connolly, S. Roman-Roman, S. Bushnell, A. Jackson, K. Call, T. Garcia and R. Baron, Genome Res., 165 (2002).

100.　　W. Huang, B. Carlsen, G.H. Rudkin, N. Shah, C. Chung, K. Ishida, D.T. Yamaguchi and T.A. Miller, Biochem. Biophys. Res. Commun., 1120 (2001).

101.　　P.H. Krebsbach, S.A. Kuznetsov, K. Satomura, R.V. Emmons, D.W. Rowe and P.G. Robey, Transplantation, 1059 (1997).

102.　　P. Bianco, M. Riminucci, S. Gronthos and P.G. Robey, Stem Cells, 180 (2001).

103. W.Y. Park, C.I. Hwang, M.J. Kang, J.Y. Seo, J.H. Chung, Y.S. Kim, J.H. Lee, H. Kim, K.A. Kim, H.J. Yoo and J.S. Seo, Biochem. Biophys. Res. Commun., 934 (2001).

104. R.N. Van Gelder, M.E. von Zastrow, A. Yool, W.C. Dement, J.D. Barchas and J.H. Eberwine, Proc. Natl. Acad. Sci. USA, 1663 (1990).

105. M. Bakay, Y.W. Chen, R. Borup, P. Zhao, K. Nagaraju and E.P. Hoffman, BMC Bioinformatics, 4 (2002).

106. M.L.T. Lee, F.C. Kuo, G.A. Whitmore and J. Sklar, Proc. Natl. Acad. Sci. USA, 9834 (2000).

107. X. Peng, C.G. Wood, E. Blalock, K. Chen, P. Landfield and A. Stromberg, BMC Bioinformatics, 26 (2003).

108. C.M. Kendziorski, Y. Zhang, H. Lan and A.D. Attie, Biostat., 465 (2003).

109. K.J. Kyng, A. May, S. Kolvraa and V.A. Bohr, Proc. Natl. Acad. Sci. USA, 12259 (2003).

110. A. Alizadeh, M.B. Eisen, R.E. Davis, C. Ma, I.S. Lossos, A. Rosenwald, J.C. Boldrick, H. Sabet, T. Tran, X. Yu, J.I. Powell, L. Yang, G.E. Marti, T. Moore, J.J. Hudson, L. Lu, D.B. Lewis, R. Tibshirani, G. Sherlock, W.C. Chan, T.C. Greiner, D.D. Weisenburger, J.O. Armitage, R.A. Warnke, R. Levy, W. Wilson, M.R. Grever, J.C. Byrd, D. Botstein, P.O. Brown and L.M. Staudt, Nature, 503 (2000).

111. J.C. Chang, E.C. Wooten, A. Tsimelzon, S.G. Hilsenbeck, M.C. Gutierrez, R. Elledge, S. Mohsin, C.K. Osborne, G.C. Chamness, D.C. Allred and P. O'Connell, Lancet, 362 (2003).

112. C. Fargeas, C.Y. Wu, H.Y. Luo, M. Sarfati, G. Delespesse and J.P. Wu, J. Immunol., 4053 (1990).

113. P. Salomon, A. Pizzimenti, A. Panja, A. Reisman and L. Mayer, Autoimmunity, 141 (1991).

114. D.V. Kuprash, V.E. Boitchenko, F.O. Yarovinsky, N.R. Rice, A. Nordheim, A. Ruhlmann and S.A. Nedospasov, Blood, 1721 (2002).

115. H.Q. Zhang, H. Lu, S. Enosawa, S. Takahara, K. Sakamoto, T. Nakajima, H. Saito and S. Suzuki, Transplant. Proc., 1757 (2002).

116. C.W. Slemenda, J.C. Christian, T. Reed, T.K. Reister, C.J. Williams and C.C. Johnston, Ann. Intern. Med., 286 (1992).

117. K.D. Ward and R.C. Klesges, Calcif. Tissue Int., 259 (2001).

118. T.R. Hughes, M.J. Marton, A.R. Jones, C.J. Roberts, R. Stoughton, C.D. Armour, H.A. Bennett, E. Coffey, H. Dai, Y.D. He, M.J. Kidd, A.M. King, M.R. Meyer, D. Slade, P.Y. Lum, S.B. Stepaniants, D.D. Shoemaker, D. Gachotte, K. Chakraburtty, J. Simon, M. Bard and S.H. Friend, Cell, 109 (2000).

119. K.D. Dahlquist, N. Salomonis, K. Vranizan, S.C. Lawlor and B.R. Conklin, Nat. Genet., 19 (2002).

120. R.A. Power, U.T. Iwaniec and T.J. Wronski, Bone, 143 (2002).

121. F. Kamme and M.G. Erlander, Curr. Opin. Drug Discov. Devel., 231 (2003).

122. F. Kamme, R. Salunga, J. Yu, D.T. Tran, J. Zhu, L. Luo, A. Bittner, H.Q. Guo, N. Miller, J. Wan and M. Erlander, J. Neurosci., 3607 (2003).

123. E. Sanz, M. Alvarez-Mon, A. Martinez and de la Hera A., Blood, 3424 (2003).

124. R.F. Klein, J. Allard, Z. Avnur, T. Nikolcheva, D. Rotstein, A.S. Carlos, M. Shea, R.V. Waters, J.K. Belknap, G. Peltz and E.S. Orwoll, Science, 229 (2004).

125. L. Anderson and J. Seilhamer, Electrophoresis, 533 (1997).

126. A. Abbott, Nature, 715 (1999).

127. S.P. Gygi, Y. Rochon, B.R. Franza and R. Aebersold, Mol. Cell. Biol., 1720 (1999).

128. T. Ideker, V. Thorsson, J.A. Ranish, R. Christmas, J. Buhler, J.K. Eng, R. Bumgarner, D.R. Goodlett, R. Aebersold and L. Hood, Science, 929 (2001).

129. V.C. Wasinger, S.J. Cordwell, A. Cerpa-Poljak, J.X. Yan, A.A. Gooley, M.R. Wilkins, M.W. Duncan, R. Harris, K.L. Williams and I. Humphery-Smith, Electrophoresis, 1090 (1995).

130. M.R. Wilkins, J.C. Sanchez, A.A. Gooley, R.D. Appel, I. Humphery-Smith, D.F. Hochstrasser and K.L. Williams, Biotechnol. Genet. Eng. Rev., 19 (1996).

131. C.H. Cho and M.E. Nuttall, Expert. Opin. Ther. Targets, 679 (2002).

132. D.J. Oliver, B. Nikolau and E.S. Wurtele, Metab. Eng., 98 (2002).

133. P.R. Graves and T.A. Haystead, Microbiol. Mol. Biol. Rev., 39 (2002).

134. U.K. Laemmli, Nature, 680 (1970).

135. A. Gorg, C. Obermaier, G. Boguth, A. Harder, B. Scheibe, R. Wildgruber and W. Weiss, Electrophoresis, 1037 (2000).

136. M. Unlu, M.E. Morgan and J.S. Minden, Electrophoresis, 2071 (1997).

137. A.L. McCormack, D.M. Schieltz, B. Goode, S. Yang, G. Barnes, D. Drubin and J.R. Yates, III, Anal. Chem., 767 (1997).

138. A.J. Link, J. Eng, D.M. Schieltz, E. Carmack, G.J. Mize, D.R. Morris, B.M. Garvik and J.R. Yates, III, Nat. Biotechnol., 676 (1999).

139. J.R. Yates, III, A.J. Link and D. Schieltz, Methods Mol. Biol., 17 (2000).

140. D. Figeys, G.L. Corthals, B. Gallis, D.R. Goodlett, A. Ducret, M.A. Corson and R. Aebersold, Anal. Chem., 2279 (1999).

141. W. Tong, A. Link, J.K. Eng and J.R. Yates, III, Anal. Chem., 2270 (1999).

142. S.P. Gygi, B. Rist, S.A. Gerber, F. Turecek, M.H. Gelb and R. Aebersold, Nat. Biotechnol., 994 (1999).

143. M. Karas and F. Hillenkamp, Anal. Chem., 2299 (1988).

144. J.B. Fenn, M. Mann, C.K. Meng, S.F. Wong and C.M. Whitehouse, Science, 64 (1989).

145. R. Aebersold and M. Mann, Nature, 198 (2003).

146. D.J. Cahill, J. Immunol. Methods, 81 (2001).

147. W.P. Blackstock and M.P. Weir, Trends Biotechnol., 121 (1999).

148. A. Sali, R. Glaeser, T. Earnest and W. Baumeister, Nature, 216 (2003).

149. N. Ban, P. Nissen, J. Hansen, P.B. Moore and T.A. Steitz, Science, 905 (2000).

150. B.T. Wimberly, D.E. Brodersen, W.M. Clemons, Jr., R.J. Morgan-Warren, A.P. Carter, C. Vonrhein, T. Hartsch and V. Ramakrishnan, Nature, 327 (2000).

151. J. Harms, F. Schluenzen, R. Zarivach, A. Bashan, S. Gat, I. Agmon, H. Bartels, F. Franceschi and A. Yonath, Cell, 679 (2001).

152. M.M. Yusupov, G.Z. Yusupova, A. Baucom, K. Lieberman, T.N. Earnest, J.H. Cate and H.F. Noller, Science, 883 (2001).

153. O. Medalia, I. Weber, A.S. Frangakis, D. Nicastro, G. Gerisch and W. Baumeister, Science, 1209 (2002).

154. A. Pandey and M. Mann, Nature, 837 (2000).

155. S. Fields and O. Song, Nature, 245 (1989).

156. P. Uetz, L. Giot, G. Cagney, T.A. Mansfield, R.S. Judson, J.R. Knight, D. Lockshon, V. Narayan, M. Srinivasan, P. Pochart, A. Qureshi-Emili, Y. Li, B. Godwin, D. Conover, T. Kalbfleisch, G. Vijayadamodar, M. Yang, M. Johnston, S. Fields and J.M. Rothberg, Nature, 623 (2000).

157. G. MacBeath, Nat. Genet., 526 (2002).

158. H. Zhu, J.F. Klemic, S. Chang, P. Bertone, A. Casamayor, K.G. Klemic, D. Smith, M. Gerstein, M.A. Reed and M. Snyder, Nat. Genet., 283 (2000).

159. H. Zhu, M. Bilgin, R. Bangham, D. Hall, A. Casamayor, P. Bertone, N. Lan, R. Jansen, S. Bidlingmaier, T. Houfek, T. Mitchell, P. Miller, R.A. Dean, M. Gerstein and M. Snyder, Science, 2101 (2001).

160. D.K. Arrell, I. Neverova and J.E. Van Eyk, Circ. Res., 763 (2001).

161. J. Macri and S.T. Rapundalo, Trends Cardiovasc. Med., 66 (2001).

162. M.A. Knepper, J. Am. Soc. Nephrol., 1398 (2002).

163. D.B. Martin and P.S. Nelson, Trends Cell Biol., S60-S65 (2001).

164. M.V. Dwek and S.L. Rawlings, Mol. Biotechnol., 139 (2002).

165. A. Sinz, M. Bantscheff, S. Mikkat, B. Ringel, S. Drynda, J. Kekow, H.J. Thiesen and M.O. Glocker, Electrophoresis, 3445 (2002).

166. H. Andersen, O.N. Jensen, E.P. Moiseeva and E.F. Eriksen, J. Bone Miner. Res., 195 (2003).

167. W.N. Pappano, B.M. Steiglitz, I.C. Scott, D.R. Keene and D.S. Greenspan, Mol. Cell. Biol., 4428 (2003).

168. C.A. Evans, R. Tonge, D. Blinco, A. Pierce, J. Shaw, Y. Lu, H.G. Hamzah, A. Gray, C.P. Downes, S.J. Gaskell, E. Spooncer and A.D. Whetton, Blood, (2004).

169. R.E. Brown and J.L. Boyle, Ann. Clin. Lab Sci., 131 (2003).

170. K. Kubota, K. Wakabayashi and T. Matsuoka, Proteomics, 616 (2003).

171. M.E. Nuttall, Cells Tissues Organs, 265 (2001).

172. H.W. Deng, H. Shen, F.H. Xu, H. Deng, T. Conway, Y.J. Liu, Y.Z. Liu, J.L. Li, Q.Y. Huang, K.M. Davies and R.R. Recker, Am. J. Med. Genet., 121 (2003).

173. D.L. Koller, G. Liu, M.J. Econs, S.L. Hui, P.A. Morin, G. Joslyn, L.A. Rodriguez, P.M. Conneally, J.C. Christian, C.C. Johnston, Jr., T. Foroud and M. Peacock, J. Bone Miner. Res., 985 (2001).

174. D.L. Koller, K.E. White, G. Liu, S.L. Hui, P.M. Conneally, C.C. Johnston, M.J. Econs, T. Foroud and M. Peacock, J. Bone Miner. Res., 1057 (2003).

175. B.D. Mitchell, C.M. Kammerer, J.L. Schneider, S.A. Cole, J.E. Hixson, R. Perez and R.L. Bauer. A quantitative trait locus on chromosome 4p influences variation in bone mineral density at the wrist and hip. J.Bone Miner.Res., 16 (2001).

176. M.L. Johnson, G. Gong, W. Kimberling, S.M. Recker, D.B. Kimmel and R.R. Recker, Am. J. Hum. Genet., 1326 (1997).

177. B.D. Mitchell, S.A. Cole, R.L. Bauer, S.J. Iturria, E.A. Rodriguez, J. Blangero, J.W. MacCluer and J.E. Hixson, J. Clin. Endocrinol. Metab., 1362 (2000).

CHAPTER 18

ANIMAL MODELS AND STUDY DESIGN FOR OSTEOPOROSIS RESEARCH

Hua Zhu Ke [1], and Xiao-Jian Li [2]

[1] *Pfizer Global Research and Development, Groton, CT, USA*
E-mail: huazhu_ke@groton.pfizer.com.

[2] *Wyeth Research, Cambridge, MA, USA*
E-mail: jli@wyeth.com

Introduction

Animal models are of major importance for understanding the pathophysiology of various human diseases. In osteoporosis pre-clinical research, animal studies can provide information on mechanism of action on tissue and cellular levels, bone efficacy and bone tolerance. Such information will provide help on selection of clinical candidates, designing clinical trials, and predictions of clinical outcome. So far, preclinical studies have been carried out in various mammalian species: mice, rats, rabbits, minipigs, ewes, dog, and monkeys. The criteria for selection of animal species include: (a) basal bone remodeling pattern is comparable to human, (b) response to osteotropic agents is similar to that observed in human, (c) relatively rapid and significant bone loss can be induced, (d) availability and price including the cost for maintenance, (e) ease of handling and experimentation, (f) cultural sensitivity. Mimetic of human condition and prediction of human reaction to therapies, hormonal and other factor are of the most important criteria for selection of an animal model (Ammann et al., 1998).

Various models have been used to induce bone loss in experimental animals: (I) ovariectomy (Kalu 1991; Wronski and Yen 1991; Frost and Jee 1992; Dempster et al., 1995; Thompson et al., 1995), (II) orchidectomy (Ke et al., 2001; Erben 2001), (III) low calcium diet animals (Shen et al., 1995), (IV) immobilization including space flight models, hindlimb immobilization, tail suspension, nerve section, spinal cord section, tendon section (Jee and Ma, 1999), and (V) knockout and transgenic animals. Since the orchidectomized model (Ke et al., 2001; Erben 2001) and the immobilization models have been describerd in great details by Jee and Ma (1999), this chapter deals only with the OVX models and its applications in pre-clinical research. Further this chapter will also describe how to characterize the transgenic mouse models.

The Ovariectomized (OVX) Rat Model

The rat OVX model is useful for studying the pathophysiology of cancellous bone osteopenia and for the evaluation of potential agents for the prevention and treatment of estrogen-deficient osteoporosis.

A few important physiological characters: The mean healthy life span for most commercial available rats is 21 to 24 months. Longitudinal bone growth dramatically slows down at important sampling sites, such as proximal tibia, distal tibia, and vertebra in female rats by age 6 to 9 months. Peak bone mass for the adult female rat skeleton occurs around 10 months of age, as periosteal expansion continues. Thus, the rat has an appreciable life span both before and after attainment of adult skeletal status. Adult female rats have a regular estrus cycle in which estradiol levels spike to 50 to 90 pg/mL for 18 hours every 4 days. During the second year of life, the fraction of female rats found in constant diestrus rises gradually, and concellous bone loss is also frequently observed. Although this is not a true menopause, spikes in estradiol cease as cancellous bone loss occurs, making a linkage of rat "menopause" to cancellous bone loss possible.

Immediate effects of OVX: Plasma levels of estradiol in rat fall rapidly within 5 days after OVX and remain at very low level thereafter. Biochemical bone turnover makers such as serum alkaline phosphatase

(ALP), osteocalcin (BGP), and urinary pyridinoline and creatinine increased beginning at 3 - 7 days following OVX. At two weeks following surgery, bone turnover is increased and bone loss is occurring at the most commonly used skeletal site, the proximal tibia metaphysis. These changes include increased osteoclast number (#OC/BS), mineral apposition rate (MAR), bone formation rate (BFR), and decreased trabecular bone volume (BV/TV). The decreased BV/TV is due to the combination of thinning and loss of individual trabeculae.

In young adult (3 – 6 months of age) female rats, the earliest response for different parameters to ovariectomy is listed in Table 1 based on the available references (Kalu 1991; Wronski and Yen 1991; Frost and Jee 1992; Dempster et al., 1995; Thompson et al., 1995; Li et al., 1997).

Table 1. The earliest response to ovariectomy in young adult female rats.

Decreased uterine wet weight	Day 2
Increased body weight	Day 7
Proximal tibial cancellous bone	
Decreased trabecular thickness	Day 7
Decreased trabecular bone volume	Day 10
Decreased trabecular number	Day 20
Decreased node number	Day 20
Increased osteoclast surface	Day 7
Increased osteoclast number	Day 14
Increased bone formation	Day 14
Increased bone turnover	Day 14
Distal femur	
Decreased bone mineral density	Day 10
Femoral neck cancellous bone	
Decreased trabecular bone volume	Day 30
Increased bone turnover	Day 30
Lumbar vertebral cancellous bone	
Decreased trabecular bone volume	Day 21
Increased bone turnover	Day 21
Increased bone turnover	Day 30

In these young adult female rats, OVX induced significant bone loss in proximal tibial metaphysis, lumbar vertebral body, femoral neck, but not in distal tibial metaphysis. In long bone shaft (tibial diaphysis or femoral diaphysis), OVX induced significant increase in endocortical bone resorption and endocortical bone loss. However, due to the increased periosteal bone formation induced by OVX in the shaft, cortical bone loss does not occur in young adult OVX rats. It has been characterized that OVX in aged (>12 months) female rats induced bone loss in the similar manner as in young adult rats. It may take longer time to induce osteopenia in aged rats than in young rats. Bone loss induced by OVX in aged rats reaches steady state level by approximately 5-6 months post-surgery. Since postmenopausal osteoporosis is, for the most part, a disease of aging, aged OVX rat model is favorite model for pre-clinical research (Ke et al., 1999).

Progressive effects of OVX: Following OVX, cancellous bone and strength gradually decline with time. The rate of bone loss is varied at different skeletal sites. The OVX rats lose ~ 50% of their cancellous bone mass in the proximal tibial metaphyses or distal femur by 30 – 60 days post-ovariectomy. Equivalent loss of cancellous bone in the femoral neck and lumbar vertebra of OVX rats does not occur until 180 and 270 days post-ovariectomy, respectively. The deterioration of cancellous bone structure is accompanied with the loss of cancellous bone mass as shown by the decreases in trabecular number and thickness and increase in trabecular separation. The increased bone turnover in OVX rats reaches its peak value at ~ 30 days and drops to lower level at ~ 60 – 90 days after surgery, then it remains significantly higher than that of sham animals afterwards. Bone loss induced by OVX in these young adult rats reaches steady state level by approximately 3 months post-surgery.

Long-term (12 months) effects of OVX: Body weight is significantly increased in OVX rats compared to sham-operated rats. The body mass analysis by DEXA at 12 months demonstrates that the increased body weight gain found in OVX rats is due entirely to increased body fat and not increased lean body mass. In contrast to those reported in postmenopausal women, total body bone mineral content (BMC) and bone area (BA) are significantly increased in OVX rats compared to sham-operated controls over the 12 months duration of the study. These differences in BMC and BA in OVX rats become apparent by 1-month post-OVX. Thus, whole body bone mineral data from study suing OVX rats lasting one month or more must be interpreted with caution (Thompson et al., 1995). However, in cancellous bone enriched sites such as distal femur and lumbar vertebra, significant decreases in bone mineral content and density are found in OVX rats compared to sham-operated controls. Histomorphometric analyses of cancellous bone in the proximal tibia metaphyses demonstrate severe concellous osteopenia in OVX rats after 12 months compared to sham-operated controls. However, by 12 months no differences in bone turnover suggesting that a new steady state in bone remodeling has been achieved (Ma et al., 2002; Ke et al., 2004).

Skeletal sites for studies: The proximal tibia and distal femur are favorite sites in OVX rat model for studies, in part, because they contain substantial cancellous bone, and they lost this bone at a fast rate, thereby permitting a study to be completed in a short period of time. However, the vertebral bodies and femoral neck of rats lose significant amount of cancellous bone following OVX and should always be included in the evaluation of therapeutic agents because they are important sites of bone loss and fracture in humans. All these bone sites are suitable for biomechanical test. In general, the diaphyses of long bone of rats are not suitable for studying cortical bone loss due to the periosteal expansion following OVX. However, total cortical bone loss associated with decreased bone strength was observed in OVX rats at one year post-surgery and the endocortical bone loss accompanied with increased bone turnover is evident as early as 3 to 4 weeks post-surgery. Thus, these bone sites are still valuable when the study is designed to investigate the response of different envelope of bone to anti-osteoporotic drugs. It has been emphasized that histomorphometric measurement of cancellous bone should be made in the secondary spongiosa due to the continuing growth of rat skeleton. This should not exclude the concomitant exploration of whether the therapy under investigation also affects the primary spongiosa if the mature rat model with still open epithyses is used. Anabolic agents for bone, which act primarily to stimulate bone formation, have also been evaluated for their efficacy as preventive therapy. Care should be exercised when anabolic agents are studied because such drugs may also increase growth plate activity in the mature rat model or reactivate the growth plate if it is not completed fused in aged rats. Increased growth plate activity can increase cancellous bone volume and confound the interpretation of findings derived from drug therapy.

Limitations of the OVX rat model: The rat OVX model restricts the evaluations to cancellous bone sites in the skeleton. For the evaluation of cortical bone or whole body bone mineral content responses to therapy, the OVX rat model may not be appropriate since the rat does not mimic the postmenopausal women in these respects.

In summary, OVX rat model mimics human condition of osteoporosis in cancellous bone. US FDA, European Regulatory Agency, Japan and other regulatory agencies recommend this model for evaluating the bone efficacy and safety of evaluating anti-osteoporosis agents.

Study Design Using Young Adult OVX Rat Model

As stated above, we can use OVX young adult rat model to test bone efficacy of potential therapeutic agents. To understand the effect of an agent in this model, both short- and long-term studies in prevention mode and restoration model are recommended. Short-term study provides the quick answer to transient effect and long-term study provides steady state effect and bone safety.

Recommendation for short-term prevention study in young adult OVX rats: This model is recommended for the evaluation of the effects of anti-resorptive agents in prevention of bone loss induced by ovariectomy. In our laboratory, we use 4 weeks as the short-term duration for prevention modes (Ke et al., 1998). In such study, treatment should be stared one to two days post-surgery. Ideally, four doses (no effect, ED50, ED100, and a 5-10 time higher than ED100 doses) should be given to the OVX rats. Proximal tibial or distal femoral metaphyseal and lumbar vertebral body cancellous bone mass, structural indices, bone resorption, bone formation, bone turnover and bone strength should be evaluated by dual energy x-ray absorptiometry (DEXA), peripheral quantitative computerized tomography (pQCT), micro-computed tomography (μCT), histomorphometry and bone biomechanical tests. If there is a need, serum bone marker and endocortical bone surface of long bone shaft should also be evaluated.

Recommendation for short-term restoration study in young adult OVX rats: This model is recommended for the evaluation of the effects of anabolic agents in restoring bone mass in established osteopenia, OVX rats. In our laboratory, we use 4 weeks as the short-term duration for restoration modes. In such study, treatment should be given 6 weeks post-surgery to allow the development of cancellous bone osteopenia prior to treatment. Ideally, four doses (no effect, ED50, ED100, and a 5-10 time higher than ED100 doses) should be given to the rats. Proximal tibial or distal femoral metaphyseal and lumbar vertebral body cancellous bone mass, structural indices, bone resorption, bone formation, bone turnover and bone strength should be evaluated by dual energy x-ray absorptiometry (DEXA), peripheral quantitative computerized tomography (pQCT), micro-computed tomography (μCT), histomorphometry and bone biomechanical tests. Long bone shaft should also be evaluated for the cortical bone response to the treatment. If there is a need, serum bone marker should also be evaluated.

Recommendation for long-term prevention study in young adult OVX rats: The "FDA Guidelines For Preclinical and Clinical Evaluation of Agents Used in the Treatment or Prevention of Postmenopausal Osteoporosis (1994)" recommend a 12 month OVX rat study for evaluating anti-resorptive agents' long-term efficacy and bone safety as measured by bone markers, bone density, bone histomorphometry and bone strength. Some anti-resorptive agents have been tested in the 12 months duration (Ma et al., 2002; Ke et al., 2004). However, to the author's experience, 6 months is more appropriate model for this purpose. Therefore, the model recommended is illustrated in the following graph. Three time-points (1, 3 and 6 months) and four doses (no effect, ED50, ED100 and ED500) should be evaluated. Treatment should be given one to two days post-surgery. Proximal tibial or distal femoral metaphyseal and lumbar vertebral body cancellous bone mass, structural indices, bone resorption, bone formation, bone turnover and bone strength should be evaluated by dual energy x-ray absorptiometry

(DEXA), peripheral quantitative computerized tomography (pQCT), histomorphometry and bone biomechanical tests. Long bone shaft should also be evaluated for the cortical bone response to the treatment. If there is a need, serum bone marker should also be evaluated.

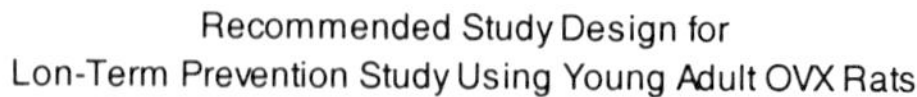
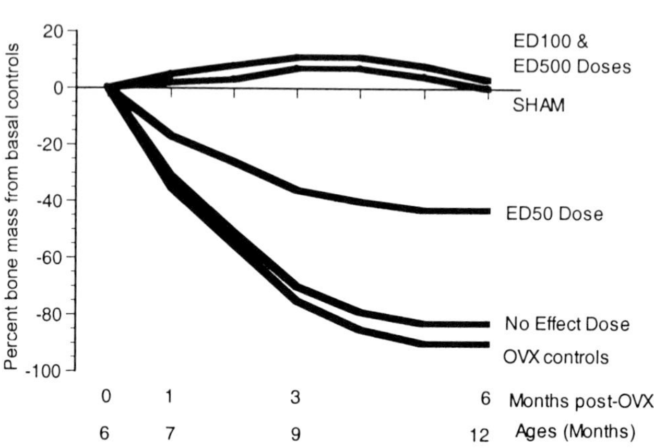

Recommendation for long-term *restoration* study in young adult OVX rats. To test the long-term efficacy and safety of **anabolic agents** in this model, the model recommended is illustrated in the following graph. Treatment should be given 3 months post-surgery to allow the development of osteopenia. Three time-points (1, 3 and 6 months post-treatment) and four doses (no effect, ED50, ED100 and ED500) should be evaluated. Proximal tibial or distal femoral metaphyseal and lumbar vertebral body cancellous bone mass, structural indices, bone resorption, bone formation, bone turnover and bone strength should be evaluated by dual energy x-ray absorptiometry (DEXA), peripheral quantitative computerized tomography (pQCT), histomorphometry and bone biomechanical tests. Long bone shaft should also be evaluated for the cortical bone response to the treatment. If there is a need, serum bone marker should also be evaluated.

The OVX Mouse Model

The adult OVX mice can also be used as a model of postmenopausal bone loss. As in rats, mice experience rapid loss of cancellous bone following OVX. As non-invasive measurement of bone mass and mechanical properties was recently adapted to mice, these animals represent an attractive model. Thus, the amount of tested drug necessary for an in vivo study could be markedly reduced in mice compared to rats.

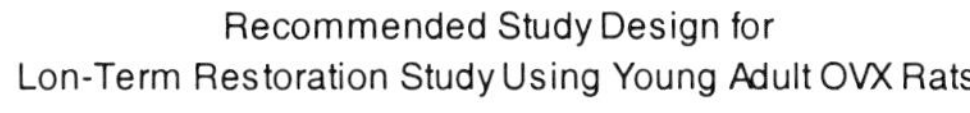

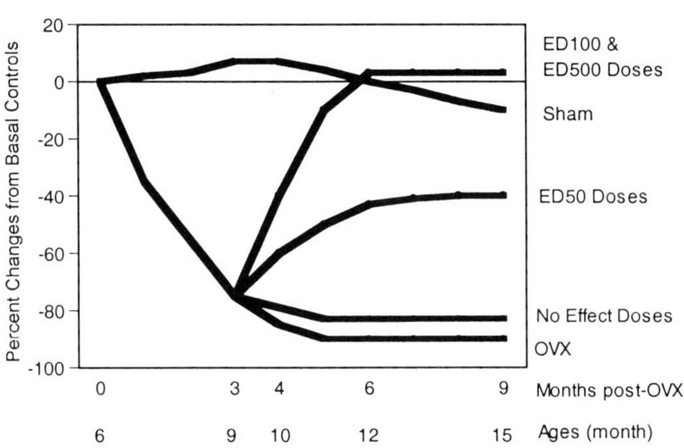

This advantage is especially appreciated with the availability or price of a drug represents a limiting factor for undertaking an in vivo investigation. Furthermore, transgenic technology makes the mouse a desirable animal model for the investigations of genetics of osteoporosis. However, several facts need to keep in mind when use mice as a model for postmenopausal osteoporosis. First, the characterization of bone loss following OVX in mice and the validation of mice as a model for osteoporosis are not as well documented. Secondary, estrogen prevents bone loss in mice mainly by stimulating bone formation in contrast to inhibiting bone resorption as in the humans. Third, there are significant stain and gender differences in aged-related bone changes in mice and its response to therapies.

The OVX Dog Model

The adult dog has always been a reliable model for the adult human skeleton. It is generally similar to the human skeleton in both metabolic and structural characteristics. Skeletal responsiveness of the adult beagle parallels the adult human for corticosteroids, uremia, bisphosphonates, and disuse. However, reports on the responses of dog skeleton to estrogen depletion are conflicting. Such conflicting has made dog as a controversial choice for studying estrogen-depletion bone loss.

The OVX Nonhuman Primate

The nonhuman primate has both growing and adult skeletal phases. It appears that peak bone mass occurs around age 10 years in cynomolgous and rhesus monkeys and baboons. Nonhuman primates have reproductive physiology and endocrinology that closely resembles that of the human females. They have a regular menstrual cycle with an approximate duration of 28 days, which is accompanied with the cycling changes in estrogen and progesterone. Primates experience a natural menopause near the end of second decade of life. More importantly, primates experience decrease bone mass with increased bone turnover following OVX. Decreases in bone mineral density (BMD) evaluated by DEXA are evident at the spine and femoral neck of cynomolgus monkeys as early as 3 to 4 months following OVX. Such decrease in BMD continues at a slower rate with time and reaches its maximum (~ 9 to 10 %) between 6 to 12 months after OVX. A 20% decrease in trabecular bone density of the proximal tibia assessed by pQCT was observed in cynomolgus monkeys. The magnitude of this change offers a large window to monitor the effects of treatment and provides a sensitivity no attainable by DEXA. Biochemical markers of bone turnover such as N-telopeptide (NTx) and skeletal alkaline phosphatase (sALP) are significantly elevated following OVX. The meaningful increase is observed at 3 months and the maximum level attained between 6 to 12 months after OVX. Similar to the findings in humans, treatments with antiresorptive agents such as estrogen and bisphosphonate suppress bone resorption and prevent bone loss in the OVX nonhuman primates.

Extreme requirement for housing and care of nonhuman primates limits their use to relatively small numbers of facilities. Large variance occurs in bone parameters in primate studies, which calls for large numbers of animals in each experimental group in order to achieve adequate statistical power. A sample size of 19 to 25 has been recommended. Acclimatization to laboratory diet is required before using if the monkeys are captured in the wild.

Other OVX Animal Models

The OVX guinea pig, ferret, pig, and sheep have been explored as animal models for postmenopausal bone loss due to the present of Haversian remodeling in these animals. However, the bone loss following OVX in these animals has not been well characterized. More data are needed to validate these animals as in vivo models of osteoporosis.

The Knockout/Transgenic Models

Generation of mice lacking or over-expression genes or growth factors provide an important tool for understanding the physiological role of each gene or growth factor in the skeletal growth, development and maintenance. Appropriate study design is essential for the characterization of the skeletal changes of these mice. At least two to three time-points are needed for the complete understanding of the effects of targeted genes in different life stages. For example, if one wants to understand the effects of targeted gene in early skeletal growth and development, the young, rapid growing phase of mice (such as younger than 3 months of age) will be needed for this purpose. If the purpose of the study is to determine the effects of target gene on peak bone mass, 5-8 month old mice will be needed. To understand the effects of target gene in age-related bone loss, mice older than 12 months will be used. In general speaking, detail characterization of mice in rapid growing (< 3 month old), maturation (5-9 months of age) and age-related bone loss phases (>13 month old) are needed to provide accurate understanding of the role of target gene in the skeleton. Furthermore, detail characterization of all bone surfaces (cancellous, periosteal, endocortical and intracortical surfaces) will provide site-specific information on the effects of target gene (Ke et al., 2002 and 2003).

Summary

There are available animal models for studying the pathophysiology of osteopenia and osteoporosis, and for evaluation of potential therapeutic agents. OVX rat model is the most common one used for such purposes. Appropriate study design is essential. It is recommended that 6- to 9-month-old female rats can be used for these studies. Duration of 4 weeks duration is recommended for the short-term study and duration of 6 months is recommended for the long-term study. Prevention ˙mode is recommended for evaluating anti-resorptive agents and restoration model is recommended for evaluating anabolic agents.

Knockout or transgenic models provide important tools to understand skeletal physiology and pathology. Different ages and different bone sites and all bone surfaces need to be evaluated to gain complete understanding of the targeted genes or factors.

REFERENCES

1.   Ammann P, Rizzoli R, Bonjour J-P Preclinical evaluation of new therapeutic agents for osteoporosis. In Meunier PJ ed., Osteoporosis: Diagnosis and Management. Martin Dunitz, London, UK. 1998, pp 257-273.

2.   Erben RG Skeletal effects of androgen withdrawal. J Musculoskel Neuron Interact 1:225-233; 2001.

3.	Frost HM, Jee WSS On the rat model of human osteopenia and osteoporosis. Bone and Mineral 18: 227-236, 1992.

4.	Jee WSS, Ma YF Animal models of immobilization osteopenia. Morphologie 83:25-34,1999.

5.	Kalu DN The ovariectomized rat model of postmenopausal bone loss. Bone and Mineral 15:175-192, 1991.

6.	Ke HZ, Crawford DT, QI H, Chidsey-Frink KL, Simmons HA, Li M, Jee WSS, Thompson DD Long-term effects of aging and orchidectomy on bone and body composition in rapidly growing male rats. J Musculoskel Neuron Interact 1:215-224; 2001.

7.	Ke HZ, Crawford DT, Qi H, Pirie CM, Simmons HA, Chidsey-Frink KL, Chen HK, Jee WSS, Thompson DD Droloxifene does not blunt bone anabolic effects of prostaglandin E2 but maintains prostaglandin E2-restored bone in aged, ovariectomized rats. Bone 24:41-47, 1999.

8.	Ke HZ, Paralkar VM, Grasser WA, Crawford DT, Qi H, Simmons HA, Pirie CM, Chidsey-Frink KL, Owen TA, Smock SL, Chen HK, Jee WSS, Cameron KO, Rosati RL, Brown TA, DaSilva-Jardine P, Thompson DD Effects of CP-336,156, a new, nonsteroidal estrogen agonist/antagonist, on bone, serum cholesterol, uterus, and body composition in rat models. Endocrinology 139:2068-2076, 1998

9.	Ke HZ, Brown TA, Chidsey-Frink KL, Qi H, Crawford DT, Simmons HA, Petersen DN, Allen MR, McNeish JD, and Thompson DD. The role of estrogen receptor-beta (ER-b) in the early age-related bone gain and later age-related bone loss in female mice. J Musculoskel Neuron Interact 2(5):479-488; 2002.

10.	Ke HZ, Qi H, Weidema AF, Zhang Q, Panupinthu N, Crawford DT, Grasser WA, Paralkar VM, Li M, Audoly LP, Gabel CA, Jee WSS, Dixon SJ, Sims SM, Thompson DD. Deletion of the P2X7 nuceotide receptor reveals its regulatory roles in bone formation and bone resorption. Molecular Endocrinology, 17:1356-1367, 2003.

11.	Ke HZ, Foley GL, Simmons HA, Shen V, Thompson DD Long-term treatment of lasofoxifene preserves bone mass and bone strength and does not adversely affect the uterus in ovariectomized rats. Endocrinology 145:1996-2005; 2004.

12.	Li M, Shen Y, Wronski TJ Time course of femoral neck osteopenia in ovariectomized rats. Bone 20:55-61, 1997.

13.	Ma YL, Bryant HU, Zeng Q, Palkowitz A, Jee WSS, Turner CH, Sato M Long-term dosing of arzoxifene lowers cholesterol, reduces bone turnover, and preserves bone quality in ovariectomized rats. J Bone Miner Res 17:2256-2264, 2002

14.   Shen V, Birchman R, Xu R, Lindsay R, Dempster DW Short-term changes in histomorphometric and biochemical turnover markers and bone mineral density in estrogen- and/or dietary calcium-deficient rats. Bone 16:149-156, 1995.

15.   Thompson DD, Simmons HA, Pirie, CM, Ke HZ FDA guidelines and animal models for osteoporosis. Bone 17: 125S-133S, 1995.

CHAPTER 19

PREVENTION AND TREATMENT OF OSTEOPOROSIS WITH TRADITIONAL HERBAL MEDICINE

QIN Ling,[1] ZHANG Ge,[1,2] SHI Yenyu,[2] LEE Kwongman,[3]
LEUNG Pingcheung[1,4]

Dept. of Orthopaedics and Traumatology, The Chinese University of Hong Kong (CUHK), Hong Kong SAR, PR China

Suguang Hospital, Shanghai University of Chinese Medicine, PR China

Lee Hysan Clinical Research Laboratory, CUHK, Hong Kong SAR, PR China

Institute of Chinese Medicine, CUHK, Hong Kong SAR, PR China

'Kidney tonifying' herbal medicine has been traditionally using in treatment of fractures, joint diseases, and gonadal dysfunctions in Asia for thousands of years. In the last 2 decades, many such herbal formulae have also been developed and evaluated clinically in small-scale trials for prevention and treatment of osteoporosis. In order to explore the potential underlying mechanisms as to how these herbs or herbal formulae work on their target cells, tissues or organs, both *in vitro* and *in vivo* experimental studies have been conduced. The related English literature is however lacking and majority of such studies are published in local journals, such as in China. Up to date, no single herb or herbal component has been found to be effective since osteoporosis is a multifactorial deteriorating skeletal condition. Phytoestrogen, found in many herbs or plants, shows structural similarities to estrogen and binds to estrogen receptors, suggesting an important pathway for maintaining bone mineral homeostasis and as a bioactive component in quality assurance. This paper provides a brief overview of the herbal preparations developed for the prevention and treatment of estrogen deficiency induced bone loss in rodent animals and postmenopausal women. The outcomes of the majority of the previous investigations are encouraging. This warrants further studies, including identification and purification of active components for development of new herbal formulae and evidence-based clinical trials in prevention and treatment of osteoporosis and its related medical conditions. The potential beneficial effects on non-skeletal elements associated with prevention of fragility fractures are also briefly mentioned. In order to enhance the quality of the research, "General Guidelines for Research & Development of Herbal Medicine and Evaluation of Its Efficacy in the Prevention and Treatment of Osteoporosis and Fragility Fractures" have therefore been proposed.

1. Introduction
2. Efficacy-driven approach in studying traditional herbal medicine
3. Preclinical studies
4. Clinical trials
5. Safety and toxicity of herbal medicine
6. General Guidelines to be established for further R&D and evaluation of tradition herbal medicine
7. Summary

1. Introduction

Epidemiological studies suggest that the incidence of osteoporosis varies among populations or ethnic groups.[1] It has been reported that the lower incidence menopausal symptoms, osteoporosis and associated fractures in Japanese women may be associated with high consumption of dietary phytoestrogens, a diverse group of compounds found in many edible plants or herbs, as compared with the rest of the industrialized world.[2-5]

Phytoestrogen has been categorized according to their chemical structures into isoflavones, lignans, and coumestants. The most estrogenically active ones are genistein and daidzein of the isoflavones.[2,3,6,7] Yin Yang Huo (YYH) (*Epimedium Leptorhizum*) is an herb used as one of the most important herbs in "kidney-tonifying' formulae in Traditional Chinese Medicine,. YYH is identified with such bioactive element (Fig. 1),[6-9] which has been developed for the treatment of fractures and joint diseases, gonadal dysfunctions and for relieving menopausal related symptoms over thousands of years.[10-12] At present, more than 40 herbs or their preparations have been claimed to be effective for the treatment of gynecological diseases including low back pain and postmenopausal osteoporosis.[3-6,10-16] Therefore, herbals with YYH as main component have been recently developed and evaluated for the prevention and treatment of osteoporosis in Asian countries like China[6,10-15] and Japan (mostly found in preclinical evaluation)[17-20]

Recent data suggests that traditional medicine has been integrated well into the health systems of many Asian countries such as China, Japan, North and South Korea, and Vietnam. In western countries such as France and Germany, there are growing number of patients rely on alternative medicine for preventive or palliative care, including the interests in herbal products for prevention of menopausal related medical conditions.[5,6,21-23]

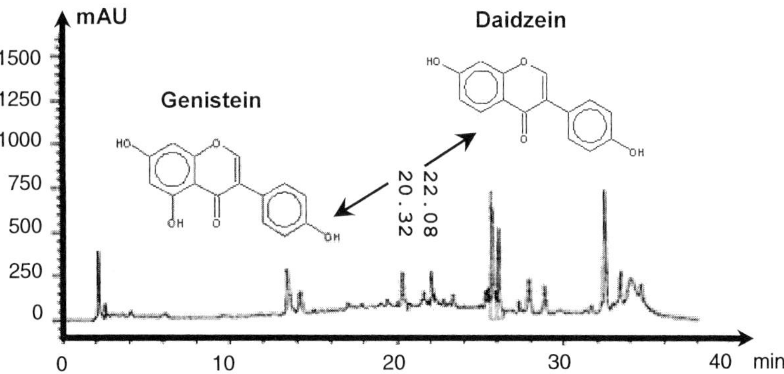

Fig. 1. The levels of phytoestrogen used for the studies reported in the references [6,7,15] are detected using high-performance liquid chromatography (HPLC). HPLC chromatograms of extracts from the herbal formula Xianlingubao (仙灵骨葆) with Yin Yang Huo (Epimedium Leptorhizum) as main component. Spiked with genistein (20.321mAU) and daidzein (22.084mAU).

2. Efficacy-driven approach in studying traditional herbal medicine

In evaluation of herbal medicine for the prevention of osteoporosis, the efficacy shall be established, i.e. a therapeutic or scientific rationale must exist for the presence of each herb in the mixture. If the active ingredients with the therapeutic activity have been identified, the preparation of these products should be standardized to contain a defined amount of the active ingredients. In addition, "in cases where it is not possible to identify the active ingredients, the whole herbal product may be considered as one active ingredient".[24] The efficacy of herbal products can be present in three aspects as recommended by WHO,[24] including

2.1. Characterizing compound (may differ from active ingredients)

A natural constituent of herbal part that may be used to assure the identity or quality of herbal preparation, but this is not necessarily responsible for the herbal biological or therapeutic activity.

2.2. Biological activity

Changes in the baseline function of an animal or part of an animal brought about by the administration of a test herbal preparation or product (e.g. phytoestrogen has been proposed as one of the major active components in herbal preparations or products for prevention or treatment of osteoporosis. As the concentration of isoflavone varies from species to species, quality control is essential.[9,25]

2.3. Therapeutic activity

An intervention that results in the amelioration of the manifestations of osteoporosis and fragility fractures of patients. Studies compared "mechanism-based research to drug development in conventional medicine" with "the proposed efficacy-driven approach advocated for the advancement of Traditional Chinese Medicine". An efficacy-driven approach can avoid basic research done on therapies that are clinically ineffective, thus sparing precious research resources.[26,27]

3. Preclinical studies

The general significance of preclinical studies involves pharmacodynamics, safety, and toxicity in research and development

(R&D) of any new agent.[24] Since many traditional herbs and their combinations or formulae have been tested in human subjects, many preclinical studies aimed at using modern science and technologies to validate or evaluate potential underlying mechanisms related to treatment efficacy of these agents using in vitro and vivo experimental models.[23,26] This also applies to evaluation of traditional herbal medicine for prevention and treatment of osteoporosis.[28]

3.1. In vivo experimental studies

A total of 123 papers related to herbal medicine and osteoporosis have been found to be published in 36 journals between 1990 and 2003 in our literature search using Chinese literature databases CMCC (Chinese Medical Current Contents; http://www.39.net/Super_DB/cmcc/cmcc.asp)" and CBMdisc (Chinese Biology Medical Disc; http://www.imicams.ac.cn/cbmdisc/cbmdisc.htm) and limited number in Medline Search that are mainly from Japanese research groups.[17-20] We evaluated oral administration of YYH preparation (Miegu Capsule) and its dosing effects in adult OVX rats.[29] The pQCT evaluation showed that 0.2g/kg oral administration of YYH preparation was effective in preventing osteoporosis in weight-bearing proximal femur and tibia of OVX rats, with a significant 13.3% and 17.8% higher trabecular BMD in proximal femur and tibia as compared with controls (Fig. 2a); while Raloxifene treatment showed preventive effects in the spine (Fig. 2b). A recent OVX rat experimental study on a phytoestrogen-rich herbal formula Xianlingubao (XLGB, 仙灵骨葆) (the general one: genistein/daidzein, 250mAU, or equivalent to Genistein510μg/g, Daidzein2500μg/g, each as shown in Figure 1; and formula specific one: Icariin9200 μg/g, Psoralen930μg/g and Isopsoralen950μg/g), showed that XLGB, calcium, and XLGB with calcium intervention had significant preventive effects against OVX induced bone loss in proximal femur, however, without significant additive effects when XLGB and calcium were combined (Fig. 3a-c), which was explained by effects on both anti-bone resorption and promoting bone formation using biochemical markers (osteocalcin and DPD/Cr levels) and hormone

                                      L. Qin et al.

levels such as PTH.[7] Studies on another commercial available herbal preparation Gushukang also showed similar effects for prevention of osteoporosis in Chinese literature.[30-32]

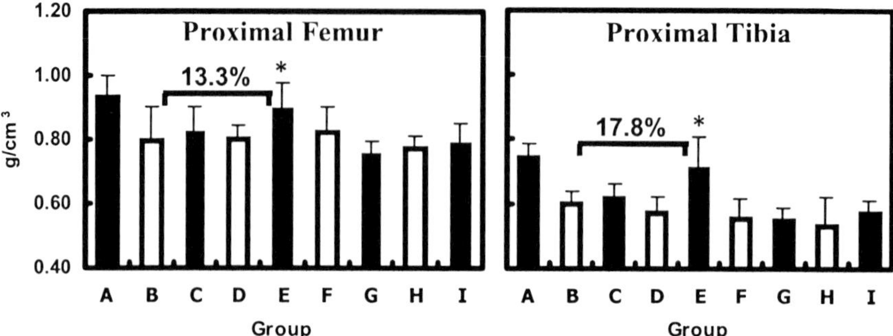

Fig. 2a: pQCT tBMD of proximal femur / proximal tibia in rats at age 11 months (evaluated 3 months after OVX and drug intervention). A: Sham; B: OVX; C: High dose herbal; D: Middle dose herbal; E: Low dose herbal; F: Raloxifene; G: VitD3; H: Total flavone extract of herbal; I: Total polysaccharide extract of herbal. (*: p<0.05 compared with other groups).

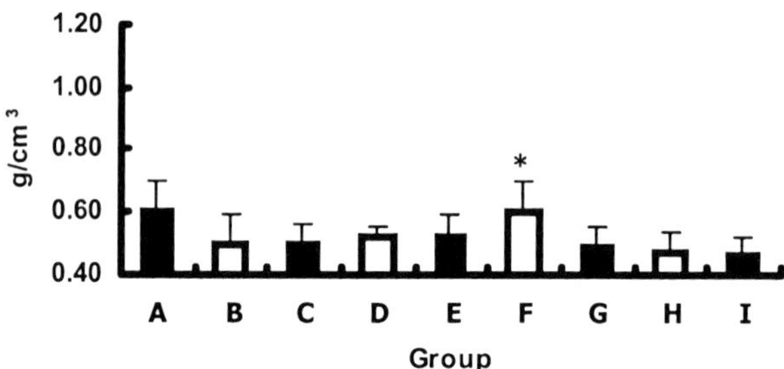

Fig. 2b. pQCT tBMD of spine (L2) in rats at age 11 months (evaluated 3 months after OVX and drug intervention). A: Sham; B: OVX; C: High dose herbal; D: Middle dose herbal; E: Low dose herbal; F: Raloxifene; G: VitD3; H: Total flavone extract of herbal; I: Total polysaccharide extract of herbal. (*: p<0.05 compared with other groups)

A most recent published study in English literature was from Xu and co-worker,[33] who examined the effects of an extract of ten medicinal herbs on estrogen deficiency bone loss in rats. BMD and mechanical strength were used as end-point measure. The urinary pyridinoline creatinine ratio, deoxypyridinoline creatinine ratio, plasma alkaline phosphatase, calcium, phosphorus and albumin were also determined to explain the potential underlying mechanism of gerbil action. The results revealed that the herbal extract developed for the study demonstrated a therapeutic effect in inhibiting bone resorption and reducing estrogen-dependent bone loss and decrease in bone strength without uterine stimulation by measuring uterine weight.

As osteoporosis and fragility fractures are closely associated with many non-skeletal intrinsic and extrinsic factors, muscle structure and function have been emphasized in the Utah paradigm mechanostat.[34,35] Our recent experimental findings showed that phytoestrogen-rich herb formula 'XLGB' prevents OVX-induced deterioration of bone and fast twitch muscles at hip in aged rats(Fig. 4-6).[36,37]

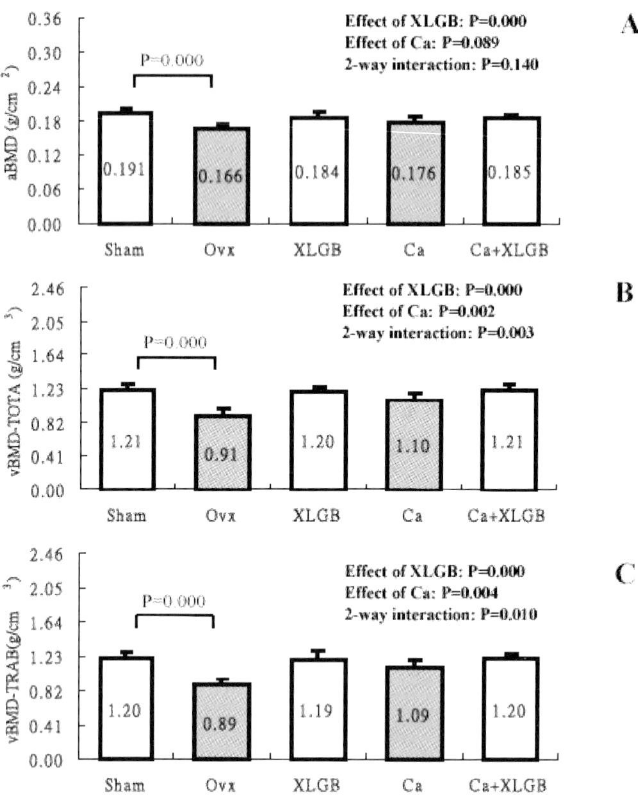

Fig. 3. 3a: aBMD (areal BMD measured by DXA); 3b: vBMD-TOTA(pQCT volumetric BMD measured within total volume of proximal femur); 3c: vBMD-TRAB(pQCT volumetric BMD measured within 50% of core volume of the proximal femur). Immediately postovariectomy, Ovariectomized rats orally received vehicle (Ovx), XLGB (250mg/kg body weight/day), Calcium Citrate (65mg/kg body weight/day) and combination of XLGB 仙灵骨葆 (250mg/kg body weight/day) and Calcium Citrate (65mg/kg body weight/day). Statistical comparisons between the vehicle-treated Sham and Ovx groups were made with a two-sided t test. The prevention effect of XLGB and Ca as well as their interaction in OVX rats were analyzed by two-way factorial ANOVA. Each bar represents the mean ± SD of 7-9 rats.

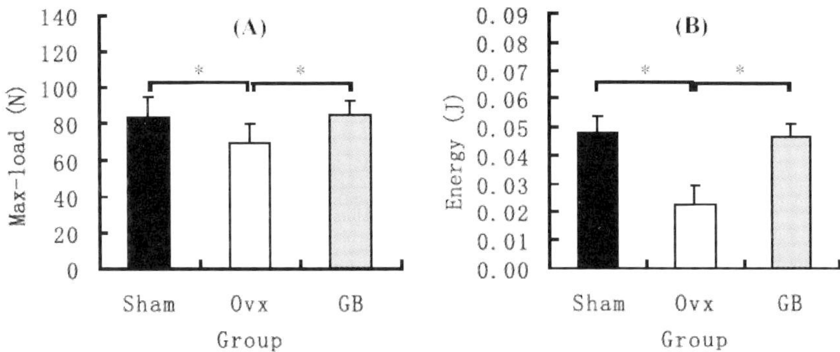

Fig. 4 (A) The effect of XLGB(GB) on Max-load (in fall configuration) of proximal femur in aged ovx rat model. * P<0.05. (n=7~9) (B) The effect of XLGB(GB) on Energy (in fall configuration) of proximal femur in aged ovx rat model. * P<0.05. (n=7~9)

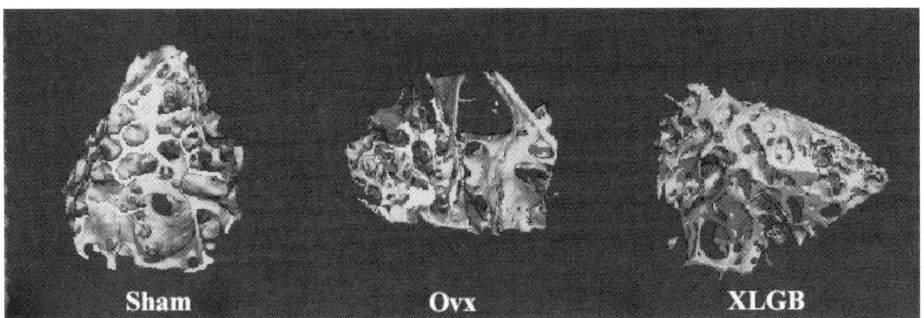

Fig. 5 3-D architecture of weight-beraing trabecular bone of aged ovx rat proximal femur in respective group, using Micro-CT (micro40, Scanco Medical, Switzerland).

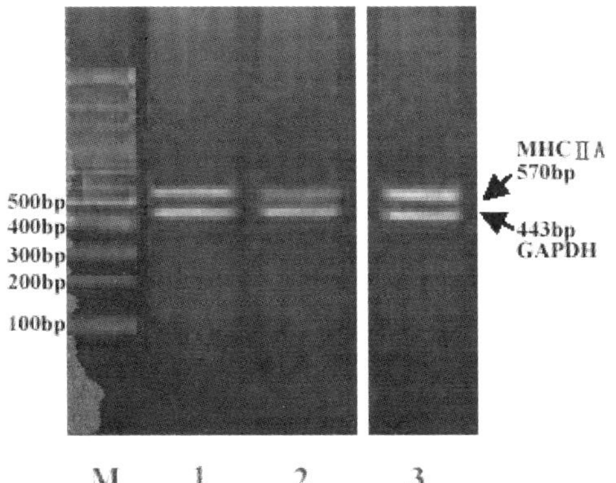

Fig. 6 Representative electrophoresis images of RT-PCR products for mRNA level of **Myosin Heavy Chain IIA** gene (typing fast twitch muscle fiber) from quadriceps muscle samples in respective group.
M: Marker, 1: Sham, 2: Ovx, 3: XLGB

3.2 In vitro mechanistic studies

In vitro studies are helpful to elaborate potential underlying mechanisms of herbal formulae using cell culture models, which may partially explain their biological functions in bone mineral homeostasis in vivo. Studies showed various potential pathways or multitargets of herbal formulae with YYH as the main component, including 1) restoration of the activities of $Ca^{2}+$ - ATPase and $Mg^{2}+$ -ATPase in erythrocyte membrane, which underlies the preventive and therapeutic effect of the drugs on osteoporosis due to kidney-asthenia.[38] 2) acceleration of secretion of collagen as well as deposition of mineral and formation of bone nodules.[39] 3) promotion of RNA synthesis in growth and maturation of osteoblasts and the activity of osteoblasts and/or anti-osteoclastic resorption.[40-43] Though the exact mechanism of the YYH herbal formulae, the prevention of estrogen deficiency induced bone loss is not well understood, its potential estrogenic function via its phytoestrogen elements seems to be important.[2-7]

4. Clinical trials

Randomized and controlled trials are required in studying efficacy of herbal medicine.[24,44] Up to date, there is no clinical trial on herbal medicine for prevention and treatment of osteoporosis and fragility fractures published in indexed English literature, except conference reports and degree thesis.[6,45,45] The available studies are found in Chinese literature, and our search using "CMCC" and "CBMdisc" databases show a total of 39 papers in 18 journals published between 1990 and 2003. These published ones were small-scale clinical trails with short duration from 4 to 24 months. They generally showed positive effects of YYH herbal formulae in prevention or retardation of postmenopausal bone loss.[6,12-15,32]

Xu[46] reported a 4-month randomization double-blinded, placebo-controlled clinical trial in 90 Chinese postmenopausal women with low BMD (lower than −1SD) at the lumbar spine. Herbal capsules composed of YYH and other four herbs were administrated orally and 3 capsules/time, 3 times/day. BMD was measured using dual energy X-ray absorptiometry (DXA) at lumbar spine at baseline and 4-month follow up. Biochemical markers were also measured. The results showed that the percentage changes of the lumbar L1-4 BMD in the placebo (n=30) were −1.9+3.6 (p<0.02), while in the groups treated by the herbal capsules (n=30) and estrogen capsules (n=30) were +0.3±2.4 and +0.1±4.0 (p<0.05 each, vs. placebo group) respectively. Herbal treatment showed a significant effect in inhibiting bone resorption via monitoring bone turnover markers. A most recent 24-month follow-up clinical trial reported by Shi demonstrated that the invigorating kidney formula resulted in an average 4.5% increase in femoral BMD of osteoporotic patients.[14,15] This increase was found to be similar to that in patients treated with hormone replacement therapy (HRT) or Vitamin D supplement. The YYH formula XLGB is one of the commercially available herbal products with 5 different herbs, which was evaluated by authors in a small case-control trail in postmenopausal women treated with 4 tablets daily oral XLGB for 1 year. Each tablet contains 0.35 g YYH formula, with a concentration $510\mu g/g$ genistein and $2500\mu g/g$ daidzein (refer to Fig. 1). Similar preventive treatment effects were found for BMD from both DXA and pQCT in both axial and extremity skeletons, except the femoral neck measured by DXA (Fig. 7a.b).[6]

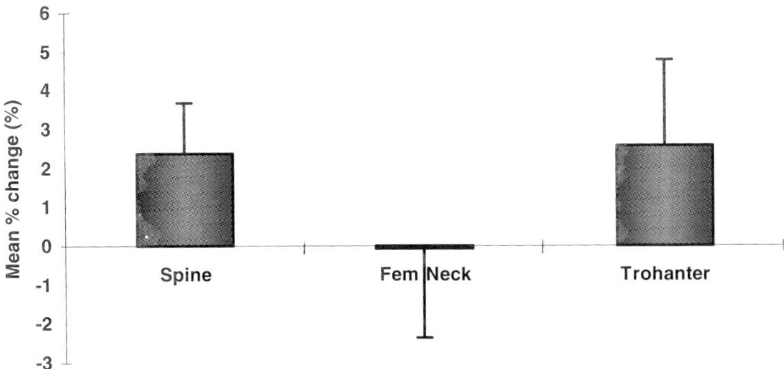

Fig. 7a. One year Xianlingubao (XLGB, 仙灵骨葆) treatment in elderly women at spin and hip: BMD maintained or increased in spin and femoral trochanter but not at femoral neck as measured by DXA. Data interpreted in percentage changes between follow-up and baseline (n=14).

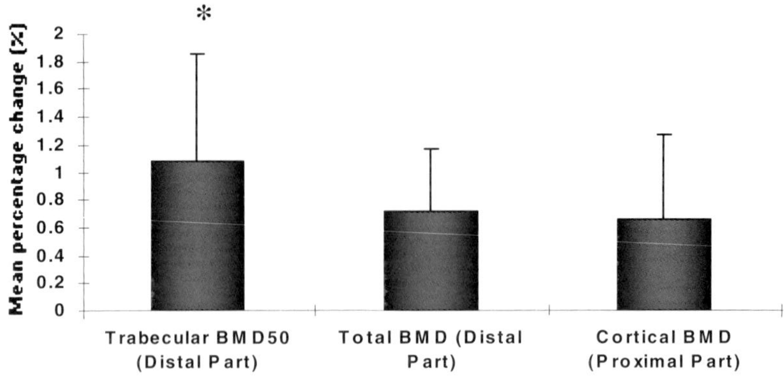

Fig. 7b. One year Xianlingubao (XLGB, 仙灵骨葆) treatment in elderly women at distal radius: BMD maintained or increased in all parts of distal radius of non-dominant forearm as measured by a multislice pQCT (Densiscan 2000) spin and femoral trochanter but not femoral neck (n=14) (*: p<0.05 as compared with baseline).

Comparing western drugs with well-defined mechanisms in increasing or at least maintaining BMD, traditional Chinese herbal products may not be able to induce significant measurable effects in terms of increase in BMD. However, when clinical complications of osteoporosis, i.e. fragility fractures are used as the end-point, risk-based approach (fragility fracture related risk factors) should be adopted.[47-49] This suggests that TCM herbal formulae, preparations or products, which may demonstrate effects, e.g. in maintaining muscle function[36,37] but may not demonstrate measurable effects in the prevention of bone loss, may be beneficial in reducing risk factors of fall (such as Dementia, arthritis/leg weakness, gait/balance problem, impaired eyesight, etc) and fall-related fragility fractures in old people.[47-49] This implies that its efficacy in overall strategy of osteoporosis prevention and treatment.[47-49]

5. Safety and toxicity of herbal preparations

Given the tremendous expansion in the use of traditional medicine worldwide, safety and efficacy as well as quality control of herbal medicines and traditional procedure-based therapies have become important concerns for both health authorities and the public.[23,24] Reported and documented side-effects of traditional herbal medicine in terms of a herb or mixture, its closely related species, constituents of the herb and its preparations or herbal products should be taken into account when decisions are made about the need for new pharmacological or toxicological studies. The absence of any reported or documented side-effect does not provide any absolute assurance of safety. However, a full range of related tests might not be necessary.[24,50]

Table 1: Heavy metals and toxic elements of YYH herbal formula as compared with HK diet standard

Heavy metal and Toxic elements	HK Standard*	YYH formula used for the reported studies.[6,7,15]
Arsenic (As$_2$O$_3$)	1.4 mg/kg	0.9mg/kg
Lead (Pb)	6.0 mg/kg	0.3mg/kg
Mercury (Hg)	0.5 mg/kg	<0.04mg/kg
Cadmium (Cd)	0.1 mg/kg	<0.04mg/kg
Chromium (Cr)	1.0 mg/kg	0.4mg/kg
Antimony (Sb)	1.0 mg/kg	0.04mg/kg
Tin (Sn)	230 mg/kg	0.1 mg/kg
Calcium (Ca)	/	3400mg/kg

*: Hong Kong Food Adulteration (Metallic Contamination) Regulations Maximum Permitted Concentration of Certain Metals present in Specified Foods (using fish or fish products or food in solid form. Note: the consumption of daily herbal preparation is 1.5g but the consumption of fish product for one meal may vary from a few grams to a few hundred grams. Therefore, the total amount of the substances in the herbal preparation listed in the table is fact much less than that as compared with consuming fish products (evaluated by SGS Hong Kong Ltd. Bio-Science Division (Member of the SGS Group).

As for herbal medicines, which have been traditionally using over thousands of years for the treatment of gynecological and bone disorders, are known to have no or low toxicity. To date, there are no reports or observations from our current research to show that the herbal preparation YYH may have side effects for the treatment of estrogen deficiency induced bone loss. The potentially toxic chemical composition of YYH preparations used for above mentioned studies[6,7,15] meet the Hong Kong standards for the concentrations of heavy metals and toxic elements in food (Table 1).

6. General guidelines to be established for further R&D and evaluation of tradition herbal medicine

Unlike the approved chemically synthesized western medicines for prevention and treatment of osteoporosis, traditional herbal preparations have large variations in compositions, even for herb YYH products from different regions.[9,24] This makes a direct comparison among the published studies difficult, especially with diversity in study design found in both experimental and clinical studies, such as, age, duration of intervention, evaluation methods used, data interpretation etc.

Western anti-osteoporosis drugs with known mechanisms have been well developed over the years to increase and maintain bone mass, setting standards for the evaluation of their efficacy in preventing osteoporosis and osteoporotic fractures. In 1998, WHO published an important document on "Guidelines for Preclinical Evaluation and Clinical Trials in Osteoporosis".[48] However, in this document, no specific considerations have been made on the role of traditional medicine in the prevention of osteoporosis and osteoporotic fractures. Two year later, WHO also finalized the "General Guidelines for Methodologies on Research and Evaluation of Traditional Medicine" at a WHO consultation held in Hong Kong in 2000,[24] but no specific guidelines were made on the application of Traditional Medicine (herbal preparations or products) in the prevention and treatment of osteoporosis and its associated complications, i.e. fragility fractures.

"In conducting research and evaluation of traditional medicine, knowledge and experience obtained through the long history of established practices should be respected".[24-27] However, we may still need to document and centralize data for peer-review and critical analysis to gain insight into the quantity and quality of the safety and efficacy issues of traditional herbal products used in the prevention and treatment of osteoporosis and fragility fractures. This suggests an urgent need to set up an expert panel to establish corresponding "General Guidelines", which have been proposed as "General Guidelines for Research & Development (R&D) of Herbal Medicine and Evaluation of Its Efficacy in the Prevention and Treatment of Osteoporosis and Fragility Fractures" and should serve as a reference source for researchers, health care providers, manufacturers, and health authorities.[28,51] The foundation to complete this ""General Guidelines" shall be based on the above-mentioned two WHO's guidelines and available Chinese Documentations related to traditional Chinese medicine.[52,53]

As osteoporosis is now generally accepted as a systemic skeletal deterioration characterized by low bone mineral density (density factor), deterioration of the bone structure (structural factor) and increased fragility (strength factor) of the bone resulting in increased risk of osteoporotic fractures,[48,49] systematic evaluations on herbal effects shall be an evidence-based approach, not only based on evaluation of its potential protective effects on skeletons using the State-of-the Art biotechnologies, including various clinical densitometry[54,55] but also on nonskeletal factors, which may be beneficial to reduce fragility fractures.

8. Summary

Chinese herbal preparations developed for the prevention and treatment of osteoporosis is generally safe and effective for retardation and prevention of estrogen deficiency induced bone loss, deterioration of the bone structure and mechanical strength. This warrants further studies, including identification and purification of active components for the development of new herbal formulae and efficacy-driven or evidence-based clinical trials in the prevention and treatment of osteoporosis and its related medical conditions, especially its role in reducing fragility fractures. In order to meet the demands of modern sciences, 'General Guidelines' related to R&D of herbal medicine and evaluation of efficacy in the prevention and treatment of osteoporosis and fragility fractures have also been proposed.

Acknowledgments

This work was supported by a grant from the Research Grants Council of the Hong Kong Special Administrative Regions, with the reference Number: RGC Earmarked CUHK4097/01M.

REFERENCES

1.   Riggs BL, Melton LJ. The world-wide problem of osteoporosis: insights afforded by epidemiology. Bone 17:505-511, 1995

2.   Ramsey LA, Ross BS, Fischer RG. Phytoestrogens and the management of menopause. Adv Nurse Practitioners 7:26-30, 1999

3.   Lien LL, Lien EJ. Hormone therapy and phytoestrogens. J Clin Pharm Therap 21(2):101-111, 1996

4.   Cohen DP. Anti-Osteoporotic Medications: Traditional and nontraditional. Clin Obst Gynecol 46(2):341-348, 2003

5.   Prestwood KM. Editorial: The search for alternative therapies for menopausal women: Estrogenic effects of herbs. J Clin Endocrinol Metabol 88(9):4075-4076, 2003

6.   Qin L. R&D of Herbal Formulae for Prevention and Treatment of Osteoporosis. Proceedings pp112-120, 2002 International Bone Research Instructional Course and Hands-on Workshop, Hong Kong, October 17-19, 2002

7.   Qin L, Zhang G, Hung WY, Dambacher MA, Leung PC. Phytoestrogen-rich herbal formula for prevention of OVX induced bone loss in rats. J Bone Miner Res 17(suppl-1):479, 2002

8.   韩立民，刘波，徐彭.淫羊藿总黄酮对成骨细胞增殖的影响.上海中医药杂志.37(6): 55-57，2003 (Han LM, Liu Bo, Xu P. Influence of herba epimedii flavone on proliferation of osteoblasts. Shanghai J Trad Chin Med 37(6):55-57, 2003)

9.   郭宝林. 中国淫羊霍属植物总黄酮含量及资源前景. 中药材 (9):13-14, 1993 (Guo BL. Contents and prospects of resource of herba epimedii flavone in China. J Chin Med Mater 16(9): 13-14, 1993)

10. Yin J, Guo L (eds). Modern Study and Clinical Applications on Chinese Materia Medica. Xue Yuan Press, Beijing, pp382-652, 1993

11. 张大新，蒋天裕，王丽丽，等.中药治疗骨质疏松症腰腿痛症状机理探讨.中国康复理论与实践.7(2):84-85，2001 (Zhang DX, Jiang TY, Wang LL, et al. Effect of Xianlinggubao tablet on bone pain resutlt from osteoporosis. Chin J Rehab Theo Prac 7(2):84-85, 2001)

12. An SJ. Effect of kidney-tonifying herbs on ovary function and bone mass in postmenopausal women. Chin J Osteoporosis 6(2):55-59, 2000

13. 李峭峰，谭朝晖，谢晓青，等.中药骨补方对骨质疏松症患者疼痛及骨密度的影响.中国临床康复.7(11):1666-1667，2003 (Li QF, Tan ZH, Xie XQ, et al. The effects of traditional bone tonifying prescription on pain and bone density in patients with osteoporosis. Chin J Clin Rehab 7(11):1666-1667, 2003)

14. Shi YY et al. Comparative study of four Chinese formulas on prevention of osteoporosis. Chin J Osteoporosis. 4(3):68-70, 1998

15. Shi YY. Summary report on Xianlingubao capsule for treatment of osteoporosis – clinical investigations. Int J Chin Orthop 2(2):18-21, 2000

16. Cheng J, Lee P, Li J, Dennehy CE, Tsourounis C. Use of Chinese herbal products in Oakland and San Francisco Chinatowns. Am J Health-System Pharma 61(7):688-694, 2004

17. Hidaka S, Okamoto Y, Nakajima K, Suekawa M, Liu SY. Preventive effects of traditional Chinese (Kampo) medicines on experimental osteoporosis induced by ovariectomy in rats. Calcif Tissue Int 61(3):239-246, 1997

18. Hidaka S, Okamoto Y, Yamada Y, Kon Y, Kimura T, A Japanese herbal medicine, Chujo-to, has a beneficial effect on osteoporosis in rats. Phytother Res 13(1):14-19, 1999

19. Sakamoto S, Sassa S, Kudo H, Suzuki S, Mitamura T, Shinoda H. Preventive effects of a herbal medicine on bone loss in rats treated with a GnRH agonist. Euro J Endocrinol 143(1):139-42, 2000

20. Sassa S, Sakamoto S, Zhou YF, Mori T, Kikuchi T, Shinoda H. Preventive effects of a Chinese herbal medicine, hochu-ekki-to, on bone loss in ovariectomized rats. In Vivo 15(1):25-8, 2001

21. Kass-Annese B. Alternative therapies for menopause. Clin Obstet Gynecol 43(1):162-183, 2000

22. WHO 1998. World Health Organization. Regulatory situation of herbal medicines: a worldwide review. Geneva, World Health Organization, 1998

23. WHO 2003: WHO Traditional Medicine Strategy 2002-2005: http://www.who.int/medicines/organization/trm/orgtrmmain.shtml. World Health Organization, 2003

24. WHO 2000. General Guidelines for Methodologies on Research and Evaluation of Traditional Medicine. Geneva, World Health Organization, 2000

25. WHO 1998. World Health Organization. Quality control methods for medical plant materials. Geneva, World Health Organization, 1998

26. Tang JL, Leung PC. An efficacy-driven approach to the research and development of traditional Chinese medicine. HK Med J 7(4):375-380, 2001

27. Lewith GT, Breen A, Filshie J, Fisher P, McIntyre M, Mathie R, Peters D. Complementary medicine: evidence base, competence to practice and regulation. Clin Med 3(3):235-240, 2003

28. Qin L. Call for establishing international standards for research & development of herbal medicine in the prevention and treatment of osteoporosis. The 2nd HOMA Awarding Ceremony & 2003 International Osteoporosis Conf Proc pp77-83, Beijing, October 19-22, 2003

29. Qin L, Shi YY, Lu HB, Zhang G, Hung YW, Leung PC. Bone mineral density and structural evaluation on preventive effects Chinese herbal preparation in oariectomy-induced osteoporosis in rats. International Symposium on Bone Biotechnology and Histotechnology, Phoenix, Arizona, USA, Proceedings p30, 2001

30. Xiong XH, Liu QS, Yu KQ. Effects of GuKang on bone Gla-protein in serum and bone mineral density in the ovariectomized rats. Chin J Trad Med Traumatol Orthop 10(2):14-16, 2002

31. Cui SQ. Prevention and treatment of osteoporosis in rats induced by retinoic acid with Gushukang combined with calcium. Chin J Osteoporosis 5(2):74-77, 1999

32. 王长海，王文，李军昌.中药骨松康治疗绝经后骨质疏松症临床疗效观察.中国骨质疏松杂志 9(2):165-166，131，2003 (Wang CH, Wang W, Li JC. Clinical efficacy of Gusongkang capsule in treatment of postmenopausal osteoporosis. Chin J Osteoporosis 9(2):165-166,131,2003)

33. Xu M, Dick IM, Day R, Randall D, Prince RL. Effects of a herbal extract on the bone density, strength and markers of bone turnover of mature ovariectomized rats. Am J Chin Med 31(1):87-101, 2003

34. Frost HM. From Wolff's law to the Utah paradigm: insights about bone physiology and its clinical applications. Anat Rec 262(4):398-419, 2001

35. Ferretti JL, Cointry GR, Capozza RF, Frost HM. Bone mass, bone strength, muscle-bone interactions, osteopenias and osteoporoses. Mechanisms Ageing Devel 124(3):269-79, 2003

36. Qin L, Zhang Z, Hung WY, Shi YY, Leung PC, Leung KS. Phytoestrogen-rich herb formula 'GB' prevents OVX-induced deterioration of muscuoloskeletal tissues at hip in aged rats. The First Asian Pacific Congress of Bone Histomorphometry, Takamatsu, Japan, June 22-24, 2004

37. Zhang Ge. Biomechanical Signaling Regulation and Control Systems: Interaction between Upper-stream muscle genes' and down-stream bone materials, structure and strength" PhD thesis, Shanghai University of Chinese Medicine, China, 2003

38. Cui JP. Effects of kidney-tonifying traditional Chinese drugs on activities of protein kinase C and Ca2+ -Mg2+ -ATPase in erythrocyte membrane. Chin J Osteoporosis 3(3):66-69, 1997

39. Xu RH. Histochemical study on effect of Radix Savial Miltorrhizae on growth of isolated cells from embryonic chicken frontal bone cultured in vitro. Chin J Traditional Western Med 11(11):668-670, 1991

40. Li H, Miyahara T, Tezuka Y, Namba T, Nemoto N, Tonami S, Seto H, Tada T, Kadota S. The effect of Kampo formulae on bone resorption in vitro and in vivo. I. Active constituents of Tsu-kan-gan. Biol Pharma Bulletin 21(12):1322-1326, 1998

41. Jin WF, Wang HF, Wei DL, Zhao YF, Shi YY. Comparative study among several Chinese herbals for proliferation of osteoblasts and mineralization – an in vitro model. Symposium on Prevention of Osteoporosis in Elderly, Proc. pp17-21, Ximan, China 2000

42. Lin YP. The effect of experimental fracture healing treated by Bu GU Su – Observation on osteoblast RNA an studies on blood biochemistry. Chin J Orthop Trauma 6(1):8-11, 1993

43. Yu S, Chen K, Li S, Zhang K. In vitro and in vivo studies of the effect of a Chinese herb medicine on osteoclastic bone resorption. Chin J Dental Res 2(1):7-11, 1999

44. Kronenberg F, Fugh-Berman A. Complementary and alternative medicine for menopausal symptoms: A review of randomized, controlled trials. Ann Int Med 137(10):805-813, 2002

45. Shi YY. Application of Chinese herbs to primary osteoporosis: Comprehensively improving the bone quality. 2002 International Bone Research Instructional Course and Hands-on Workshop. Proc. pp104-111, Hong Kong, October 17-19, 2002

46.   Xu M. Treatment and prevention of postmenopausal osteoporosis with Chinese herbs. Doctoral thesis, The University of Western Australia, 2000

47.   Albrand G. Independent predictors of all osteoporosis-related fractures in healthy postmenopausal women: The OFELY Study. Bone. 32(1):78-85, 2003

48.   WHO 1998. Guidelines for preclinical evaluation and clinical trials in osteoporosis. Geneva; 1998

49.   NIH: NIH statement on Osteoporosis Prevention, Diagnosis, and Therapy can be accessed on http://consensus.nih.gov/cons/cons.htm

50.   Ernst E. Harmless herbs? A review of the recent literature. Am J Med 104(2):170-178, 1998

51.   秦岭, 石印玉, 建立防治骨质疏松症传统药物研发和有效性检证准. 中国骨质疏松杂志 (3): 2004 (in print) (Qin L, Shi YY. Establishing international standards for research & development of herbal medicine in the prevention and treatment of osteoporosis. Chin J Osteoporosis 10(3): 2004 (in print)

52.   郑筱芋主编 《中药新药指导原则》中国医药科技出版社, 2002 (Zhen XY.Guideline for New Drug R & D of Chinese herb. Science & Technology Publishing company of Chinese Medicamentc 2002)

53.   中国国家药品和食品监督管理局 《新药研究管理办法》中国国家药品和食品监督管理局, 2002 (Bureau of the Chinese State Food and Drug Administration. Administration for R & D of New Drugs, 2002)

54.   Qin L, Yeung HY, Zhang M. State-of the Art technologies for bone and mineral research. Proc. p 62-64, 2nd Int Con. On Bone and Mineral Research & 4th Int Osteoporosis Symposium & First WHO-Collaborating Center Asian Regional Conf on Osteoporosis. Guilin, China, March 26-31, 2004

55.   The Writing Group for the ISCD Position Development Conference. Position statement: introduction, methods, and participants. The Writing Group for the International Society for Clinical Densitometry (ISCD) Position Development Conference. J Clin Densitometry. 7(1):13-6, 2004

APPENDIX

AN INTRODUCTION TO HOLOGIC TECHNOLOGY

Discover the Difference 10 Seconds Makes:

The new standard in point-of-care fracture risk assessment.

Now with Express BMD.

The revolutionary Discovery – the latest addition to the Hologic QDR Series –

Combine the proven clinical value of bone mineral density (BMD) measurement with Instant Vertebral Assessment (IVA), enabling the fastest point-of-care evaluation of the two most definitive factors associated with osteoporotic fracture: low BMD and the presence of vertebral fracture.

Utilizing OnePass single-sweep scanning technology, Discovery raises the standard of bone densitometry with features that include:

- 10-second Express BMD – Regional spine and hip BMD results in just 10 seconds with better than 1% precision.

- 10-second Instant Vertebral Assessment – single-energy imaging of the spine (L4-T4) with exceptional image quality in only 10 seconds.

- e-Reporting – Advanced remote interpretation and reporting software, including speech recognition compatibility.

- CADfx – Computer-aided fracture assessment tool quantifies degree of vertebral compression and simplifies IVA interpretation.

- QDR Mobility – An exclusive package of mobile reporting tools, enabling physicians to receive BMD studies and generate reports using a wireless network.

See specifications data sheet for available features on specific Discovery models.